Advances in Experimental Medicine and Biology

Volume 1280

Advances in Experimental Medicine and Biology provides a platform for scientific contributions in the main disciplines of the biomedicine and the life sciences. This series publishes thematic volumes on contemporary research in the areas of microbiology, immunology, neurosciences, biochemistry, biomedical engineering, genetics, physiology, and cancer research. Covering emerging topics and techniques in basic and clinical science, it brings together clinicians and researchers from various fields.

Advances in Experimental Medicine and Biology has been publishing exceptional works in the field for over 40 years, and is indexed in SCOPUS, Medline (PubMed), Journal Citation Reports/Science Edition, Science Citation Index Expanded (SciSearch, Web of Science), EMBASE, BIOSIS, Reaxys, EMBiology, the Chemical Abstracts Service (CAS), and Pathway Studio.

2019 Impact Factor: 2.450 5 Year Impact Factor: 2.324.

More information about this series at http://www.springer.com/series/5584

Shen Hu
Editor

Cancer Metabolomics

Methods and Applications

Springer

Editor
Shen Hu
University of California, Los Angeles
Los Angeles, CA, USA

ISSN 0065-2598 ISSN 2214-8019 (electronic)
Advances in Experimental Medicine and Biology
ISBN 978-3-030-51651-2 ISBN 978-3-030-51652-9 (eBook)
https://doi.org/10.1007/978-3-030-51652-9

This Springer imprint is published by the registered company Springer Nature Switzerland AG
The registered company address is: Gewerbestrasse 11, 6330 Cham, Switzerland

To my father, Liangbin Hu, who has always encouraged me to edit a book.

Contents

Contributors

Yang D. Chai School of Dentistry and Jonsson Comprehensive Cancer Center, University of California, Los Angeles, CA, USA

Hong Chen Oil Crops Research Institute of the Chinese Academy of Agricultural Sciences, Key Laboratory of Biology and Genetic Improvement of Oil Crops, Ministry of Agriculture, Wuhan, People's Republic of China

Hubei Key Laboratory of Lipid Chemistry and Nutrition, Wuhan, China

Maria Emilia Dueñas Department of Chemistry, Iowa State University, Ames, IA, USA

Biosciences Institute, Newcastle University, Newcastle upon Tyne, UK

Naseim Elzakra School of Dentistry, University of California Los Angeles, Los Angeles, CA, USA

Sizhe Feng Institute of Neuroscience and Division of Neurosurgery, General Hospital of Northern Theater Command, Shenyang, China

G. A. Nagana Gowda Northwest Metabolomics Research Center, Anesthesiology and Pain Medicine, University of Washington, Seattle, WA, USA

Rui Guo Key Laboratory of Systems Biomedicine (Ministry of Education), Shanghai Center for Systems Biomedicine, Shanghai Jiao Tong University, Shanghai, China

Wei Guo Department of Otolaryngology Head and Neck Surgery, Beijing Tongren Hospital, Key Laboratory of Otolaryngology Head and Neck Surgery, Ministry of Education, Capital Medical University, Beijing, China

Xianlin Han Barshop Institute for Longevity and Aging Studies, San Antonio, TX, USA

Department of Medicine – Diabetes, University of Texas Health Science Center at San Antonio, San Antonio, TX, USA

Haiping Hao Key Laboratory of Drug Metabolism and Pharmacokinetics, State Key Laboratory of Natural Medicines, China Pharmaceutical University, Nanjing, China

School of Pharmacy, China Pharmaceutical University, Nanjing, China

Jing Huang School of Pharmaceutical Science and Technology, Dalian University of Technology, Dalian, China

Junwei Huang Department of Otolaryngology Head and Neck Surgery, Beijing Tongren Hospital, Key Laboratory of Otolaryngology Head and Neck Surgery, Ministry of Education, Capital Medical University, Beijing, China

Zhigang Huang Department of Otolaryngology Head and Neck Surgery, Beijing Tongren Hospital, Key Laboratory of Otolaryngology Head and Neck Surgery, Ministry of Education, Capital Medical University, Beijing, China

Rui Hu State Key Laboratory of Magnetic Resonance and Atomic Molecular Physics, Key Laboratory of Magnetic Resonance in Biological Systems, National Center for Magnetic Resonance in Wuhan, Wuhan National Laboratory for Optoelectronics, Wuhan Institute of Physics and Mathematics, Chinese Academy of Sciences, Wuhan, China

Shen Hu School of Dentistry and Jonsson Comprehensive Cancer Center, University of California, Los Angeles, CA, USA

Eoon Hye Ji School of Dentistry and Jonsson Comprehensive Cancer Center, University of California, Los Angeles, CA, USA

Zhenning Jin School of Dentistry and Jonsson Comprehensive Cancer Center, University of California, Los Angeles, CA, USA

Wroocha Kadam UCLA School of Dentistry, Los Angeles, CA, USA

Yong Kim School of Dentistry, University of California Los Angeles, Los Angeles, CA, USA

Laboratory of Stem Cell and Cancer Epigenetics, Center for Oral Oncology Research, UCLA School of Dentistry, Los Angeles, CA, USA

UCLA's Jonsson Comprehensive Cancer Center, Los Angeles, CA, USA

Broad Stem Cell Research Institute, Los Angeles, CA, USA

Ashok Kumar Department of Biochemistry, All India Institute of Medical Sciences (AIIMS), Bhopal, Madhya Pradesh, India

Dhruv Kumar Amity Institute of Molecular Medicine & Stem Cell Research, Amity University, Noida, Uttar Pradesh, India

Jason Lee School of Dentistry and Jonsson Comprehensive Cancer Center, University of California, Los Angeles, CA, USA

Young Jin Lee Department of Chemistry, Iowa State University, Ames, IA, USA

Feng Li UCLA School of Dentistry, Los Angeles, CA, USA

Liang Li Department of Chemistry, University of Alberta, Edmonton, AB, Canada

Tao Li State Key Laboratory of Magnetic Resonance and Atomic Molecular Physics, Key Laboratory of Magnetic Resonance in Biological Systems, National Center for Magnetic Resonance in Wuhan, Wuhan National Laboratory for Optoelectronics, Wuhan Institute of Physics and Mathematics, Chinese Academy of Sciences, Wuhan, China

University of Chinese Academy of Sciences, Beijing, China

Baodong Liu State Key Laboratory of Environmental Chemistry and Ecotoxicology, Research Center for Eco-Environmental Sciences, Chinese Academy of Sciences, Beijing, China

University of Chinese Academy of Sciences, Beijing, China

Jianzhou Liu School of Pharmaceutical Science and Technology, Dalian University of Technology, Dalian, China

Lian Liu School of Biomedical Sciences, Faculty of Health, Queensland University of Technology, Brisbane, Australia

Yutong Liu Department of Pharmacology, Shenyang Pharmaceutical University, Shenyang, China

Haitao Lu Key Laboratory of Systems Biomedicine (Ministry of Education), Shanghai Center for Systems Biomedicine, Shanghai Jiao Tong University, Shanghai, China

Wenjie Lu Key Laboratory of Drug Metabolism and Pharmacokinetics, State Key Laboratory of Natural Medicines, China Pharmaceutical University, Nanjing, China

Xialin Luo Key Laboratory of Systems Biomedicine (Ministry of Education), Shanghai Center for Systems Biomedicine, Shanghai Jiao Tong University, Shanghai, China

Xin Lv Oil Crops Research Institute of the Chinese Academy of Agricultural Sciences, Key Laboratory of Biology and Genetic Improvement of Oil Crops, Ministry of Agriculture, Wuhan, People's Republic of China

Hubei Key Laboratory of Lipid Chemistry and Nutrition, Wuhan, China

Craig McClain University of Louisville Alcohol Research Center, University of Louisville, Louisville, KY, USA

University of Louisville Hepatobiology & Toxicology Program, University of Louisville, Louisville, KY, USA

Department of Pharmacology & Toxicology, University of Louisville, Louisville, KY, USA

Department of Medicine, University of Louisville, Louisville, KY, USA

Robley Rex Louisville VAMC, Louisville, KY, USA

Md Aminul Islam Prodhan Department of Chemistry, University of Louisville, Louisville, KY, USA

University of Louisville Alcohol Research Center, University of Louisville, Louisville, KY, USA

University of Louisville Hepatobiology & Toxicology Program, University of Louisville, Louisville, KY, USA

Center for Regulatory and Environmental Analytical Metabolomics, University of Louisville, Louisville, KY, USA

Zuojian Qin Oil Crops Research Institute of the Chinese Academy of Agricultural Sciences, Key Laboratory of Biology and Genetic Improvement of Oil Crops, Ministry of Agriculture, Wuhan, People's Republic of China

Hubei Key Laboratory of Lipid Chemistry and Nutrition, Wuhan, China

Daniel Raftery Northwest Metabolomics Research Center, Anesthesiology and Pain Medicine, University of Washington, Seattle, WA, USA

Department of Chemistry, University of Washington, Seattle, WA, USA

Fred Hutchinson Cancer Research Center, Seattle, WA, USA

Sibi Raj Amity Institute of Molecular Medicine & Stem Cell Research, Amity University, Noida, Uttar Pradesh, India

Chang Shao Pharmacy Department, Shenzhen Luohu People's Hospital, Shenzhen, China

School of Pharmacy, China Pharmaceutical University, Nanjing, China

Yuan Tian State Key Laboratory of Magnetic Resonance and Atomic Molecular Physics, Key Laboratory of Magnetic Resonance in Biological Systems, National Center for Magnetic Resonance in Wuhan, Wuhan National Laboratory for Optoelectronics, Wuhan Institute of Physics and Mathematics, Chinese Academy of Sciences, Wuhan, China

Department of Veterinary and Biomedical Sciences, Pennsylvania State University, University Park, PA, USA

Chunyan Wang Barshop Institute for Longevity and Aging Studies, San Antonio, TX, USA

Hailin Wang State Key Laboratory of Environmental Chemistry and Ecotoxicology, Research Center for Eco-Environmental Sciences, Chinese Academy of Sciences, Beijing, China

University of Chinese Academy of Sciences, Beijing, China

Jianing Wang Barshop Institute for Longevity and Aging Studies, San Antonio, TX, USA

Xijun Wang National Chinmedomics Research Center, Sino-America Chinmedomics Technology Collaboration Center, National TCM Key Laboratory of Serum Pharmacochemistry, Harbin, China

Bowen Wei UCLA School of Medicine, Los Angeles, CA, USA

Fang Wei Oil Crops Research Institute of the Chinese Academy of Agricultural Sciences, Key Laboratory of Biology and Genetic Improvement of Oil Crops, Ministry of Agriculture, Wuhan, People's Republic of China

Hubei Key Laboratory of Lipid Chemistry and Nutrition, Wuhan, China

Bangfu Wu Oil Crops Research Institute of the Chinese Academy of Agricultural Sciences, Key Laboratory of Biology and Genetic Improvement of Oil Crops, Ministry of Agriculture, Wuhan, People's Republic of China

Hubei Key Laboratory of Lipid Chemistry and Nutrition, Wuhan, China

Zongyuan Wu Oil Crops Research Institute of the Chinese Academy of Agricultural Sciences, Key Laboratory of Biology and Genetic Improvement of Oil Crops, Ministry of Agriculture, Wuhan, People's Republic of China

Hubei Key Laboratory of Lipid Chemistry and Nutrition, Wuhan, China

Gary Guishan Xiao School of Pharmaceutical Science and Technology, Dalian University of Technology, Dalian, China

Center of Functional Genomics and Proteomics, Creighton University Medical Center, Omaha, NE, USA

Ya Xie Oil Crops Research Institute of the Chinese Academy of Agricultural Sciences, Key Laboratory of Biology and Genetic Improvement of Oil Crops, Ministry of Agriculture, Wuhan, People's Republic of China

Hubei Key Laboratory of Lipid Chemistry and Nutrition, Wuhan, China

Xu Xin Key Laboratory of Systems Biomedicine (Ministry of Education), Shanghai Center for Systems Biomedicine, Shanghai Jiao Tong University, Shanghai, China

National Chinmedomics Research Center, Sino-America Chinmedomics Technology Collaboration Center, National TCM Key Laboratory of Serum Pharmacochemistry, Harbin, China

Xiangdong Xu School of Public Health and Key Laboratory of Environment and Human Health, Hebei Medical University, Shijiazhuang, China

Yunhuang Yang State Key Laboratory of Magnetic Resonance and Atomic Molecular Physics, Key Laboratory of Magnetic Resonance in Biological Systems, National Center for Magnetic Resonance in Wuhan, Wuhan National Laboratory for Optoelectronics, Wuhan Institute of Physics and Mathematics, Chinese Academy of Sciences, Wuhan, China

Hui Ye Key Laboratory of Drug Metabolism and Pharmacokinetics, State Key Laboratory of Natural Medicines, China Pharmaceutical University, Nanjing, China

Gaofei Yin Department of Otolaryngology Head and Neck Surgery, Beijing Tongren Hospital, Key Laboratory of Otolaryngology Head and Neck Surgery, Ministry of Education, Capital Medical University, Beijing, China

Bi-Feng Yuan Key Laboratory of Analytical Chemistry for Biology and Medicine (Ministry of Education), Department of Chemistry, Wuhan University, Wuhan, China

Limin Zhang State Key Laboratory of Magnetic Resonance and Atomic Molecular Physics, Key Laboratory of Magnetic Resonance in Biological Systems, National Center for Magnetic Resonance in Wuhan, Wuhan National Laboratory for Optoelectronics, Wuhan Institute of Physics and Mathematics, Chinese Academy of Sciences, Wuhan, China

Xiang Zhang Department of Chemistry, University of Louisville, Louisville, KY, USA

University of Louisville Alcohol Research Center, University of Louisville, Louisville, KY, USA

University of Louisville Hepatobiology & Toxicology Program, University of Louisville, Louisville, KY, USA

Center for Regulatory and Environmental Analytical Metabolomics, University of Louisville, Louisville, KY, USA

Department of Pharmacology & Toxicology, University of Louisville, Louisville, KY, USA

Shuang Zhao Department of Chemistry, University of Alberta, Edmonton, AB, Canada

About the Editor

Shen Hu is a Tenured Full Professor at the University of California, Los Angeles, and currently directs the Oral Biology Graduate Program. He received his PhD in Bioanalytical Chemistry from Wuhan University and MBA from the Anderson School of Management at the University of California, Los Angeles. Dr. Hu's research interests are in cancer metabolomics, stem cell biology and single cell analysis. His laboratory is developing diagnostic tools for early cancer detection and therapeutic drugs targeting the metabolic pathways of cancer.

Chemical Isotope Labeling LC-MS for Metabolomics

Shuang Zhao and Liang Li

1 LC-MS for Metabolomics: Conventional Approach

The main goal of metabolomics is to characterize the metabolome by qualitative and quantitative analysis of as many metabolites as possible [1, 2]. Achieving this goal requires highly sensitive metabolite detection, accurate relative or absolute quantification, and confident metabolite identification. In conventional LC-MS-based metabolomics approach, increasing the number of metabolites detected and quantified (i.e., metabolomic coverage) is achieved by the use of different instrumental platforms and methods to analyze the same samples [3, 4]. The combined results from individual analyses represent the overall metabolome covered. These individual analyses are usually carried out according to the metabolites' physical and chemical properties. In a typical LC-MS workflow, after sample collection and pretreatment (e.g., protein removal, metabolite extraction, etc.), reversed phase (RP) LC is used for separating hydrophobic metabolites, while hydrophilic interaction LC (HILIC) is used for separating more polar compounds [5]. In each case, the eluted analytes are ionized in positive ion mode and negative ion mode. In this way, four LC-MS runs are required to analyze one sample. The main advantage of this approach is that it is easy to implement by using readily available LC and MS instruments to collect data and commercial or freely available software to process the resultant data. The major limitation of this approach is that the metabolome coverage is still low even after combining all the multiple analysis data. Although tens of thousands of features can be detected in LC-MS analysis of a metabolome sample, only a small fraction of them (hundreds) are originated from unique metabolites. Many redundant peaks, such as adduct ions and fragment ions, are detected from one metabolite. This is not surprising considering that electrospray ionization (ESI), the most widely used method for LC-MS, does not offer the same ionization efficiency for all metabolites. In fact, a large number of metabolites cannot be ionized with high efficiency. The combined low ionization efficiency and low metabolite concentration result in low or no MS signals.

Another challenge in conventional LC-MS for metabolome analysis is on quantification which relies on the use of internal standards to correct for sample loss, instrument drift, matrix effect, and ion suppression in the whole workflow. Compared with chemical structural analogue, stable isotope labeled (SIL) internal standard is a better choice due to its nearly identical physical and chemical properties to the analyte of interest. However, SIL internal standards are generally

S. Zhao · L. Li (✉)
Department of Chemistry, University of Alberta, Edmonton, AB, Canada
e-mail: liang.li@ualberta.ca

S. Hu (ed.), *Cancer Metabolomics*, Advances in Experimental Medicine and Biology 1280,
https://doi.org/10.1007/978-3-030-51652-9_1

expensive and their availability is limited. Particularly in metabolomics area, it is impossible to purchase or synthesize isotopic internal standards for all the metabolites. Thus, conventional LC-MS is widely used for quantification of a small number of metabolites with SIL (i.e., targeted analysis). Untargeted analysis of metabolites without using SIL offers limited quantification precision and accuracy.

2 Stable Isotope Labeling LC-MS for Metabolomics

In order to perform quantitative metabolomics using LC-MS, methods that can simultaneously introduce stable isotopes into many metabolites have been developed. In one approach, cells are cultured with a stable isotope-labeled substrate (e.g., D, ^{13}C, ^{15}N, etc.) in growth medium. During cultivation, the substrate-related metabolites and metabolic networks are "in vivo" labeled with enriched heavy isotopes. As a result, each heavy-isotope-labeled metabolite can potentially serve as the internal standard. This cell-culture-based metabolic isotope labeling (MIL) is not only useful for quantitative metabolite measurement but also an important tool for metabolic flux analysis [6]. For example, growing cells using ^{13}C-glucose or ^{13}C- or ^{15}N-glutamine as main energy sources can be used for monitoring and analyzing many cellular pathways, such as glycolysis and pentose phosphate pathway [6, 7]. This MIL approach is particularly convenient for metabolomic analysis of cells or organisms that can be cultured in isotope-enriched media, including microbial, yeast, some mammalian cell cultures [7] or plants [8]. However, this approach is not easily applicable for samples that cannot be readily cultured, such as human biofluids including urine, blood, etc. [9] In addition, this approach does not alter the chemical and physical property of a metabolite to improve its detectability in LC-MS. Metabolites that are not ionized efficiently will still not be detected. In other words, MIL can improve quantification in analyzing special types of samples, but cannot overcome the limitation of low coverage.

An alternative approach to create isotope internal standards for LC-MS-based quantitative metabolomics is to use chemical-reaction-based isotope labeling or chemical isotope labeling (CIL), which is, in principle, suitable for all categories of samples. In contrast to MIL, biological samples are "in vitro" labeled in CIL using a reagent which targets a specific chemical functional group. Ideally, all the metabolites containing the same functional group react with the reagent to form the corresponding derivatized metabolites. Many reagents can incorporate one or more isotopic atoms (e.g., H/D, $^{12}C/^{13}C$, $^{14}N/^{15}N$, etc.) in the molecular structure, thereby introducing the isotopic moiety into the labeled metabolites after chemical derivatization. The metabolites derivatized by a heavy isotope reagent can serve as the internal standards for light isotope reagent labeled metabolites. This CIL strategy has been widely used in relative quantification for untargeted metabolomics as well as absolute quantification for targeted metabolomics.

3 Chemical Isotope Labeling LC-MS Metabolomics Workflow

The general workflow using CIL LC-MS for metabolomics is shown in Fig. 1. In this workflow, for metabolome profiling or relative quantification in two comparative groups of samples, a control sample (e.g., a pooled sample) is labeled by a heavy isotope reagent, while individual samples are derivatized by a light isotope reagent. Then the two derivatized samples are mixed and injected into LC-MS for analysis. Since the light-labeled derivative and heavy-labeled derivative of a metabolite have nearly identical properties, they elute out at the same time from LC. In the mass spectra, the two derivatives of the same metabolite are shown as a peak pair. The relative amount of the metabolite can be determined from the comparison of peak areas of two derivatives. Combined with database identification and statistical analysis, this approach has been successfully used for biological studies and biomarker discovery [10].

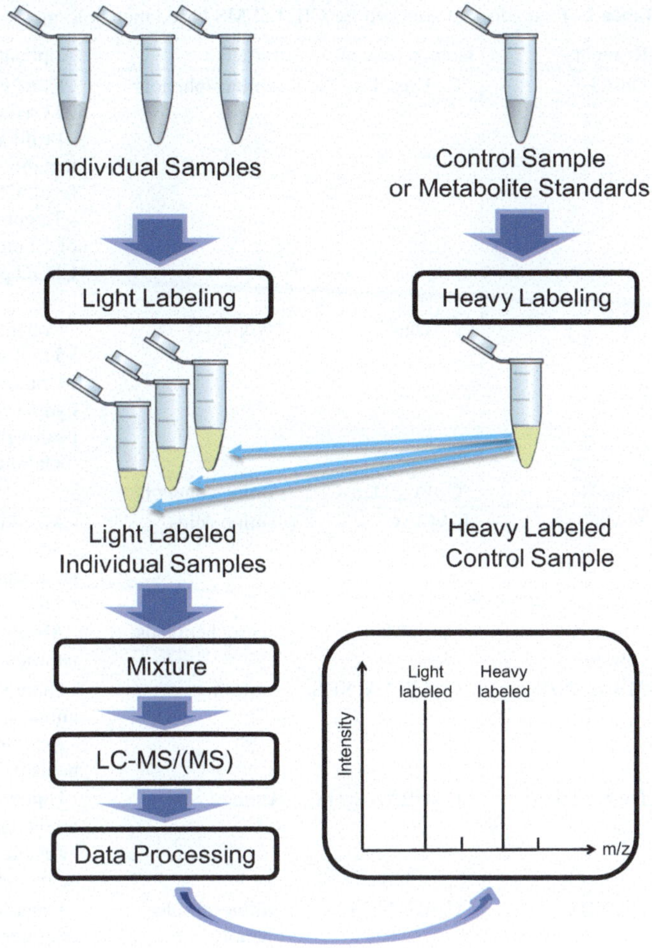

Fig. 1 General workflow of CIL LC-MS-based metabolomic analysis

For absolute quantification of metabolites in samples, similar to the above-described method, samples are derivatized with a light isotope labeling reagent and the analyte standards of known concentrations are labeled with a heavy isotope reagent. The resulting heavy derivatives are used as CIL internal standards for performing quantification with MS. For absolute quantification of a small number of metabolites of interest, tandem MS can also be used to increase sensitivity and quantification dynamic range by using selected reaction monitoring (SRM) or multiple reaction monitoring (MRM).

4 Derivatization Reagents for CIL LC-MS Metabolomics

Many derivatization reagents are developed for different functional groups and have been widely used for biological studies. Table 1 lists a number of reagents that are used for CIL LC-MS-based metabolomics. We highlight some examples of reagents below. Detailed information for each reagent can be found in the references listed in the table.

For amine-containing metabolites, sulfonyl chloride, acyl chloride, NHS esters, and isothio-

Table 1 Reagents that are used for CIL LC-MS based metabolomics

Reagent	Isotope reagent	Targets	Applications	References
DnsCl	$^{13}C_2$-DnsCl	Amines/phenols	- Constructed library containing 273 dansylated metabolites - Profiled and positively identified metabolites in urine, blood, serum, fecal, CSF, cells - Targeted absolute quantification of 19 metabolites as asthma/CPOD potential biomarkers	Guo and Li [27], Chen et al. [44], Han et al. [10], Xu et al. [47], Guo et al. [46] and Khamis et al. [42]
	$^{13}C_2$-DnsCl	Hydroxyls	- Constructed library containing 85 hydroxyl standards - Untargeted profiled urinary hydroxyl submetabolome and positively identified 20 metabolites	Zhao et al. [22]
DensCl	$^{13}C_2$/$^{13}C_4$-DensCl	Amines/phenols		Zhou et al. [52]
MASC	d_3-MASC	Amino acids	- Absolute quantification of amino acids and monoamine neurotransmitters using MRM mode	Song et al. [53] and Zheng et al. [54]
Benzoyl chloride	$^{13}C_6$-BzCl	Neurochemicals	- Absolute quantification of 70 neurochemicals	Wong et al. [11]
MBAA-NHS	$^{13}C_2$-MBAA-NHS	Amines	- Untargeted profiling of urinary amine submetabolome - Absolute quantification of amino acids in human urine	Zhou et al. [55]
DBAA-NHS	$^{13}C_2$-DBAA-NHS	Amines	- Untargeted profiling of urinary amine submetabolome - Absolute quantification of amino acids in human urine	Zhou et al. [55]
BZ-NHS	$^{13}C_6$-BZ-NHS	Amines/thiols/phenols	- Untargeted metabolome profiling of cell extracts - Positively identified 10 metabolites	Wagner et al. [56]
DIPP-L-Ala-NHS	$^{18}O_2$-DIPP-L-Ala-NHS	Amines	- Determination of 20 L-amino acids and 10 D-amino acids	Zhang et al. [57]
iTRAQ	iTRAQ	Amines	- Analysis of 44 amino acids in plasma, urine and tissue	Takach et al. [35]
DiLeu	4-plex DiLeu	Amines	- Profiling and relative quantification of amine submetabolome of mouse urine	Hao et al. [58]
DMAP	d_4-DMAP	Amines	- Constructed library containing 118 amine compounds - Positively identified 46 amine metabolites in fecal sample	Yuan et al. [34]
Cyanuric chloride/methylamine	Methyl-d_3-amine	Amines	- Determined concentrations of 27 metabolites in HepG2 cells	Lee and Chang [59]
Acetone	d_6-acetone	Phosphatidyl-ethanolamine	- Identified and quantified 45 PE species in rat livers using double neutral loss scan.	Wang et al. [60]
MPBS	d_3-MPBS	Amino acids	- Analysis of amino acids in newborn bloodspot	Johnson [28]

(continued)

Table 1 (continued)

Reagent	Isotope reagent	Targets	Applications	References
DMABS	d_3/d_6-DMABS	Amino acids	- Analysis of amino acids in newborn bloodspot	Johnson [28]
C_n-NA-NHS	C_4d_9-NA-NHS	Amines		Yang et al. [61]
Methyl acetimidate	$^{13}C_2$-methyl acetimidate	Amines	- Relative quantification of primary and secondary amines in Arabidopsis seed extracts	Shortreed et al. [62]
Formaldehyde	^{13}C-formaldehyde	Amines	- Analysis of 20 amino acids and 15 amines - Profiling human urine amine-containing metabolites	Guo et al. [63]
Acetyaldehyde	d_4-acetaldehyde	Monoamine neurotransmitters	- Determination of neurotransmitters in brain microdialysate	Ji et al. [64]
PEG-OPFP	^{13}C-PEG-OPFP	Primary amines	- Quantification of intracellular amino acids	Abello et al. [65]
TAHS	d_3-TAHS	Amino acids	- Determination of amino acids in rat plasma	Shimbo et al. [66]
L-PGA-OSu	L-PGA(d_5)-OSu	Chiral amines	- Differential analysis of DL-amino acids in serum and yogurt	Mochizuki et al. [67]
DMED	d_4-DMED	Carboxylic acids	- Constructed library containing 184 carboxyl metabolites - Positively identification of 83 carboxyl metabolites	Yuan et al. [34]
Cholamine	d_9-cholamine	Carboxylic acids	- Relative quantification of fatty acids from hydrolyzed egg lipid using nanoLC	Lamos et al. [68]
	^{15}N-cholamine	Carboxylic acids	- Analysis of 48 carboxylic acids	Tayyari et al. [69]
3-NPH	$^{13}C_6$-3-NPH	Short-chain fatty acids	- Quantification of short-chain fatty acids in human feces	Han et al. [14]
Butanolic HCl	d_9-butanol	Carboxylic acids	- Profiling and relative quantification of human plasma metabolites	O'Maille et al. [16]
Aniline	$^{13}C_6$-aniline	Carbonyl, phosphoryl, and carboxyl	- Quantification 33 intermediate metabolites in central carbon and energy metabolism	Yang et al. [21]
BAMP/HAMP	d_9-BMAP	Carboxylic acids	- Metabolome profiling of rat urine sample and positively identified 32 metabolites	Yang et al. [70]
BMP/CMP	d_3-CMP	Fatty acids	- Metabolome profiling, relative quantification and absolute quantification of human serum	Yang et al. [71]
DmPA bromide	$^{13}C_2$-DMPA	Carboxylic acids	- Constructed library containing 113 carboxylic acid - Positively identified 51 metabolites in urine	Guo and Li [17]
HMEP	d_5-HMEP	Fatty acids	- Monitored changes of metabolite levels in plasma of individuals	Koulman et al. [72]
DBD-PZ-NH2	d_6-DBD-PZ-NH2	Carboxylic acid	- Determination and relative quantification of fatty acids in plasma	Tsukamoto et al. [73]

(continued)

Table 1 (continued)

Reagent	Isotope reagent	Targets	Applications	References
DMPP	d_6-DMPP	Carboxylic acid	- Determined trace free fatty acids in human urine and thyroid tissues	Leng et al. [74] and Leng et al. [75]
T3	d_{20}-T3	Fatty acids	- Relative quantification of FAs with general MRM conditions. - Discovered FA species related to the ageing process	Tie et al. [76]
HIQB	d_7-HIQB	Carbonyls	- Constructed library containing 147 carbonyl compounds - Untargeted profiling of carbonyl submetabolome of human serum and fecal sample using double precursor ion scan. 12 and 50 metabolites were positively identified, respectively	Guo et al. [77] and Yuan et al. [34].
4-APC	d_4-4-APC	Aldehydes	- Profiled aldehyde submetabolome using double neutral loss scan of urine, beer, and wine samples	Zheng et al. [78], and Yu et al. [79]
DnsHz	$^{13}C_2$-DnsHz	Carbonyls	- Constructed library containing 78 carbonyl compounds - Profiling of urinary carbonyl submetabolome and positive identification of 33 metabolites	Zhao et al. [37]
Aniline	$^{13}C_6$-aniline	Carbonyls, phosphoryls and carboxyls	- Quantification of 33 intermediate metabolites in central carbon and energy metabolism	Yang et al. [21]
Girard P	d_5-GP	Steroid hormones	- Quantified steroid hormones in human follicular fluid	Guo et al. [29]
	d_5-GP/isobaric mass	Sterols/oxysterols	- Profiled plasma sterols/ oxysterols to identify inborn errors	Crick et al. [80]
HMP	d_3-HMP	Neurosteroids	- Relative and absolute quantification of allopregnanolene and pregnenolone levels in brain	Higashi et al. [81]
T3	D3 (d_{20}-T3)	Fatty aldehydes	- Globally profiling of fatty aldehyde in plasma and brain tissue	Tie et al. [82]
QAO	d_3-QAO	Ketosterols	- Absolute quantification of ketosterol in very small volumes of plasma	DeBarber et al. [83]
DMBA	d_4-DMBA	Hydroxyl-containing steroid hormones	- Measurement of 17 derivatized free steroid hormones in urine	Dai et al. [23]
MDMAES	$^{13}C_4$-MDMAES	Steroids	- Quantitative and comparative analysis of SIRS and sepsis clinical samples	O'Maille et al. [16]
Acetone	d_6-acetone	Ribonucleosides	- Profiled urinary metabolome and positively identified 56 ribonucleosides - Metal oxide-based dispersive SPE applied for enrichment of ribonucleosides	Li et al. [33], and Chu et al. [84]

(continued)

Table 1 (continued)

Reagent	Isotope reagent	Targets	Applications	References
Pyridine and Tf2O	d_5-pyridine	Steroids, fatty alcohols and carbohydrates	- Ten pairs of d_0/d_5 ion peaks were identified as cholesterol and fatty alcohols	Wang et al. [85], and Wang et al. [86],
BQB	d_7-BQB	Thiols and oxidized thiols	- Constructed library containing 27 thiol metabolites - Profiled thiol submetabolome in urine, beer and fecal samples - Positively identified 14 and 8 thiol metabolites in fecal and urine, respectively	Yuan et al. [34],, Huang et al. [87], and Liu et al. [26]

cyanates are used for CIL. For example, Kennedy's group developed a method targeting 70 neurochemicals using LC-MS/MS and benzoyl chloride (BzCl) derivatization [11]. The commercially available ^{13}C-BzCl was used for labeling internal standards. The reagent offers very fast reaction (seconds at room temperature). This approach has been proved to be effective in various matrix, including tissue, serum, CSF, and microdialysate [12].

Many reactions for labeling carboxylic acids are based on condensation reaction with amines. In this type of reaction, carboxyl groups in metabolites are activated by a condensation reagent (e.g., carbodiimide), followed by reacting with amine groups in the labeling reagents, generating a stable amide bond [13]. The method of using ^{12}C/^{13}C-3-nitrophenylhydrazine (3-NPH) to analyzed carboxylic acids was reported. The labeled metabolites gain significant enhancement of detection in negative ion mode. It has been successfully applied in the detection and quantitation of many important categories of acids, including carboxylic acids in central carbon metabolism [13], short-chain fatty acids [14] and bile acids [15]. In addition, esterification reaction was also used to derivatize carboxyl group [16, 17].

Various hydrazine or hydrazide reagents have been proven to be effective on labeling ketones or aldehydes, such as Girard reagents. Girard's reagent P was used in quantitative glycomics with its pentadeuterated (d_5-) counterpart [18]. In this method, reducing glycans were labeled with either nondeuterated (d_0-) or deuterated (d_5-) Girard's reagent P, followed by online HILIC-MS analysis to achieve rapid and sensitive relative quantitation of reducing glycans between two comparative groups. It was also used for analyzing oxysterol [19, 20]. The signal enhancement factor after Girard derivatization was more than 30-folds. Several amine-containing reagents are also developed for carbonyl group derivatization, such as $^{12}C_6/^{13}C_6$-aniline [21].

For hydroxyl group, which is a weaker nucleophile compared with amine groups, electrophilic reagents were also used for chemical isotope labeling, such as sulfonyl chloride (e.g., ^{12}C-/^{13}C-dansyl chloride [22]) or carboxylic acids (e.g., d_0/d_4-(dimethylamino)-benzoic acid [23]).

At last, thiol groups are easily oxidized by autoxidation and disulfide formation during the sample preparation process [24]. Several reagents were reported to be useful in both isotopic labeling and stabilizing for thiol-containing metabolites [25, 26].

5 Key Features of High-Performance CIL LC-MS

In addition to the introduction of isotopic moiety into metabolites to create isotope internal standards, many CIL LC-MS methods also provide enhancement in other aspects of the LC-MS analysis, including detection and separation. Therefore, using a rationally designed labeling reagent with proper structure can improve the overall performance of LC-MS analysis for a complex metabolomic system.

Improving metabolite detectability is a common advantage of many CIL LC-MS methods. This is achieved by introducing permanent charge or easily ionizable moiety to metabolites in order to increase their ionization efficiency. For example, ^{13}C-/^{12}C-dansyl chloride (DnsCl) was developed as a high-performance CIL reagent for derivatizing amine-, phenol- [27] and hydroxyl-containing metabolites [22]. The dimethylamino structure is an easily ionizable group and can increase the detection ability by 10–1000-folds compared with unlabeled metabolites. Figure 2 shows the ion chromatograms comparison between dansyl-labeled and unlabeled human urine. Enhancement of detection can be clearly observed. The presence of permanently charged moieties can also greatly improve ionization efficiency of labeled molecules, such as quaternary ammonium [28], pyridinium [29] and phosphonium [30] salts for positive ion mode detection. After labeling, the labeled metabolites can be charged readily in ESI, requiring only positive ion mode detection.

Improvement of separation is another important feature of high-performance CIL LC-MS. In conventional LC-MS metabolomics, RPLC and HILIC are usually used to separate complex metabolome. However, this approach suffers from poor retention of polar compounds on RPLC, less-than-ideal reproducibility of HILIC separation [31] and requirement of multiple instruments or changing of columns. Some high-performance CIL methods have been proved to be effective to overcome these problems by improving the separation ability of a complex biological sample. If the introduced moiety dur-

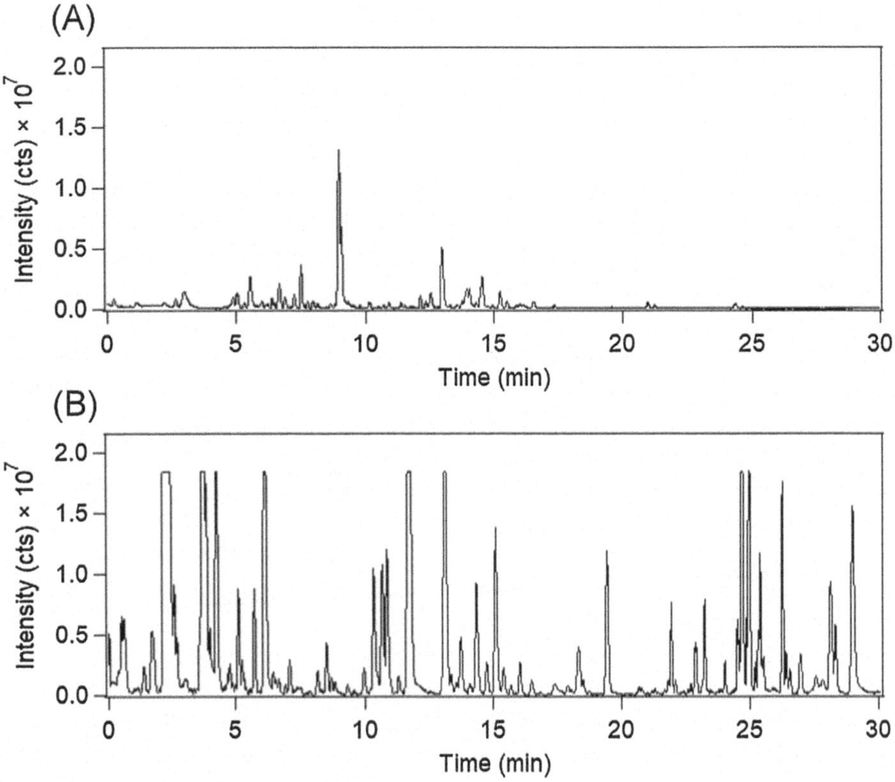

Fig. 2 Comparison of ion chromatograms obtained from (**a**) unlabeled human urine with the injection of 5 μL of sample containing 5 μL of the original urine and (**b**) dansyl-labeled human urine with the injection of 2 μL of sample containing 0.48 μL of the original urine. Despite the injection of 10.4-fold less sample in (**b**), the labeled urine sample gave significantly higher intensities with peaks distributed along the entire gradient elution window

ing derivatization contains an aromatic ring (e.g., dansyl chloride for amine/phenol/hydroxyl group derivatization [22, 27]), an alkyl chain (e.g., N,N′-dimethylethylenediamine for carboxyl group derivatization [32]), or parts that can block polar groups (e.g., acetone for ribonucleosides derivatization [33]), the hydrophobicity of the labeled metabolites would increase, resulting in better retention and peak shapes in RPLC. As a result, polar metabolites in a biological sample can be retained and separated effectively only using RPLC. We note that the consideration of retention properties of metabolites on RPLC favors the use of a reagent without a permanently charged moiety to labeled metabolites. A reagent with permanent charges will increase the hydrophilicity of labeled metabolites and thus poor retention on RPLC. The use of HILIC or other mode LC is required for separation. For the convenience of a user to perform LC-MS, sticking with one mode of separation (i.e., RPLC) for all sample analyses offers a significant advantage.

Introduction of hydrophobic moiety into metabolites also increases the detection ability. This is because the labeled metabolites will elute out at higher composition of organic phase on RP column, leading to more efficient desolvation process and less surface tension of droplets in ESI. In the meantime, increased hydrophobicity prompts metabolite molecules to reside on the surface of the droplets. Both of them benefit the ionization process.

Another significant improvement in metabolite detection offered by CIL is that adding one or more labeling moieties or tags increases the mass of the analyte, thereby avoiding severe interferences in the low m/z region from the low mass impurities and backgrounds in solvents and reagents.

Finally, CIL allows data processing to be done relatively easier with much higher confidence in determining true metabolite peaks, compared to analyzing LC-MS data of unlabeled samples. If differential isotope labeling (e.g., mixture of heavy-labeled pooled sample and light-labeled individual sample) is used for CIL LC-MS metabolome profiling, all metabolite peaks are detected in pairs of light-labeled and heavy-labeled metabolite ions. Impurity and background peaks are detected in singlet peaks. Thus, special software program can be developed to filter out the singlet peaks to improve the data quality. For example, IsoMS was developed to pick the peak pairs from all the peaks detected in mass spectra, followed by removing redundant peaks such as adduct ions, dimers, multimers, etc. These redundant peaks are detected as peak pairs with different m/z values in the same mass spectrum as the peak pair of $[M + H]^+$. A simple algorithm can be used to filter these additional peak pairs to retain only one peak pair for one labeled metabolite.

Instead of directly extracting peak pairs from MS spectra, using common MS/MS fragmentation pattern is another approach to recognize metabolite peaks. For example, Feng and coworkers developed stable isotope labeling combined with double precursor ion scan/double neutral loss scan in MS to selectively analyze a particular group of metabolites [34].

The isobaric tag for relative and absolute quantification (iTRAQ) reagents has been widely used in proteomics. These reagents have been applied for analyzing amino acids [35] and other amine-containing metabolites. Unlike the reagents used in MS-based peak pair detection, iTRAQ reagent consists of a reporter group, a mass balance group, and an amine-reactive group which could be NHS ester. Two differential iTRAQ reagents use different isotope coding patterns in both reporter group and balance group; however, the overall mass of the reagents keeps constant. In derivatization for absolute quantification, metabolites of a sample will be labeled by the reagent containing a light reporter group and a heavy mass balance group. The metabolite standards are labeled by the reagent containing a heavy reporter group and a light mass balance group, which are spiked into the labeled sample as internal standards for LC-MS analysis. The labeled standards and corresponding metabolites in the sample elute out at the same time and have the same m/z in mass spectra. Upon MS/MS fragmentation, the reporter group will be cleaved from the labeled compounds and produce unique product ions, which can be quantified in the SRM mode to reflect the metabolite quantity in a sample.

6 Multichannel CIL LC-MS Metabolome Analysis

In CIL LC-MS-based metabolomics approach, several different submetabolomes targeting different groups of metabolites can be analyzed separately, and the combined datasets can be used to represent the entire metabolome. Zhao et al. have recently reported a study of analyzing the chemical structures of compound entries in several well-used databases to determine the distributions of chemical groups in each database [36]. Because of the interest in studying endogenous metabolites of a metabolome, they removed the lipids, inorganic species, and other molecules that are unique to drug, food, plant, and environmental origins from database compound entries. They found that five groups, namely, amine, phenol, hydroxyl, carboxyl, and carbonyl, are the dominant classes in the remaining endogenous metabolites. In the databases of MCID (2683 filtered metabolites), HMDB (5506), KEGG (11,598), YMDB (1107), and ECMDB (1462), 94.7%, 85.7%, 86.4%, 85.7%, and 95.8% of the filtered metabolites were found to be belonging to one or more of the five groups, respectively. Figure 3 shows an example of the chemical group distribution analysis for the 2683 filtered metabolites in MCID. Thus, in-depth analysis of these five groups of metabolites can result in a very high coverage of a metabolome.

Zhao et al. described a 4-channel high-performance CIL LC-MS approach (Fig. 4) for targeting amine/phenol- [27], carboxyl- [17], carbonyl- [, 37] and hydroxyl-containing metabolites [22] using dansyl and DmPA labeling reagents (Fig. 5) [36]. They showed the detection of a total of 7431 peak pairs with 6109 unique-mass pairs in labeled human plasma using 4-channel CIL LC-MS. Among them, 670 peak pairs (9.0%) could be identified with high confidence and 6256 (84.3%) could be mass-matched to metabolome database entries. In the case of yeast samples, a total of 5629 pairs with 4955 unique-mass pairs were detected. There were 431 peak pairs (7.6%) identified with high confidence and 4836 peak pairs (85.7%) mass-matched to database entries. These results illustrated that the combined datasets from the analyses of four submetabolomes can detect many metabolites. While four different labeling methods were used for profiling four submetabolomes, the LC-MS setup

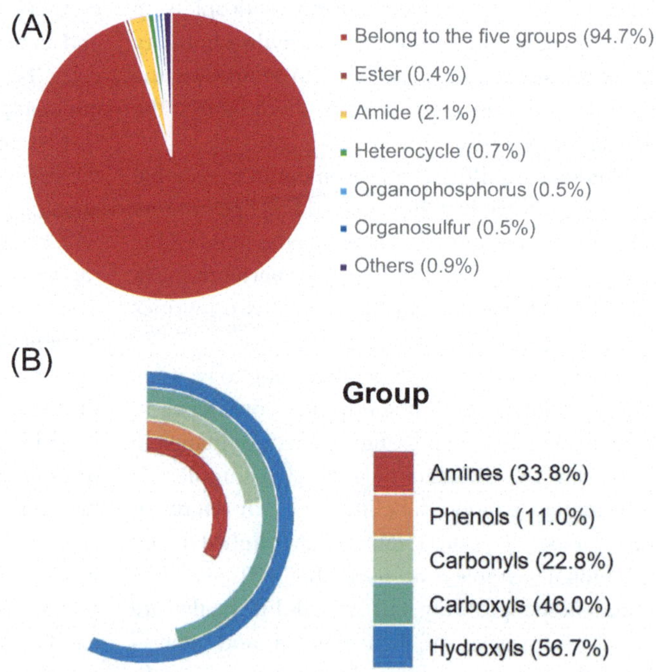

Fig. 3 (a) Classification of chemical groups of 2683 known human endogenous metabolites from the MyCompoundID library. (b) Percent distributions of metabolites belonging to the five groups

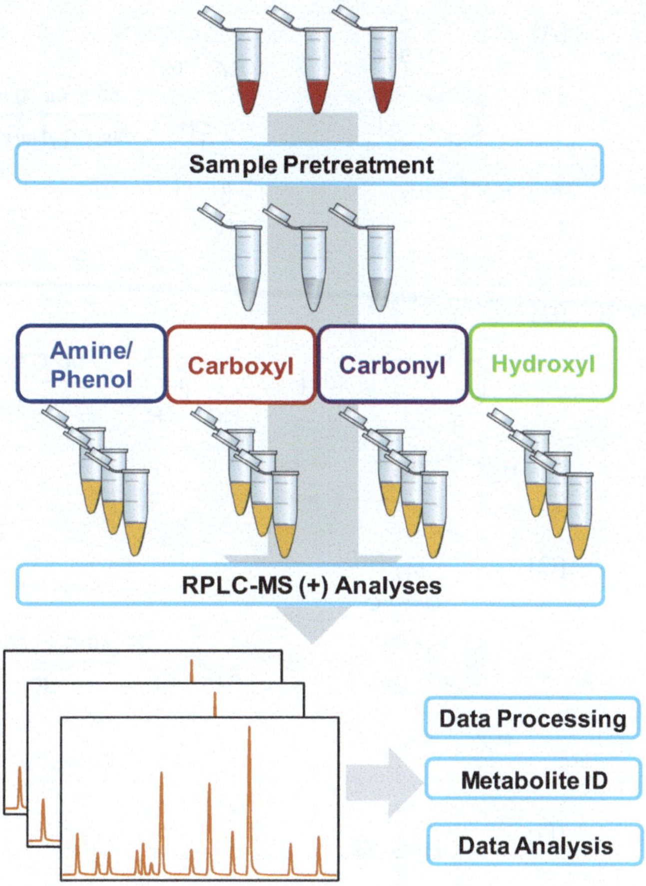

Fig. 4 Workflow of 4-channel high-performance CIL LC-MS-based metabolomics

remained to be the same; all labeled samples were analyzed using RPLC-MS with positive ion detection.

In a similar way, Yu-Qi Feng's group reported profiling of mice fecal samples using integrated derivatization combined LC-MS strategy [34]. In their study, different reagents targeting amine-, carboxyl-, carbonyl-, and thiol-submetabolome were applied. 2302 metabolite candidates were detected and 308 metabolites were further confirmed.

7 Limitations and Future Direction of CIL LC-MS Metabolomics

One presumed weakness of CIL LC-MS is the requirement of performing chemical derivatization. However, due to the need of carrying out multiple steps in a typical sample workup procedure leading to LC-MS analysis, the addition of a chemical labeling step does not necessarily increase the workload significantly. If a very robust and convenient labeling method is used, the chemical derivatization step can be viewed like those of other sample handling steps, such as methanol precipitation of proteins used for analyzing serum samples, creatinine measurement sample normalization in urine sample analysis, cell lysis and metabolite extraction in cellular metabolomics, etc. Thus, developing a reproducible labeling procedure that can be easily implemented in a laboratory and carried out by personnel with little chemistry expertise is critical for wide usage of CIL LC-MS in metabolomics.

Although the reactions that are chosen for derivatization have relatively rapid reaction speed, the required time for many reactions is in still in hours to ensure that the complex subme-

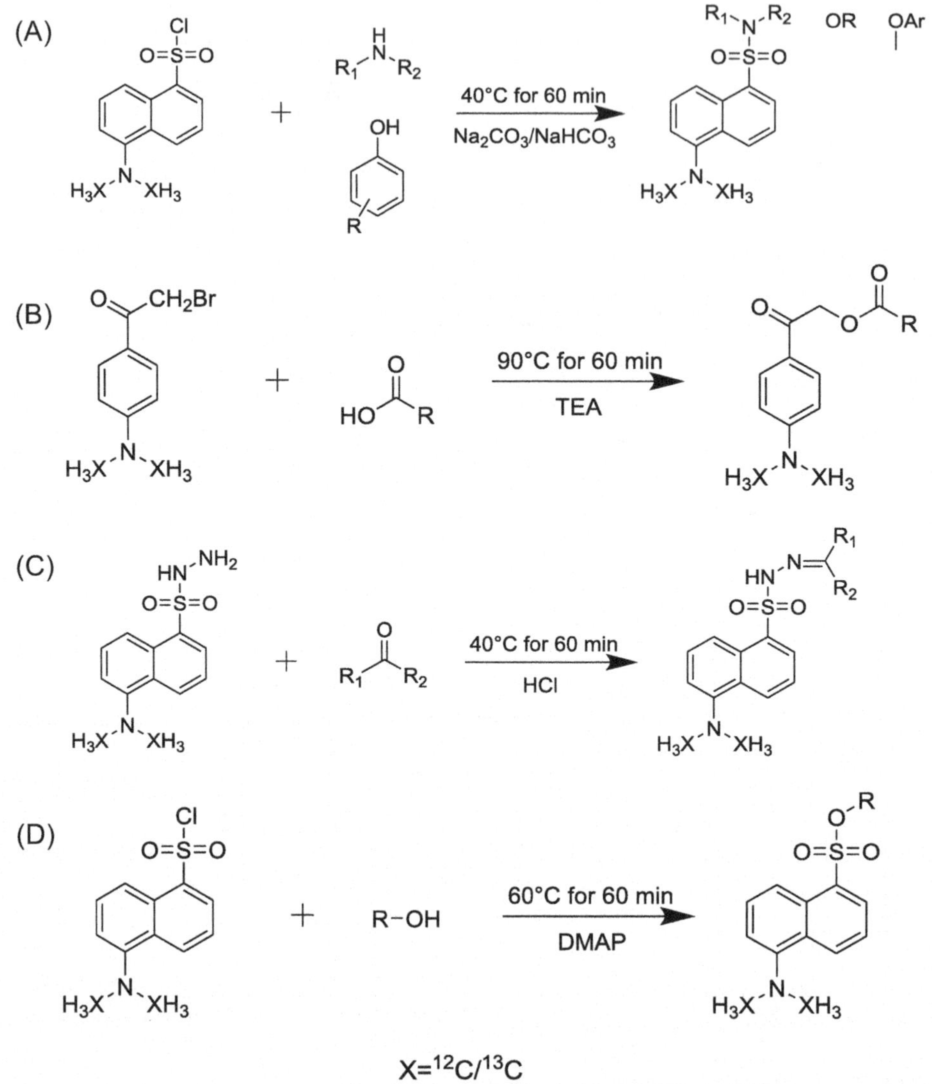

Fig. 5 Reaction schemes of (**a**) dansylation labeling for amine/phenol-containing metabolites; (**b**) DmPA bromide labeling for carboxyl-containing metabolites; (**c**) dansylhydrazine labeling for carbonyl-containing metabolites; (**d**) base-activated dansylation labeling for hydroxyl-containing metabolites

tabolome can be fully labeled and analyzed. One way to address this is to develop and employ reaction conditions that can achieve very fast derivatization. For example, Bian et al. used cholamine derivatization coupled with LC-MS to determine long-chain free fatty acids in complex biological samples [38]. The derivatization step can be finished within 1 min at room temperature. Increase in 2000-fold of sensitivity was obtained and the limits of detection of femtogram level were achieved. The feasibility of one-minute derivatization has been validated using both targeted quantification and untargeted profiling approach with serum samples. Further the authors discovered several metabolites that have significantly differences between healthy and asthma groups. We note that while fast reaction is beneficiary for some applications, parallel labeling of multiple samples can be done, and thus the labeling step is usually not the rate-limiting step in determining the overall sample analysis throughput in metabolomics.

Using robotic liquid handling systems to automatically perform derivatization can be very helpful to achieve high throughput. For example, an autosampler-in-needle-derivatization technique was reported by Siegel et al. [39]. The authors used p-toluenesulfonylhydrazine to derivatize aldehydes and ketones in a UHPLC autosampler. The labeling reagents and samples were consecutively drawn into the autosampler needle and mixed. The complete derivatization can be finished within 10 min and the solution is ready to be injected for analysis. This automatic derivatization approach has been proved to be useful in simultaneously quantifying and identifying molecules containing carbonyl groups.

Relative quantification by CIL LC-MS can be very accurate as the same metabolite in the pooled sample and an individual sample would encounter the same matrix (e.g., urine matrix for urine metabolome analysis). Moreover, the concentration of the metabolite in a pool should be similar to that in an individual sample (usually less than ten-fold changes among different samples). If we perform the labeling of the pool and an individual sample in parallel, the minor differences in matrix effect and labeling efficiency can be accounted for using the intensity ratio of a peak pair of the same metabolite in LC-MS. However, for absolute quantification using CIL LC-MS, we need to be aware of potential pitfalls. In conventional LC-MS-based quantification approach, an internal standard, either SIL or chemical structural analogue, is added to the sample at the very beginning of the sample workup process. Therefore, the internal standard and analyte share the identical preparation steps and, theoretically, the same recovery rate. However, an internal standard created by CIL is usually added to the sample just before the instrumental analysis. Thus, the analyte recovery rate from a sample is assumed to be 100%. Moreover, sample matrix effect, if any, on the labeling efficiency is not accounted for; labeling the internal standard dissolved in a clean solvent may be more or less efficient than labeling the analyte with the presence of many other components in a sample. To address these issues, sample pretreatment procedures need be optimized to obtain high recovery rates of analytes. Matrix effect on labeling efficiency should be measured. Another approach is to use the standard addition method for quantification. However, this method has a low throughput for quantifying many metabolites in a metabolomic sample.

Another potential pitfall of using CIL internal standards is the isotope effect in chromatography when using deuterium [40, 41]. The retention of deuterium derivatized species is generally less than its hydrogen coded counterpart on RPLC column due to weaker hydrophobic interactions with the stationary phase. The lack of co-elution leads to different matrix for ionization, which may be detrimental for quantification. The isotope effect of ^{13}C-, ^{18}O-, or ^{15}N- is usually negligible. Thus, in high-performance CIL methods, these isotope atoms are preferred; however, the synthesis of the reagents containing these isotopes may be more expensive than making the deuterium-coded reagents.

Finally, current CIL methods do not cover all chemical groups. There are several chemical groups such as amides and esters that require the development of efficient and robust labeling methods. Prior to the available of these methods, targeted analysis using LC-MRM-MS may be used to analyze some important metabolites that are not covered with current labeling methods.

8 Applications of CIL LC-MS for Cancer Metabolomics

Because of the possibility of performing highly accurate relative quantification of many different metabolites in metabolome samples, CIL LC-MS is a powerful technique in many metabolomics applications, including cancer metabolomics. For example, dansylation isotope labeling LC-MS has been widely used in various metabolomics studies. Dansyl chloride is one of the most commonly used reagents to derivatize primary, secondary amines, phenol [27] and alcoholic hydroxyl [22]. It provides all the features mentioned above that improve the analytical power for metabolome analysis. In addition, the concentration of dansyl-labeled metabolites can be determined using UV absorbance, which can be very useful for sample normalization. The workflow of using DnsCl for metabolites profiling and biomarker discovery in various samples have been developed, including urine [42, 43], blood [44], serum [10], sweat [45], cerebrospinal fluid [46], faces [43, 47] and cell extracts [48, 49]. This method has been used for cancer biomarker discovery research.

One example is the work reported by Huan et al. describing a method of metabolomic profiling of prostate tissue samples using DnsCl labeling and conducted a proof-of-principle study for metabolic classification of prostate cancer [50]. In this study, the authors presented a typical workflow of high-performance CIL LC-MS method for metabolomics biomarker discovery of disease. In this workflow, metabolites were first extracted from prostate needle biopsies using molecular preservation by extraction and fixation techniques. Then samples from patients were individually labeled with ^{12}C-dansyl chloride and the total concentration of the labeled metabolites was determined using LC-UV. Based on the total concentration information, the same amount of ^{13}C-labeled universal metabolome standard generated from a pooled tissue extract was spiked into each labeled individual sample, served as internal standard for metabolome comparison. The generated ^{12}C-/^{13}C- mixtures were analyzed by RPLC-QTOF-MS. The data were then processed using a set of in-house programs in batch mode, including peak pair picking and chromatographic peak ratio measurement. Metabolite identification was performed either using labeled standard library [51] for definitive identification or other metabolite database (e.g., HMDB, MyCompoundID) for putative matches. At last, various statistical tools were used to visualize the separation between groups, find significant metabolites, and understand biological meanings.

Using this workflow, three batches of samples were analyzed. In the first batch of experiment, 2900 metabolites were consistently detected in more than 50% of the samples and 88 metabolites were positively identified. Then the panel of significant metabolites was refined using the second batch of samples. Receiver operating characteristic (ROC) analysis showed area under the curve (AUC) of 0.896 with sensitivity of 84.6% and specificity of 83.3% using 7 metabolites. At last, a blind study of validation samples was conducted, providing specificity of 90.9% and sensitivity of 84.6%. Although the sample numbers in this proof-of-concept studies is limited (in total 85 samples), it was still a good example showing the analysis power of high-performance chemical isotope labeling LC-MS method in disease biomarker discovery.

9 Conclusions

CIL LC-MS is a very powerful method for improving metabolomic coverage and quantification accuracy and precision. The presumed disadvantage of adding an extra step of performing chemical labeling of samples in the metabolome analysis workflow is often outweighed by the benefits offered by CIL. We envisage a wide use of this method for comprehensive and quantitative metabolomics in many areas of applications including discovery studies of biomarkers and therapeutic targets. For technical development, work on expanding the labeled standard library to identify more metabolites is needed. In addition, developing new labeling methods targeting chemical groups that are not covered by the current methods will further increase the overall metabolome coverage.

References

1. Peng, B., Li, H., & Peng, X. X. (2015). Functional metabolomics: From biomarker discovery to metabolome reprogramming. *Protein & Cell, 6*(9), 628–637.
2. Caldwell, G. W., & Leo, G. C. (2017). Can untargeted metabolomics be utilized in drug discovery/development? *Current Topics in Medicinal Chemistry, 17*(24), 2716–2739.
3. Aretz, I., & Meierhofer, D. (2016). Advantages and pitfalls of mass spectrometry based metabolome profiling in systems biology. *International Journal of Molecular Sciences, 17*(5), 14.
4. Ortmayr, K., Causon, T. J., Hann, S., & Koellensperger, G. (2016). Increasing selectivity and coverage in

LC-MS based metabolome analysis. *Trac-Trends Analitical Chemistry, 82*, 358–366.
5. Tang, D. Q., Zou, L., Yin, X. X., & Ong, C. N. (2016). HILIC-MS for metabolomics: An attractive and complementary approach to RPLC-MS. *Mass Spectrometry Reviews, 35*(5), 574–600.
6. Antoniewicz, M. R. (2018). A guide to C-13 metabolic flux analysis for the cancer biologist. *Experimental & Molecular Medicine, 50*, 13.
7. Nilsson, R., & Jain, M. (2016). Simultaneous tracing of carbon and nitrogen isotopes in human cells. *Molecular BioSystems, 12*(6), 1929–1937.
8. Freund, D. M., & Hegeman, A. D. (2017). Recent advances in stable isotope-enabled mass spectrometry-based plant metabolomics. *Current Opinion in Biotechnology, 43*, 41–48.
9. Sun, R. C., Fan, T. W. M., Deng, P., Higashi, R. M., Lane, A. N., Le, A. T., Scott, T. L., Sun, Q. S., Warmoes, M. O., & Yang, Y. (2017). Noninvasive liquid diet delivery of stable isotopes into mouse models for deep metabolic network tracing. *Nature Communications, 8*, 10.
10. Han, W., Sapkota, S., Camicioli, R., Dixon, R. A., & Li, L. (2017). Profiling novel metabolic biomarkers for Parkinson's disease using in-depth Metabolomic analysis. *Movement Disorders, 32*(12), 1720–1728.
11. Wong, J. M. T., Malec, P. A., Mabrouk, O. S., Ro, J., Dus, M., & Kennedy, R. T. (2016). Benzoyl chloride derivatization with liquid chromatography-mass spectrometry for targeted metabolomics of neurochemicals in biological samples. *Journal of Chromatography. A, 1446*, 78–90.
12. Mohebi, A., Pettibone, J. R., Hamid, A. A., Wong, J.-M. T., Vinson, L. T., Patriarchi, T., Tian, L., Kennedy, R. T., & Berke, J. D. (2019). Dissociable dopamine dynamics for learning and motivation. *Nature, 570*(7759), 65–70.
13. Han, J., Gagnon, S., Eckle, T., & Borchers, C. H. (2013). Metabolomic analysis of key central carbon metabolism carboxylic acids as their 3-nitrophenylhydrazones by UPLC/ESI-MS. *Electrophoresis, 34*(19), 2891–2900.
14. Han, J., Lin, K., Sequeira, C., & Borchers, C. H. (2015). An isotope-labeled chemical derivatization method for the quantitation of short-chain fatty acids in human feces by liquid chromatography-tandem mass spectrometry. *Analytica Chimica Acta, 854*, 86–94.
15. Han, J., Liu, Y., Wang, R. X., Yang, J. C., Ling, V., & Borchers, C. H. (2015). Metabolic profiling of bile acids in human and mouse blood by LC-MS/MS in combination with phospholipid-depletion solid-phase extraction. *Analytical Chemistry, 87*(2), 1127–1136.
16. O"Maille, G., Go, E. P., Hoang, L., Want, E. J., Smith, C., O'Maille, P., Nordstrom, A., Morita, H., Qin, C., Uritboonthai, W., Apon, J., Moore, R., Garrett, J., & Siuzdak, G. (2008). Metabolomics relative quantitation with mass spectrometry using chemical derivatization and isotope labeling. *Spectroscopy an International Journal, 22*(5), 327–343.
17. Guo, K., & Li, L. (2010). High-performance isotope labeling for profiling carboxylic acid-containing metabolites in biofluids by mass spectrometry. *Analytical Chemistry, 82*(21), 8789–8793.
18. Wang, C. J., Wu, Z. Y., Yuan, J. B., Wang, B., Zhang, P., Zhang, Y., Wang, Z. F., & Huang, L. J. (2014). Simplified quantitative Glycomics using the stable isotope label Girard's reagent P by electrospray ionization mass spectrometry. *Journal of Proteome Research, 13*(2), 372–384.
19. Griffiths, W. J., Hornshaw, M., Woffendin, G., Baker, S. F., Lockhart, A., Heidelberger, S., Gustafsson, M., Sjoall, J., & Wang, Y. Q. (2008). Discovering oxysterols in plasma: A window on the metabolome. *Journal of Proteome Research, 7*(8), 3602–3612.
20. DeBarber, A. E., Sandlers, Y., Pappu, A. S., Merkens, L. S., Duell, P. B., Lear, S. R., Erickson, S. K., & Steiner, R. D. (2011). Profiling sterols in cerebrotendinous xanthomatosis: Utility of Girard derivatization and high resolution exact mass LC-ESI-MSn analysis. *Journal of Chromatography B, 879*(17–18), 1384–1392.
21. Yang, W. C., Sedlak, M., Regnier, F. E., Mosier, N., Ho, N., & Adamec, J. (2008). Simultaneous quantification of metabolites involved in central carbon and energy metabolism using reversed-phase liquid chromatography-mass spectrometry and in vitro C-13 labeling. *Analytical Chemistry, 80*(24), 9508–9516.
22. Zhao, S., Luo, X., & Li, L. (2016). Chemical isotope labeling LC-MS for high coverage and quantitative profiling of the hydroxyl submetabolome in metabolomics. *Analytical Chemistry, 88*(21), 10617–10623.
23. Dai, W. D., Huang, Q., Yin, P. Y., Li, J., Zhou, J., Kong, H. W., Zhao, C. X., Lu, X., & Xu, G. W. (2012). Comprehensive and highly sensitive urinary steroid hormone profiling method based on stable isotope-labeling liquid chromatography mass spectrometry. *Analytical Chemistry, 84*(23), 10245–10251.
24. Comini, M. A. (2016). Measurement and meaning of cellular thiol:Disufhide redox status. *Free Radical Research, 50*(2), 246–271.
25. Ortmayr, K., Schwaiger, M., Hann, S., & Koellensperger, G. (2015). An integrated metabolomics workflow for the quantification of sulfur pathway intermediates employing thiol protection with N-ethyl maleimide and hydrophilic interaction liquid chromatography tandem mass spectrometry. *Analyst, 140*(22), 7687–7695.
26. Liu, P., Huang, Y. Q., Cai, W. J., Yuan, B. F., & Feng, Y. Q. (2014). Profiling of thiol-containing compounds by stable isotope labeling double precursor ion scan mass spectrometry. *Analytical Chemistry, 86*(19), 9765–9773.
27. Guo, K., & Li, L. (2009). Differential C-12/C-13-isotope Dansylation labeling and fast liquid chromatography/mass spectrometry for absolute and relative quantification of the metabolome. *Analytical Chemistry, 81*(10), 3919–3932.

28. Johnson, D. W. (2011). Free amino acid quantification by LC-MS/MS using derivatization generated isotope-labelled standards. *Journal of Chromatography B, 879*(17–18), 1345–1352.
29. Guo, N., Liu, P., Ding, J., Zheng, S. J., Yuan, B. F., & Feng, Y. Q. (2016). Stable isotope labeling - liquid chromatography/mass spectrometry for quantitative analysis of androgenic and progestagenic steroids. *Analytica Chimica Acta, 905*, 106–114.
30. Woo, H. K., Go, E. P., Hoang, L., Trauger, S. A., Bowen, B., Siuzdak, G., & Northen, T. R. (2009). Phosphonium labeling for increasing metabolomic coverage of neutral lipids using electrospray ionization mass spectrometry. *Rapid Communications in Mass Spectrometry, 23*(12), 1849–1855.
31. Buszewski, B., & Noga, S. (2012). Hydrophilic interaction liquid chromatography (HILIC)-a powerful separation technique. *Analytical and Bioanalytical Chemistry, 402*(1), 231–247.
32. Zhu, Q. F., Hao, Y. H., Liu, M. Z., Yue, J., Ni, J., Yuan, B. F., & Feng, Y. Q. (2015). Analysis of cytochrome P450 metabolites of arachidonic acid by stable isotope probe labeling coupled with ultra high-performance liquid chromatography/mass spectrometry. *Journal of Chromatography. A, 1410*, 154–163.
33. Li, S. F., Jin, Y. B., Tang, Z., Lin, S. H., Liu, H. X., Jiang, Y. Y., & Cai, Z. W. (2015). A novel method of liquid chromatography-tandem mass spectrometry combined with chemical derivatization for the determination of ribonucleosides in urine. *Analytica Chimica Acta, 864*, 30–38.
34. Yuan, B. F., Zhu, Q. F., Guo, N., Zheng, S. J., Wang, Y. L., Wang, J., Xu, J., Liu, S. J., He, K., Hu, T., Zheng, Y. W., Xu, F. Q., & Feng, Y. Q. (2018). Comprehensive profiling of fecal metabolome of mice by integrated chemical isotope labeling-mass spectrometry analysis. *Analytical Chemistry, 90*(5), 3512–3520.
35. Takach, E., O'Shea, T., & Liu, H. L. (2014). High-throughput quantitation of amino acids in rat and mouse biological matrices using stable isotope labeling and UPLC-MS/MS analysis. *Journal of Chromatography B, 964*, 180–190.
36. Zhao, S., Li, H., Han, W., Chan, W., & Li, L. (2019). Metabolomic coverage of chemical-group-submetabolome analysis: Group classification and 4-channel chemical isotope labeling LC-MS. *Analytical Chemistry*.
37. Zhao, S., Dawe, M., Guo, K., & Li, L. (2017). Development of high-performance chemical isotope labeling LC-MS for profiling the carbonyl submetabolome. *Analytical Chemistry, 89*(12), 6758–6765.
38. Bian, X. Q., Sun, B. Q., Zheng, P. Y., Li, N., & Wu, J. L. (2017). Derivatization enhanced separation and sensitivity of long chain-free fatty acids: Application to asthma using targeted and non-targeted liquid chromatography-mass spectrometry approach. *Analytica Chimica Acta, 989*, 59–70.
39. Siegel, D., Meinema, A. C., Permentier, H., Hopfgartner, G., & Bischoff, R. (2014). Integrated quantification and identification of aldehydes and ketones in biological samples. *Analytical Chemistry, 86*(10), 5089–5100.
40. Turowski, M., Yamakawa, N., Meller, J., Kimata, K., Ikegami, T., Hosoya, K., Tanaka, N., & Thornton, E. R. (2003). Deuterium isotope effects on hydrophobic interactions: The importance of dispersion interactions in the hydrophobic phase. *Journal of the American Chemical Society, 125*(45), 13836–13849.
41. Szarka, S., Prokai-Tatrai, K., & Prokai, L. (2014). Application of screening experimental designs to assess chromatographic isotope effect upon isotope-coded derivatization for quantitative liquid chromatography-mass spectrometry. *Analytical Chemistry, 86*(14), 7033–7040.
42. Khamis, M. M., Adamko, D. J., & El-Aneed, A. (2017). Development of a validated LC-MS/MS method for the quantification of 19 endogenous asthma/COPD potential urinary biomarkers. *Analytica Chimica Acta, 989*, 45–58.
43. Su, X. L., Wang, N., Chen, D. Y., Li, Y. N., Lu, Y. F., Huan, T., Xu, W., Li, L., & Li, L. J. (2016). Dansylation isotope labeling liquid chromatography mass spectrometry for parallel profiling of human urinary and fecal submetabolomes. *Analytica Chimica Acta, 903*, 100–109.
44. Chen, D. Y., Han, W., Su, X. L., Li, L., & Li, L. J. (2017). Overcoming sample matrix effect in quantitative blood metabolomics using chemical isotope labeling liquid chromatography mass spectrometry. *Analytical Chemistry, 89*(17), 9424–9431.
45. Hooton, K., Han, W., & Li, L. (2016). Comprehensive and quantitative profiling of the human sweat submetabolome using high-performance chemical isotope labeling LC-MS. *Analytical Chemistry, 88*(14), 7378–7386.
46. Guo, K., Bamforth, F., & Li, L. A. (2011). Qualitative metabolome analysis of human cerebrospinal fluid by C-13-/C-12-isotope Dansylation labeling combined with liquid chromatography Fourier transform ion cyclotron resonance mass spectrometry. *Journal of the American Society for Mass Spectrometry, 22*(2), 339–347.
47. Xu, W., Chen, D. Y., Wang, N., Zhang, T., Zhou, R. K., Huan, T., Lu, Y. F., Su, X. L., Xie, Q., Li, L., & Li, L. J. (2015). Development of high-performance chemical isotope labeling LC-MS for profiling the human fecal metabolome. *Analytical Chemistry, 87*(2), 829–836.
48. Luo, X., & Li, L. (2017). Metabolomics of small numbers of cells: Metabolomic profiling of 100, 1000, and 10000 human breast Cancer cells. *Analytical Chemistry, 89*(21), 11664–11671.
49. Luo, X., Zhao, S., Huan, T., Sun, D. F., Friis, R. M. N., Schultz, M. C., & Li, L. (2016). High-performance chemical isotope labeling liquid chromatography mass spectrometry for profiling the Metabolomic reprogramming elicited by ammonium limitation in yeast. *Journal of Proteome Research, 15*(5), 1602–1612.

50. Huan, T., Troyer, D. A., & Li, L. (2016). Metabolite analysis and histology on the exact same tissue: Comprehensive Metabolomic profiling and metabolic classification of prostate Cancer. *Scientific Reports, 6*, 13.
51. Huan, T., Wu, Y. M., Tang, C. Q., Lin, G. H., & Li, L. (2015). DnsID in MyCompoundID for rapid identification of Dansylated amine- and phenol-containing metabolites in LC-MS-based metabolomics. *Analytical Chemistry, 87*(19), 9838–9845.
52. Zhou, R. K., Guo, K., & Li, L. (2013). 5-Diethylamino-naphthalene-1-sulfonyl chloride (DensCl): A novel triplex isotope labeling reagent for quantitative metabolome analysis by liquid chromatography mass spectrometry. *Analytical Chemistry, 85*(23), 11532–11539.
53. Song, C. H., Zhang, S. J., Ji, Z. Y., Li, Y. P., & You, J. M. (2015). Accurate determination of amino acids in serum samples by liquid chromatography-tandem mass spectrometry using a stable isotope labeling strategy. *Journal of Chromatographic Science, 53*(9), 1536–1541.
54. Zheng, L. F., Zhao, X. E., Zhu, S. Y., Tao, Y. D., Ji, W. H., Geng, Y. L., Wang, X. A., Chen, G. A., & You, J. M. (2017). A new combined method of stable isotope-labeling derivatization-ultrasound-assisted dispersive liquid-liquid microextraction for the determination of neurotransmitters in rat brain microdialysates by ultra high performance liquid chromatography tandem mass spectrometry. *Journal of Chromatography B, 1054*, 64–72.
55. Zhou, R., Huan, T., & Li, L. (2015). Development of versatile isotopic labeling reagents for profiling the amine submetabolome by liquid chromatography-mass spectrometry. *Analytica Chimica Acta, 881*, 107–116.
56. Wagner, M., Ohlund, L. B., Shiao, T. C., Vezina, A., Annabi, B., Roy, R., & Sleno, L. (2015). Isotope-labeled differential profiling of metabolites using N-benzoyloxysuccinimide derivatization coupled to liquid chromatography/high-resolution tandem mass spectrometry. *Rapid Communications in Mass Spectrometry, 29*(18), 1632–1640.
57. Zhang, S. S., Shi, J. W., Shan, C. K., Huang, C. T., Wu, Y. L., Ding, R., Xue, Y. H., Liu, W., Zhou, Q., Zhao, Y. F., Xu, P. X., & Gao, X. (2017). Stable isotope N-phosphoryl amino acids labeling for quantitative profiling of amine-containing metabolites using liquid chromatography mass spectrometry. *Analytica Chimica Acta, 978*, 24–34.
58. Hao, L.; Zhong, X. F.; Greer, T.; Ye, H.; Li, L. J., Relative quantification of amine-containing metabolites using isobaric N,N-dimethyl leucine (DiLeu) reagents via LC-ESI-MS/MS and CE-ESI-MS/MS. Analyst 2015, **140** (2), 467–475.
59. Lee, D. Y., & Chang, G. D. (2015). Quantitative liquid chromatography-electrospray ionization-mass spectrometry analysis of amine-containing metabolites derivatized with cyanuric chloride and methylamine isotopologues. *Journal of Chromatography. A, 1388*, 60–68.
60. Wang, X., Wei, F., Xu, J. Q., Lv, X., Dong, X. Y., Han, X. L., Quek, S. Y., Huang, F. H., & Chen, H. (2016). Profiling and relative quantification of phosphatidylethanolamine based on acetone stable isotope derivatization. *Analytica Chimica Acta, 902*, 142–153.
61. Yang, W. C., Mirzaei, H., Liu, X. P., & Regnier, F. E. (2006). Enhancement of amino acid detection and quantification by electrospray ionization mass spectrometry. *Analytical Chemistry, 78*(13), 4702–4708.
62. Shortreed, M. R., Lamos, S. M., Frey, B. L., Phillips, M. F., Patel, M., Belshaw, P. J., & Smith, L. M. (2006). Ionizable isotopic labeling reagent for relative quantification of amine metabolites by mass spectrometry. *Analytical Chemistry, 78*(18), 6398–6403.
63. Guo, K., Ji, C. J., & Li, L. (2007). Stable-isotope dimethylation labeling combined with LC-ESI MS for quantification of amine-containing metabolites in biological samples. *Analytical Chemistry, 79*(22), 8631–8638.
64. Ji, C. J., Li, W. L., Ren, X. D., El-Kattan, A. F., Kozak, R., Fountain, S., & Lepsy, C. (2008). Diethylation labeling combined with UPLC/MS/MS for simultaneous determination of a panel of monoamine neurotransmitters in rat prefrontal cortex microdialysates. *Analytical Chemistry, 80*(23), 9195–9203.
65. Abello, N., Geurink, P. P., van der Toorn, M., van Oosterhout, A. J. M., Lugtenburg, J., van der Marel, G. A., Kerstjens, H. A. M., Postma, D. S., Overkleeft, H. S., & Bischoff, R. (2008). Poly(ethylene glycol)-based stable isotope labeling reagents for the quantitative analysis of low molecular weight metabolites by LC-MS. *Analytical Chemistry, 80*(23), 9171–9180.
66. Shimbo, K., Yahashi, A., Hirayama, K., Nakazawa, M., & Miyano, H. (2009). Multifunctional and highly sensitive Precolumn reagents for amino acids in liquid chromatography/tandem mass spectrometry. *Analytical Chemistry, 81*(13), 5172–5179.
67. Mochizuki, T., Todoroki, K., Inoue, K., Min, J. Z., & Toyo'oka, T. (2014). Isotopic variants of light and heavy L-pyroglutamic acid succinimidyl esters as the derivatization reagents for DL-amino acid chiral metabolomics identification by liquid chromatography and electrospray ionization mass spectrometry. *Analytica Chimica Acta, 811*, 51–59.
68. Lamos, S. M., Shortreed, M. R., Frey, B. L., Belshaw, P. J., & Smith, L. M. (2007). Relative quantification of carboxylic acid metabolites by liquid chromatography - mass spectrometry using isotopic variants of cholamine. *Analytical Chemistry, 79*(14), 5143–5149.
69. Tayyari, F., Gowda, G. A. N., Gu, H. W., & Raftery, D. (2013). N-15-Cholamine-a smart isotope tag for combining NMR- and MS-based metabolite profiling. *Analytical Chemistry, 85*(18), 8715–8721.
70. Yang, W. C., Regnier, F. E., & Adamec, J. (2008). Comparative metabolite profiling of carboxylic acids in rat urine by CE-ESI MS/MS through positively pre-charged and H-2-coded derivatization. *Electrophoresis, 29*(22), 4549–4560.
71. Yang, W. C., Adamec, J., & Regnier, F. E. (2007). Enhancement of the LC/MS analysis of fatty acids

through derivatization and stable isotope coding. *Analytical Chemistry, 79*(14), 5150–5157.
72. Koulman, A., Petras, D., Narayana, V. K., Wang, L., & Volmer, D. A. (2009). Comparative high-speed profiling of carboxylic acid metabolite levels by differential isotope-coded MALDI mass spectrometry. *Analytical Chemistry, 81*(18), 7544–7551.
73. Tsukamoto, Y.; Santa, T.; Yoshida, H.; Miyano, H.; Fukushima, T.; Hirayama, K.; Imai, K.; Funatsu, T., Synthesis of the isotope-labeled derivatization reagent for carboxylic acidsr 7-(N,N-dimethylaminosulfonyl)-4-(aminoethyl)piperazino-2,1,3-benzoxadiaz ole (d(6)) DBD-PZ-NH2 (D) , and its application to the quantification and the determination of relative amount of fatty acids in rat plasma samples by high-performance liquid chromatography/mass spectrometry. *Biomed. Chromatogr.* **2006,** *20* (4), 358–364.
74. Leng, J. P., Wang, H. Y., Zhang, L., Zhang, J., Wang, H., & Guo, Y. L. (2013). A highly sensitive isotope-coded derivatization method and its application for the mass spectrometric analysis of analytes containing the carboxyl group. *Analytica Chimica Acta, 758*, 114–121.
75. Leng, J. P., Guan, Q., Sun, T. Q., Wang, H. Y., Cui, J. L., Liu, Q. H., Zhang, Z. X., Zhang, M. Y., & Guo, Y. L. (2015). Direct infusion electrospray ionization-ion mobility-mass spectrometry for comparative profiling of fatty acids based on stable isotope labeling. *Analytica Chimica Acta, 887*, 148–154.
76. Tie, C., Hu, T., Zhang, X. X., Zhou, J., & Zhang, J. L. (2014). HPLC-MRM relative quantification analysis of fatty acids based on a novel derivatization strategy. *Analyst, 139*(23), 6154–6159.
77. Guo, N., Peng, C. Y., Zhu, Q. F., Yuan, B. F., & Feng, Y. Q. (2017). Profiling of carbonyl compounds in serum by stable isotope labeling double precursor ion scan - mass spectrometry analysis. *Analytica Chimica Acta, 967*, 42–51.
78. Zheng, S. J., Wang, Y. L., Liu, P., Zhang, Z., Yu, L., Yuan, B. F., & Feng, Y. Q. (2017). Stable isotope labeling-solid phase extraction-mass spectrometry analysis for profiling of thiols and aldehydes in beer. *Food Chemistry, 237*, 399–407.
79. Yu, L., Liu, P., Wang, Y. L., Yu, Q. W., Yuan, B. F., & Feng, Y. Q. (2015). Profiling of aldehyde-containing compounds by stable isotope labelling-assisted mass spectrometry analysis. *Analyst, 140*(15), 5276–5286.
80. Crick, P. J., Bentley, T. W., Abdel-Khalik, J., Matthews, I., Clayton, P. T., Morris, A. A., Bigger, B. W., Zerbinati, C., Tritapepe, L., Iuliano, L., Wang, Y. Q., & Griffiths, W. J. (2015). Quantitative charge-tags for sterol and oxysterol analysis. *Clinical Chemistry, 61*(2), 400–411.
81. Higashi, T., Aiba, N., Tanaka, T., Yoshizawa, K., & Ogawa, S. (2016). Methods for differential and quantitative analyses of brain neurosteroid levels by LC/MS/MS with ESI-enhancing and isotope-coded derivatization. *Journal of Pharmaceutical and Biomedical Analysis, 117*, 155–162.
82. Tie, C., Hu, T., Jia, Z. X., & Zhang, J. L. (2016). Derivatization strategy for the comprehensive characterization of endogenous fatty aldehydes using HPLC-multiple reaction monitoring. *Analytical Chemistry, 88*(15), 7762–7768.
83. DeBarber, A. E., Luo, J., Star-Weinstock, M., Purkayastha, S., Geraghty, M. T., Chiang, J., Merkens, L. S., Pappu, A. S., & Steiner, R. D. (2014). A blood test for cerebrotendinous xanthomatosis with potential for disease detection in newborns. *Journal of Lipid Research, 55*(1), 146–154.
84. Chu, J. M., Qi, C. B., Huang, Y. Q., Jiang, H. P., Hao, Y. H., Yuan, B. F., & Feng, Y. Q. (2015). Metal oxide-based selective enrichment combined with stable isotope labeling-mass spectrometry analysis for profiling of ribose conjugates. *Analytical Chemistry, 87*(14), 7364–7372.
85. Wang, H., Wang, H. Y., Zhang, L., Zhang, J., & Guo, Y. L. (2011). N-Alkylpyridinium isotope quaternization for matrix-assisted laser desorption/ionization Fourier transform mass spectrometric analysis of cholesterol and fatty alcohols in human hair. *Analytica Chimica Acta, 690*(1), 1–9.
86. Wang, H., Wang, H. Y., Zhang, L., Zhang, J., Leng, J. P., Cai, T. T., & Guo, Y. L. (2011). Improvement and extension of the application scope for matrix-assisted laser desorption/ionization mass spectrometric analysis-oriented N-alkylpyridinium isotope quaternization. *Analytica Chimica Acta, 707*(1), 100–106.
87. Huang, Y. Q., Ruan, G. D., Liu, J. Q., Gao, Q., & Feng, Y. Q. (2011). Use of isotope differential derivatization for simultaneous determination of thiols and oxidized thiols by liquid chromatography tandem mass spectrometry. *Analytical Biochemistry, 416*(2), 159–166.

NMR-Based Metabolomics

G. A. Nagana Gowda and Daniel Raftery

1 Metabolomics

The field of metabolomics involves the quantitative and simultaneous analysis of large numbers of metabolites in biological systems. Metabolites provide information on action, inaction, or over action of the upstream molecular species such as genes, transcripts, and proteins, in health and diseases. Analysis of complex metabolite data in combination with univariate and multivariate statistical methods, as well as mapping of altered pathways, enables understanding of biological phenotypes, deciphering mechanisms, and identifying biomarkers or drug targets for a variety of conditions [1-5]. Applications of metabolomics span a wide range of disciplines including health and various diseases, pharmacology, drug development, toxicology, environment, plants, and food and nutrition. However, a majority of the studies are focused on improving the mechanistic understanding, along with prevention, early diagnosis, and management of human health and diseases.

2 Analytical Methods for Metabolomics

Development of analytical methods represents a major component of metabolomics research. Numerous types of analytical techniques have been used; however, nuclear magnetic resonance (NMR) spectroscopy and mass spectrometry (MS) are the two most commonly employed methods in the metabolomics field. MS is a highly sensitive method and it enables the analysis of several hundreds to thousands of metabolites from a single measurement and on a routine basis. In MS analysis, often, metabolites are subjected to chromatographic separation using liquid chromatography, gas chromatography, or capillary electrophoresis prior to detection. A variety of MS methods are often used for analysis of different classes of metabolites from the same samples to achieve a wider coverage of the metabolome. NMR spectroscopy, on the other hand, is often used without combining with any sample preprocessing or separation techniques and provides data complementary to MS. Peaks in the NMR

G. A. Nagana Gowda (✉)
Northwest Metabolomics Research Center, Anesthesiology and Pain Medicine, University of Washington, Seattle, WA, USA
e-mail: ngowda@uw.edu

D. Raftery
Northwest Metabolomics Research Center, Anesthesiology and Pain Medicine, University of Washington, Seattle, WA, USA

Department of Chemistry, University of Washington, Seattle, WA, USA

Fred Hutchinson Cancer Research Center, Seattle, WA, USA
e-mail: draftery@uw.edu

S. Hu (ed.), *Cancer Metabolomics*, Advances in Experimental Medicine and Biology 1280,
https://doi.org/10.1007/978-3-030-51652-9_2

spectra can be reliably assigned to specific metabolites and peak intensities are directly proportional to the number of contributing nuclei. Thus, NMR provides a wealth of information on both the identity and quantity of many metabolites in parallel.

3 Characteristics of NMR Spectroscopy

NMR spectroscopy exhibits numerous unique characteristics that are beneficial to the field of metabolomics [6-8]. Some of these important characteristics include:

1. It is highly reproducible and quantitative.
2. A single internal reference is sufficient for absolute quantitation of all metabolites in a spectrum.
3. It enables establishment of the identity for unknown metabolites, which is important considering that advances in analytical technologies have enabled the detection of an increasing number of signals in complex biological mixtures and many of them are unknown.
4. It enables the analysis of intact biofluids and tissue with no need for sample separation or preparation, which is important considering that sample preparation and separation processes contribute significantly to the analytical variability.
5. It is nondestructive, which means the sample remains intact after the analysis and can be used for reanalysis using NMR at a later time or other methods such as MS.
6. It enables tracing of metabolic pathways and measuring metabolic fluxes utilizing a variety of stable isotope-labeled precursors.
7. It has the ability to detect metabolites through one or more types of atomic nuclei such as ^{1}H, ^{13}C, ^{31}P, or ^{15}N.
8. It does not involve harsh sample treatment prior to or during the analysis, which is important for analysis of metabolites such as glutamine and coenzymes that are fragile or sensitive to ionization voltage as used in the MS analysis [9-13].

4 Workflow for NMR-Based Metabolomics

Figure 1 shows a schematic diagram for a general workflow involved in NMR-based metabolomics. Biological samples from humans (e.g., plasma or serum, urine, and tissue), animal models, or cell lines can be used for NMR-based metabolomics studies. Important steps involved are detection of metabolite signals, metabolite identification using a combination of 1D and 2D NMR methods, database searching and spiking with authentic compounds, and finally quantifying the identified metabolites using a single internal or external standard. Metabolite concentrations are then used for distinguishing diseases from controls; this is done generally based on univariate or multivariate statistical analysis, developing and validating classification models, and testing the sensitivity and specificity of the models based on the area under the receiver operating characteristic (ROC) curve. Additionally, metabolite concentrations are used for identifying altered metabolic pathways, which help provide a mechanistic understanding of cellular function including information on drug targets for therapeutic development and translational opportunities for preventing or curing diseases.

5 Biological Samples

NMR-based metabolomics studies use a wide variety of biological specimens. The most widely used biological specimen for investigation of virtually all human diseases is blood. The clinical relevance of blood arises from its close association with essentially every living cell in the human body combined with its relatively easy access for routine investigations. Generally, blood samples from overnight fasted subjects are preferred to avoid confounding effects from the diet. Conventional metabolomics studies of serum or plasma samples provide a wealth of metabolic information on health and diseases [14, 10, 15]. However, serum and plasma metabolomics lacks the ability to measure and evaluate important metabolites such as redox and energy

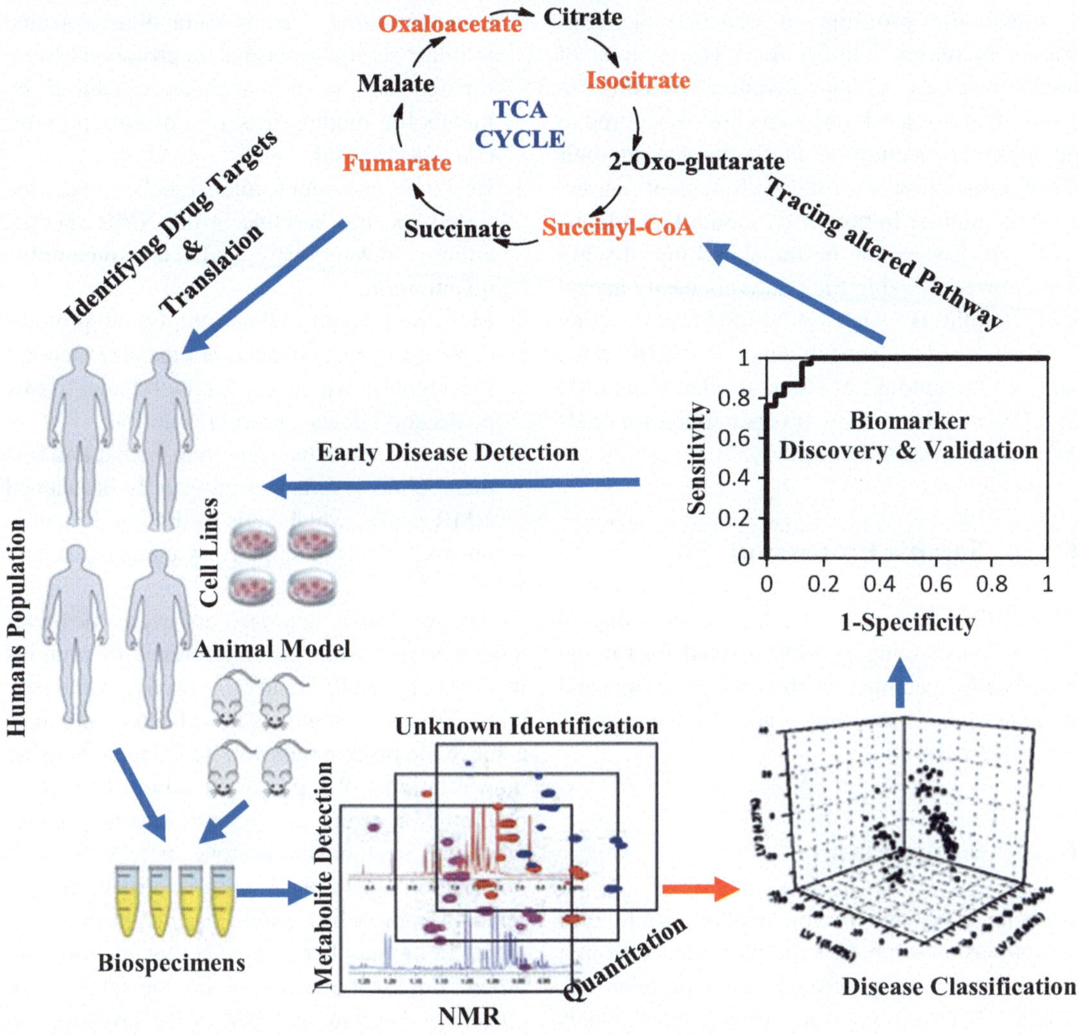

Fig. 1 Schematic diagram describing the workflow of NMR based metabolomics

coenzymes, as well as antioxidants, which are generally present in high concentrations in red blood cells. An important alternative to serum/plasma metabolomics is a whole blood metabolomics approach using NMR [16]. Whole blood metabolomics enables access to a wider and complementary pool of metabolites and also avoids the potential confounding effects of hemolysis often encountered in serum/plasma metabolite analysis.

Other biological specimens used in NMR-based metabolomics include urine [17, 18], saliva [19], cerebrospinal fluid [20], gut aspirate [21], bile [22], amniotic fluid [23], synovial fluid [24], exhaled breath condensate [25], intact tissue [26], and tissue extracts [27]. Specimens from animal models, cell lines, yeast [28], bacteria [29], tumor cells [30], and tumor spheroids have also been analyzed by NMR [31].

Urine is the most widely used biological specimen, apart from blood. Interest in using urine for NMR-based metabolomics stems from the fact that it is a rich source of disease biomarkers and the sample can be obtained noninvasively. In addition, unlike blood, urine has a relatively low concentration of proteins and a large number of low molecular weight compounds (metabolites); hence metabolomics studies of urine are relatively simple in terms of both sample preparation and NMR analysis.

Metabolite profiling of intact tissues has gained increased interest for investigations of human diseases. A major advantage of using tissues is that disease biomarkers are considered to be highly concentrated in tissue due to their close association with the pathological source, such as tumors. Importantly, biomarkers identified from tissues can be translated into disease detection tools using the relatively easily accessible biofluids such as blood and urine. Technological advancements in NMR have reduced the amount of tissue needed to as little as a few nanoliters, which is beneficial for analysis of mass limited samples [32].

6 Sample Processing

One of the advantages of NMR is its ability to analyze intact samples with no need for sample processing. Specimens such as serum/plasma and urine have thus been widely used for the analysis without processing.

6.1 Serum/Plasma

A major challenge for metabolite profiling of serum/plasma samples is the interference from a massive amount of serum/plasma proteins (6–8 g/dL). The unwanted macromolecular signals from proteins are typically suppressed prior to NMR experiments that use a T_2 (transverse relaxation) filter, such as the CPMG sequence [14]; metabolites generally exhibit longer T_2 relaxation times compared to macromolecules, and hence they are selectively retained by the CPMG sequence. The CPMG-based NMR experiments have thus long been exploited for serum and plasma metabolomics. While the analysis of intact serum/plasma samples is attractive, numerous limitations as shown below make this approach less suitable for metabolomics studies:

1. The number of metabolites detected using intact serum/plasma is restricted to about 30 or less, which is far fewer compared to the actual number of blood metabolites present in the sample [15].
2. Concentrations of many metabolites detected in intact serum or plasma are grossly underestimated due to the attenuation caused by metabolite binding to serum/plasma proteins (Fig. 2a) [33-36].
3. Residual macromolecule signals cause distorted spectral baseline in the NMR spectra, which deleteriously affects metabolite quantitation.
4. Massive amounts of serum/plasma proteins cause reduced T_2 relaxation times for metabolite signals, which results in broader NMR peaks and affects spectral resolution.
5. The exchange between protein-bound and free metabolites results in significantly broadened NMR peaks, which adds to the line broadening and affects quantitative accuracy.

An alternative approach to overcome challenges arising from the interference of proteins involves physically removing serum/plasma proteins. Numerous methods have been explored to achieve the protein removal, which include using ultrafiltration, solid phase extraction, or protein precipitation using an organic solvent such as methanol, acetonitrile, acetone, perchloric acid, or trichloroacetic acid [37-40]. Such protein removal approaches enable significant improvements in the number of metabolites identified in blood. For example, based on the analysis of ultrafiltered serum, as a part of the investigation of the human serum metabolome, 49 metabolites could be analyzed [15]. In another study, based on ultrafiltered human plasma from NIST SRM (National Institute of Standards and Technology Standard Reference Material), 39 metabolites were identified [41].

Realizing the need to process serum/plasma before the analysis, additional efforts were focused on the development of a method for both optimal recovery of metabolites and expanding the number of quantifiable metabolites. A detailed quantitative assessment of the performance of protein precipitation methods and the ultrafiltration approach was made based on a comprehensive analysis using various NMR techniques. Both methods (protein precipitation and ultrafiltration) allowed the detection of metabolites with comparable

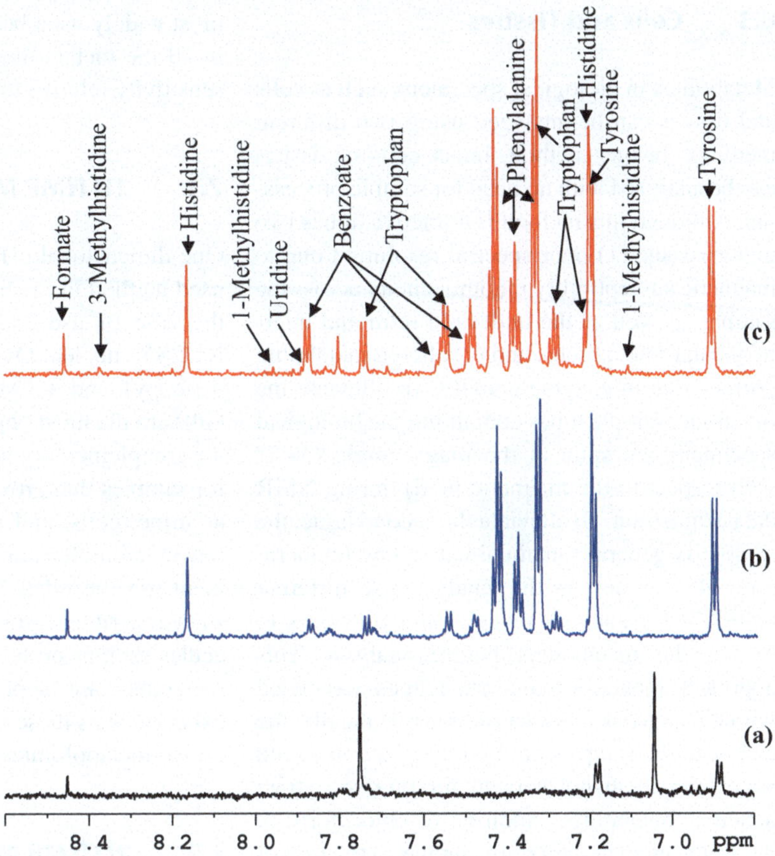

Fig. 2 Comparison of portions of ^{1}H NMR spectra of the same pooled human serum sample obtained by suppressing protein signals by (**a**) T_2 filtering using the CPMG pulse sequence, (**b**) ultrafiltration using a 3 kDa molecular weight cutoff filter, and (**c**) protein precipitation using methanol (1:2 v/v). In (**a**) most of the metabolite signals are missing or significantly attenuated, while in (**b**) many metabolites including tryptophan, benzoate, and formate are significantly attenuated when compared to (**c**). (Reproduced with permission from [35])

reproducibility. However, nearly half of the metabolites in ultrafiltered serum exhibited 10–75% lower concentrations [35] (Fig. 2). Further experiments indicated that protein precipitation using methanol offers a more optimal approach for NMR-based metabolomics of serum/plasma. In addition, comparison of the serum NMR spectra obtained after protein precipitation using methanol and acetonitrile revealed a surprisingly poor performance for protein precipitation using acetonitrile [10]. Nearly one-third of the detected metabolites were attenuated up to nearly 70% compared to methanol precipitation at the same solvent to serum ratio of 2:1 (v/v). A further attenuation of nearly two-thirds of the metabolites (by up to 65%) was observed upon increasing acetonitrile to serum ratio to 4:1 (v/v). Therefore, precipitation using a methanol to serum/plasma ratio of 2:1 (v/v) is recommended for NMR-based metabolomics studies.

6.2 Urine

For urine analysis, no sample preprocessing is required due to the absence of macromolecules, and hence, intact urine samples are generally used. The pH of normal human urine varies widely, from approximately 5 to 8 [42-44]. Many peaks in the urine NMR spectra are sensitive to the pH variation, and sample to sample variation in pH is therefore a major challenge in the analysis of urine. Therefore, urine samples are generally mixed with a buffer solution in D_2O, typically in a 1:1 (v/v) ratio (at pH = 7.4). A detailed procedure for urine analysis by NMR is provided in a comprehensive article published previously [14].

6.3 Cells and Tissues

Metabolites in biological specimens such as cells and tissues can be analyzed using two different methods. In one method, intact cells or tissues can be analyzed with no need for sample processing. Although this method is attractive, it has two major issues: (1) poor spectral resolution due to magnetic susceptibility inhomogeneity across the sample, as well as the undesired intra and intermolecular interactions, and (2) altered metabolite profiles due to enzyme activity. To alleviate the first issue, sample tubes containing the biological specimens are spun at the magic angle (54.7° with respect to the magnetic field) during NMR data acquisition. To alleviate the second issue, the sample is generally maintained at low temperature (4° C) during the analysis. A different approach for analysis of cells and tissues is to extract the metabolites before analysis. This approach alleviates major challenges associated with the analysis of intact samples. Typically, the cell or tissue samples are homogenized in a cold water and methanol solvent mixture to extract aqueous metabolites. Addition of chloroform to the water-methanol mixture enables extraction of both aqueous and lipid metabolites, in a single step. This three solvent mixture forms two phases; aqueous metabolites dissolve in the top phase, which contains water and methanol, whereas lipid metabolites are dissolved in the bottom phase, which contains methanol and chloroform. The two phases are separated and solvents removed by drying. The dried residue containing aqueous metabolites is then dissolved in D_2O, whereas the residue containing lipids is dissolved in a mixture of deuterated chloroform ($CDCl_3$), deuterated methanol (CD_3OD), and water (D_2O) typically in 16:7:1 (v/v/v) ratio (which does not phase separate) for analysis using NMR.

7 NMR Experiments

Many NMR active nuclei such as ^1H, ^{13}C, ^{31}P, and ^{15}N can be used to analyze metabolites in biological mixtures [45, 8, 46-48]. However, ^1H NMR is most widely used because ^1H is present virtually in all the metabolites, and it has a higher NMR sensitivity relative to other nuclei.

7.1 1D NMR Methods

One-dimensional (1D) NMR is the most widely used method in the metabolomics field, owing to the ease of use and high throughput. The 1D NOESY (nuclear Overhauser enhancement spectroscopy) and CPMG (Carr-Purcell-Meiboom-Gill) are the most popular NMR experiments and are complementary in nature. 1D NOESY is used for samples that provide narrow line shapes such as urine, cells, and tissue extracts, due to their low macromolecular content. The CPMG experiment, on the other hand, is useful for samples such as serum/plasma, which contain macromolecules such as proteins. Signals from the macromolecules are suppressed selectively by this experiment as these signals are often not of interest for metabolomics studies.

7.2 2D NMR Methods

Two-dimensional (2D) NMR experiments are increasingly used in metabolomics. Two major areas of 2D NMR applications are unknown metabolite identification and improved metabolite quantitation. Unknown metabolite identification is a major issue in the metabolomics field and NMR represents a gold standard method. Two-dimensional NMR experiments are particularly well suited for the identification of unknown compounds. In addition, due to the fact that 2D NMR experiments significantly improve the spectral resolution and alleviate the peak overlap problem for complex biological samples, 2D NMR offers improved accuracy for metabolite quantitation. Statistically relevant changes in low abundant metabolites can be better characterized using 2D NMR compared to 1D NMR [49]. The most commonly used 2D NMR experiments involving only ^1H nuclei are correlation spectroscopy (COSY) and total correlation spectroscopy (TOCSY). Two-dimensional *J*-resolved spectroscopy is another type of 2D experiment used in metabolomics; it provides no additional peaks compared to 1D NMR, unlike COSY and TOCSY, but it greatly simplifies the NMR spectrum. Important 2D experiments that involve heteronuclei such as ^{13}C or ^{15}N are heteronuclear single quantum coherence spectroscopy (HSQC), heteronuclear multiple quantum correlation spectroscopy (HMQC), and heteronuclear multiple bond correction spectroscopy (HMBC). A challenge for heteronuclear 2D experiments is the low natural abundance of the ^{13}C and ^{15}N; while the 2D experiments involving the natural abundance ^{13}C require significantly increased data acquisition time, those involving the natural abundance ^{15}N are currently largely impractical to use in the metabolomics field owing to its extremely lower sensitivity. Nevertheless, isotope-labeled experiments (described below) do provide opportunities to measure ^{15}N containing compounds. When compared to 1D NMR, 2D NMR experiments generally involve longer data acquisition times, larger data size, and less convenience for data analysis.

7.3 NMR Techniques for Analysis of Mass Limited Samples

Use of micro-coil probes offer additional sensitivity for NMR detection and are particularly useful for mass limited samples [50-53]. Various analysis methods using micro-coil NMR include online detection of eluted fractions from the liquid chromatography (LC), LC followed by online pre-concentration and micro-coil NMR detection, and LC followed by offline detection [54-56]. Commercially available micro-coil probes integrated with automation enable high throughout analysis and are well suited for large cohorts of small volume samples. Recently, as an important alternative to conventional 5 mm and 3 mm NMR probes, a commercially available 1.7 mm micro-coil probe is gaining interest for metabolomic applications. Cryoprobes offer further enhancement to the sensitivity by a factor of 3–4 compared to room temperature probes. A combination of cryoprobe and micro-coil technologies offers an order of magnitude reduction in the data acquisition time. It is important, however, to remember that sample preparation for micro-coil NMR experiments can be challenging as sample pre-concentration can result in the loss of linear response among the metabolites due to their varied solubilities [51]. Thus, while the use of micro-coil NMR offers significant enhancement in sensitivity, care should be exercised while concentrating samples, online or offline, for enhancing the sensitivity.

7.4 Fast Data Acquisition Methods

A number of approaches have been used to speed the acquisition of NMR data. Important developments in fast acquisition methods include nonlinear sampling and forward maximum entropy reconstruction, which offers significant reduction in data acquisition times [57, 58]. Using this approach for 2D HSQC experiments, a reduction in acquisition time of an order of magnitude was achieved [57]. Separately, nonlinear sampling and forward maximum entropy reconstruction was applied to 2D HSQC experiments in combination with J-compensation to achieve more than a 20-fold reduction in data acquisition time [59]. Another approach that speeds up the data acquisition is the SOFAST (band-selective optimized flip angle short transient) technique, in which 2D data are acquired in a few seconds; fast acquisition in SOFAST is achieved through the enhancement of the steady-state magnetization by combining an accelerated T_1 relaxation time and optimized flip angle [60, 61]. SOFAST HMQC with its capability to acquire data within 15 s enables real-time metabolism studies in live cells [62]. Somewhat recently, the SOFAST HMQC was combined with nonlinear sampling to acquire serum and urine spectra at natural ^{13}C abundance with sevenfold reduced time compared to the conventional heteronuclear 2D experiment [63]. Covariance NMR spectroscopy is another fast acquisition approach, which provides high resolution 2D NMR spectra with minimal data points in the indirect dimension [64]. An altogether different class of NMR experiments that speeds up the data acquisition is the so-called ultrafast NMR techniques. The 2D NMR spectrum is acquired in a single scan with a sub-second data acquisition based on the application of field gradients that divide the sample into different segments; the NMR signals from these segments are then acquired in parallel using magnetic resonance imaging type of acquisition. Applications of this approach to areas including metabolomics have been demonstrated [65].

7.5 Ultrasensitive NMR Methods

Hyperpolarization methods such as optical pumping of ^{3}He or ^{129}Xe, parahydrogen-induced polarization (PHIP), and dynamic nuclear polarization (DNP) are shown to boost NMR sensitivity by several orders of magnitude. Of these, PHIP and DNP have been shown to be promising for metabolomics applications. Parahydrogen produced by PHIP can be transferred to other spins by chemical synthesis using an unsaturated compound or by transfer of magnetization to metabolites via a catalyst [66, 67]. PASADENA (parahydrogen and synthesis allow dramatically enhanced nuclear alignment) is a commonly used PHIP method [68-70]. DNP is an especially promising signal enhancement method for metabolomic applications because, unlike PHIP, DNP enables hyperpolarization of a very wide range of substrates. DNP uses paramagnetic centers to transfer polarization from electron spins to nuclear spins of substrates [71-73]. The dissolution DNP approach starts with nuclear spin polarization in the solid state at low temperature, after which the sample is liquified, transported, and then injected into a high-resolution NMR spectrometer for detection. This approach promises new avenues for real-time metabolism studies [74, 75]. Some drawbacks of DNP are the long hyperpolarization preparation time, the need for an expensive polarizer, and short relaxation times of a number of biologically interesting substrates, which limit signal intensities for metabolite tracer studies. Progress is being made on multi-sample polarization approaches that promise high-throughput studies using dissolution DNP [74].

8 Isotope Labeling Methods

NMR methods involving isotope incorporation in vivo or ex vivo offer unique opportunities to the metabolomics field. These methods offer a combination of selectivity, sensitivity, and resolution and alleviate major challenges in NMR experiments involving low natural abundant nuclei. Numerous isotope labeling studies using nuclei such as ^{13}C, ^{15}N, ^{2}H, and/or ^{31}P have so far been reported.

8.1 Isotope Labeling in Flux Measurements

Isotope labeling in vivo enables the tracing of metabolic pathways and measurement of fluxes through specific pathways. Using this approach, the same metabolite that flows through multiple pathways can be identified with a particular flux or pathway, unlike the traditional metabolic profiling approach that measures the overall metabolite intensity and lacks such an ability. As an illustration, lactate can be formed by the catabolism of glucose or through pathways unconnected to glycolysis. Pyruvate arising from glycolysis can be distinguished from that arising from several other pathways by treating cells with ^{13}C-labeled glucose, for example, and measuring the ^{13}C-labeled pyruvate. Numerous pathways including glycolysis, glutaminolysis, and TCA cycle can thus be investigated using NMR- and isotope-labeled substrates such as ^{13}C-glucose and ^{13}C/^{15}N-glutamine [76-78]. Understanding the alterations of these pathways under different conditions and diseases is important owing to the fact that catabolism of glucose and glutamine is critical for the viability and growth of mammalian cells [79, 80]. Cancer cells have been shown to depend on high rates of glucose and/or glutamine uptake and metabolism to maintain their viability [81, 78]. While in vivo isotope-labeled studies using cell line models enable understanding of metabolic pathways under controlled conditions, the use of animal models or humans can translate the findings from cellular studies to the pathogenesis in the relevant organs [82- 85].

8.2 Isotope Labeling in Plants/Organisms

Generally, the high level of biological complexity continually demands new approaches for unraveling such complexity. NMR methods combined with isotope labeling in vivo in plants and organisms such as bacteria and yeast offer significant enhancement to spectral resolution and the detection sensitivity [86-89]. In particular, in vivo labeling enables a systematic analysis of a large number of metabolites (including novel metabolites) using conventional high-resolution 2D NMR experiments such as HSQC. In addition, owing to the uniform labeling of metabolites using nuclei such as ^{13}C, the approach also enables characterization of metabolites based on homonuclear 2D ^{13}C NMR experiments, whereas it is generally impractical to perform such experiments under natural ^{13}C abundance. Carbon-bond topology networks obtainable from the homonuclear 2D ^{13}C experiments provide additional avenues for unknown metabolite identification [86, 88].

8.3 Ex Vivo Isotope Labeling

Isotope labeling ex vivo selectively targets different classes of metabolites based on the specific functional group [45, 46, 48]. Derivatization of metabolites using substrates containing isotope-labeled nuclei, such as ^{13}C, ^{15}N, and ^{31}P offers benefits in terms of both sensitivity and resolution, owing to the high isotopic abundance and wide chemical shift dispersion of tagged heteronuclei (Fig. 3). 2D NMR experiments involving heteronuclei generally provide a single peak for each tagged metabolite, devoid of multiplicity, which further adds to the sensitivity and resolution. Numerous substrates for isotope tagging have been used to date focusing on metabolite classes such as amines, carboxylic acids, and hydroxyls [45, 46, 48]. The "smart isotope tag" ^{15}N-cholamine targets carboxylic acids containing metabolites and can detect the same metabolites using both NMR and MS methods [47]. This is because the smart isotope tag possesses an NMR sensitive isotope (^{15}N) that offers good chemical shift dispersion and a permanent positive charge that improves MS sensitivity. Use of this smart isotope tag approach enables direct comparison of NMR and MS data for the same samples and hence allows exploitation of the combined strengths of the two analytical platforms.

9 Data Analysis

Analysis of complex NMR data in metabolomics is made using one of the two major approaches: One is a global chemometric analysis and the other is quantitative analysis, referred to as quantitative metabolomics [90].

9.1 Chemometric Analysis

Chemometric analysis is a traditional method in untargeted or global metabolomics, in which metabolites are not identified initially. Instead, the complex data are directly used for statistical analysis. Prior to the analysis, the data are subjected to preprocessing such as baseline correction, peak alignment, and solvent peak removal. Finally, the data are subjected to multivariate analysis. A challenge to the chemometric approach, however, is that often sample classes are differentiated based on minor spectral features, which needs to be addressed by appropriate data scaling or filtering. In addition, imperfect peak alignments and spectral baselines pose significant challenges to the analysis. Peak misalignment is particularly pronounced for biological samples such urine, for which peak positions are sensitive to sample conditions such as pH, ionic strength, temperature, and concentration of metabolites [91, 92].

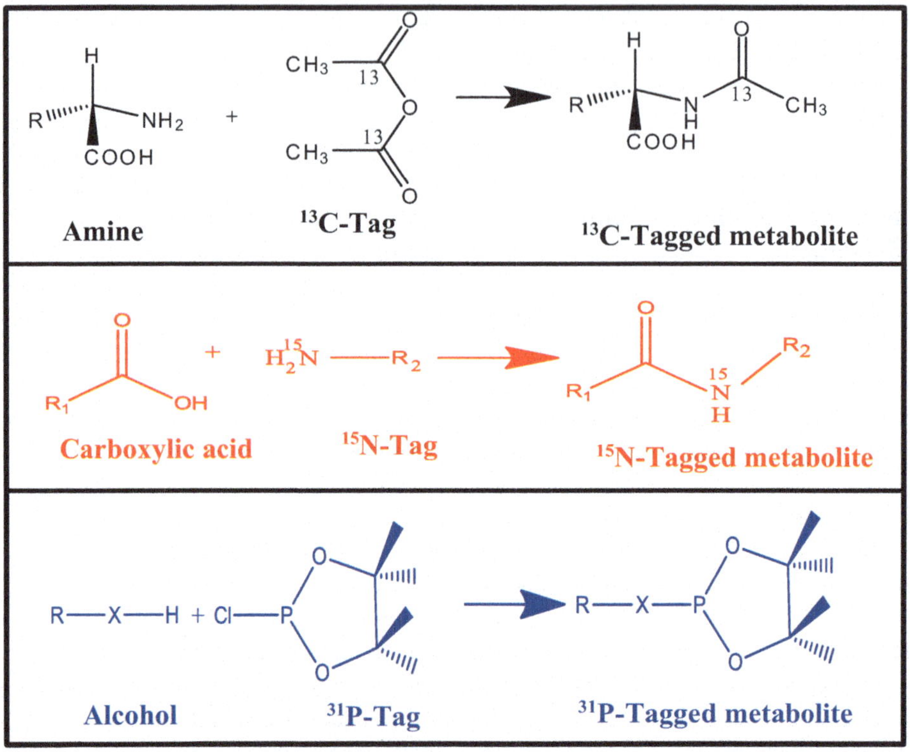

Fig. 3 Reaction schemes for chemical derivatization using ^{13}C, ^{15}N, or ^{31}P tags to target amine, carboxylic acid, or hydroxyl group containing metabolites in complex biological mixtures that enable detection of metabolites by NMR with enhanced resolution and sensitivity. (Reproduced with permission from [7])

Multivariate statistical approaches are broadly classified into two categories: unsupervised analysis and supervised analysis. In unsupervised analysis, the sample class identity is not known, whereas in supervised methods the sample class information (e.g., disease or control) is provided as an input prior to the analysis. Detailed descriptions of multivariate statistical analyses are widely available [93-96].

9.1.1 Unsupervised Analysis

Unsupervised analysis is often used in the exploratory research for hypothesis generation. Several methods including principal component analysis (PCA), hierarchical cluster analysis (HCA), k-nearest neighbor (KNN), and factor analysis are often used [97]. However, PCA is the most widely used among these in the metabolomics field [98]. Using PCA, it is relatively straightforward to detect potential outliers and clusters in the whole sample set. It transforms metabolites data into a set of ranked principal components (PCs). The variance in PCs can then be visualized through the "scores" plot, and specific variables that cause such variance are visualized through the "loadings" plot. The variables' identities may not be known and hence further analysis can be required to establish their identities [99]. HCA, another unsupervised method, is most useful for comparing a small number of variables. It defines natural clusters based on the distances between pairs of samples or variables within the data set. The smallest distances between samples imply that this subset of samples share similar metabolite levels and signify that the samples exhibit similar physiological properties or disease states.

9.1.2 Supervised Analysis

Supervised statistical analysis methods are used for developing predictive models; they take into account the sample class (e.g., disease versus control), which are used as dependent variables, as well as the metabolites used as independent variables. Partial least squares discriminant analysis (PLS-DA) [100], often combined with orthogonal signal correction [101], is by far the most popular method used in metabolomics. This is in part because PLS-DA can handle well the inherent correlation among metabolite variables. Other methods, such as logistic regression, soft independent modeling of class analogies (SIMCA), random forests, and neural networks are also used as supervised methods in metabolomics. Somewhat similar to PCA, in PLS-DA, each orthogonal axis is referred to as a latent variable (LV) and the LVs contain the combinations of weights of each metabolite variable. Based on the LVs, putative biomarker variables can be identified. Supervised methods need extensive validation using a "set-aside" part of the same data set or, ideally, a separate data set to test the predictive model. The model is evaluated, typically, by single or multiple cross-validation steps, to test the robustness of putative variables (biomarker candidates) [102]. The successful use of additional sets of samples, preferably from independent sources, which are sufficiently large to yield statistically significant results, is a current challenge in metabolomics.

9.2 Quantitative Analysis

Quantitative analysis, on the other hand, involves metabolite identification and quantitation, which may then be followed by multivariate statistical analysis. Pathway analyses are also made based on the obtained metabolite levels. Quantitative analysis is generally a targeted method wherein the metabolites are first identified based on the literature or databases of standard compounds. The identified metabolite peaks are then quantified using internal or external reference compounds. Such quantitative data become the input variables for multivariate statistical analysis. A major benefit of the quantitative analysis approach compared to global chemometric analysis is that it can reduce potential errors arising from factors such as baseline distortions, strong solvent signals, and peak misalignments. Hence the quantitative metabolomics approach promises numerous benefits including reliable insights into the mechanistic understanding of diseases.

Recent advances have expanded the pool of metabolites quantifiable by NMR in various biological specimens including serum/plasma, whole blood, tissue and cells, thus offering new avenues in the quantitative metabolomics field.

9.2.1 Quantitative Analysis of Metabolites in Serum, Plasma, and Whole Blood

Metabolite profiling of human serum/plasma is of major interest for the investigations of virtually all human diseases. Despite its significance, for many years, metabolomics analysis of blood was largely restricted to serum/plasma. A significant challenge for widespread quantitative metabolomics of blood by NMR was limited number of metabolites that could be identified and quantified. Limited resolution and sensitivity combined with the challenges associated with unknown metabolite identification have long restricted both the number and quantitative accuracy of measuring blood metabolites. The origin for such a limitation was due to the practice of performing serum/plasma analysis in their intact form, which invariably met with interference from a vast amount of serum/plasma proteins. In contrast, removal of the proteins, physically, prior to the analysis improved resolution and sensitivity, dramatically [37-40], and enabled significant improvement to quantitation in terms of the number of metabolites. Subsequent developments have enabled optimized protein removal methods [35] (Fig. 2). Use of this optimized method has resulted in the identification of the vast majority of peaks in the NMR spectrum and identification and quantitation of nearly 70 serum/plasma metabolites from a single 1D NMR experiment [10]. Characteristic peaks for the identified metabolites were annotated in the NMR spectra to enable their identification and quantitation, routinely, even for beginners to the metabolomics field (Fig. 4). The ability to analyze such a vast pool of metabolites by NMR, quantitatively, promises significant

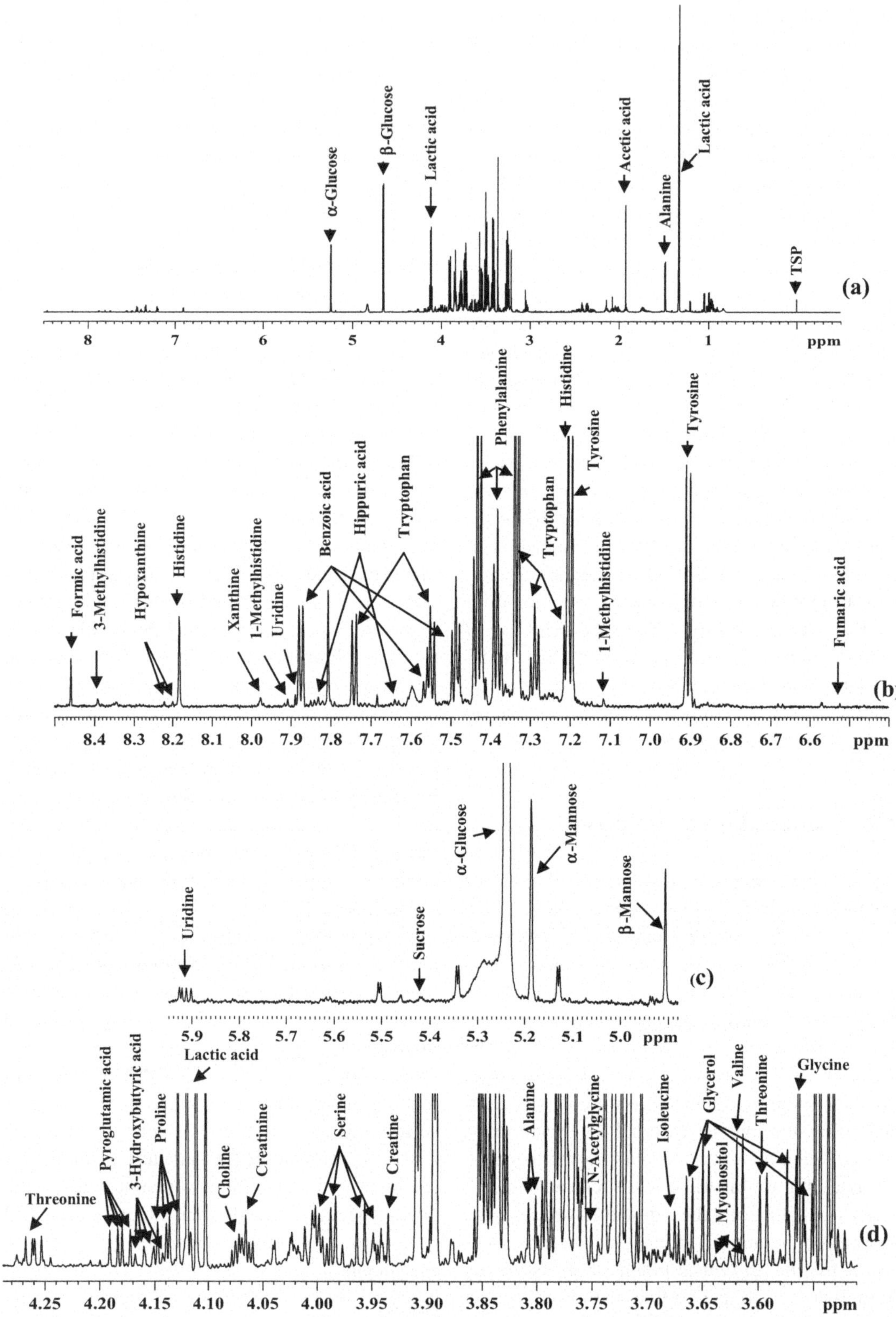

Fig. 4 (**a**) A typical 800 MHz 1D CPMG ^{1}H NMR spectrum of a human serum obtained after protein precipitation using methanol with expanded regions (**b** – **h**) and annotations for all identified metabolites. (Modified from [10])

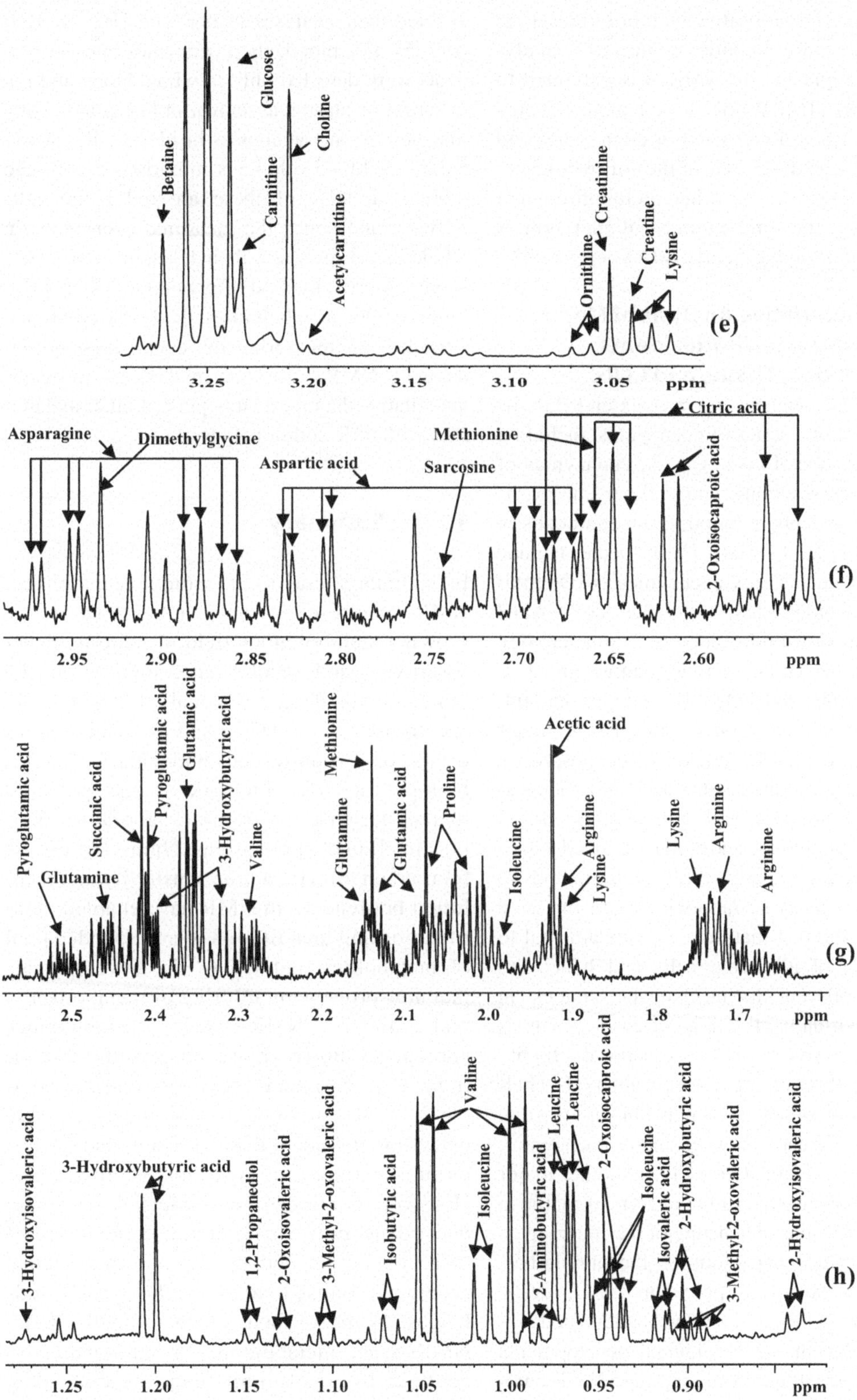

Fig. 4 (continued)

advances in the quantitative metabolomics area. Further, and more recently, quantitative analysis of serum/plasma by NMR was extended to whole blood [16]. Whole blood analysis now enables analysis of many major coenzymes and antioxidants, as described in the following section, in addition to the other metabolites, and has extended the total number of metabolites quantified in blood to nearly 80.

9.2.2 Quantitative Analysis of Major Coenzymes/Antioxidants in Blood, Tissue, and Cells

Recently, NMR analysis has been extended to the measurement of a series of coenzymes, including coenzyme A, acetyl coenzyme A, coenzymes of cellular redox reactions, and cellular energy, as well as antioxidants in blood, tissue, and cells in one step [103, 16, 11, 104]. These species include the major cellular redox coenzymes NAD^+ (oxidized nicotinamide adenine dinucleotide), NADH (reduced nicotinamide adenine dinucleotide), $NADP^+$ (oxidized nicotinamide adenine dinucleotide phosphate), and NADPH (reduced nicotinamide adenine dinucleotide phosphate); major energy coenzymes ATP (adenosine triphosphate), ADP (adenosine diphosphate), and AMP (adenosine monophosphate); and antioxidants GSSG (oxidized glutathione) and GSH (reduced glutathione). Increased interest to develop methods to analyze the coenzymes/antioxidants in one step stems from the fact that they are fundamental to the function of all living cells and hence are extremely relevant to mechanistic studies in health and virtually all human diseases. Analysis of these coenzymes in one step using the highly sensitive method of mass spectrometry is challenging owing to factors such as ion suppression, unit mass difference between many coenzymes, and in-source fragmentation [11]. Another major challenge unconnected to the analytical platform is the extremely unstable nature of the coenzymes; many coenzymes, depending on the sample harvesting and extraction procedure used, evade detection altogether or their levels attenuated significantly. Recent methodological developments in sample harvesting, processing, and NMR analysis have alleviated the major challenges and enabled their analyses in one step [16, 11, 104] (Fig. 5). For blood, the coenzymes and antioxidants were detected only in whole blood and not in serum or plasma as shown in Fig. 5 indicating that they are endogenous to the blood cells. Nearly half of the blood volume is comprised of cells and more than 99% of these are red blood cells (RBCs), and hence the measured coenzymes in whole blood represent their levels in RBCs. The newly reported method offers numerous opportunities in the metabolomics field. An additional advantage of measuring the coenzymes/antioxidants by NMR is that the method also provides quantitative data for a large pool of other metabolites with little additional effort.

10 Summary

In summary, due to its unique capabilities, NMR spectroscopy plays a key role in the growing metabolomics field, despite its lower sensitivity and resolution compared to the other widely used analytical platform, mass spectrometry. NMR-based metabolomics offers opportunities to understand systems biology, discover biomarkers and potential therapy targets, and translate laboratory findings to clinical applications. Numerous efforts focused on alleviating the sensitivity and resolution bottlenecks in NMR have enabled identification and quantitation of an expanded pool of metabolites and led to the developments that now promise monitoring of metabolism in real time. NMR-based metabolomics approaches, however, are not devoid of limitations. Owing to the increasingly realized complexity of biological mixtures, reliable detection, unknown identification, and quantitation continue to pose major challenges. However, continued, multifaceted efforts to boost sensitivity, resolution, and the speed of data acquisition and to improve quantitative accuracy promise to alleviate the current challenges. With constant advances in the field, NMR-based metabolomics is anticipated to continue to greatly impact the understanding of systems biology and to help make progress

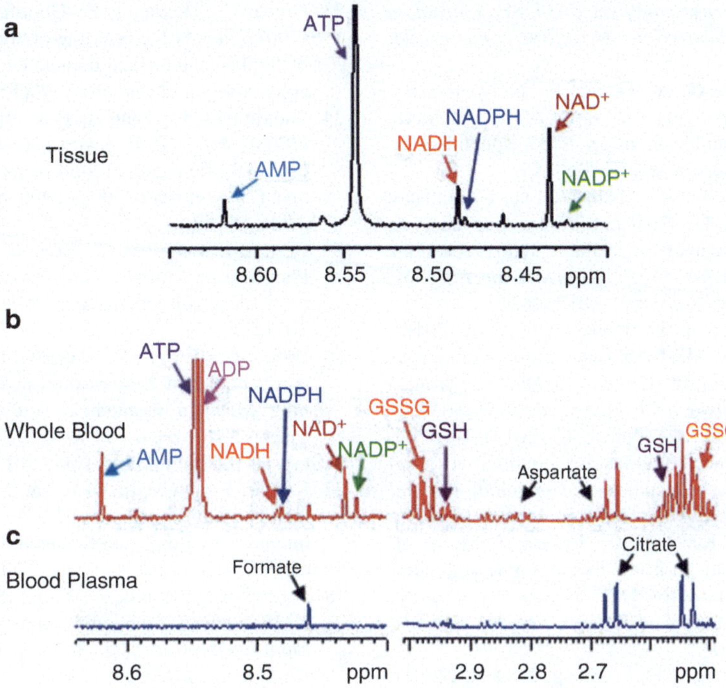

Fig. 5 Portions of typical 800 MHz ^{1}H NMR spectra of extracts of (**a**) mouse heart tissue, (**b**) whole blood, and (**c**) blood plasma. Identification of redox and energy coenzymes and antioxidant in the extract of whole blood/tissue is indicated. *NAD*$^{+}$ nicotinamide adenine dinucleotide, oxidized, *NADH* nicotinamide adenine dinucleotide, reduced, *NADP*$^{+}$ nicotinamide adenine dinucleotide phosphate, oxidized, *NADPH* nicotinamide adenine dinucleotide phosphate, reduced, *ATP* adenosine triphosphate, *ADP* adenosine diphosphate, *AMP* adenosine monophosphate, *GSH* glutathione, reduced, and *GSSG* glutathione, oxidized. Note: none of these compounds were detected in blood plasma

in the treatment and management of a range of human diseases.

Acknowledgments We gratefully acknowledge the financial support from NIH grants P30CA015704 and RO1GM131491.

References

1. Dang, N. H., Singla, A. K., Mackay, E. M., et al. (2014). Targeted cancer therapeutics: Biosynthetic and energetic pathways characterized by metabolomics and the interplay with key cancer regulatory factors. *Current Pharmaceutical Design, 20*, 2637–2647.
2. Griffin, J. L., Atherton, H., Shockcor, J., et al. (2011). Metabolomics as a tool for cardiac research. *Nature Reviews. Cardiology, 8*, 630–643.
3. Lindon, J. C., & Nicholson, J. K. (2014). The emergent role of metabolic phenotyping in dynamic patient stratification. *Expert Opinion on Drug Metabolism & Toxicology, 10*, 915–919.
4. Nagana Gowda, G. A., & Raftery, D. (2013). Biomarker discovery and translation in metabolomics. *Current Metabolomics, 1*, 227–240.
5. Rhee, E. P., & Gerszten, R. E. (2012). Metabolomics and cardiovascular biomarker discsovery. *Clinical Chemistry, 58*, 139–147.
6. Nagana Gowda, G. A., Raftery, D. (2014) *Advances in NMR based metabolomics, in fundamentals of advanced Omics technologies: From genes to metabolites, comprehensive analytical chemistry*, Eds. Carolina Simo´ Alejandro Cifuentes, Virginia Garcı'a-Can˜ as, Elsvier, New York, 63:187–211.
7. Nagana Gowda, G. A., & Raftery, D. (2015). Can NMR solve some significant challenges in metabolomics? *Journal of Magnetic Resonance, 260*, 144–160.
8. Nagana Gowda, G. A., & Raftery, D. (2017). Recent advances in NMR-based metabolomics. *Analytical Chemistry, 89*(1), 490–510.
9. Kumar, M., Chatterjee, A., Khedkar, A. P., et al. (2013). Mass spectrometric distinction of in-source and in-solution pyroglutamate and succinimide

in proteins: A case study on rhG-CSF. *Journal of the American Society for Mass Spectrometry, 24*, 202–212.
10. Nagana Gowda, G. A., Gowda, Y. N., & Raftery, D. (2015). Expanding the limits of human blood metabolite quantitation using NMR spectroscopy. *Analytical Chemistry, 87*(1), 706–715.
11. Nagana Gowda, G. A., Abell, L., Lee, C. F., Tian, R., & Raftery, D. (2016). Simultaneous analysis of major coenzymes of cellular redox reactions and energy using ex vivo (1)H NMR spectroscopy. *Analytical Chemistry, 88*(9), 4817–4824.
12. Purwaha, P., Silva, L. P., Hawke, D. H., et al. (2014). An artifact in LC-MS/MS measurement of glutamine and glutamic acid: In-source cyclization to pyroglutamic acid. *Analytical Chemistry, 86*, 5633–5637.
13. Trammell, S. A. J., & Brennera, C. (2013). Targeted, LCMS-based metabolomics for quantitative measurement of NAD+ metabolites. *Computational and Structural Biotechnology Journal, 4*, e201301012.
14. Beckonert, O., Keun, H. C., Ebbels, T. M., et al. (2007). Metabolic profiling, metabolomic and metabonomic procedures for NMR spectroscopy of urine, plasma, serum and tissue extracts. *Nature Protocols, 2*(11), 2692–2703.
15. Psychogios, N., Hau, D. D., Peng, J., et al. (2011). The human serum metabolome. *PLoS One, 6*(2), e16957.
16. Nagana Gowda, G. A., & Raftery, D. (2017). Whole blood metabolomics by 1H NMR spectroscopy provides a new opportunity to evaluate coenzymes and antioxidants. *Analytical Chemistry, 89*(8), 4620–4627.
17. Emwas, A. H., Luchinat, C., Turano, P., et al. (2015). Standardizing the experimental conditions for using urine in NMR-based metabolomic studies with a particular focus on diagnostic studies: A review. *Metabolomics, 11*(4), 872–894.
18. Emwas, A. H., Roy, R., McKay, R. T., et al. (2016). Recommendations and standardization of biomarker quantification using NMR-based metabolomics with particular focus on urinary analysis. *Journal of Proteome Research, 15*(2), 360–373.
19. Aimetti, M., Cacciatore, S., Graziano, A., et al. (2012). Metabonomic analysis of saliva reveals generalized chronic periodontitis signature. *Metabolomics, 8*(3), 465–474.
20. Wishart, D. S., Lewis, M. J., Morrissey, J. A., et al. (2008). The human cerebrospinal fluid metabolome. *Journal of Chromatography B-Analytical Technologies in the Biomedical and Life Sciences, 871*(2), 164–173.
21. Bala, L., Ghoshal, U. C., Ghoshal, U., et al. (2006). Malabsorption syndrome with and without small intestinal bacterial overgrowth: A study on upper-gut aspirate using 1H NMR spectroscopy. *Magnetic Resonance in Medicine, 56*(4), 738–744.
22. Nagana Gowda, G. A. (2011). NMR spectroscopy for discovery and quantitation of biomarkers of disease in human bile. *Bioanalysis, 3*(16), 1877–1890.
23. Graca, G., Duarte, I. F., Goodfellow, B. J., et al. (2008). Metabolite profiling of human amniotic fluid by hyphenated nuclear magnetic resonance spectroscopy. *Analytical Chemistry, 80*(15), 6085–6092.
24. Lacitignola, L., Fanizzi, F. P., Francios, E., et al. (2008). H-1 NMR investigation of normal and osteoarthritic synovial fluid in the horse. *Veterinary and Comparative Orthopaedics and Traumatology, 21*(1), 85–88.
25. Bertini, I., Luchinat, C., Miniati, M., et al. (2014). Phenotyping COPD by H-1 NMR metabolomics of exhaled breath condensate. *Metabolomics, 10*(2), 302–311.
26. Dietz, C., Ehret, F., Palmas, F., et al. (2017). Applications of high-resolution magic angle spinning MRS in biomedical studies II-Human diseases. *NMR in Biomedicine, 30*(11). https://doi.org/10.1002/nbm.3784. Epub 2017 Sep 15. Review.
27. Kumar, V., Dwivedi, D. K., & Jagannathan, N. R. (2014). High-resolution NMR spectroscopy of human body fluids and tissues in relation to prostate cancer. *NMR in Biomedicine, 27*(1), 80–89.
28. Airoldi, C., Tripodi, F., Guzzi, C., et al. (2015). NMR analysis of budding yeast metabolomics: A rapid method for sample preparation. *Molecular BioSystems, 11*(2), 379–383.
29. Lussu, M., Camboni, T., Piras, C., et al. (2017). ^{1}H NMR spectroscopy-based metabolomics analysis for the diagnosis of symptomatic E. coli-associated urinary tract infection (UTI). *BMC Microbiology, 17*(1), 201. https://doi.org/10.1186/s12866-017-1108-1.
30. Lane, A. N., Tan, J., Wang, Y., et al. (2017). Probing the metabolic phenotype of breast cancer cells by multiple tracer stable isotope resolved metabolomics. *Metabolic Engineering, 43*(Pt B), 125–136.
31. Kalfe, A., Telfah, A., Lambert, J., et al. (2015). Looking into living cell systems: Planar waveguide microfluidic NMR detector for in vitro metabolomics of tumor spheroids. *Analytical Chemistry, 87*(14), 7402–7410.
32. Wong, A., Jiménez, B., Li, X., et al. (2012). Evaluation of high resolution magic-angle coil spinning NMR spectroscopy for metabolic profiling of nanoliter tissue biopsies. *Analytical Chemistry, 84*(8), 3843–3848.
33. Bell, J. D., Brown, J. C., Kubal, G., et al. (1988). NMR-invisible lactate in blood plasma. *FEBS Letters, 235*, 81–86.
34. Chatham, J. C., & Forder, J. R. (1999). Lactic acid and protein interactions: Implications for the NMR visibility of lactate in biological systems. *Biochimica et Biophysica Acta, 1426*(1), 177–184.
35. Nagana Gowda, G. A., & Raftery, D. (2014). Quantitating metabolites in protein precipitated serum using NMR spectroscopy. *Analytical Chemistry, 86*(11), 5433–5440.
36. Nicholson, J. K., & Gartland, K. P. (1989). 1H NMR studies on protein binding of histidine, tyrosine and phenylalanine in blood plasma. *NMR Biomed, 2*(2), 77–82.

37. Daykin, C. A., Foxall, P. J., Connor, S. C., et al. (2002). The comparison of plasma deproteinization methods for the detection of low-molecular-weight metabolites by (1)H nuclear magnetic resonance spectroscopy. *Analytical Biochemistry, 304*(2), 220–230.
38. Fan, T. W. (2012). In T. W. Fan, R. M. Higashi, & A. N. Lane (Eds.), *The handbook of metabolomics, methods in pharmacology and toxicology* (pp. 7–27). New York: Springer.
39. Tiziani, S., Emwas, A. H., Lodi, A., et al. (2008). Optimized metabolite extraction from blood serum for 1H nuclear magnetic resonance spectroscopy. *Analytical Biochemistry, 377*(1), 16–23.
40. Wevers, R. A., Engelke, U., & Heerschap, A. (1994). High-resolution 1H-NMR spectroscopy of blood plasma for metabolic studies. *Clinical Chemistry, 40*(7 Pt 1), 1245–1250.
41. Simón-Manso, Y., Lowenthal, M. S., Kilpatrick, L. E., et al. (2013). Metabolite profiling of a NIST standard reference material for human plasma (SRM 1950): GC-MS, LC-MS, NMR, and clinical laboratory analyses, libraries, and web-based resources. *Analytical Chemistry, 85*(24), 11725–11731.
42. Hernandez, M. E., Lopez, A. C., Calatayud, A. G., et al. (2001). Vesical uric acid lithiasis in a child with renal hypouricemia. *Anales Espanoles de Pediatria, 55*(3), 273–276.
43. Rylander R, . Remer T, Berkemeyer S et al (2006) Acid–base status affects renal magnesium losses in healthy, elderly persons. Journal of Nutrition 136(9):2374–2377.
44. Welch, A. A., Mulligan, A., Bingham, S. A., et al. (2008). Urine pH is an indicator of dietary acid-base load, fruit and vegetables and meat intakes: Results from the European prospective investigation into Cancer and nutrition (EPIC)- Norfolk population study. *British Journal of Nutrition, 99*(6), 1335–1343.
45. DeSilva, M. A., Shanaiah, N., Nagana Gowda, G. A., et al. (2009). Application of 31P NMR spectroscopy and chemical derivatization for metabolite profiling of lipophilic compounds in human serum. *Magnetic Resonance in Chemistry, 47*(Suppl 1), S74–S80.
46. Shanaiah, N., Desilva, M. A., Nagana Gowda, G. A., et al. (2007). Class selection of amino acid metabolites in body fluids using chemical derivatization and their enhanced 13C NMR. *Proceedings of the National Academy of Sciences of the United States of America, 104*(28), 11540–11544.
47. Tayyari, F., Nagana Gowda, G. A., Gu, H., et al. (2013). Raftery D. 15N-cholamine--a smart isotope tag for combining NMR- and MS-based metabolite profiling. *Analytical Chemistry, 85*(18), 8715–8721.
48. Ye, T., Mo, H., Shanaiah, N., et al. (2009). Chemoselective 15N tag for sensitive and high-resolution nuclear magnetic resonance profiling of the carboxyl-containing metabolome. *Analytical Chemistry, 81*(12), 4882–4888.
49. Van, Q. N., Issaq, H. J., Jiang, Q., et al. (2008). Comparison of 1D and 2D NMR spectroscopy for metabolic profiling. *Journal of Proteome Research, 7*(2), 630–639.
50. Bird, S. S., Sheldon, D. P., Gathungu, R. M., et al. (2012). Structural characterization of plasma metabolites detected via LC-electrochemical coulometric array using LC-UV fractionation, MS, and NMR. *Analytical Chemistry, 84*(22), 9889–9898.
51. Grimes, J. H., & O'Connell, T. M. (2011). The application of micro-coil NMR probe technology to metabolomics of urine and serum. *Journal of Biomolecular NMR, 49*(3–4), 297–305.
52. Lacey, M. E., Subramanian, R., Olson, D. L., et al. (1999). High-resolution NMR spectroscopy of sample volumes from 1 nL to 10 μL. *Chemical Reviews, 99*(10), 3133–3152.
53. Ravi, K. C., Henry, I. D., Park, G. H. J., et al. (2010). New solenoidal microcoil NMR probe using zero-susceptibility wire Conc. *Magnetic Resonance Part B: Magnetic Resonance Engineering, 37B*, 13–19.
54. Cloarec, O., Campbell, A., Tseng, L. H., et al. (2007). Virtual chromatographic resolution enhancement in cryoflow LC-NMR experiments via statistical total correlation spectroscopy. *Analytical Chemistry, 79*(9), 3304–3311.
55. Djukovic, D., Liu, S., Henry, I., et al. (2006). Signal enhancement in HPLC/micro-coil NMR using automated column trapping. *Analytical Chemistry, 78*(20), 7154–7160.
56. Djukovic, D., Appiah-Amponsah, E., Shanaiah, N., et al. (2008). Ibuprofen metabolite profiling using a combination of SPE/column-trapping and HPLC-micro-coil NMR. *Journal of Pharmaceutical and Biomedical Analysis, 47*(2), 328–334.
57. Hyberts, S. G., Heffron, G. J., Tarragona, N. G., et al. (2007). Ultrahigh-resolution (1)H-(13)C HSQC spectra of metabolite mixtures using nonlinear sampling and forward maximum entropy reconstruction. *American Chemical Society, 129*(16), 5108–5116.
58. Hyberts, S. G., Arthanari, H., & Wagner, G. (2012). Applications of non-uniform sampling and processing. *Topics in Current Chemistry, 316*, 125–148.
59. Rai, R. K., & Sinha, N. (2012). Fast and accurate quantitative metabolic profiling of body fluids by nonlinear sampling of 1H–13C two-dimensional nuclear magnetic resonance spectroscopy. *Analytical Chemistry, 84*(22), 10005–10011.
60. Ernst, R. R., Bodenhausen, G. & Wokaun, A. (1987). Oxford University Press: Oxford.
61. Pervushin, K., Vögeli, B., & Eletsky, A. (2002). Longitudinal (1)H relaxation optimization in TROSY NMR spectroscopy. *Journal of the American Chemical Society, 124*(43), 12898–12902.
62. Motta, A., Paris, D., & Melck, D. (2010). Monitoring real-time metabolism of living cells by fast two-dimensional NMR spectroscopy. *Analytical Chemistry, 82*(6), 2405–2411.
63. Ghosh, S., Sengupta, A., & Chandra, K. (2017). SOFAST-HMQC-an efficient tool for metabolomics.

Analytical and Bioanalytical Chemistry, 409(29), 6731–6738.
64. Bruschweiler, R., & Zhang, F. (2004). Covariance nuclear magnetic resonance spectroscopy. *The Journal of Chemical Physics, 120*, 5253–5260.
65. Giraudeau, P., & Frydman, L. (2014). Ultrafast 2D NMR: An emerging tool in analytical spectroscopy. *Annual Review of Analytical Chemistry (Palo Alto Calif), 7*, 129–161.
66. Adams, R. W., Aguilar, J. A., Atkinson, K. D., et al. (2009). Reversible interactions with Para-hydrogen enhance NMR sensitivity by polarization transfer. *Science, 323*(5922), 1708–1711.
67. Reile, I., Eshuis, N., Hermkens, N. K., et al. (2016). NMR detection in biofluid extracts at sub-μM concentrations via Para-H2 induced hyperpolarization. *The Analyst, 141*(13), 4001–4005.
68. Bhattacharya, P., Chekmenev, E. Y., Perman, W. H., et al. (2007). Towards hyperpolarized (13) C-succinate imaging of brain cancer. *Journal of Magnetic Resonance, 186*, 150–155.
69. Chekmenev, E. Y., Norton, V. A., Weitekamp, D. P., et al. (2009). Hyperpolarized 1H NMR employing low γ nucleus for spin polarization storage. *Journal of the American Chemical Society, 131*, 3164–3165.
70. Shchepin, R. V., Coffey, A. M., Waddell, K. W., et al. (2012). PASADENA hyperpolarized 13C phospholactate. *Journal of the American Chemical Society, 134*(9), 3957–3960.
71. Frydman, L., & Blazina, D. (2007). Ultrafast two-dimensional nuclear magnetic resinance spectroscopy of hyperpolarized solutions. *Nature Physics, 3*, 415–419.
72. Mishkovsky, M., & Frydman, L. (2008). Progress in hyperpolarized ultrafast 2D NMR spectroscopy. *ChemPhysChem, 9*, 2340–2348.
73. Saunders, M. G., Ludwig, C., & Gunther, U. L. (2008). Optimizing the signal enhancement in cryogenic ex situ DNP-NMR spectroscopy. *Journal of the American Chemical Society, 130*, 6914–6915.
74. Ardenkjaer-Larsen, J. H. (2016). On the present and future of dissolution-DNP. *Journal of Magnetic Resonance, 264*, 3–12.
75. Ardenkjaer-Larsen, J. H., Fridlund, B., Gram, A., et al. (2003). Increase in signal-to-noise ratio of > 10,000 times in liquid-state NMR. *Proceedings of the National Academy of Sciences of the United States of America, 100*, 10158–10163.
76. Lane, A. N., & Fan, T. W. (2007). Quantification and identification of isotopomer distributions of metabolites in crude cell extracts using 1H TOCSY. *Metabolomics, 3*, 79–86.
77. Lloyd, S. G., Zeng, H., Wang, P., et al. (2004). Lactate isotopomer analysis by 1H NMR spectroscopy: Consideration of long-range nuclear spin-spin interactions. *Magnetic Resonance in Medicine, 51*, 1279–1282.
78. Wise, D. R., DeBerardinis, R. J., Mancuso, A., et al. (2008). Myc regulates a transcriptional program that stimulates mitochondrial glutaminolysis and leads to glutamine addiction. *Proceedings of the National Academy of Sciences of the United States of America, 105*, 18782–18787.
79. Coles, N. W., & Johnstone, R. M. (1962). Glutamine metabolism in Ehrlich ascites carcinoma cells. *The Biochemical Journal, 83*, 284–291.
80. Eagle, H. (1955). Nutrition needs of mammalian cells in tissue culture. *Science, 122*, 501–514.
81. DeBerardinis, R. J., Mancuso, A., Daikhin, E., et al. (2007). Beyond aerobic glycolysis: Transformed cells can engage in glutamine metabolism that exceeds the requirement for protein and nucleotide synthesis. *Proceedings of the National Academy of Sciences of the United States of America, 104*, 19345–19350.
82. Fan, T. W., Lane, A. N., Higashi, R. M., et al. (2011). Stable isotope resolved metabolomics of lung cancer in a SCID mouse model. *Metabolomics, 7*, 257–269.
83. Fan, T. W., Lane, A. N., Higashi, R. M., et al. (2009). Altered regulation of metabolic pathways in human lung cancer discerned by (13)C stable isotope-resolved metabolomics (SIRM). *Molecular Cancer, 8*, 41.
84. Lane, A. N., Fan, T. W., Bousamra, M., II, et al. (2011). Stable Isotope-Resolved Metabolomics (SIRM) in Cancer Research with Clinical Application to NonSmall Cell Lung Cancer OMICS. *A Journal of Integrative Biology, 15*, 173–182.
85. Locasale, J. W., Grassian, A. R., Melman, T., et al. (2011). Phosphoglycerate dehydrogenase diverts glycolytic flux and contributes to oncogenesis. *Nature Genetics, 43*, 869–874.
86. Bingol, K., Zhang, F., Bruschweiler-Li, L., et al. (2012). Carbon backbone topology of the metabolome of a cell. *Journal of the American Chemical Society, 134*, 9006–9011.
87. Bingol, K., Zhang, F., Bruschweiler-Li, L., et al. (2013). Quantitative analysis of metabolic mixtures by two-dimensional 13C constant-time TOCSY NMR spectroscopy. *Analytical Chemistry, 85*, 6414–6420.
88. Chikayama, E., Suto, M., Nishihara, T., et al. (2008). Systematic NMR analysis of stable isotope labeled metabolite mixtures in plant and animal systems: Coarse grained views of metabolic pathways. *PLoS One, 3*, e3805.
89. Zhang, F., Bruschweiler-Li, L., & Brüschweiler, R. (2012). High-resolution homonuclear 2D NMR of carbon-13 enriched metabolites and their mixtures. *Journal of Magnetic Resonance, 225*, 10–13.
90. Djukovic, D., Nagana Gowda, G. A., & Raftery, D. (2013). Mass spectrometry and NMR spectroscopy-based quantitative metabolomics. In H. J. Issaq & T. D. Veenstra (Eds.), *Proteomic and Metabolomic approaches to biomarker discovery* (pp. 279–297). New York: Elsevier.
91. Asiago, V., Nagana Gowda, G. A., Zhang, S., et al. (2008). Use of EDTA to minimize ionic strength and pH dependent frequency shifts in the ^{1}H NMR spectra of urine. *Metabolomics, 3*, 328–336.

92. Lauridsen, M., Hansen, S. H., Jaroszewski, J. W., et al. (2007). Human urine as test material in 1H NMR-based metabonomics: Recommendations for sample preparation and storage. *Analytical Chemistry, 79*, 1181–1186.
93. Brereton, R. G. (2010). *Chemometrics: Data analysis for the laboratory and chemical plant*. Hoboken: Wiley.
94. Johnson, R. A., & Wichern, D. W. (2007). In Prentice Hall (Ed.), *Applied multivariate statistical analysis* (56th ed.). Upper Saddle River.
95. Krzanowksi, W. J. (2000). *Principals of multivariate analysis: A users perspective*. Oxford, UK: Oxford University Press.
96. Zhou, X. H., Obuchowski, N. A., & McClish, D. K. (2001). *Statistical methods in diagnostic medicine*. Hoboken: Wiley.
97. Brereton, R. G. (2003). *Chemometrics: Data analysis for the laboratory and chemical plant*. Wiley. ISBN: 978-0-471-48978-8.
98. Lindon, J. C., Holmes, E., & Nicholson, J. K. (2001). Pattern recognition methods and applications in biomedical magnetic resonance. *Progress in Nuclear Magnetic Resonance, 39*, 1–40.
99. Gu, H., Chen, H., Pan, Z., et al. (2007). Monitoring diet effects via biofluids and their implications for metabolomics studies. *Analytical Chemistry, 79*(1), 89–97.
100. Barker, M., & Rayens, W. (2003). Partial least squares for discrimination. *Journal of Chemometrics, 17*, 166–173.
101. Beckwith-Hall, B. M., Brindle, J. T., Barton, R. H., Coen, M., Holmes, E., Nicholson, J. K., & Antti, H. (2002). Application of orthogonal signal correction to minimise the effects of physical and biological variation in high resolution ^{1}H NMR spectra of biofluids. *The Analyst, 127*, 1283–1288.
102. Johnson, R. A., & Wichern, D. W. (1999). *Applied multivariate statistical analysis*. Upper Saddle River: Prentice Hall.
103. Nagana Gowda, G. A. (2018). Profiling redox and energy coenzymes in whole blood, tissue and cells using NMR spectroscopy. *Metabolites, 8*(2), 1–12.
104. Nagana Gowda, G. A., Abell, L., & Tian, R. (2019). Extending the scope of 1H NMR spectroscopy for the analysis of cellular coenzyme A and acetyl coenzyme A. *Analytical Chemistry, 91*(3), 2464–2471.

Mass Spectrometry-Based Shotgun Lipidomics for Cancer Research

Jianing Wang, Chunyan Wang, and Xianlin Han

Acronyms

APCI	atmospheric pressure chemical ionization
APPI	atmospheric pressure photoionization
CID	collision-induced dissociation
CL	cardiolipin
CoA	coenzyme A
DAG	diacylglycerol
DESI	desorption electrospray ionization
ESI	electrospray ionization
FTICR	Fourier-transform ion cyclotron resonance
IS	internal standard
LIPID MAPS	lipid metabolites and pathway strategy
MAG	monoacylglycerol
MALDI	matrix-assisted laser desorption/ionization
MDMS-SL	multidimensional MS-based shotgun lipidomics
MS	mass spectrometry
MS/MS	tandem MS
NEFA	non-esterified fatty acid
NLS	neutral loss scan
PA	phosphatidic acid
PC	phosphatidylcholine
PE	phosphatidylethanolamine
PG	phosphatidylglycerol
PI	phosphatidylinositol
PIS	precursor ion scan
PS	phosphatidylserine
QqQ	triple quadrupole
Q-TOF	quadrupole time-of-flight
S1P	sphingosine-1-phosphate
SIM	selected ion monitoring
SIMS	secondary ion mass spectrometry
S/N	signal-to-noise
SM	sphingomyelin
SRM/MRM	selected/multiple reaction monitoring
ST	sulfatide
TAG	triacylglycerol

J. Wang · C. Wang
Barshop Institute for Longevity and Aging Studies, San Antonio, TX, USA

X. Han (✉)
Barshop Institute for Longevity and Aging Studies, San Antonio, TX, USA

Department of Medicine – Diabetes, University of Texas Health Science Center at San Antonio, San Antonio, TX, USA
e-mail: hanx@uthscsa.edu

S. Hu (ed.), *Cancer Metabolomics*, Advances in Experimental Medicine and Biology 1280,
https://doi.org/10.1007/978-3-030-51652-9_3

1 Introduction

Lipids are a class of small molecules that differ in their structural properties and are largely insoluble in water, but soluble in organic solutions. Lipids are either hydrophobic or amphiphilic. The most common forms are fatty acids and their derivatives. According to the structural characteristics of lipid molecules and their building blocks (ketoacyl and isoprene subunits) utilized in biochemical synthesis in vivo, the lipid metabolites and pathway strategy (LIPID MAPS) consortium funded by the National Institutes of Health in 2003 classifies cellular lipids into eight categories. They include 1) fatty acyls, 2) glycerolipids, 3) glycerophospholipids, 4) sphingolipids, 5) saccharolipids, 6) polyketides, 7) sterol lipids, and 8) prenol lipids [1, 2]. The number of lipid species is enormous. More than 43,000 unique lipid structures have been recorded in the LIPID MAPS Structure Database (LMSD), excluding the various forms of oxidation, regioisomers, and modifications [3].

Lipids are the main components of the cell membrane, the secretory vesicles, and lipoproteins. Lipids play numerous essential roles in cellular functions such as energy storage and utilization, molecular transportation, signaling, and cell cycle regulation [4]. Therefore, abnormalities in lipid content, composition, and metabolism could lead to disorders in physiological functions of organisms and are associated with the pathogeneses of many diseases, such as diabetes, neurodegenerative diseases, cardiovascular diseases, and cancer [4–10]. A comprehensive analysis and understanding of the changes in total lipid entities (i.e., lipidome) of organisms under different pathophysiological conditions can effectively achieve the biomarker discovery and the understanding of disease mechanisms.

Shotgun lipidomics is an analytical approach for large-scale and systematic analysis of the composition, structure, and quantity of cellular lipids directly from lipid extracts of biological samples by mass spectrometry (MS) [11, 12]. This approach has the advantages of high throughput and quantitative accuracy (especially in absolute quantification) compared to the online separation-detection lipidomics approaches such as liquid chromatography-mass spectrometry (LC-MS) [13]. The effectiveness of this approach has led to great advances in biomedical research, including a variety of metabolic-related diseases such as diabetes, neurodegenerative diseases, cardiovascular diseases, and cancer [14, 15]. In cancer research, as the focus on metabolic reprogramming increases, so do the application and demand for lipidomic analysis.

At present, lipidomics has become one of the most important branches of omics and is a very active research field [15]. However, analytical methods of lipidomics are less mature than those of proteomics or metabolomics for water-soluble metabolites [16]. This is mainly hindered by the development of MS methods for nonaqueous biological samples. Moreover, the foundation of shotgun lipidomics is very different from those of other "omics" analyses. Shotgun lipidomics takes full advantage of the structural and chemical properties of lipid molecules, as well as the physics of MS, and focuses on the ability for quantitative analysis [17, 18]. Development of shotgun lipidomics has helped the lipidomics discipline become an independent one from metabolomics. However, owing to the complexity of individual lipid structures and lipid class diversities, there is still room for evolving and improving the lipidomic approaches—from sample preparation to MS analysis and data processing [19–21].

A shotgun lipidomics workflow usually consists of the following processes (Fig. 1): the introduction of lipid molecules from lipid extracts, biological matrix, or a tissue section into the mass spectrometer (i.e., direct infusion or desorption in the case of MS imaging); data acquisition and lipid identification and quantification; and data mining and bioinformatic analysis. In step two, there are three major and intensively developed MS data acquisition strategies, including tandem MS-based shotgun lipidomics, high mass accuracy-based shotgun lipidomics, and multidimensional MS-based shotgun lipidomics (MDMS-SL). MS imaging is another pseudo-approach of shotgun lipidomics. Although the analytical capabilities for quantification and structural identification are limited, imaging

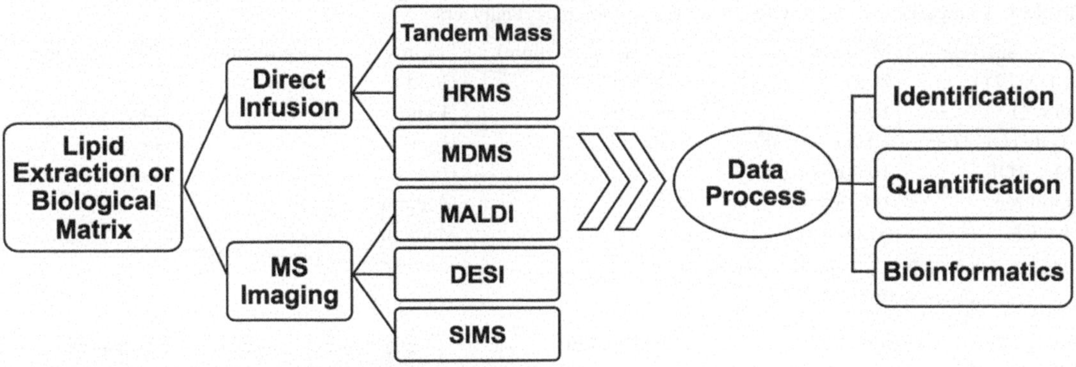

Fig. 1 A schematic workflow of MS-based shotgun lipidomics. HRMS, high-resolution mass spectrometry; MDMS, multidimensional mass spectrometry; MALDI, matrix-assisted laser desorption/ionization; DESI, desorption electrospray ionization; and SIMS, secondary ion mass spectrometry

methods can provide spatial information on lipid distribution and are important for biomedical studies. In this chapter, we will introduce the principles, approaches, and applications of shotgun lipidomics for cancer research.

2 MS-Based Shotgun Lipidomic Approaches

2.1 Mass Spectrometers and Ionization Methods

The development of biological MS is the technical basis of lipidomics. The standard triple quadrupole (QqQ) instrument plays a central role in shotgun lipidomic analysis due to its quantitative analysis power. At the same time, high-resolution MS has expanded the capabilities for lipid identification and discovery. Table 1 shows a comparison of the representative mass spectrometers frequently used in shotgun lipidomics.

The variety of ionization methods fundamentally determines the detectable range of lipid species (Fig. 2). Currently, the frequently used ionization methods in MS for lipidomics include electrospray ionization (ESI), desorption electrospray ionization (DESI), matrix-assisted laser desorption/ionization (MALDI), atmospheric pressure chemical ionization (APCI), atmospheric pressure photoionization (APPI), and secondary ion mass spectrometry (SIMS). DESI is a variant of ESI, where the ionized solvent droplets sprayed separately from the analyte provide it to be suitable for in situ analysis. APCI uses a corona discharge method to produce high-energy metastable ions that react with the analyte to accomplish ionization. APPI uses energy from a vacuum-ultraviolet lamp to directly or indirectly (chemical reaction of metastable ions) ionize the analyte. APCI and APPI are necessary additions to the ESI source. They work well with solvents of very low polarity. APCI is a soft ionization source that is more suitable for ionizing low-polarity molecules. Compared with APCI or ESI, APPI is a relatively hard ionization source, but it can increase the ionization efficiency of samples that are not easily ionized under APCI and ESI. SIMS utilizes the focused high-energy ion (the primary ion) to bombard the analyte, causing the ionization (often accompanied with severe fragmentation) of the analytes (the secondary ion). MALDI can ionize molecules of a wide range of properties under laser excitation employing the energy transfer of the matrix. Despite the availability of multiple ionization methods, the most widely used methods are ESI (including DESI) and MALDI. Since MALDI, DESI, and SIMS are often used in MS imaging for lipidomics, we will discuss them separately in Sect. 2.3.

Table 1 Comparison of the features of some common mass analyzers

Mass analyzer	Mass resolution[a]	Mass accuracy (ppm)	Sensitivity	Identification	Quantification
LTQ (LIT)	2000	100–500	Good	++	+
Q-q-Q	1000	100–1500	High	+	+++
TOF/TOF-TOF	10,000–40,000	5–50	High	++	++
Q-q-TOF	10,000–60,000	5–50	High	++	+++
Orbitrap	100,000–800,000	<5	Medium	+++	++
FTICR	>1,000,000	<1	Medium	+++	++

[a]Mass resolution at full width half maximum

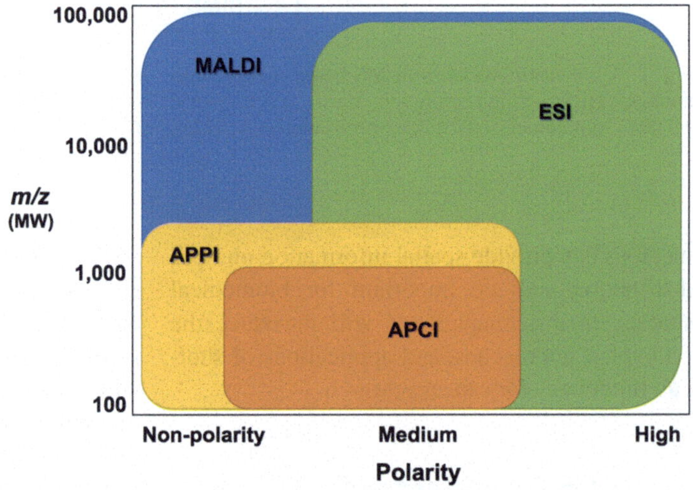

Fig. 2 The relationship between ionization methods and applicable analysis range

2.2 Direct Infusion-Based Shotgun Lipidomics

2.2.1 Introduction

In most circumstances, shotgun lipidomics is also referred to as direct infusion-based lipidomics. The lipids are not separated by chromatography, and the continuously injected lipid extract mixture is ionized directly from solution (e.g., ESI) under a constant lipid concentration [17]. Although there is no chromatographic separation, lipid sample preparation can be carried out by multiplexed extraction strategies according to the diversity in hydrophobicity, acid/base stability, and reactivity among the lipid classes and subclasses [22]. The most commonly used ionization methods in this approach are ESI, and then APCI, APPI, and MALDI.

An important feature of shotgun lipidomics is to employ a selective ionization strategy (Fig. 3). Different lipid classes have different charged properties in solution due to their distinctive structures (e.g., different polar head groups in polar lipids). These different lipids can be selectively ionized in the ion source under a given solution condition, referred to as intrasource separation [23, 24]. The concept of the pseudo-separation in the ion source is analogous to the electrophoresis of different compounds with different pI values.

Shotgun lipidomics maximizes the original information of a biological sample. A long-term MS analysis time is possible via a low flow rate of continuous direct injection, allowing multiple acquisitions in different MS scan modes for the analysis of the same component in a sample [18]. Usually, shotgun lipidomics is not suitable for analyzing low-abundance or less-ionizable lipids due to ion suppression. However, it can be improved by derivatization or multiplex extraction [25–27]. Since there is no change of lipid concentrations and solvent composition during the analysis, it is possible to achieve a high signal-to-noise (S/N) ratio by long-time acquisi-

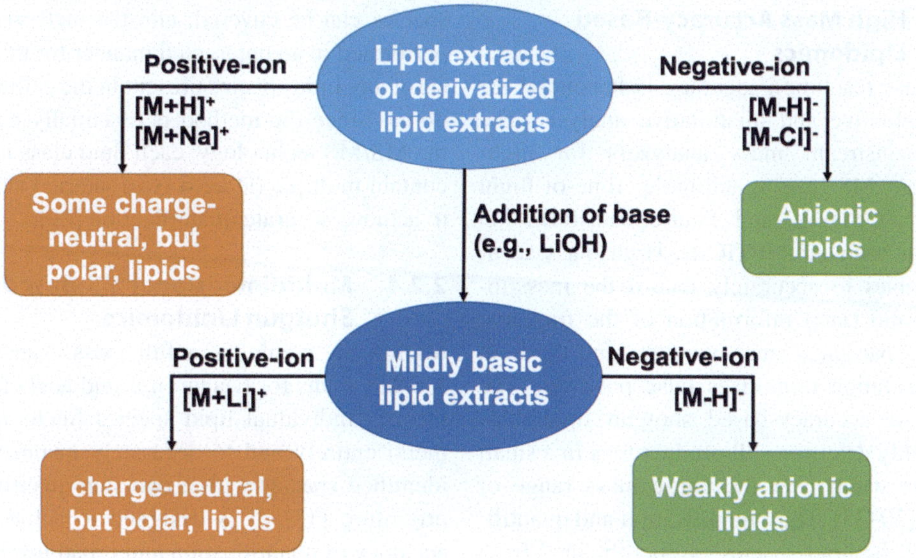

Fig. 3 Scheme of a typical experimental strategy based on the concept of intrasource separation for measurement of different categories of lipids from lipid extracts to achieve maximal lipidomics coverage

tion, which ensures accurate quantification using internal standards [18].

Currently, there are three well-developed and widely used approaches in shotgun lipidomics: tandem MS (MS/MS)-based shotgun lipidomics, high mass accuracy-based shotgun lipidomics, and multidimensional MS-based shotgun lipidomics (MDMS-SL).

2.2.2 Tandem MS-Based Shotgun Lipidomics

Lipid molecules contain structural building blocks that reflect their chemical characteristics. In MS/MS of lipids, especially for polar lipids, there are individual fragments related to their head groups. A lipid class can be specifically identified by a neutral loss scan (NLS) or precursor ion scan (PIS) of the specific fragment. According to the structural features of each lipid class, researchers should design a shotgun-based MS/MS scanning that "isolates" a category of lipid species of interest from a lipid mixture employing a unique NLS or PIS [24]. The filtered head group fragments that detected by PIS or NLS are used to classify lipid classes, and the PIS or NLS of fatty acyl chains is used to identify the exact molecular species in a lipid class [28]. Orders of magnitude of S/N ratio can be increased through this MS/MS double-filtering process. In general, QqQ mass spectrometers are the most common instrument (usually because of their multiple acquisition modes, high dynamic range, and low cost) to detect all species in a lipid class directly from total lipid extracts in one MS/MS acquisition.

The benefits of the MS/MS-based approach include its simplicity, high sensitivity, easy to use, and low cost. However, there are some limitations to this approach. For example, the length and unsaturation of the fatty acyl chain of lipid species are usually not determined. The specificities of individual fragments used in MS/MS scans may not be sufficient, which may introduce some false-positive results. Since the signal responses of the fragment to different species of a lipid class are not fundamentally constant, accurate quantification of the identified lipid species may be difficult. It requires at least two internal standards to accomplish accurate measurements for each lipid class [29], which increases the difficulty of internal standard selection.

2.2.3 High Mass Accuracy-Based Lipidomics

High mass resolution/accuracy is beneficial for both qualitative and quantitative analysis. The three mainstream mass analyzers for high-resolution MS are quadrupole time-of-flight (Q-TOF), Orbitrap, and Fourier-transform ion cyclotron resonance (FTICR). High mass accuracy enables to accurately record the mass-to-charge ratio (*m/z*) information of the fragment ions in a particular mass window, and the high mass resolution minimizes false positives. The high mass accuracy-based shotgun lipidomics can quickly determine all product ions in a small mass bin width over the entire mass range of interest [30–33]. Thus, qualification and quantification of the lipid species can be obtained from the product ion mass spectral set. This full range of coverage of a product ion scan is referred to as "top-down lipidomics" or "bottom-up shotgun lipidomics" [34, 35].

A high mass accuracy-based shotgun lipidomics can perform data-independent analysis due to its high mass resolution and high mass accuracy [36–38]. MS/MS^{all} is a data-independent analytical method that has been applied in lipidomic analysis [37, 39, 40]. In MS/MS^{all}, parallel scanning over the quadrupole is done across the full mass range, with 1 Da as the mass window. The selected precursor ions (usually with a quadrupole analyzer) are injected to collision cell, and then all fragment ions are detected with a high-resolution mass analyzer. This method could provide more comprehensive coverage of identification than that provided by data-dependent analysis, with better reproducibility and sensitivity. It theoretically maximizes the fragmentation information of the sample, if fragmentation of the lipid species in the mass range does not depend too much on CID energy, and provides a large data pool for data mining, including the distinguishment of isomers and the identification of unknown species.

The high mass accuracy-based shotgun lipidomic approach can provide highly efficient, adaptable, and sensitive determinations of lipid species. Within the dynamic range allowed by the instrument, all of the potentially existing lipid species can be covered, and the method can be performed in an untargeted manner for the analysis of any lipid species present in the cellular lipidome. Since the method is essentially based on the MS/MS technology, each lipid class needs to contain multiple (at least two) internal standards to achieve accurate quantification [29].

2.2.4 Multidimensional MS-Based Shotgun Lipidomics

MDMS-SL combines a full mass scan and all MS/MS scans for headgroups and acyl chains to identify individual lipid species (including isomers) entirely and to accurately quantify these identified species with a two-step quantification procedure [13]. It is designed to achieve high accuracy of quantification and broad linear range of quantification.

In MDMS-SL, the unique structural building blocks of the lipid molecules are fully applied to identify individual lipid species [5, 12]. A two-dimensional (2D) mass map can be constructed from MDMS-SL, with the *m/z* range as the first dimension and all spectra (including a full scan and unit-by-unit NLS and PIS scans) as the second dimension [18]. As can be deduced from the description in the MS/MS method, the NLS and PIS scans over the mass range of interest can provide sufficient data to distinguish the class and the fatty acyl chain length that are required for characterization of the lipid species. Typically, for identification of a specific class of lipids, it is adequate to selectively scan the structurally specific building blocks and fatty acyl chains by PIS or NLS or both (Fig. 4). Currently, this approach is capable of analyzing thousands of lipids from a small amount of biological sample, covering around 50 lipid classes. The total coverage has exceeded 95% of the mass content of a cellular lipidome [13, 19].

Moreover, the direct acquisition of multidimensional spectra provides much more information that can be mined for reliable identification and quantification of lipid species, including isomers with different fatty acyl chains and regioisomers with identical fatty acyl chains at different linked position with glycerol. Accurate absolute quantification can be achieved with two-step

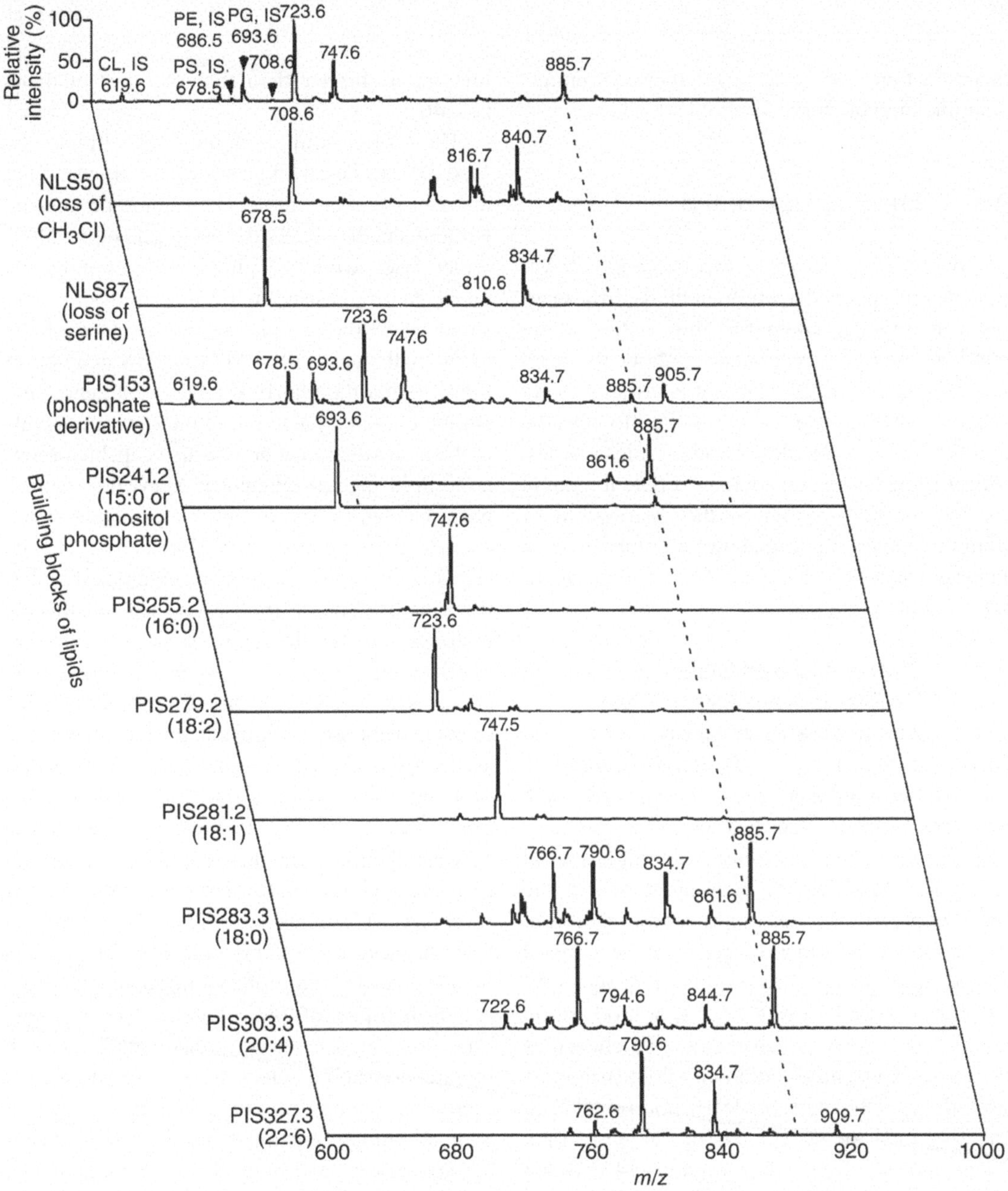

Fig. 4 A 2D mass spectrum of rat myocardial lipid extract in negative ion electrospray ionization for analysis of phospholipids. As shown, the first dimension represents the mass range from *m/z* 600 to 1000. The second dimension, composed of different PIS and NLS analyses, shows specific fragment (building block) information about these species. For example, the ion at *m/z* 885.7 was present in the negative ion full scan (the most top one), as well as PIS153, PIS241.2, PIS283.3, and PIS303.3 spectra. This indicates that this molecular ion is an anionic phospholipid and can yield fragments at *m/z* 153, 241.2, 283.3, and 303.3 corresponding to the building blocks of dehydrated glycerophosphate, inositol phosphate, and carboxylate ions of stearic acid (18:0) and arachidonic acid (20:4), respectively. These building blocks plus their intensities allow us to identify the ion as PI (18:0–20:4). Similarly, the 2D analysis identifies the ion peaks at *m/z* 619.6, 678.5, 693.6, and 708.6 as the internal standards (IS) of CL (14:0/14:0/14:0/14:0), PS (14:0/14:0), PG (15:0/15:0), and PC (14:1/14:1), respectively, which were added prior to lipid extraction for quantification. The peaks at *m/z* 723.6 and 747.6 were also apparently identified as CL (18:2/18:2/18:2/18:2) and PG (16:0/18:1), respectively, which are the major species of lipids present in rat myocardium. The identified major species could be quantified in the full MS scan mode in comparison to the corresponding IS. By using these quantified species plus IS, the low abundance lipid species can be quantified by using PIS/NLS spectra

quantification (see Sect. 3.2), which is a unique quantification method for MDMS-SL [13].

2.3 Imaging Lipidomics

Although the sensitivity of MS imaging is lower than that of optical detection methods, MS imaging can directly obtain the information about hundreds of lipid compounds without the need for labeling [41, 42]. Because it is difficult to get specific labeling tags or antibodies to observe specific lipid molecules through microscopes, MS imaging has become the most potent method for large-scale profiling of the distribution of lipid molecules. Table 2 shows a comparison of the characteristics of various MS imaging methods used in lipidomics.

2.3.1 Matrix-Assisted Laser Desorption/Ionization-Mass Spectrometry Imaging

MALDI-MS imaging is an effective label-free method that simultaneously detects a wide range of biomolecules, identifies unknown species, and displays their distribution in high spatial resolution. MALDI-MS imaging is one of the most popularly applied approaches in current development [43] mainly because the method can achieve both high-resolution and high-sensitivity imaging by using laser spot modulation and a wide variety of substrates to be chosen as matrices. Currently, commercial instruments provide a stable and reliable 10-micron level of imaging and achieve imaging at less than 1-micron resolution in the laboratory [44]. Since MALDI can be modulated with the energy of a laser source, the sensitivity in high-resolution imaging is higher than that of other methods [45, 46].

The successful imaging of lipids by MALDI-MS largely depends on the choice of the matrix. The lipid molecule cannot be ionized without a matrix under the excitation of the ultraviolet laser while keeping the lipid molecule intact. Matrix-assisted ionization allows the sensitive detection of lipid molecules. One of the main challenges for the MALDI-MS imaging of lipids is that the matrix should avoid generating strong, cluttered background interference signals in the detection range and be also capable of ionizing lipid species efficiently. Many efforts have been devoted to find or optimize suitable matrices and their imaging procedures [47–51]. The requirement of analysis for the complex distribution and diversity of lipid species leads to diverse matrices for MS imaging of lipids. Different matrices can be used to ionize the target lipid classes selectively [52]. Based on the knowledge of the distribution of lipid classes in different tissue sections or organs, the reasonable selection of a suitable matrix can maximize data acquisition [51, 53–55]. For example, N-(1-naphthyl) ethylenediamine dihydrochloride is a highly selective and sensitive matrix for ionization of glycerophospholipids [51], whereas 9-aminoacridine is highly selective for analysis of sulfatides [53]. In order to improve the coverage of the lipids of interest and reduce unnecessary interference from other lipid classes, researchers should select the appropriate matrix according to the selectivity or preference.

In addition to organic matrices, nanomaterial-based matrices have been a focused research area in recent years in order to eliminate the effects of the matrix background on interference [56]. This

Table 2 Comparison of the features of major MS imaging approaches

	MALDI	DESI	SIMS
Typical spatial resolution	5–100 μm	100–200 μm	50 nm-2 μm
Mass range (*m/z*)	Full range	< 2000	< 1500
Mass analyzer	TOF/TOF, Q-TOF, FTICR, Orbitrap	Q-TOF, Orbitrap	TOF, magnetic section
Sample preparation	Tissue section; dehydration; matrix coating	No pretreatment	Tissue section; dehydration; fixation (optional)

is because many inorganic nanomaterials are stable under laser irradiation and do not have the propensity to generate fragmentation and free radicals. Nanomaterial matrices include the following categories: nano-metal oxides (e.g., TiO_2, WO_3, and ZnO) [57], nano-metal particles (e.g., platinum, gold, and silver) [58–60], nano-carbon materials (carbon dots, graphene, and diamond) [61–63], and 2D nanosheets (e.g., hBN nanosheet, MoS_2 nanosheet, and tellurium nanosheet) [64–66]. The nanomaterial matrices are the beneficial complementarity to organic matrices due to the advantage of low or free background interference. However, the detection sensitivity of nanomaterial matrices still lags behind that of organic matrices.

2.3.2 Desorption Electrospray Ionization Imaging

DESI imaging is a widely used ambient-MS imaging technique [67]. In the DESI process, charged primary organic droplets impact on the sample surface with specific kinetic energy, and the secondary droplets that are dissolving sample molecules are sputtered from the surface upon impact. The charged nanometer-scale sputtered sample droplets then undergo a desolvent and charge transfer process (similar to ESI) under the potential of the electric field to guide the generated ions into the mass spectrometer. It can be understood from the principle of DESI that although its spatial resolution and sensitivity are not as good as those of MALDI-MS, real-time or native imaging can be achieved by maintaining the original state of the sample because no pretreatment is required [68]. Accordingly, DESI imaging has some advantages that MALDI imaging cannot replace, such as intraoperative assessment, assisted diagnosis, and the surface analysis for forensic samples [69–72].

2.3.3 Secondary Ion Mass Spectrometry Imaging

SIMS imaging is performed by point-by-point bombarding a beam of highly focused high-energy ions onto the sample surface to produce secondary ions. Its concept is similar to that of electron microscopy, except that ions are excited and monitored instead of electrons. The most important feature of SIMS imaging is that it can reach the spatial resolution to an optical microscopy level, which is currently not possible for any other MS imaging methods. SIMS imaging has been used for single-cell lipid imaging [73]. Since it is not a soft ionization method, it is currently hard to obtain rich intact lipid peaks without accompanying fragments.

3 Quantification Methods

3.1 Principles and Single-Step Quantification

The quantification of shotgun lipidomics is performed in the absence of chromatographic separation. The requirements for relative quantification and absolute quantification are similar. Both quantifications need the addition of internal standards, and the quantity cannot be derived from the ion count [74]. This is because the matrix effects of the samples on different groups may be very different. This feature makes it easier to perform relative quantification in chromatographic separation-based lipidomics [75, 76], while shotgun lipidomics is more conducive to an accurate absolute quantification.

Absolute quantification measures the amount of each lipid component under a specific physical unit reference, such as nanomole per milligram (nmol/mg) of protein. The absolute quantification of lipids is critical for elucidation of lipid metabolism pathways/network. In addition, absolute quantification is also beneficial for batch-to-batch studies. The most common absolute quantification method is the one that spikes the sample with internal standard(s) and thereby directly compares the relative signal relationship between the analytes and the internal standard(s) under identical experimental conditions. It is assumed that the concentration of the sample is proportional to the signal (i.e., a constant response factor). This proportional relationship is established by subtracting the baseline effect, avoiding lipid aggregation, and being detected within the linear dynamic range of the MS system [29].

Individual species of polar lipids have nearly identical ionization efficiencies (i.e., same response factor) in the low concentration range after correction for different ^{13}C isotope distributions [12, 77]. It is because the MS signal response factors of polar lipids are mainly determined by the polar groups, whereas the length and number of unsaturation of the fatty acyl chains have minimal effects on the signal under the same conditions. This property makes it easy to quantify lipid species with internal standards. However, for nonpolar lipids, the signal response is affected by the structure of the fatty acyl chain. The signal response factors between the analytes and the spiked internal standard are not identical, even in the low concentration region. The response factors of nonpolar lipids should be precorrected or derivatization should be conducted to ensure accurate quantification [78, 79]. Similarly, for the PIS and NLS spectra, lipid structures, such as molecular weight, acyl chain length, and unsaturation, also affect the reaction channel of the collision dissociation. Thus, correction for the signal response factors among internal standards is needed.

The quantitative methods of high mass accuracy and MS/MS approaches are both based on this principle. Ultrahigh-resolution MS increases the accuracy of quantification by reducing the overlapping effect of the isobaric peaks.

3.2 Two-Step Quantification by MDMS-Based Shotgun Lipidomics

The first step of the two-step quantification is based on the principle described in the previous section, which is to quantify high-abundance lipids in a full-scan mass spectrum. Therefore, any of the quantified lipid molecules can be used as a new internal standard for the quantitative analysis of the rest lipid species in this lipid class. In the second step of quantification, newly determined "internal standards" can be used to correct PIS and NLS signal responses for different structures to quantify low abundance lipids [23].

In MDMS-SL, the lipid molecules identified by intrasource separation and MDMS screening are typically quantified using a two-step quantification procedure [13, 17]. The two-step quantification method makes MDMS-SL particularly useful for accurate quantification of low-abundance lipids and peaks overlapping with lipid species from other lipid classes. In the MDMS scan, comprehensive PIS and NLS information can be collected. The first step of the two-step quantification process is to use the spiked internal standard of a class to directly and ratiometrically compare full-scan MS peaks of other lipid species in the class that have both high abundance and no interference. The quantitative results are corrected by baseline subtraction and ^{13}C deisotoping. The second step of quantification is based on the results of the first quantification step, where the low-abundance peaks and the peaks that overlapped with other lipid classes are quantified. Since the signal response factors of different species are different in the PIS or NLS mass spectrum, the strategy is to use both the structural representative species quantified in the first step plus the originally spiked internal standard as the standard set for the second step quantification. Usually, the correction utilizes an algorithm based on multivariate least-square regression. PIS and NLS scanning improves the S/N ratio of the low-abundance peaks and excludes interference from other lipid classes. By using the second step of quantification, which is used as a dynamic range relay, it is possible to achieve a linear dynamic range of more than 5000-fold for many lipid classes.

4 Bioinformatics for Shotgun Lipidomics

The lipidomic analysis produces a large amount of data. Without proper computational tools and effective data mining, it is difficult to recognize the biological significance of the dataset. Therefore, bioinformatics has become a critical component of lipidomics [80].

4.1 Lipid Identification Tools and Databases

Many software packages can be applied for large-scale analysis of lipids in an automated or semi-automated manner. These tools use the fragment information generated by CID to identify and quantify lipid species and chain lengths. LipidBlast [28] is an in silico tandem mass spectral database containing hundreds of thousands of possible lipid structures. This library is very helpful for spectral annotation and lipid identification. MDMS-SL requires a theoretical database based on the concept of building blocks, covering all lipids and including all possible structural building block combinations [13]. Other typical representatives of these tools are LipidFinder [81, 82], LipidProfiler [31], LipidInspector [32], and ALEX [83].

The LIPID MAPS website covers structural information of a wide range of lipid classes, as well as a variety of bioinformatics tools for lipid analysis [3]. Its main contents involve several aspects, including structural classification and nomenclature, experimental verified and in-silicon generated lipid database, and computer-aided spectral comparisons. These tools can help build and predict possible lipid structures from mass spectra. Similarly, both the METLIN Metabolomics Database [84] and the Human Metabolome Database (HMDB) [85] are large, comprehensive metabolite databases (including lipids) that provide rich functional information and cross-indexed links to facilitate metabolic pathway studies. Among them, HMDB provides a number of mass spectra measured under different conditions that are helpful for lipid identification.

4.2 Biostatistics and Data Interpretation

The analysis and interpretation of the data require the use of statistical analysis. Descriptive statistics and hypothesis testing are basic data analysis methods [86]. There are many general statistical packages in this area, for example, GraphPad and Minitab. Advanced statistical methods, such as multivariate statistical analysis and biomarker discovery, are also widely used in lipidomics studies. MetaboAnalyst is a set of online tools for metabolomics data analysis and interpretation [87]. It provides a variety of analytical tools, including descriptive statistics, multivariate statistical analysis, biomarker discovery, and metabolic pathway analysis. Its numerous statistical tools are easy to understand and continent to use. However, MetaboAnalyst may not be able to meet the requirements of more advanced and complex statistics or highly customized visual output. For example, to support vector machine analysis, only two sets of comparisons are supported in MetaboAnalyst. For sophisticated data mining, some statistical software such as SIMCA (especially for multivariate analysis) and SPSS (general and comprehensive), and even fully programmable software such as SAS and R, provide powerful functions.

Biostatistics tools can reveal major changes in variables in samples. However, how these changes reflect or explain the disease mechanism, and to exclude interference of the irrational changes caused by hidden variables, data interpretation employing knowledge of lipid metabolism is required. The continuous accumulation of metabolic pathways and lipidomics data has detailed information on lipid metabolism, transformation, and regulatory pathways, such as KEGG [88] and VENTED [89]. Based on this type of information, the researcher can use the quantitative results obtained from lipidomics analysis to construct the changed pathways of the research object. It should be noted that the model pathways provided by various databases explain the overall pathways of the entire lipid class, but not the individual species of a class. However, the target of lipidomics research does not stop at this point. Analysis of factors for specific lipid species changes is also a goal of lipidomics. This level of knowledge accumulation and the database are still limited.

5 Application of Shotgun Lipidomics for Cancer Research

Lipids play a key role in the crucial processes for tumor development [90]. Table 3 shows the cellular function of the major cellular lipid classes. Tumors alter the cell cycle, function, differentiation, morphology, homeostasis, and the dependence of energy metabolism, so almost all types of lipid classes are affected and changed at different stages of tumor development [91–96].

Shotgun lipidomics plays an important role in revealing the changes in lipid homeostasis underlying the cancer progression to support mechanism studies or assessment of tumor margins [69, 97]. This type of lipidomic analysis, especially MS imaging analysis, provides an intraoperative assessment of tumor surgeon at shorter intervals than existing methods, and a more efficient and automated analysis system can be established by pattern recognition [98]. In addition, MS imaging analysis of early tumor development, especially the homeostasis of small tumor foci, provides important reference information for the study of tumor metastasis and potential therapeutic targets [51, 99, 100].

Table 3 Cellular functions of major lipid classes

Cellular functions	Lipid classes[a]
Membrane structural component	PC, PE, PI, PS, PG, PA, SM, CL, cholesterol, cerebroside, glycolipids, ST, gangliosides, etc.
Energy storage and metabolism	NEFA, TAG, DAG, MAG, acyl CoA, acylcarnitine, etc.
Signaling	All lysolipids, DAG, MAG, acyl CoA, acylcarnitine, NEFA, eicosanoids, and other oxidized FA, ceramide, sphingosine, S1P, psychosine, steroids, *N*-acyl ethanolamine, etc.
Other special functions	Plasmalogen (antioxidant), acylcarnitine (transport), CL (respiration), PS (cofactors, substrate of PE synthesis), etc.

[a]The full name of abbreviations can be found in the list of acronyms

Another active research at present is concentrated on the biomarker discovery and facilitating early diagnosis or prognosis. For example, numerous studies have shown that altered glycerophospholipids can be considered biomarkers for cancer diagnosis [101–103]. In early diagnosis, the discovery of protein markers is much more difficult than lipid markers. This is mainly because a small number of changes in protein species may have a substantial chance of triggering a wider range of phenotype changes [104, 105]. Less developed research areas relevant to cancer research are the lipidomics-assisted studies on the functions of microRNAs and long noncoding RNAs [106–108] and drug efficacy tests [109]. Overall, changes of lipid species are a valuable analytical window for early diagnosis and intervention of tumors and broad areas of cancer research.

6 Summary

In short, lipidomic analysis is the basis of biomedical science, as a limited understanding of the composition of biological systems often puts biomedical research in a state of inefficiency or even based on accidental discovery. Due to the extraordinary complexity of the lipidome, unlike the predictable proteome from the nucleic acid sequence, we do not know how many lipid species are present in the cellular lipidome. Consequently, a comprehensive chemical analysis, including both qualitative and quantitative aspects, is essential for the mapping of lipidomes and the study of their metabolism. In addition, statistical tools, such as those that facilitate data interpretation and visualization of lipid metabolism pathways, are still at an underdeveloped stage. Combining the results of lipidomics with clinical pathology and pharmacology will become increasingly desirable. The future development of lipidomics should significantly facilitate our understanding of the biological mechanisms of diseases including human cancers.

Acknowledgments This work was partially supported by NIH/NIA (RF1 AG061872), intramural institutional research funds from the University of Texas Health Science Center at San Antonio (UT Health SA), the Mass Spectrometry Core Facility of UT Health SA, and the Methodist Hospital Foundation endowment.

References

1. Fahy, E., Subramaniam, S., Murphy, R. C., Nishijima, M., Raetz, C. R., Shimizu, T., Spener, F., van Meer, G., Wakelam, M. J., & Dennis, E. A. (2009). Update of the LIPID MAPS comprehensive classification system for lipids. *Journal of Lipid Research, 50*(Suppl), S9–S14.
2. Fahy, E., Subramaniam, S., Brown, H. A., Glass, C. K., Merrill, A. H., Jr., Murphy, R. C., Raetz, C. R., Russell, D. W., Seyama, Y., Shaw, W., Shimizu, T., Spener, F., van Meer, G., VanNieuwenhze, M. S., White, S. H., Witztum, J. L., & Dennis, E. A. (2005). A comprehensive classification system for lipids. *Journal of Lipid Research, 46*, 839–861.
3. Sud, M., Fahy, E., Cotter, D., Brown, A., Dennis, E. A., Glass, C. K., Merrill, A. H., Jr., Murphy, R. C., Raetz, C. R., Russell, D. W., & Subramaniam, S. (2007). LMSD: LIPID MAPS structure database. *Nucleic Acids Research, 35*, D527–D532.
4. van Meer, G., Voelker, D. R., & Feigenson, G. W. (2008). Membrane lipids: Where they are and how they behave. *Nature Reviews. Molecular Cell Biology, 9*, 112–124.
5. Han, X. (2007). Neurolipidomics: Challenges and developments. *Frontiers in Bioscience, 12*, 2601–2615.
6. Shevchenko, A., & Simons, K. (2010). Lipidomics: Coming to grips with lipid diversity. *Nature Reviews. Molecular Cell Biology, 11*, 593–598.
7. Gross, R. W., & Han, X. (2011). Lipidomics at the interface of structure and function in systems biology. *Chemistry & Biology, 18*, 284–291.
8. Yang, K., & Han, X. (2016). Lipidomics: Techniques, applications, and outcomes related to biomedical sciences. *Trends in Biochemical Sciences, 41*, 954–969.
9. Loizides-Mangold, U., Perrin, L., Vandereycken, B., Betts, J. A., Walhin, J. P., Templeman, I., Chanon, S., Weger, B. D., Durand, C., Robert, M., Paz Montoya, J., Moniatte, M., Karagounis, L. G., Johnston, J. D., Gachon, F., Lefai, E., Riezman, H., & Dibner, C. (2017). Lipidomics reveals diurnal lipid oscillations in human skeletal muscle persisting in cellular myotubes cultured in vitro. *Proceedings of the National Academy of Sciences of the United States of America, 114*, E8565–E8574.
10. Ji, J., Kline, A. E., Amoscato, A., Samhan-Arias, A. K., Sparvero, L. J., Tyurin, V. A., Tyurina, Y. Y., Fink, B., Manole, M. D., Puccio, A. M., Okonkwo, D. O., Cheng, J. P., Alexander, H., Clark, R. S., Kochanek, P. M., Wipf, P., Kagan, V. E., & Bayir, H. (2012). Lipidomics identifies cardiolipin oxidation as a mitochondrial target for redox therapy of brain injury. *Nature Neuroscience, 15*, 1407–1413.
11. Han, X., & Gross, R. W. (2003). Global analyses of cellular lipidomes directly from crude extracts of biological samples by ESI mass spectrometry: A bridge to lipidomics. *Journal of Lipid Research, 44*, 1071–1079.
12. Han, X., & Gross, R. W. (2005). Shotgun lipidomics: Multidimensional MS analysis of cellular lipidomes. *Expert Review of Proteomics, 2*, 253–264.
13. Yang, K., Cheng, H., Gross, R. W., & Han, X. (2009). Automated lipid identification and quantification by multidimensional mass spectrometry-based shotgun lipidomics. *Analytical Chemistry, 81*, 4356–4368.
14. Ferreri, C., & Chatgilialoglu, C. (2015). *Membrane lipidomics for personalized health*. Chichester\West Sussex\Hoboken: Wiley.
15. Han, X. (2016). Lipidomics for studying metabolism. *Nature Reviews. Endocrinology, 12*, 668–679.
16. Griffiths, W. J., & Wang, Y. (2009). Mass spectrometry: From proteomics to metabolomics and lipidomics. *Chemical Society Reviews, 38*, 1882–1896.
17. Han, X., & Gross, R. W. (2005). Shotgun lipidomics: Electrospray ionization mass spectrometric analysis and quantitation of cellular lipidomes directly from crude extracts of biological samples. *Mass Spectrometry Reviews, 24*, 367–412.
18. Han, X., Yang, K., & Gross, R. W. (2012). Multi-dimensional mass spectrometry-based shotgun lipidomics and novel strategies for lipidomic analyses. *Mass Spectrometry Reviews, 31*, 134–178.
19. Wang, M., Wang, C., Han, R. H., & Han, X. (2016). Novel advances in shotgun lipidomics for biology and medicine. *Progress in Lipid Research, 61*, 83–108.
20. Rustam, Y. H., & Reid, G. E. (2018). Analytical challenges and recent advances in mass spectrometry based Lipidomics. *Analytical Chemistry, 90*, 374–397.
21. Cajka, T., & Fiehn, O. (2016). Toward merging untargeted and targeted methods in mass spectrometry-based metabolomics and Lipidomics. *Analytical Chemistry, 88*, 524–545.
22. Jiang, X., Cheng, H., Yang, K., Gross, R. W., & Han, X. (2007). Alkaline methanolysis of lipid extracts extends shotgun lipidomics analyses to the low-abundance regime of cellular sphingolipids. *Analytical Biochemistry, 371*, 135–145.
23. Han, X., Yang, K., Yang, J., Fikes, K. N., Cheng, H., & Gross, R. W. (2006). Factors influencing the electrospray intrasource separation and selective ionization of glycerophospholipids. *Journal of the American Society for Mass Spectrometry, 17*, 264–274.
24. Brugger, B., Erben, G., Sandhoff, R., Wieland, F. T., & Lehmann, W. D. (1997). Quantitative analysis of biological membrane lipids at the low picomole level by nano-electrospray ionization tandem mass spectrometry. *Proceedings of the National Academy*

of Sciences of the United States of America, 94, 2339–2344.
25. Wang, M., Han, R. H., & Han, X. (2013). Fatty acidomics: Global analysis of lipid species containing a carboxyl group with a charge-remote fragmentation-assisted approach. *Analytical Chemistry, 85*, 9312–9320.
26. Wang, C., Wang, M., & Han, X. (2015). Comprehensive and quantitative analysis of lysophospholipid molecular species present in obese mouse liver by shotgun lipidomics. *Analytical Chemistry, 87*, 4879–4887.
27. Wang, C., Palavicini, J. P., Wang, M., Chen, L., Yang, K., Crawford, P. A., & Han, X. (2016). Comprehensive and quantitative analysis of Polyphosphoinositide species by shotgun Lipidomics revealed their alterations in db/db mouse brain. *Analytical Chemistry, 88*, 12137–12144.
28. Kind, T., Liu, K. H., Lee, D. Y., DeFelice, B., Meissen, J. K., & Fiehn, O. (2013). LipidBlast in silico tandem mass spectrometry database for lipid identification. *Nature Methods, 10*, 755–758.
29. Wang, M., Wang, C., & Han, X. (2017). Selection of internal standards for accurate quantification of complex lipid species in biological extracts by electrospray ionization mass spectrometry-what, how and why? *Mass Spectrometry Reviews, 36*, 693–714.
30. Ekroos, K., Chernushevich, I. V., Simons, K., & Shevchenko, A. (2002). Quantitative profiling of phospholipids by multiple precursor ion scanning on a hybrid quadrupole time-of-flight mass spectrometer. *Analytical Chemistry, 74*, 941–949.
31. Ejsing, C. S., Duchoslav, E., Sampaio, J., Simons, K., Bonner, R., Thiele, C., Ekroos, K., & Shevchenko, A. (2006). Automated identification and quantification of glycerophospholipid molecular species by multiple precursor ion scanning. *Analytical Chemistry, 78*, 6202–6214.
32. Schwudke, D., Oegema, J., Burton, L., Entchev, E., Hannich, J. T., Ejsing, C. S., Kurzchalia, T., & Shevchenko, A. (2006). Lipid profiling by multiple precursor and neutral loss scanning driven by the data-dependent acquisition. *Analytical Chemistry, 78*, 585–595.
33. Cajka, T., & Fiehn, O. (2014). Comprehensive analysis of lipids in biological systems by liquid chromatography-mass spectrometry. *Trends in Analytical Chemistry, 61*, 192–206.
34. Schuhmann, K., Herzog, R., Schwudke, D., Metelmann-Strupat, W., Bornstein, S. R., & Shevchenko, A. (2011). Bottom-up shotgun lipidomics by higher energy collisional dissociation on LTQ Orbitrap mass spectrometers. *Analytical Chemistry, 83*, 5480–5487.
35. Schwudke, D., Hannich, J. T., Surendranath, V., Grimard, V., Moehring, T., Burton, L., Kurzchalia, T., & Shevchenko, A. (2007). Top-down lipidomic screens by multivariate analysis of high-resolution survey mass spectra. *Analytical Chemistry, 79*, 4083–4093.
36. Holewinski, R. J., Parker, S. J., Matlock, A. D., Venkatraman, V., & Van Eyk, J. E. (2016). Methods for SWATH: Data independent acquisition on TripleTOF mass spectrometers. *Methods in Molecular Biology, 1410*, 265–279.
37. Simons, B., Kauhanen, D., Sylvanne, T., Tarasov, K., Duchoslav, E., & Ekroos, K. (2012). Shotgun Lipidomics by sequential precursor ion fragmentation on a hybrid Quadrupole time-of-flight mass spectrometer. *Metabolites, 2*, 195–213.
38. Bilbao, A., Varesio, E., Luban, J., Strambio-De-Castillia, C., Hopfgartner, G., Muller, M., & Lisacek, F. (2015). Processing strategies and software solutions for data-independent acquisition in mass spectrometry. *Proteomics, 15*, 964–980.
39. Chen, J., & Nichols, K. K. (2018). Comprehensive shotgun lipidomics of human meibomian gland secretions using MS/MS(all) with successive switching between acquisition polarity modes. *Journal of Lipid Research, 59*, 2223–2236.
40. Gao, F., McDaniel, J., Chen, E. Y., Rockwell, H., Lynes, M. D., Tseng, Y. H., Sarangarajan, R., Narain, N. R., & Kiebish, M. A. (2016). Monoacylglycerol analysis using MS/MSALL quadruple time of flight mass spectrometry. *Metabolites, 6*, 25.
41. Norris, J. L., & Caprioli, R. M. (2013). Analysis of tissue specimens by matrix-assisted laser desorption/ionization imaging mass spectrometry in biological and clinical research. *Chemical Reviews, 113*, 2309–2342.
42. Berry, K. A., Hankin, J. A., Barkley, R. M., Spraggins, J. M., Caprioli, R. M., & Murphy, R. C. (2011). MALDI imaging of lipid biochemistry in tissues by mass spectrometry. *Chemical Reviews, 111*, 6491–6512.
43. Ellis, S. R., Paine, M. R. L., Eijkel, G. B., Pauling, J. K., Husen, P., Jervelund, M. W., Hermansson, M., Ejsing, C. S., & Heeren, R. M. A. (2018). Automated, parallel mass spectrometry imaging and structural identification of lipids. *Nature Methods, 15*, 515–518.
44. Zavalin, A., Yang, J., Hayden, K., Vestal, M., & Caprioli, R. M. (2015). Tissue protein imaging at 1 mu m laser spot diameter for high spatial resolution and high imaging speed using transmission geometry MALDI TOF MS. *Analytical and Bioanalytical Chemistry, 407*, 2337–2342.
45. Baker, T. C., Han, J., & Borchers, C. H. (2017). Recent advancements in matrix-assisted laser desorption/ionization mass spectrometry imaging. *Current Opinion in Biotechnology, 43*, 62–69.
46. Buchberger, A. R., DeLaney, K., Johnson, J., & Li, L. J. (2018). Mass spectrometry imaging: A review of emerging advancements and future insights. *Analytical Chemistry, 90*, 240–265.
47. Flinders, B., Huizing, L. R. S., van Heerden, M., Cuyckens, F., Neumann, U. P., van der Laan, L. J. W., Damink, S. W. M. O., Heeren, R. M. A., Schaap, F. G., & Vreeken, R. J. (2018). Cross-species molecular imaging of bile salts and lipids

in liver: Identification of molecular structural markers in health and disease. *Analytical Chemistry, 90*, 11835–11846.
48. Ibrahim, H., Jurcic, K., Wang, J. S. H., Whitehead, S. N., & Yeung, K. K. C. (2017). 1,6-Diphenyl-1,3,5-hexatriene (DPH) as a novel matrix for MALDI MS imaging of fatty acids, phospholipids, and sulfatides in brain tissues. *Analytical Chemistry, 89*, 12828–12836.
49. Wang, X. D., Han, J., Chou, A., Yang, J. C., Pan, J. X., & Borchers, C. H. (2013). Hydroxyflavones as a new family of matrices for MALDI tissue imaging. *Analytical Chemistry, 85*, 7566–7573.
50. Calvano, C. D., Monopoli, A., Cataldi, T. R. I., & Palmisano, F. (2018). MALDI matrices for low molecular weight compounds: An endless story? *Analytical and Bioanalytical Chemistry, 410*, 4015–4038.
51. Wang, J., Qiu, S., Chen, S., Xiong, C., Liu, H., Wang, J., Zhang, N., Hou, J., He, Q., & Nie, Z. (2015). MALDI-TOF MS imaging of metabolites with a N-(1-naphthyl) ethylenediamine dihydrochloride matrix and its application to colorectal cancer liver metastasis. *Analytical Chemistry, 87*, 422–430.
52. Wang, J., Wang, C., & Han, X. (2018). Enhanced coverage of lipid analysis and imaging by matrix-assisted laser desorption/ionization mass spectrometry via a strategy with an optimized mixture of matrices. *Analytica Chimica Acta, 1000*, 155–162.
53. Cheng, H., Sun, G., Yang, K., Gross, R. W., & Han, X. (2010). Selective desorption/ionization of sulfatides by MALDI-MS facilitated using 9-aminoacridine as matrix. *Journal of Lipid Research, 51*, 1599–1609.
54. Shanta, S. R., Zhou, L. H., Park, Y. S., Kim, Y. H., Kim, Y., & Kim, K. P. (2011). Binary matrix for MALDI imaging mass spectrometry of phospholipids in both ion modes. *Analytical Chemistry, 83*, 1252–1259.
55. Schroter, J., Fulop, A., Hopf, C., & Schiller, J. (2018). The combination of 2,5-dihydroxybenzoic acid and 2,5-dihydroxyacetophenone matrices for unequivocal assignment of phosphatidylethanolamine species in complex mixtures. *Analytical and Bioanalytical Chemistry, 410*, 2437–2447.
56. Lu, M., Yang, X., Yang, Y., Qin, P., Wu, X., & Cai, Z. (2017). Nanomaterials as assisted matrix of laser desorption/ionization time-of-flight mass spectrometry for the analysis of small molecules. *Nanomaterials, 7*, 87.
57. Yagnik, G. B., Hansen, R. L., Korte, A. R., Reichert, M. D., Vela, J., & Lee, Y. J. (2016). Large scale nanoparticle screening for small molecule analysis in laser desorption ionization mass spectrometry. *Analytical Chemistry, 88*, 8926–8930.
58. Shrivas, K., Agrawal, K., & Wu, H. F. (2011). Application of platinum nanoparticles as affinity probe and matrix for direct analysis of small biomolecules and microwave digested proteins using matrix-assisted laser desorption/ionization mass spectrometry. *Analyst, 136*, 2852–2857.
59. Spencer, M. T., Furutani, H., Oldenburg, S. J., Darlington, T. K., & Prather, K. A. (2008). Gold nanoparticles as a matrix for visible-wavelength single-particle matrix-assisted laser desorption/ionization mass spectrometry of small biomolecules. *Journal of Physical Chemistry C, 112*, 4083–4090.
60. Niziol, J., & Ruman, T. (2013). Surface-transfer mass spectrometry imaging on a Monoisotopic silver nanoparticle enhanced target. *Analytical Chemistry, 85*, 12070–12076.
61. Dong, X. L., Cheng, J. S., Li, J. H., & Wang, Y. S. (2010). Graphene as a novel matrix for the analysis of small molecules by MALDI-TOF MS. *Analytical Chemistry, 82*, 6208–6214.
62. Lu, M. H., Lai, Y. Q., Chen, G. N., & Cai, Z. W. (2011). Matrix interference-free method for the analysis of small molecules by using negative ion laser desorption/ionization on graphene flakes. *Analytical Chemistry, 83*, 3161–3169.
63. Chen, S. M., Zheng, H. Z., Wang, J. N., Hou, J., He, Q., Liu, H. H., Xiong, C. Q., Kong, X. L., & Nie, Z. X. (2013). Carbon Nanodots as a matrix for the analysis of low-molecular-weight molecules in both positive- and negative-ion matrix-assisted laser desorption/ionization time-of-flight mass spectrometry and quantification of glucose and uric acid in real samples. *Analytical Chemistry, 85*, 6646–6652.
64. Chen, Y. S., Ding, J., He, X. M., Xu, J., & Feng, Y. Q. (2018). Synthesis of tellurium nanosheet for use in matrix assisted laser desorption/ionization time-of-flight mass spectrometry of small molecules. *Microchimica Acta, 185*, 368.
65. Zhao, Y., Tang, M., Liao, Q., Li, Z., Li, H., Xi, K., Tan, L., Zhang, M., Xu, D., & Chen, H. Y. (2018). Disposable MoS2-arrayed MALDI MS Chip for high-throughput and rapid quantification of sulfonamides in multiple real samples. *ACS Sensors, 3*, 806–814.
66. Wang, J., Sun, J., Wang, J., Liu, H., Xue, J., & Nie, Z. (2017). Hexagonal boron nitride nanosheets as a multifunctional background-free matrix to detect small molecules and complicated samples by MALDI mass spectrometry. *Chemical Communications, 53*, 8114–8117.
67. Pirro, V., Guffey, S. C., Sepulveda, M. S., Mahapatra, C. T., Ferreira, C. R., Jarmusch, A. K., & Cooks, R. G. (2016). Lipid dynamics in zebrafish embryonic development observed by DESI-MS imaging and nanoelectrospray-MS. *Molecular BioSystems, 12*, 2069–2079.
68. Henderson, F., Jones, E., Denbeigh, J., Christie, L., Batey, M. A., Claude, E., Williams, K. J., & McMahon, A. (2018). Automated, high-throughput 3D desorption electrospray ionization (DESI) mass spectrometry imaging of a xenograft model of glioblastoma. *Cancer Research, 78*, 33–33.
69. Pirro, V., Alfaro, C. M., Jarmusch, A. K., Hattab, E. M., Cohen-Gadol, A. A., & Cooks, R. G. (2017). Intraoperative assessment of tumor margins during glioma resection by desorption electrospray

ionization-mass spectrometry. *Proceedings of the National Academy of Sciences of the United States of America, 114*, 6700–6705.
70. Calligaris, D., Caragacianu, D., Liu, X. H., Norton, I., Thompson, C. J., Richardson, A. L., Golshan, M., Easterling, M. L., Santagata, S., Dillon, D. A., Jolesz, F. A., & Agar, N. Y. R. (2014). Application of desorption electrospray ionization mass spectrometry imaging in breast cancer margin analysis. *Proceedings of the National Academy of Sciences of the United States of America, 111*, 15184–15189.
71. Jarmusch, A. K., Pirro, V., Baird, Z., Hattab, E. M., Cohen-Gadol, A. A., & Cooks, R. G. (2016). Lipid and metabolite profiles of human brain tumors by desorption electrospray ionization-MS. *Proceedings of the National Academy of Sciences of the United States of America, 113*, 1486–1491.
72. Zhou, Z. P., & Zare, R. N. (2017). Personal information from latent fingerprints using desorption electrospray ionization mass spectrometry and machine learning. *Analytical Chemistry, 89*, 1369–1372.
73. Bich, C., Touboul, D., & Brunelle, A. (2014). Cluster TOF-SIMS imaging as a tool for micrometric histology of lipids in tissue. *Mass Spectrometry Reviews, 33*, 442–451.
74. Milac, T. I., Randolph, T. W., & Wang, P. (2012). Analyzing LC-MS/MS data by spectral count and ion abundance: Two case studies. *Statistics and Its Interface, 5*, 75–87.
75. Smith, C. A., Want, E. J., O'Maille, G., Abagyan, R., & Siuzdak, G. (2006). XCMS: Processing mass spectrometry data for metabolite profiling using nonlinear peak alignment, matching, and identification. *Analytical Chemistry, 78*, 779–787.
76. Benton, H. P., Wong, D. M., Trauger, S. A., & Siuzdak, G. (2008). XCMS2: Processing tandem mass spectrometry data for metabolite identification and structural characterization. *Analytical Chemistry, 80*, 6382–6389.
77. Koivusalo, M., Haimi, P., Heikinheimo, L., Kostiainen, R., & Somerharju, P. (2001). Quantitative determination of phospholipid compositions by ESI-MS: Effects of acyl chain length, unsaturation, and lipid concentration on instrument response. *Journal of Lipid Research, 42*, 663–672.
78. Han, X., & Gross, R. W. (2001). Quantitative analysis and molecular species fingerprinting of triacylglyceride molecular species directly from lipid extracts of biological samples by electrospray ionization tandem mass spectrometry. *Analytical Biochemistry, 295*, 88–100.
79. Bowden, J. A., Shao, F., Albert, C. J., Lally, J. W., Brown, R. J., Procknow, J. D., Stephenson, A. H., & Ford, D. A. (2011). Electrospray ionization tandem mass spectrometry of sodiated adducts of cholesteryl esters. *Lipids, 46*, 1169–1179.
80. Checa, A., Bedia, C., & Jaumot, J. (2015). Lipidomic data analysis: Tutorial, practical guidelines and applications. *Analytica Chimica Acta, 885*, 1–16.
81. O'Connor, A., Brasher, C. J., Slatter, D. A., Meckelmann, S. W., Hawksworth, J. I., Allen, S. M., & O'Donnell, V. B. (2017). LipidFinder: A computational workflow for discovery of lipids identifies eicosanoid-phosphoinositides in platelets. *JCI Insight, 2*, e91634.
82. Fahy, E., Alvarez-Jarreta, J., Brasher, C. J., Nguyen, A., Hawksworth, J. I., Rodrigues, P., Meckelmann, S., Allen, S. M., & O'Donnell, V. B. (2019). LipidFinder on LIPID MAPS: Peak filtering, MS searching and statistical analysis for lipidomics. *Bioinformatics, 35*, 685–687.
83. Husen, P., Tarasov, K., Katafiasz, M., Sokol, E., Vogt, J., Baumgart, J., Nitsch, R., Ekroos, K., & Ejsing, C. S. (2013). Analysis of lipid experiments (ALEX): A software framework for analysis of high-resolution shotgun Lipidomics data, *Plos one, 8*, e79736.
84. Guijas, C., Montenegro-Burke, J. R., Domingo-Almenara, X., Palermo, A., Warth, B., Hermann, G., Koellensperger, G., Huan, T., Uritboonthai, W., Aisporna, A. E., Wolan, D. W., Spilker, M. E., Benton, H. P., & Siuzdak, G. (2018). METLIN: A technology platform for identifying Knowns and unknowns. *Analytical Chemistry, 90*, 3156–3164.
85. Wishart, D. S., Tzur, D., Knox, C., Eisner, R., Guo, A. C., Young, N., Cheng, D., Jewell, K., Arndt, D., Sawhney, S., Fung, C., Nikolai, L., Lewis, M., Coutouly, M. A., Forsythe, I., Tang, P., Shrivastava, S., Jeroncic, K., Stothard, P., Amegbey, G., Block, D., Hau, D. D., Wagner, J., Miniaci, J., Clements, M., Gebremedhin, M., Guo, N., Zhang, Y., Duggan, G. E., Macinnis, G. D., Weljie, A. M., Dowlatabadi, R., Bamforth, F., Clive, D., Greiner, R., Li, L., Marrie, T., Sykes, B. D., Vogel, H. J., & Querengesser, L. (2007). HMDB: the Human Metabolome Database. *Nucleic Acids Research, 35*, D521–D526.
86. Ali, Z., & Bhaskar, S. B. (2016). Basic statistical tools in research and data analysis. *Indian Journal of Anaesthesia, 60*, 662–669.
87. Xia, J., Sinelnikov, I. V., Han, B., & Wishart, D. S. (2015). MetaboAnalyst 3.0--making metabolomics more meaningful. *Nucleic Acids Research, 43*, W251–W257.
88. Kanehisa, M., & Goto, S. (2000). KEGG: Kyoto encyclopedia of genes and genomes. *Nucleic Acids Research, 28*, 27–30.
89. Junker, B. H., Klukas, C., & Schreiber, F. (2006). VANTED: A system for advanced data analysis and visualization in the context of biological networks. *BMC Bioinformatics, 7*, 109.
90. Santos, C. R., & Schulze, A. (2012). Lipid metabolism in cancer. *The FEBS Journal, 279*, 2610–2623.
91. DeBerardinis, R. J., & Chandel, N. S. (2016). Fundamentals of cancer metabolism. *Science Advances, 2*, e1600200.
92. Liberti, M. V., & Locasale, J. W. (2016). The Warburg effect: How does it benefit Cancer cells? *Trends in Biochemical Sciences, 41*, 211–218.

93. Fhaner, C. J., Liu, S., Ji, H., Simpson, R. J., & Reid, G. E. (2012). Comprehensive lipidome profiling of isogenic primary and metastatic colon adenocarcinoma cell lines. *Analytical Chemistry, 84*, 8917–8926.
94. Hu, Q., Wang, M., Cho, M. S., Wang, C., Nick, A. M., Thiagarajan, P., Aung, F. M., Han, X., Sood, A. K., & Afshar-Kharghan, V. (2016). Lipid profile of platelets and platelet-derived microparticles in ovarian cancer. *BBA Clinical, 6*, 76–81.
95. Marien, E., Meister, M., Muley, T., Fieuws, S., Bordel, S., Derua, R., Spraggins, J., Van de Plas, R., Dehairs, J., Wouters, J., Bagadi, M., Dienemann, H., Thomas, M., Schnabel, P. A., Caprioli, R. M., Waelkens, E., & Swinnen, J. V. (2015). Non-small cell lung cancer is characterized by dramatic changes in phospholipid profiles. *International Journal of Cancer, 137*, 1539–1548.
96. Kiebish, M. A., Han, X., Cheng, H., Chuang, J. H., & Seyfried, T. N. (2008). Cardiolipin and electron transport chain abnormalities in mouse brain tumor mitochondria: Lipidomic evidence supporting the Warburg theory of cancer. *Journal of Lipid Research, 49*, 2545–2556.
97. Zhang, J., Feider, C. L., Nagi, C., Yu, W., Carter, S. A., Suliburk, J., Cao, H. S. T., & Eberlin, L. S. (2017). Detection of metastatic breast and thyroid cancer in lymph nodes by desorption electrospray ionization mass spectrometry imaging. *Journal of the American Society for Mass Spectrometry, 28*, 1166–1174.
98. Eberlin, L. S., Tibshirani, R. J., Zhang, J., Longacre, T. A., Berry, G. J., Bingham, D. B., Norton, J. A., Zare, R. N., & Poultsides, G. A. (2014). Molecular assessment of surgical-resection margins of gastric cancer by mass-spectrometric imaging. *Proceedings of the National Academy of Sciences of the United States of America, 111*, 2436–2441.
99. Gharpure, K. M., Pradeep, S., Sans, M., Rupaimoole, R., Ivan, C., Wu, S. Y., Bayraktar, E., Nagaraja, A. S., Mangala, L. S., Zhang, X., Haemmerle, M., Hu, W., Rodriguez-Aguayo, C., McGuire, M., Mak, C. S. L., Chen, X., Tran, M. A., Villar-Prados, A., Pena, G. A., Kondetimmanahalli, R., Nini, R., Koppula, P., Ram, P., Liu, J., Lopez-Berestein, G., Baggerly, K., Eberlin, S. L., & Sood, A. K. (2018). FABP4 as a key determinant of metastatic potential of ovarian cancer. *Nature Communications, 9*, 2923.
100. Marien, E., Meister, M., Muley, T., Gomez Del Pulgar, T., Derua, R., Spraggins, J. M., Van de Plas, R., Vanderhoydonc, F., Machiels, J., Binda, M. M., Dehairs, J., Willette-Brown, J., Hu, Y., Dienemann, H., Thomas, M., Schnabel, P. A., Caprioli, R. M., Lacal, J. C., Waelkens, E., & Swinnen, J. V. (2016). Phospholipid profiling identifies acyl chain elongation as a ubiquitous trait and potential target for the treatment of lung squamous cell carcinoma. *Oncotarget, 7*, 12582–12597.
101. Perez, O., Margolis, M., Santander, A. M., Martinez, M., Bhattacharya, S., & Torroella-Kouri, M. (2014). Breast cancer and obesity impact the lipid composition of breast adipose tissue: A preliminary study using shotgun lipidomics. *Cancer Research, 74*. Abstract # 3496.
102. Min, H. K., Lim, S., Chung, B. C., & Moon, M. H. (2011). Shotgun lipidomics for candidate biomarkers of urinary phospholipids in prostate cancer. *Analytical and Bioanalytical Chemistry, 399*, 823–830.
103. Farrokhi Yekta, R., Rezaie Tavirani, M., Arefi Oskouie, A., Mohajeri-Tehrani, M. R., & Soroush, A. R. (2017). The metabolomics and lipidomics window into thyroid cancer research. *Biomarkers, 22*, 595–603.
104. Mayers, J. R., Wu, C., Clish, C. B., Kraft, P., Torrence, M. E., Fiske, B. P., Yuan, C., Bao, Y., Townsend, M. K., Tworoger, S. S., Davidson, S. M., Papagiannakopoulos, T., Yang, A., Dayton, T. L., Ogino, S., Stampfer, M. J., Giovannucci, E. L., Qian, Z. R., Rubinson, D. A., Ma, J., Sesso, H. D., Gaziano, J. M., Cochrane, B. B., Liu, S., Wactawski-Wende, J., Manson, J. E., Pollak, M. N., Kimmelman, A. C., Souza, A., Pierce, K., Wang, T. J., Gerszten, R. E., Fuchs, C. S., Heiden, M. G. V., & Wolpin, B. M. (2014). Elevation of circulating branched-chain amino acids is an early event in human pancreatic adenocarcinoma development. *Nature Medicine, 20*, 1193–1198.
105. Skotland, T., Ekroos, K., Kauhanen, D., Simolin, H., Seierstad, T., Berge, V., Sandvig, K., & Llorente, A. (2017). Molecular lipid species in urinary exosomes as potential prostate cancer biomarkers. *European Journal of Cancer, 70*, 122–132.
106. Mazar, J., Zhao, W., Khalil, A. M., Lee, B., Shelley, J., Govindarajan, S. S., Yamamoto, F., Ratnam, M., Aftab, M. N., Collins, S., Finck, B. N., Han, X., Mattick, J. S., Dinger, M. E., & Perera, R. J. (2014). The functional characterization of long noncoding RNA SPRY4-IT1 in human melanoma cells. *Oncotarget, 5*, 8959–8969.
107. Zhao, Y., Ling, Z., Hao, Y., Pang, X., Han, X., Califano, J. A., Shan, L., & Gu, X. (2017). MiR-124 acts as a tumor suppressor by inhibiting the expression of sphingosine kinase 1 and its downstream signaling in head and neck squamous cell carcinoma. *Oncotarget, 8*, 25005–25020.
108. Sahoo, A., Lee, B., Boniface, K., Seneschal, J., Sahoo, S. K., Seki, T., Wang, C., Das, S., Han, X., Steppie, M., Seal, S., Taieb, A., & Perera, R. J. (2017). MicroRNA-211 regulates oxidative phosphorylation and energy metabolism in human vitiligo. *The Journal of Investigative Dermatology, 137*, 1965–1974.
109. Muth, A., Pandey, V., Kaur, N., Wason, M., Baker, C., Han, X., Johnson, T. R., Altomare, D. A., & Phanstiel, O. (2014). Synthesis and biological evaluation of antimetastatic agents predicated upon dihydromotuporamine C and its carbocyclic derivatives. *Journal of Medicinal Chemistry, 57*, 4023–4034.

Comprehensive Two-Dimensional Gas Chromatography Mass Spectrometry-Based Metabolomics

Md Aminul Islam Prodhan, Craig McClain, and Xiang Zhang

1 Introduction

The metabolome is composed of all metabolites in an organism. Those metabolites form a large network of metabolic reactions. The outputs from one enzymatic reaction are inputs to the others. Compared with genome and proteome, the metabolome is much more dynamic and complex because each metabolite is biochemically, spatially, and temporally defined [1, 2]. Metabolomics is the systematic study of metabolites and is usually divided into targeted metabolomics and untargeted metabolomics. Targeted metabolomics analyzes a limited number of known metabolites [3], while untargeted metabolomics aims to comprehensively analyze all metabolites present in a biological sample [4, 5].

Metabolites have a wide range of molecular weights and large variations in concentration. They can be polar or nonpolar as well as organic or inorganic. To date, the number of metabolites in a biological sample remains unknown even though it is estimated that at least thousands of metabolites should be detectable. As the chemical diversity of metabolites is so broad and the types of metabolites are huge, the analytical technologies needed to analyze metabolites are inherently complex, and there is not a singular

M. A. I. Prodhan
Department of Chemistry, University of Louisville, Louisville, KY, USA

University of Louisville Alcohol Research Center, University of Louisville, Louisville, KY, USA

University of Louisville Hepatobiology & Toxicology Program, University of Louisville, Louisville, KY, USA

Center for Regulatory and Environmental Analytical Metabolomics, University of Louisville, Louisville, KY, USA

C. McClain
University of Louisville Alcohol Research Center, University of Louisville, Louisville, KY, USA

University of Louisville Hepatobiology & Toxicology Program, University of Louisville, Louisville, KY, USA

Department of Pharmacology & Toxicology, University of Louisville, Louisville, KY, USA

Department of Medicine, University of Louisville, Louisville, KY, USA

Robley Rex Louisville VAMC, Louisville, KY, USA

X. Zhang (✉)
Department of Chemistry, University of Louisville, Louisville, KY, USA

University of Louisville Alcohol Research Center, University of Louisville, Louisville, KY, USA

University of Louisville Hepatobiology & Toxicology Program, University of Louisville, Louisville, KY, USA

Center for Regulatory and Environmental Analytical Metabolomics, University of Louisville, Louisville, KY, USA

Department of Pharmacology & Toxicology, University of Louisville, Louisville, KY, USA
e-mail: xiang.zhang@louisville.edu

S. Hu (ed.), *Cancer Metabolomics*, Advances in Experimental Medicine and Biology 1280,
https://doi.org/10.1007/978-3-030-51652-9_4

instrument capable of analyzing all types of metabolites [6–10].

Currently, multiple analytical platforms such as liquid chromatography–mass spectrometry (LC-MS), gas chromatography–mass spectrometry (GC-MS), and nuclear magnetic resonance (NMR) spectroscopy have been used in metabolomics. Among those analytical platforms, biological samples are frequently analyzed by LC-MS and/or GC-MS to achieve higher metabolite coverage, while NMR is generally best suited to quantitatively measure the most abundant metabolites or for molecular structure elucidation [11, 12]. Some other techniques such as capillary electrophoresis-mass spectrometry (CE-MS) are also used in metabolomics [13].

2 GC × GC-MS System and Its Operation

Due to the limited peak capacity of a single column, a one-dimensional separation method in GC-MS can only resolve a limited number of metabolites in a biological sample [14]. In order to increase the analytic power of GC-MS, multidimensional gas chromatography (MDGC) has been used for decades. Conventional MDGC technique uses the "heart cutting" method where selected portions of analytes eluted from the first dimension (^{1}D) column are transferred to the second dimension (^{2}D) column for further separation to achieve enhanced resolution for the heart-cutting zone [15]. This technique is unsuitable for untargeted metabolomics owing to its limited peak capacity and long analysis time. Comprehensive two-dimensional gas chromatography-mass spectrometry (GC × GC-MS) is the latest development to enhance the GC separation power.

A GC × GC-MS system has four major components: a ^{1}D column, a modulator, a ^{2}D column, and a mass spectrometer. The two columns ^{1}D and ^{2}D are connected in series by a modulator. After the sample is injected into the system through an injector, metabolites are initially separated on the ^{1}D column. Metabolites eluted from the ^{1}D column within a certain period of time, termed as modulation period P_M, are collected as a fraction by the modulator and then subjected to the ^{2}D column for further separation. After the separation on the ^{2}D column, metabolites are transferred to the mass spectrometer for measurement. This process is sequential and continuous throughout the analysis until all fractions collected from the ^{1}D column are analyzed by the ^{2}D column and mass spectrometer. Therefore, the GC × GC-MS offers a much more increased peak capacity and resolution.

2.1 Modulator

Modulator is a critical component in GC × GC-MS that isolates the elute from the ^{1}D column into multiple fractions, focuses, and injects each fraction to the ^{2}D column for further separation [16–20]. Modulators can be classified in two major categories: valve-based modulator and thermal modulator. In a valve-based modulator, a flow of gas is used to isolate portions of the elute from the ^{1}D column as a fraction and injects it to the ^{2}D column for further separation. A thermal modulator works by controlling the temperature to trap the elute from the ^{1}D column and then injects it to the ^{2}D column. While all types of modulators provide the common task of isolating a portion of elute from the ^{1}D column, refocusing and transferring it to the ^{2}D column for further separation, thermal modulators have fundamental advantages over the other types of modulators, by providing increased detection sensitivity and signal-to-noise (*S/N*) ratio due to its high duty cycle. The thermal modulators can be further subdivided into heater-based modulators and cryogenic modulators. Cryogenic modulators have been proven to be highly reliable, but costly.

To get optimal separation by GC × GC-MS, the modulation period (P_M) should be optimized based on experimental design, but generally, it lies between 2 and 10 s. The ideal P_M should be sufficient to resolve the unresolved peaks from the ^{1}D column with minimum loss of the ^{1}D separation. A large P_M value reduces the resolution of the ^{1}D separation, while a small P_M value may not provide enough ^{2}D separation and can give rise to a wraparound problem.

2.2 Column Configuration

The true power of a GC × GC-MS system lies in its orthogonal separation on the two columns [21]. In general, those two columns are mutually exclusive in their stationary phase and column dimension. The ^{1}D column is usually a conventional GC column with a nonpolar stationary phase, e.g., 100% dimethyl polysiloxane, 5% diphenyl-95% dimethylpolysiloxane, (5% phenyl)-polycarborane-siloxane, 5% diphenyl-dimethylpolysiloxane, etc. The stationary phase of the ^{2}D column is usually polar, e.g., polyethylene glycol (PEG), 100% bicyanopropyl polysiloxane, dimethyl polysiloxane, 70% cyanopropyl polysilphenylene-siloxane, etc. [17, 22].

A highly polar ^{2}D column can provide maximum orthogonality in separation if the ^{1}D column has nonpolar stationary phase. However, a polar column is usually not thermally stable and its upper temperature limit is only about 225 °C. In addition, trace levels of oxygen and water can degrade the polar column. Therefore, columns with middle polarity and higher temperature coverage are also used as the ^{2}D column. For instance, the column with a stationary phase of 50% phenyl, 50% methylpolysiloxane has high temperature coverage ranging from 40 °C to 320/340 °C. Furthermore, a mid-polarity column provides sufficient polarity and temperature range for derivatized metabolites because the polarity of a metabolite is usually reduced after derivatization.

In general, the optimal column combination is project dependent. Trial-and-error testing is the most popular way to find the optimal column combination. Since the ^{1}D column separation is generally boiling point separation, a long column is preferable. To get the maximum separation, a short and comparatively narrow-bore column relative to the ^{1}D column is often used as the ^{2}D column. The ^{1}D column has a typical length of 30–60 m with an inner diameter of 0.25–0.3 mm and film thickness of 0.25–1 μm. The ^{2}D column is typically 1–3 m long with an inner diameter of 0.10–0.25 mm and film thickness of 0.1–0.25 μm [23–25]. While the most used column combination is a nonpolar column connected to a polar (or a mid-polar) column, numerous applications have used a reverse order, i.e., a polar or mid-polar column followed by a nonpolar column [26–29].

To maintain the orthogonal separation in GC × GC-MS, the temperature program rate is generally kept lower, i.e., 0.5–5 °C to allow the production of a relatively broad ^{1}D peak to provide the adequate modulation for ^{2}D separation [17, 23]. However, a lower ramp rate needs a longer modulation period, and a longer modulation causes some loss of the resolution of the ^{1}D separation. The two columns are usually put in two different ovens under the same temperature-programed rate, but the ^{2}D oven is kept with a 10–30 °C offset from the ^{1}D oven to maximize the separations. The flow rate of the gas is related to the column dimension. Several papers have been dedicated to optimizing these parameters of GC × GC-MS [23, 30, 31].

2.3 Mass Spectrometer

Any mass spectrometers applicable for conventional GC-MS can be used in GC × GC-MS. Quadrupole mass spectrometer (qMS) has been hyphenated with the GC × GC system. However, qMS has a slow acquisition rate, e.g., 33–50 Hz [31–33]. The most widely used mass spectrometer in GC × GC-MS is a time-of-flight mass spectrometer (TOF-MS) equipped with an electron ionization (EI) source in which energetic electrons interact with gas phase molecules to fragment all metabolites eluted from the ^{2}D column. The fragment ions are then separated by TOF and measured by a detector. The TOF-MS operates under a snapshot technique with a very high acquisition rate, e.g., 500 Hz. Most importantly, the TOF-MS can distinguish chromatographically co-eluted metabolites if their EI mass spectra are different with a unique mass and have a small difference in their chromatographic peaks [34, 35].

High-resolution time-of-flight mass spectrometry (HRTOF-MS) has also been hyphenated with the GC × GC system. A HRTOF-MS gives superior resolution compared to the qMS and the unit mass resolution TOF-MS. The most important feature of HRTOF-MS is its capability to obtain the elemental composition of a metabolite from its precisely determined molecular ion m/z value. For that reason, a chemical ionization (CI) source is also available in HRTOF-MS [36].

3 Sample Preparation for GC × GC-MS

GC × GC-MS can only analyze volatile and thermally stable metabolites. A biological sample contains both volatile and nonvolatile metabolites. The volatile metabolites are usually extracted from a biological sample by solid phase microextraction (SPME) and then analyzed by GC × GC-MS, while the nonvolatile metabolites must be extracted from the biological sample, derivatized by a derivatization reagent, and then analyzed by GC × GC-MS.

Metabolites containing functional groups with active hydrogens (e.g., -COOH, -OH, -NH, and -SH) are of primary concern in GC × GC-MS analysis. For instance, these functional groups can form intermolecular hydrogen bonds and affect the inherent volatility of metabolites containing them. Therefore, derivatization is usually achieved by substituting the active hydrogen in a metabolite with another group such as $-Si(CH_3)_3$. Silylation, acylation, alkylation, and coordination complexation can all serve the purpose; of these, silylation is the most commonly used method. Nearly all functional groups can be derivatized by silylation reagents, and the derivatives are generally less polar, more volatile, and more thermally stable. The introduction of a silyl group can also enhance the mass spectrometric properties of derivatives by producing either more favorable diagnostic fragmentation patterns or characteristic ions.

Derivatization is a two-step procedure, methoxymation and derivatization. Some metabolites are thermally unstable even after derivatization. For example, the enol forms of aldehydes and ketones have an acidic hydrogen and can therefore be derivatized to trimethylsilyl (TMS) ethers, which can be thermally and hydrolytically unstable. Methoxymation prior to silylation can convert those functional groups to oximes or alkyloximes. In addition, direct derivatization without methoxymation can cause incomplete derivatization and result in multiple peaks for one metabolite in GC × GC-MS data. Incomplete derivatization also makes subsequent quantitation inaccurate. The most commonly used methoxymation reagent is O-methoxylamine hydrochloride in pyridine.

The second step of the derivatization is to add the silylation reagent to the methoxymated sample. Trimethylchlorosilane (TMCS) can be used to catalyze the silylation reaction. The popular silylation reagents include N-(tert-butyldimethylsily))-N-methyltrifluoroacetamide (MTBSTFA), N, O-bis(trimethylsilyl trifluoroacetamide (BSTFA), and N-methyl-N-(trimethylsilyl) trifluoroacetamide (MSTFA). Those reagents lead to the formation of either tert-butyldimethylsilyl (TBS) or TMS derivatives. The TBS derivatives are often preferred because they are more stable and sensitive than the TMS derivatives [37–39].

4 Data Analysis

GC × GC-MS data contain four pieces of information for each metabolite, the first dimension retention time ${}^{1}t_R$, the second dimension retention time ${}^{2}t_R$, parent ion or fragment ion m/z value, and its intensity. The m/z values of fragment ions and their corresponding intensities form the mass spectrum of that metabolite. The general workflow for analysis of GC × GC-MS data in metabolomics includes spectrum deconvolution, metabolite identification, cross-sample alignment, normalization, and statistical analysis.

4.1 Spectrum Deconvolution and Metabolite Identification

While the GC × GC-MS system has greatly increased peak capacity, metabolites often coelute from the ^{2}D column owing to the high complexity of biological samples. If the GC × GC-MS is equipped with an EI source, the co-eluting metabolites are simultaneously fragmented and all fragments form one mass spectrum. In that case, the mass spectrum acquired by GC × GC-MS is actually generated by the co-eluting metabolites. Spectral deconvolution distinguishes the signal arising from the instrumental noise and quantitatively deconvolutes the mass spectrum of those co-eluting metabolites into multiple mass spectra, each of which is the EI mass spectrum of one metabolite. Several software packages such as ChromaTOF, parallel factor analysis (PRAFAC), and GC Image have been developed for spectrum deconvolution.

Metabolite identification in the analysis of GC × GC-MS data is usually achieved by matching a query spectrum (i.e., an experimental mass spectrum) to the mass spectra of compound standards recorded in a reference library. A metabolite in the reference library with the highest spectral similarity measure is usually considered as the metabolite giving rise to the query spectrum. This process is called mass spectrum matching [40]. Many algorithms have been developed for spectrum matching, including composite similarity [41], probability-based matching system [42], cosine correlation [43–46], and Hertz similarity index [47].

A large mass spectral reference library increases the chance that the mass spectrum of the true metabolite is present in the library, but it also increases the chance that highly similar mass spectra from other metabolites are also present. Furthermore, multiple metabolites in a biological sample may have similar mass spectra, resulting in some metabolites in the mass spectral library having multiple mass spectrum-matched peaks in the experimental data. In addition, the mass spectrum represents only partial information concerning the molecular structure of a metabolite. Identifying metabolites based solely on mass spectrum matching has inherent limitations. Therefore, additional molecular information such as metabolite separation information (i.e., retention time) has been employed to increase identification confidence.

The magnitude of retention time depends heavily on experiment conditions. Therefore, the retention time is always converted into a retention index using the retention of reference compounds such as *n*-alkanes. Both the mass spectrum and the retention index have been used for metabolite identification in GC × GC-MS [48–50]. Most of the existing methods employ the retention index as a filter to remove the potential false-positive identifications generated by mass spectrum matching. Such an analysis strategy uses the retention index and mass spectrum in two separate analysis steps. The sequential nature of the two-step analysis strategy increases the risk of introducing errors from each independent stage since there is no way to correct the errors caused in the previous step. To improve the identification accuracy, a SimMR method was developed to simultaneously evaluate the mass spectrum similarity and the retention index distance using an empirical mixture score function [51]. It was demonstrated that the SimMR method improved the overall identification accuracy up to 1.53% compared to the sequential mass spectrum matching and retention index filtering. To identify metabolites from the GC × GC-MS data, the second-dimension retention index is not yet widely used in metabolomics because large variations are introduced during the process of calculating the second-dimension retention index [52].

4.2 Cross-Sample Alignment and Normalization

To increase the statistic power in metabolomics, multiple samples with the same treatment are usually analyzed on an instrument. Owing to some uncontrollable experimental conditions, such as the differences in temperature or pressure, matrix effects on samples, and stationary phase degradation, there is always a shift in the ${}^{1}t_R$ and ${}^{2}t_R$ of a metabolite between samples. This problem is generally overcome by cross-sample alignment. To date, cross-sample alignment has been done either directly using the instrumental data (profile alignment) or using peak lists deconvoluted from the instrumental data (peak alignment). Four profile alignment methods have been reported using the two-dimensional retention times: the rank annihilation method [53], a correlation-optimized shifting method [54], a piecewise retention time alignment [55], and a two-dimensional correlation optimized warping [56]. Aligning metabolite peaks solely based on the two-dimensional retention times may introduce a high rate of false-positive alignment because some metabolites with similar chemical functional groups have similar retention times in both GC dimensions. For this reason, methods such as MSort [57], DISCO [58], mSPA [59], and SWPA [60] were developed to perform peak list alignment using both the two-dimensional retention times and mass spectrum similarity.

After cross-sample alignment, the aligned data are generally normalized to reduce the technical variations while preserving the biological variations among samples. Several normalization algorithms have been used in metabolomics, including scaling and transformation. For instance, the auto-scaling method considers the z score of each data point rather than its initial value. Pareto scaling is a variation of auto-scaling, whereas the scaling factor is the square root of the standard deviation [61]. A common power transformation method is the one parameter Box-Cox transformation [62]. The other normalization methods include cyclic loess [63] and contrast-based normalization [64], among others.

4.3 Statistical Analysis

Two types of statistical analysis are usually performed in metabolomics, classification and statistical significance tests. The purpose of classification is to investigate the overall metabolite abundance profile, i.e., the abundance of all detected metabolites, between groups. The statistical significance tests check the difference of abundance levels of each metabolite between groups.

While different dimension reduction and classification methods, such as principal component analysis (PCA) and random forests, can be used to analyze metabolomic data, partial least squares discriminant analysis (PLS-DA) is the one most widely used in the field. PLS-DA combines dimensionality reduction and discriminant analysis into one algorithm. It sharpens the separation between groups to obtain a maximum separation among groups and to understand which variables carry the class separating information. The variable importance in projection (VIP) in PLS-DA is used to calculate the importance of individual metabolites among groups. Orthogonal signal correction PLS-DA (O-PLS-DA) is an extension of PLS-DA that seeks to maximize the explained variance between groups in a single dimension or the first latent variable and to separate the within group variance into orthogonal latent variables.

While the VIP in PLS-DA can be used to calculate the importance of individual metabolites among groups, statistical significance tests are also widely used in metabolomics to investigate whether a metabolite has different abundance levels between groups. For example, Student t-test checks whether the abundance levels of a metabolite have different means among groups. Other methods for statistical significance tests include Kolmogorov–Smirnov test, Wilcoxon rank sum test, Kruskal–Wallis H test, and others, depending on whether or not the data are parametric. The false discovery rate (FDR) is usually performed to adjust the p-value for multiple comparisons.

5 Applications of GC × GC-MS in Metabolomics

GC × GC-TOF MS has been employed in metabolomics for analysis of volatile organic compounds (VOCs). Testing of VOCs in breath is an exciting tool for rapid and noninvasive diagnosis. Phillips et al. detected around 2000 VOCs in normal human breath by GC × GC-TOF MS, of which many had not been detected before [65]. They further discovered a set of volatile biomarkers of radiation in human subjects receiving radiation therapy [66]. The same group also used the Göttingen minipig as an animal model and identified candidate biomarkers linked with external gamma radiation exposure [67]. Das et al. analyzed the breath of male and female subjects by GC × GC-TOF MS and discovered eleven exhaled breath VOCs that can differentiate the genders [68]. Recently, Beccarial et al. used GC × GC-TOF MS in combination with machine learning to investigate the possibility of using human breath for the diagnosis of active tuberculosis (TB) among TB suspect patients [69].

GC × GC-TOF MS has been also used in liver metabolomics. Shi et al. studied the effects of chronic arsenic exposure in a mouse model and discovered that distinct hepatic metabolomic profiles were associated with eating a high-fat diet, drinking arsenic-contaminated water, and the combination of the two [70]. They also studied the effects of *Lactobacillus rhamnosus* GG (LGG) on alcoholic liver disease (ALD) in mice, showing that LGGs alleviate alcohol-induced fatty liver by mechanisms involving increasing intestinal and decreasing hepatic fatty acids and increasing amino acid concentration [71]. Warner et al. found that ethanol and unsaturated dietary fat induced unique patterns of hepatic ω-6 and ω-3 polyunsaturated fatty acid (PUFA) oxylipins in a mouse model of ALD [72]. Schmidt et al. analyzed liver tissue by GC × GC-TOF MS and found that olanzapine administration increases weight and adiposity, promotes hepatic lipid accumulation, modifies hepatic expression of metabolism-regulating genes, and affects the hepatic metabolome [73].

GC × GC-TOF MS has been used to study the fecal metabolome. Nonalcoholic fatty liver disease (NAFLD) is the most common liver disease. Wei et al. analyzed rat feces to assess the effects of different dietary doses of copper combined with high fructose feeding on the homeostasis of intestine luminal metabolites [74]. Kirpich et al. analyzed the mouse fecal samples to evaluate the effects of different types of dietary fat and ethanol on the gut microbiota composition and metabolic activity and found that diet enriched in unsaturated fats enhanced alcohol-induced liver injury and caused major fecal metagenomic and metabolomic changes [75].

GC × GC-TOF MS has also been used for plasma metabolomics. In order to identify biomarkers of *Salmonella* carriage, Näsström et al. performed metabolite profiling on human plasma samples and discovered that *Salmonella* carriers could be distinguished from noncarrier controls by five metabolites, suggesting the potential of those metabolites as diagnostic markers for detecting chronic *Salmonella* carriers [76]. In another study, the same team used GC × GC-TOF MS for plasma metabolic profiling and showed that enteric fever induces distinct and reproducible metabolite profiles in the plasma of enteric fever patients [77]. Recently, Miyazaki et al. examined temporal changes in serum metabolites of neonatal calves after first ingestion of colostrum by GC × GC-TOF MS [78].

Cancer cell metabolomes have also been studied by GC × GC-TOF MS. Altered metabolism is considered as a key hallmark of cancer. Carlisle et al. explored the polar metabolome differences between MDA-MB-231 breast cancer cells expressing different levels of NAT1 activity using an untargeted metabolomics approach [79]. Dhakshinamoorthy et al. used GC × GC-TOF MS to identify systems-scale changes in metabolic dynamics that are distinct from changes induced in noncancerous cells or by other chemotherapeutics and found that phosphoethanolamine was one of the most significantly affected metabolites [80].

Weinert et al. successfully equipped a GC × GC system with a fast-scanning quadrupole mass spectrometer to analyze human urine samples and proved that GC × GC-qMS could be applicable for large-scale metabolome analyses [81]. Vasquez et al. analyzed children's urines using GC × GC-qMS. They also compared the GC × GC-qMS results with the GC-qMS and found 92 additional metabolites [82]. Luies et al. analyzed urinary metabolomes using GC × GC-TOF MS, to compare and differentiate between the culture-confirmed active TB-positive and TB-negative healthy control groups and identified 12 metabolites that could be used for explaining the differences occurring between those groups [83]. Loureiro et al. used GC × GC-TOF MS for urinary metabolite profiling to reveal the relation between oxidative stress extension, eosinophilic inflammation, and disease severity in asthmatic patients [84].

6 Conclusions

Compared with GC-MS, GC × GC-MS provides greatly increased peak capacity, resolution, and sensitivity for analysis of complex biological samples. In the last decade, GC × GC-MS has been increasingly used in metabolomics for metabolite biomarker discovery and elucidation of disease mechanisms. The recent development of coupling GC × GC with a high-resolution mass spectrometer further accelerates the applications of GC × GC-MS in metabolomics. However, metabolite derivatization and complicated data analysis remains as the two factors that prevent the wider use of GC × GC-MS in metabolomics.

References

1. Wishart, D. S. (2011). Advances in metabolite identification. *Bioanalysis, 3*, 1769–1782.
2. Kind, T., Scholz, M., & Fiehn, O. (2009). How large is the metabolome? A critical analysis of data exchange practices in chemistry. *PLoS One, 44*(5), e5440.
3. Gates, S. C., & Sweeley, C. C. (1978). Quantitative metabolic profiling based on gas chromatography. *Clinical Chemistry, 24*, 1663–1673.
4. Aharoni, A., et al. (2002). Nontargeted metabolome analysis by use of Fourier transform ion cyclotron mass spectrometry. *Omics: A Journal of Integrative Biology, 6*, 217–234.
5. Ellis, D. I., Dunn, W. B., Griffin, J. L., Allwood, J. W., & Goodacre, R. (2007). Metabolic fingerprinting as a diagnostic tool. *Pharmacogenomics, 8*(9), 1243–1266.
6. De Souza, A. G., MacCormack, T. J., Wang, N., Li, L., & Goss, G. G. (2009). Large-scale proteome profile of the zebrafish (Danio rerio) gill for physiological and biomarker discovery studies. *Zebrafish, 6*, 229–238.
7. Dunn, W. B., Bailey, N. J., & Johnson, H. E. (2005). Measuring the metabolome: Current analytical technologies. *Analyst, 130*, 606–625.
8. Wishart, D. S., et al. (2008). The human cerebrospinal fluid metabolome. *Journal of Chromatography B, 871*, 164–173.
9. Psychogios, N., et al. (2011). The human serum metabolome. *PLoS One, 6*, e16957.
10. van der Werf, M. J., Overkamp, K. M., Muilwijk, B., Coulier, L., & Hankemeier, T. (2007). Microbial metabolomics: Toward a platform with full metabolome coverage. *Analytical Biochemistry, 370*, 17–25.
11. Reo, N. V. (2002). NMR-based metabolomics. *Drug and Chemical Toxicology, 25*, 375–382.
12. Fan, T. W. M., & Lane, A. N. (2016). Applications of NMR spectroscopy to systems biochemistry. *Progress in Nuclear Magnetic Resonance Spectroscopy, 92–93*, 18–53.
13. Ramautar, R., Mayboroda, O. A., Somsen, G. W., & de Jong, G. J. (2011). CE-MS for metabolomics: Developments and applications in the period 2008–2010. *Electrophoresis, 32*, 52–65.
14. Stoll, D. R., & Carr, P. W. (2017). Two-dimensional liquid chromatography: A state of the art tutorial. *Analytical Chemistry, 89*(1), 519–531.
15. Bertsch, W. (1999). Two-dimensional gas chromatography. Concepts, instrumentation, and applications–part 1: Fundamentals, conventional two-dimensional gas chromatography, selected applications. *Journal of High Resolution Chromatography, 22*, 647–665.
16. Mondello, L., Tranchida, P. Q., Dugo, P., & Dugo, G. (2008). Comprehensive two-dimensional gas chromatography-mass spectrometry: A review. *Mass Spectrometry Reviews, 27*, 101–124.
17. Dallüge, J., Beens, J., & Udo, A. (2003). Comprehensive two-dimensional gas chromatography: A powerful and versatile analytical tool. *Journal of Chromatography. A, 1000*, 69–108.
18. Tranchida, P. Q., Purcaro, G., Dugo, P., & Mondello, L. (2011). Modulators for comprehensive two-dimensional gas chromatography. *TrAC Trends in Analytical Chemistry, 30*, 1437–1461.
19. Bahaghighat, H. D., Freye, C. E., & Synovec, R. E. (2018). Recent advances in modulator technology for comprehensive two dimensional gas chromatography. *TrAC Trends in Analytical Chemistry, 113*, 379–391.
20. Tranchida, P. Q. (2018). Comprehensive two-dimensional gas chromatography: A perspective on processes of modulation. *Journal of Chromatography. A, 1536*, 2–5.
21. Giddings, J. (1987). Concepts and comparisons in multidimensional separation. *Journal of High Resolution Chromatography, 10*, 319–323.
22. Weldegergis, B. T., et al. (2011). Characterisation of volatile components of Pinotage wines using comprehensive two-dimensional gas chromatography coupled to time-of-flight mass spectrometry (GC × GC–TOFMS). *Food Chemistry, 129*, 188–199.
23. Mostafa, A., Edwards, M., & Górecki, T. (2012). Optimization aspects of comprehensive two-dimensional gas chromatography. *Journal of Chromatography. A, 1255*, 38–55.
24. Dallüge, J., van Rijn, M., Beens, J., Vreuls, R. J. J., & Brinkman, U. A. T. (2002). Comprehensive two-dimensional gas chromatography with time-of-flight mass spectrometric detection applied to the determination of pesticides in food extracts. *Journal of Chromatography. A, 965*, 207–217.
25. Shellie, R., Marriott, P., & Morrison, P. (2001). Concepts and preliminary observations on the triple-dimensional analysis of complex volatile samples by using GC × GC–TOFMS. *Analytical Chemistry, 73*, 1336–1344.

26. Adahchour, M., Beens, J., Vreuls, R. J. J., & Brinkman, U. A. T. (2006). Recent developments in comprehensive two-dimensional gas chromatography (GC×GC): I. Introduction and instrumental set-up. *TrAC Trends in Analytical Chemistry, 25*, 438–454.
27. Dimandja, J.-M. D., et al. (2003). Standardized test mixture for the characterization of comprehensive two-dimensional gas chromatography columns: The Phillips mix. *Journal of Chromatography. A, 1019*, 261–272.
28. Cordero, C., Rubiolo, P., Sgorbini, B., Galli, M., & Bicchi, C. (2006). Comprehensive two-dimensional gas chromatography in the analysis of volatile samples of natural origin: A multidisciplinary approach to evaluate the influence of second dimension column coated with mixed stationary phases on system orthogonality. *Journal of Chromatography. A, 1132*, 268–279.
29. Dimandja, J.-M. D. (2004). Peer Reviewed: GC X GC. *Analytical Chemistry, 76*, 167 A–174 A.
30. Yu, Z., et al. (2017). Optimizing 2D gas chromatography mass spectrometry for robust tissue, serum and urine metabolite profiling. *Talanta, 165*, 685–691.
31. Adahchour, M., Beens, J., & Brinkman, U. A. T. (2008). Recent developments in the application of comprehensive two-dimensional gas chromatography. *Journal of Chromatography. A, 1186*, 67–108.
32. Adahchour, M., et al. (2005). Comprehensive two-dimensional gas chromatography coupled to a rapid-scanning quadrupole mass spectrometer: Principles and applications. *Journal of Chromatography. A, 1067*, 245–254.
33. Purcaro, G., et al. (2010). Evaluation of a rapid-scanning quadrupole mass spectrometer in an apolar × ionic-liquid comprehensive two-dimensional gas chromatography system. *Analytical Chemistry, 82*, 8583–8590.
34. Focant, J.-F., et al. (2004). High-throughput analysis of human serum for selected polychlorinated biphenyls (PCBs) by gas chromatography-isotope dilution time-of-flight mass spectrometry (GC-IDTOFMS). *Analyst, 129*, 331–336.
35. Focant, J.-F., Sjödin, A., & Patterson, D. G. (2003). Qualitative evaluation of thermal desorption-programmable temperature vaporization-comprehensive two-dimensional gas chromatography–time-of-flight mass spectrometry for the analysis of selected halogenated contaminants. *Journal of Chromatography. A, 1019*, 143–156.
36. Tranchida, P. Q., Franchina, F. A., Dugo, P., & Mondello, L. (2016). Comprehensive two-dimensional gas chromatography-mass spectrometry: Recent evolution and current trends. *Mass Spectrometry Reviews, 35*, 524–534.
37. Halket, J. M., & Zaikin, V. G. (2003). Derivatization in mass spectrometry—1. Silylation. *European. Journal of Mass Spectrometry, 9*, 1–21.
38. Zaikin, V. G., & Halket, J. M. (2003). Derivatization in mass spectrometry—2. Acylation. *European Journal of Mass Spectrometry, 9*, 421–434.
39. Zaikin, V., & Halket, J. M. (2009). *A handbook of derivatives for mass spectrometry*. Chichester: IM Publications.
40. Stein, S. E. (1999). An integrated method for spectrum extraction and compound identification from gas chromatography/mass spectrometry data. *Journal of the American Society for Mass Spectrometry, 10*, 770–781.
41. Stein, S. E., & Scott, D. R. (1994). Optimization and testing of mass spectral library search algorithms for compound identification. *Journal of the American Society for Mass Spectrometry, 5*, 859–866.
42. Atwater, B. L., Stauffer, D. B., Mclafferty, F. W., & Peterson, D. W. (1985). Reliability ranking and scaling improvements to the probability based matching system for unknown mass-spectra. *Analytical Chemistry, 57*, 899–903.
43. Tabb, D. L., MacCoss, M. J., Wu, C. C., Anderson, S. D., & Yates, J. R. (2003). Similarity among tandem mass spectra from proteomic experiments: Detection, significance, and utility. *Analytical Chemistry, 75*, 2470–2477.
44. Beer, I., Barnea, E., Ziv, T., & Admon, A. (2004). Improving large-scale proteomics by clustering of mass spectrometry data. *Proteomics, 4*, 950–960.
45. Craig, R., Cortens, J. C., Fenyo, D., & Beavis, R. C. (2006). Using annotated peptide mass spectrum libraries for protein identification. *Journal of Proteome Research, 5*, 1843–1849.
46. Frewen, B. E., Merrihew, G. E., Wu, C. C., Noble, W. S., & MacCoss, M. J. (2006). Analysis of peptide MS/MS spectra from large-scale proteomics experiments using spectrum libraries. *Analytical Chemistry, 78*, 5678–5684.
47. Hertz, H. S., Hites, R. A., & Biemann, K. (1971). Identification of mass spectra by computer-searching a file of known spectra. *Analytical Chemistry, 43*, 681.
48. Lisec, J., Schauer, N., Kopka, J., Willmitzer, L., & Fernie, A. R. (2006). Gas chromatography mass spectrometry-based metabolite profiling in plants. *Nature Protocols, 1*, 387–396.
49. Dunn, W. B., et al. (2011). Procedures for large-scale metabolic profiling of serum and plasma using gas chromatography and liquid chromatography coupled to mass spectrometry. *Nature Protocols, 6*, 1060–1083.
50. Zhang, J., et al. (2011). iMatch: A retention index tool for analysis of gas chromatography-mass spectrometry data. *Journal of Chromatography A, 1218*, 6522–6530.
51. Wei, X. L., Koo, I., Kim, S., & Zhang, X. (2014). Compound identification in GC-MS by simultaneously evaluating the mass spectrum and retention index. *Analyst, 139*, 2507–2514.
52. Prodhan, M. A. I., Yin, X., Kim, S., McClain, C., & Zhang, X. (2018). Surface fitting for calculating the second dimension retention index in comprehensive two-dimensional gas chromatography mass spectrometry. *Journal of Chromatography. A, 1539*, 62–70.

53. Fraga, C. G., Prazen, B. J., & Synovec, R. E. (2001). Objective data alignment and Chemometric analysis of comprehensive two-dimensional separations with run-to-run peak shifting on both dimensions. *Analytical Chemistry, 73*, 5833–5840.
54. van Mispelaar, V. G., Tas, A. C., Smilde, A. K., Schoenmakers, P. J., & van Asten, A. C. (2003). Quantitative analysis of target components by comprehensive two-dimensional gas chromatography. *Journal of Chromatography. A, 1019*, 15–29.
55. Pierce, K. M., Wood, L. F., Wright, B. W., & Synovec, R. E. (2005). A comprehensive two-dimensional retention time alignment algorithm to enhance Chemometric analysis of comprehensive two-dimensional separation data. *Analytical Chemistry, 77*, 7735–7743.
56. Zhang, D., Huang, X., Regnier, F. E., & Zhang, M. (2008). Two-dimensional correlation optimized warping algorithm for aligning GC×GC–MS data. *Analytical Chemistry, 80*, 2664–2671.
57. Oh, C., Huang, X., Regnier, F. E., Buck, C., & Zhang, X. (2008). Comprehensive two-dimensional gas chromatography/time-of-flight mass spectrometry peak sorting algorithm. *Journal of Chromatography. A, 1179*, 205–215.
58. Wang, B., et al. (2010). DISCO: Distance and Spectrum correlation optimization alignment for two-dimensional gas chromatography time-of-flight mass spectrometry-based metabolomics. *Analytical Chemistry, 82*, 5069–5081.
59. Kim, S., Fang, A., Wang, B., Jeong, J., & Zhang, X. (2011). An optimal peak alignment for comprehensive two-dimensional gas chromatography mass spectrometry using mixture similarity measure. *Bioinformatics (Oxford, England), 27*, 1660–1666.
60. Kim, S., Koo, I., Fang, A., & Zhang, X. (2011). Smith-waterman peak alignment for comprehensive two-dimensional gas chromatography-mass spectrometry. *BMC Bioinformatics, 12*, 235.
61. Eriksson, L. (1999). *Introduction to multi-and megavariate data analysis using projection methods (PCA & PLS)*, (Umetrics AB, 1999).
62. Sakia, R. (1992). The box-cox transformation technique: A review. *The Statistician, 41*, 169–178.
63. Dudoit, S., Yang, Y. H., Callow, M. J., & Speed, T. P. (2002). Statistical methods for identifying differentially expressed genes in replicated cDNA microarray experiments. *Statistica Sinica, 12*, 111–139.
64. Wei, X., et al. (2013). MetPP: A computational platform for comprehensive two-dimensional gas chromatography time-of-flight mass spectrometry-based metabolomics. *Bioinformatics, 29*, 1786–1792.
65. Phillips, M., et al. (2013). Detection of an extended human volatome with comprehensive two-dimensional gas chromatography time-of-flight mass spectrometry. *PLoS One, 8*, e75274.
66. Phillips, M., et al. (2013). Detection of volatile biomarkers of therapeutic radiation in breath. *Journal of Breath Research, 7*, 036002.
67. Phillips, M., et al. (2015). Breath biomarkers of whole-body gamma irradiation in the Göttingen minipig. *Health Physics, 108*, 538–546.
68. Das, M. K., et al. (2014). Investigation of gender-specific exhaled breath Volatome in humans by GCxGC-TOF-MS. *Analytical Chemistry, 86*, 1229–1237.
69. Beccaria, M., et al. (2018). Preliminary investigation of human exhaled breath for tuberculosis diagnosis by multidimensional gas chromatography – Time of flight mass spectrometry and machine learning. *Journal of Chromatography B, 1074-1075*, 46–50.
70. Shi, X., et al. (2013). Metabolomic analysis of the effects of chronic arsenic exposure in a mouse model of diet-induced fatty liver disease. *Journal of Proteome Research, 13*, 547–554.
71. Shi, X., et al. (2015). Hepatic and fecal metabolomic analysis of the effects of Lactobacillus rhamnosus GG on alcoholic fatty liver disease in mice. *Journal of Proteome Research, 14*, 1174–1182.
72. Warner, D. R., et al. (2018). Ethanol and unsaturated dietary fat induce unique patterns of hepatic ω-6 and ω-3 PUFA oxylipins in a mouse model of alcoholic liver disease. *PLoS One, 13*, e0204119.
73. Schmidt, R. H., et al. (2013). Olanzapine activates hepatic mammalian target of Rapamycin: New mechanistic insight into metabolic dysregulation with atypical antipsychotic drugs. *Journal of Pharmacology and Experimental Therapeutics, 347*, 126.
74. Wei, X., et al. (2015). Effects of dietary different doses of copper and high fructose feeding on rat fecal metabolome. *Journal of Proteome Research, 14*, 4050–4058.
75. Kirpich, I. A., et al. (2016). Saturated and unsaturated dietary fats differentially modulate ethanol-induced changes in gut microbiome and metabolome in a mouse model of alcoholic liver disease. *The American Journal of Pathology, 186*, 765–776.
76. Näsström, E., et al. (2018). Diagnostic metabolite biomarkers of chronic typhoid carriage. *PLoS Neglected Tropical Diseases, 12*, e0006215.
77. Näsström, E., et al. (2014). Salmonella Typhi and Salmonella Paratyphi A elaborate distinct systemic metabolite signatures during enteric fever. *eLife, 3*, e03100.
78. Miyazaki, T., Okada, K., Yamashita, T., & Miyazaki, M. (2017). Two-dimensional gas chromatography time-of-flight mass spectrometry-based serum metabolic fingerprints of neonatal calves before and after first colostrum ingestion. *Journal of Dairy Science, 100*, 4354–4364.
79. Carlisle, S. M., et al. (2016). Untargeted polar metabolomics of transformed MDA-MB-231 breast cancer cells expressing varying levels of human arylamine N-acetyltransferase 1. *Metabolomics, 12*, 111.
80. Dhakshinamoorthy, S., Dinh, N.-T., Skolnick, J., & Styczynski, M. P. (2015). Metabolomics identifies the intersection of phosphoethanolamine with menaquinone-triggered apoptosis in an in vitro model of leukemia. *Molecular BioSystems, 11*, 2406–2416.

81. Weinert, C. H., Egert, B., & Kulling, S. E. (2015). On the applicability of comprehensive two-dimensional gas chromatography combined with a fast-scanning quadrupole mass spectrometer for untargeted large-scale metabolomics. *Journal of Chromatography. A, 1405*, 156–167.
82. Vasquez, N. P., et al. (2015). Advances in the metabolic profiling of acidic compounds in children's urines achieved by comprehensive two-dimensional gas chromatography. *Journal of Chromatography B, 1002*, 130–138.
83. Luier, L., & Loots, D. T. (2016). Tuberculosis metabolomics reveals adaptations of man and microbe in order to outcompete and survive. *Metabolomics, 12*, 40.
84. Loureiro, C., et al. (2016). Urinary metabolomic profiling of asthmatics can be related to clinical characteristics. *Allergy, 71*, 1362–1365.

Single-Cell Metabolomics by Mass Spectrometry Imaging

Maria Emilia Dueñas and Young Jin Lee

1 Introduction to Mass Spectrometry Imaging

Exploring the metabolic differences directly on cells and tissues is essential for the comprehensive understanding of how multicellular organisms function. An improved understanding of the metabolism relies on analytical capabilities for accurate identification and quantification of metabolites, and metabolomics has largely addressed this through the development of mass spectrometry (MS) approaches, as well as separation techniques and computational tools [1, 2]. Most of the analysis performed by these methodologies provide excellent qualitative and quantitative information about chemical composition, but disregard information regarding the spatial distribution of these metabolites. Multicellular organisms, such as plants and animals, achieve their complex living activities through the highly organized metabolic interplay of a three-dimensional array of individual cells and tissues. Therefore, data regarding the original spatial distribution of metabolites in situ is necessary for in-depth understanding of biology in action.

Single-cell metabolomics is an emerging research field to understand heterogeneity and stochastic nature in cellular populations [3–5]. However, it is mostly accomplished by single-cell analysis of cultured cells and not directly applicable to multicellular organisms to understand intercellular interactions. In recent decades, mass spectrometry imaging (MSI) has demonstrated enormous potential in many fields, from mapping metabolites and other biomolecules in tissues [6–8] to drug research and development [9, 10]. This analytical tool enables untargeted as well as targeted analysis to discover biomarkers [11] or to understand biological systems at the metabolite level [12]. MSI can achieve chemical specificity and sensitivity, does not require labeling so that any compound present on the tissue can be analyzed, and allows for simultaneous imaging of hundreds of compounds. Most importantly, MSI can be used to spatially resolve the distribution of endogenous and exogenous species in tissue sections down to single-cell level resolution.

The MSI process is schematically presented in Fig. 1. In a traditional MSI experiment, the tissue sample is interrogated by a sampling beam (i.e., laser, solvent stream, ion beam) where analytes are desorbed from the surface. Matrix-assisted laser desorption/ionization (MALDI) [13],

M. E. Dueñas (✉)
Department of Chemistry, Iowa State University, Ames, IA, USA

Biosciences Institute, Newcastle University, Newcastle upon Tyne, UK
e-mail: maria.duenas@newcastle.ac.uk

Y. J. Lee
Department of Chemistry, Iowa State University, Ames, IA, USA
e-mail: yjlee@iastate.edu

S. Hu (ed.), *Cancer Metabolomics*, Advances in Experimental Medicine and Biology 1280,
https://doi.org/10.1007/978-3-030-51652-9_5

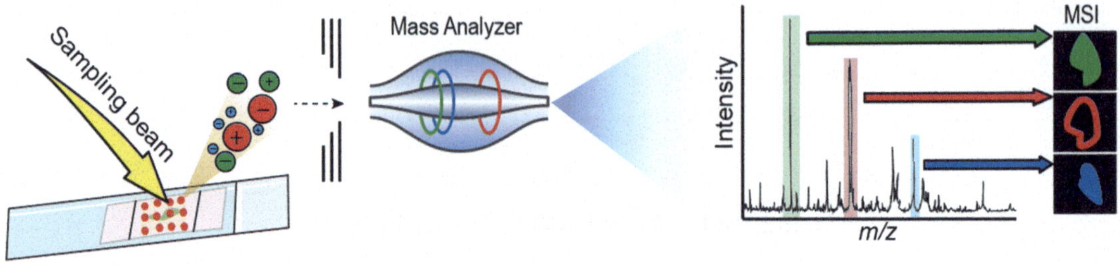

Fig. 1 Schematic representation of the MSI process

secondary ion mass spectrometry (SIMS) [14], laser ablation electrospray ionization (LAESI) [15], liquid extraction surface analysis (LESA) [16], and desorption electrospray ionization (DESI) [17] are the main sampling/ionization techniques used for MSI measurements. The ions are then introduced into a mass analyzer and sorted on the basis of their mass to charge ratios (*m/z*). A series of mass spectra are obtained by rastering the sampling beam or moving the sample plate across hundreds of *x* and *y* positions. An ion density map can then be produced for each *m/z* value detected showing where certain compounds are localized in the tissue sample, which can be correlated to an optical image of the sample.

MALDI-MSI is an attractive technique towards single-cell level resolution due to its soft ionization (compared to SIMS) and small sampling size (compared to DESI, LESA, or LAESI). Although nanoDESI has been developed and can reduce the sampling size down to ~10 μm, it is not readily available due to its delicate instrumentation [18, 19]. LESA coupled with liquid chromatography (LC)-MS is compatible with traditional metabolomics and can be integrated into MSI workflows, but is critically limited to a spatial resolution of ~400 μm for routine use and requires long data acquisition times [20].

Recently, MS images with spatial resolution of 1–5 μm have been obtained [6, 21–24] which enables the study of the molecular distribution of metabolites at cellular and subcellular levels. Although MALDI-MSI provides high-spatial-resolution information that is unprecedented in traditional metabolomics, it has fundamental limitations including the lack of chromatographic separation, the limited number of molecules available in a small sampling size, and matrix-dependent analyte selectivity, which has stalled the ability to visualize metabolites at the metabolomics scale. Many efforts are under way to overcome these limitations, and we envision that MSI-enabled metabolomics could be achieved at the single-cell resolution in the near future.

Here, we highlight the recent developments in the field of MSI, focused on single-cell level resolution metabolomics directly on tissue, particularly using MALDI-MSI. First, we present the advancements in instrumentation for MSI to achieve single-cell resolution. Second, we illustrate the advances and applications towards metabolomics scale imaging. Finally, we provide a future outlook in the field of single-cell metabolomics directly on tissue.

2 Technological Advances in High-Spatial-Resolution MALDI-MSI

The spatial resolution in MALDI-MSI is largely governed by the laser spot size as it determines the sampling size. Several efforts have been made to reduce the laser spot size including the use of a small-diameter optical fiber [25], an expanded laser beam focused close to sample specimens [26–28], and transmission geometry setups [28]. Jun et al. achieved laser spot size of ~12 μm by replacing 200 μm inner diameter optical fiber with a 25 μm core multimode optical fiber [25]. Using this modification, surface lipids from multiple tissue organs of a whole *Arabidopsis* flower were visualized at single-cell

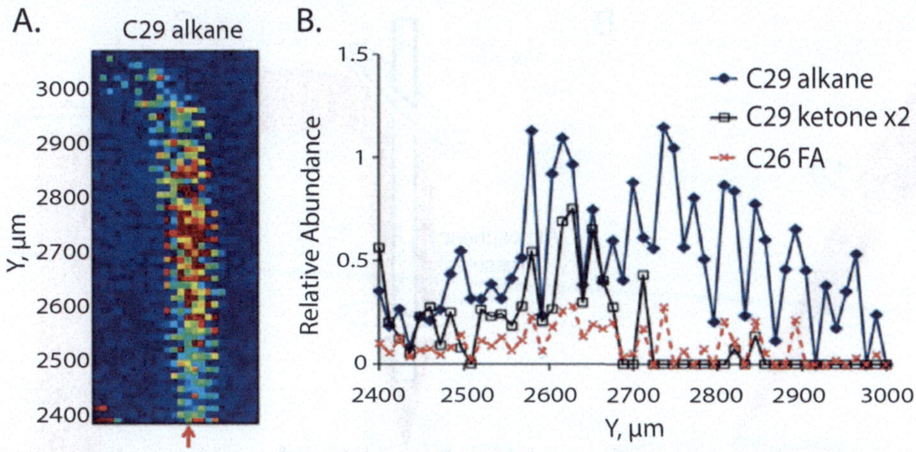

Fig. 2 Demonstration of single-cell level spatial resolution: (**a**) MS image of a stamen in *Arabidopsis* flower for C29 alkane detected as silver adduct (*m/z* 515); (**b**) the profiles of the relative ion abundance for C29 alkane, C29 ketone, and C26 fatty acid (FA) as silver ion adducts (*m/z* 515, 529, and 503, respectively) normalized to the silver dimer, $[^{107}Ag + ^{109}Ag]^+$ (*m/z* 216), along the series of single pixels vertically at the X position indicated by the arrow in (**a**). Pixel size is 12 µm. (Reproduced with the permission of American Chemical Society [25])

resolution. Figure 2 illustrates that MSI can indeed provide single-cell resolution information from the profiles of ion signals along a stamen; i.e., the periodic fluctuation of ion signals, typically every two or three pixels, matches with longitudinal epidermal cell size of ~30 µm on a stamen filament. It is difficult, however, to achieve a smaller laser spot size using optical fibers, especially because the fibers can be easily damaged at higher laser density.

Multimode homogeneous laser beams, such as Smart Beam™ [29] or TopHat [30], provide homogeneous distribution of laser beam profiles over the sampling area, but cannot be focused to a very small spot size. The direct delivery of a Gaussian shape laser profile (e.g., Nd:YAG laser) is better suited to achieve minimum laser spot size for MALDI experiments. For a Gaussian shape laser beam, the diffraction-limited spot size is defined by the following equation [23]:

$$D_s = M^2 \frac{4}{\pi} \lambda \frac{f}{D_b} \frac{1}{\cos\theta}$$

where D_s is the diffraction-limited spot size, M^2 is the beam quality factor, λ is the laser wavelength, f is the focal length of the focusing lens, D_b is the input beam diameter, and θ represents the incident angle of the laser beam on the sample. Although some of the parameters (λ, θ) can be difficult to modify in a given instrument, other parameters (M^2, f, D_b) can be altered to achieve a small laser spot size.

Three major instrumental setups, as illustrated in Fig. 3, have been developed over the years to achieve a small laser spot size. Using a large beam diameter (D_b) with a beam expander and a relatively simple modification to make the focus lens (f) close to the sample surface, a small laser spot size (D_s) can be obtained in a commercial MALDI-MS as represented in Fig. 3a. Due to the mass spectrometry ion optics occupying in front of the sample surface, however, the focus lens cannot be made any closer than ~60 mm, limiting the laser spot size of ~4–5 µm [6, 21, 23, 24]. The Spengler group overcame this limitation with atmospheric pressure MALDI-MS using a focus lens with the center bored for ion transfer capillary (Fig. 3b). In this setup, the focus lens can be as close as ~40 mm to achieve laser spot size of ~2–3 µm. An even smaller laser spot size of ~0.5–1 µm [28] can be achieved with transmission geometry as shown in Fig. 3c. In this setup, a much closer focal length can be achieved without interfering with the mass spectrometry ion

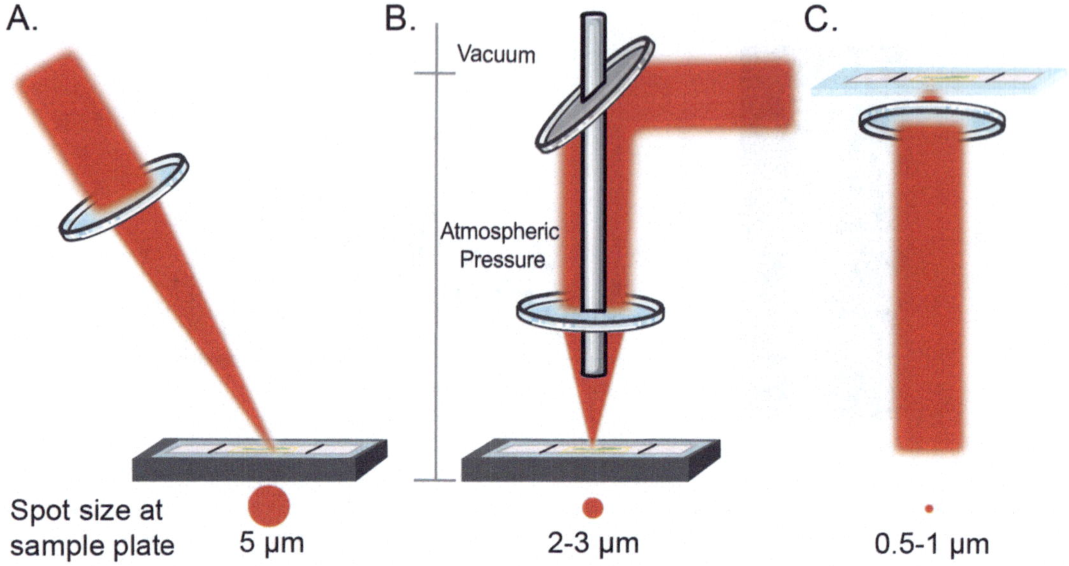

Fig. 3 Three major instrumentation setups developed to reduce the laser spot size: (**a**) a commercial MALDI-MS with a modified laser optics system to use a larger diameter beam at close distance to the sample, (**b**) atmospheric pressure MALDI to make a focus lens closer using a center-bored focus lens, and (**c**) transmission geometry without interfering ion optics

optics, since the laser beam is coming from the back of the transparent sample slide.

The Lee group improved the spatial resolution to 5–10 μm for a commercial MALDI-ion trap-Orbitrap [6, 21, 31] and has demonstrated the visualization of the distribution of a number of different metabolites in various plant tissues [21, 32–37]. A study by Korte et al. [6] revealed that molecular distributions of metabolites and lipids may be heterogeneous even among cells of the same tissue type (Fig. 4a). For example, 2,4-dihydroxy-7-methoxy-1,4-benzoxazin-3-one glucoside (DIMBOA-Glc) and 2-hydroxy-7-methoxy-1,4-benzoxazin-3-one glucoside (HMBOA-Glc) are known to be present in mesophyll cells of maize, but these compounds were not detected in all mesophyll cells but only between each pair of vascular bundles. In contrast, sulfoquinovosyl diacylglycerol (SQDG) 34:3 was found in all photosynthetic cells. Additionally, DIMBOA-Glc and HMBOA-Glc have almost no overlap with SQDG because of their different subcellular localization; i.e., DIMBOA-Glc and HMBOA-Glc are located in vacuole while SQDG in chloroplast. This platform was also applied to explore the quantitative fatty acyl distribution of thylakoid membrane lipids along the developmental gradient of maize leaves of four inbred lines of maize [33]. This study demonstrated that high-spatial resolution MALDI-MSI analysis can be directly applied to multicellular plant tissues to uncover cell-specific metabolic biology. For example, certain thylakoid membrane lipids (e.g., phosphatidylglycerol (PG) 32:0) displayed genotype-specific differences in cellular distribution. Inbred B73 showed preferential localization of PG 32:0 in bundle sheath cells, while a more uniform distribution between bundle sheath and mesophyll cells in inbred Mo17. Subcellular localization was also demonstrated in other studies. For example, Hansen et al. demonstrated that Arabidopside A (blue) is localized to the chloroplast as it is present only when pheophytin *a* (green, chlorophyll *a* without Mg^{2+}) is present, as illustrated in Fig. 4b [36].

Using atmospheric pressure scanning microprobe MALDI (AP-SMALDI) (Fig. 3b), the Spengler group visualized the subcellular localiza-

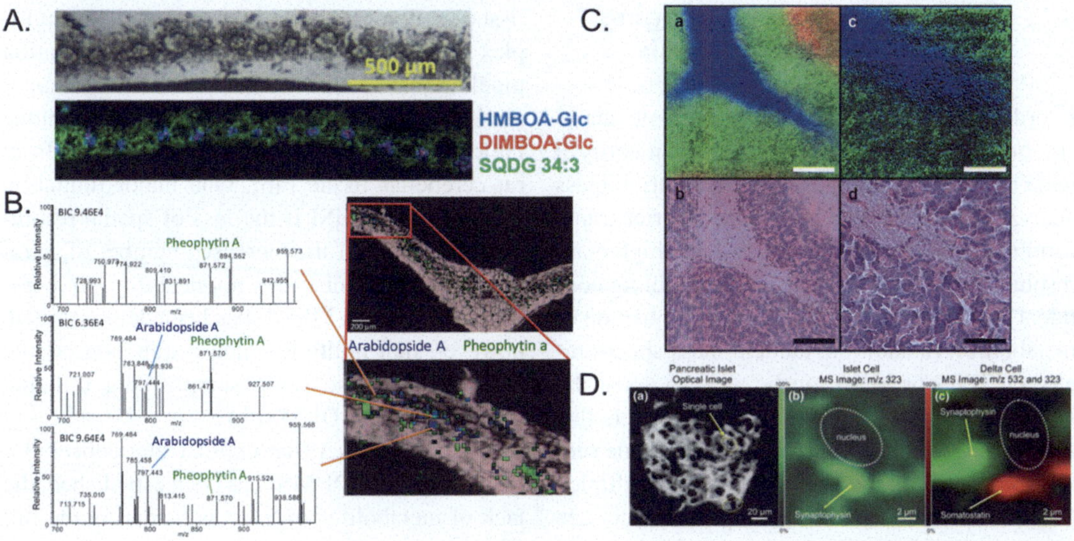

Fig. 4 (**a**) Optical (top) and selected MS images (bottom) of maize cross section obtained with 5 µm spatial resolution. Reproduced with permission of Springer Berlin Heidelberg [6]. (**b**) Five micron spatial resolution MSI of a non-wounded feronia mutant leaf cross section (right) and mass spectra of selected single pixels (left). Reproduced with permission of John Wiley and Sons Ltds [36]. (**c**) Cerebellar region of mouse brain obtained with (a) 2 µm and (c) 1 µm step size using AP-MALDI-MSI. (b,d) Optical image of the H&E stained tissue section after MSI measurement. $[PC(40:6) + K]^+$ (*m/z* 872.5570; red), $[PC(38:6) + K]^+$ (*m/z* 844.5254; green), and $[PC(36:1) + K]^+$ (*m/z* 826.5725; blue). Scale bars, 100 µm (a,b) or 50 µm (c, d). Reproduced with permission of Springer Nature [22]. (**d**) Double labelling by targeted IMS of synaptophysin (*m/z* 323) and somatostatin (*m/z* 532) in single cells. (a) Optical image of islet cells. (b) Targeted IMS of an immunoreactive islet cell for synaptophysin. (c) Targeted MSI of a delta cell for synaptophysin (green) and somatostatin (red), showing them located in different cellular structures. (Reproduced with permission of Springer-Verlag [41])

tion of lipids, metabolites, and peptides [22, 39]. This atmospheric pressure MSI platform enabled images with 1 or 2 µm spatial resolution of mouse cerebellum cross sections (Fig. 4c), allowing the visualization of phospholipids at subcellular level. Moreover, an autofocusing operation mode can be incorporated in the AP-SMALDI system to simultaneously obtain topographic and chemical information at subcellular resolution [40]. This system keeps the MALDI laser focus, fluence, and ablation spot size constant over sample height variety, thus providing high spatial resolution of <10 µm for nonplanar surfaces.

The Caprioli group [23, 24] has been developing high-spatial-resolution MSI down to 0.5–5 µm using both reflection (Fig. 3a) and transmission geometries (Fig. 3c). In transmission geometry, the laser beam can be irradiated from the back side of the sample to achieve molecular images down to 1 µm spatial resolution [41, 28]; this system is limited by the transparent substrate thickness. This platform was used for targeted imaging of human pancreatic islet at subcellular spatial resolution (Fig. 4d) for insulin, synaptophysin, and somatostatin in pancreatic islet cells. This demonstrated that targeted MSI in transmission geometry can be used to image a single mammalian cell.

A critical limitation of any "micro-probe" mode high-spatial-resolution MSI is the data acquisition time; acquiring MSI with smaller sampling size dramatically increases the data acquisition time. A next-generation high-speed MALDI imaging platform, Bruker rapifleX MALDI Tissuetyper™, uses Smartbeam™ 3D, which is capable of rapidly generating data by moving the laser and the stage independently [42]. This system also uses two rotating mirrors to rapidly scan a laser beam within a pixel to ensure homogeneous sampling. With 20–50 times faster speed, higher-spatial-resolution imaging is now practically possible for a large tissue area.

3 Mass Spectrometry Imaging for Metabolomic Analysis

In order to advance MSI for metabolomic analysis, one must detect and confidently identify a wide range of compounds. High-resolution mass analyzers, such as the Orbitrap or Fourier transform ion cyclotron resonance, provide high mass resolution and high mass accuracy enabling confident assignment of the chemical composition of metabolites. In addition, tandem mass spectrometry (MS/MS or MS^n) can be used to assist the identification of the metabolites; however, this typically needs to be done on separate tissue sections. To overcome this limitation, a "multiplex MSI method" has been developed by the Lee group to allow multiple data acquisition types to be incorporated in a single instrument run [43]. Using a hybrid linear ion trap-Orbitrap mass spectrometer, each raster step is split into several spiral steps, and each spiral step is assigned to a different scan type (high-resolution mass spectrometry (HRMS), MS/MS, etc.) [43]. The various scan types are then repeated at each raster step over the entire imaging area. This allows the collection of chemical composition from HRMS and structural information from MS/MS in a single MSI run. Polarity switching can also be incorporated in multiplex imaging to obtain both positive and negative ion mode data on a single tissue section [44]. Ellis et al. adopted this multiplex strategy for an automated lipid-identification pipeline, based on the ALEX[123] software framework [45], to identify and validate 104 unique molecular lipids and their spatial location from rat cerebellar tissue [46]. One major limitation with multiplex MSI is the loss of spatial resolution as a result of the increased number of spiral steps, which limits the applicability to high-spatial resolution MSI. It has been demonstrated, however, that multiplex data acquisition can be performed on the same sample spot utilizing overlapped MALDI-MSI [47].

Despite the fact that cellular and subcellular resolution MALDI-MSI has been established, the lack of metabolite coverage is hindering the full realization of this technique to visualize metabolites at the metabolomic scale. To overcome this limitation, Feenstra et al. proposed a MSI methodology that combines multiplex MSI data acquisition with multiple matrices on consecutive tissue sections [48]. In this proof-of-concept experiment, multiple matrices were used for consecutive tissue sections to increase the diversity of chemical compounds that could be visualized and a multiplex MSI method was used to improve the compound identification. With this approach, the visualization of many compounds is possible in a metabolic pathway, such as in the TCA cycle, as shown in Fig. 5a.

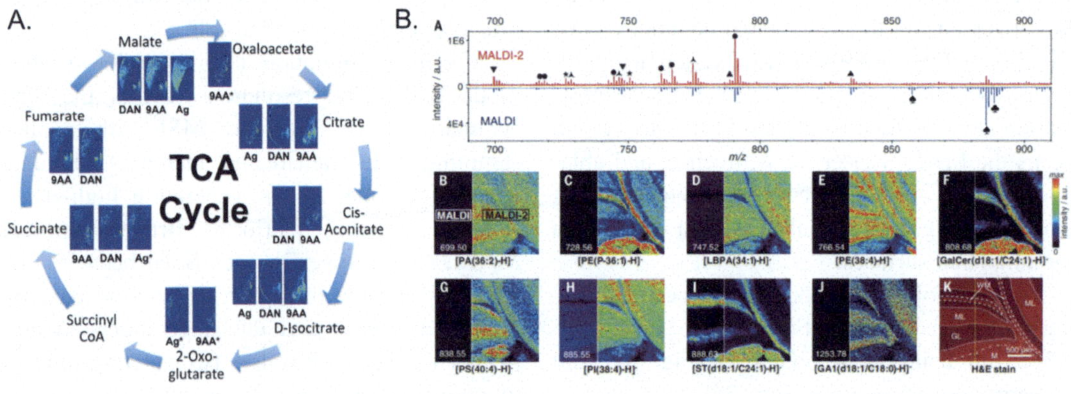

Fig. 5 (**a**) MS images of metabolites involved in TCA cycle in germinating maize seeds. Reproduced with permission of Royal Society of Chemistry [48]. (**b**) Mass spectra and MS images recorded from mouse cerebellum comparing MALDI vs MALDI-2. (Reproduced with permission of the American Association for the Advancement of Science [49])

Although this approach can eventually lead to untargeted metabolomics analysis, one critical limitation is the lack of sensitivity for some metabolites due to the inherent low ionization efficiency, especially when combined with a low number of analytes in a small sampling size. This limitation can be resolved by performing on-tissue chemical derivatization to selectively enhance targeted classes of metabolites. For example, as amphiprotic species, amino acids have variability in their protonation or deprotonation efficiency, depending on its *pKa* and local *pH*. On-tissue chemical derivatization has been developed to dramatically improve the sensitivity of amino acids and neurotransmitters using (i) coniferyl aldehyde [38], (ii) pyrylium salt [50], or (iii) *p*-*NNN*-trimethylammonioanilyl *N*-hydroxysuccinimidyl carbamate iodide [51]. As for other on-tissue chemical modifications, Girard's reagent T has been used to derivatize ketones and aldehydes [52, 53], and 2-picolylamine has been used for carboxyl acids [54]. We have recently proposed that multiple chemical reactions can be combined to enable the visualization of different classes of compounds in an untargeted manner [55]. Over six hundred new metabolite features could be detected by combining three derivatization reactions, dramatically improving metabolic coverage.

One drawback in MALDI-MSI is the fact that less than 1 out of 1000 desorbed molecules is on averaged ionized [56, 57]. To overcome this limitation, "MALDI-2" has been developed to enhance analyte signals for high-spatial-resolution MALDI-MSI (as shown in Fig. 5b). In this strategy, a second laser initiates an additional ionization process in the gas phase laser plume produced by the first MALDI process [49]. This allows for an increase in ion yields for numerous classes of compounds, by up to two orders of magnitude. Moreover, MALDI-2 can be combined with transmission geometry laser optics to compensate for the low number metabolites available in small sampling areas [58, 59].

4 Metabolite Identification and Localization

The advancements above have shown that metabolomic-scale MSI can add benefits of allowing differentiation of metabolites at a cellular and subcellular level. Currently, the identification of unknown compounds is a bottleneck that needs to be addressed in order to achieve metabolomic-scale MSI in a robust manner. Public MS/MS libraries, such as METLIN [60], have been broadly used to help identify metabolites or any other chemical entities. However, the number of molecules available in experimental MS/MS databases is limited and grows slowly due to the limited availability of authentic standards. To overcome this limitation, there has been a surge in software tool developments such as MetFrag, CSI:Finger ID, CFM-ID, iMet, ALEX^{123}, and MS-Finder that prove useful for confident metabolite identification [61–64]. Using these tools, one can search experimental MS/MS spectra against in silico MS/MS fragmentation databases with millions of chemical entries.

MetFrag can be used to obtain a candidate list, from compound libraries or from user defined structure data files, based on the precursor mass, subsequently ranked by the agreement between measured and in silico fragments [64, 65]. After in silico fragmentation, the candidate list gets filtered and scored on criteria such as reference information, retention time information, and occurrence of certain elements/substructures. iMet, a network-based computational tool, annotates metabolites for which there are no chemical structures available. This tool uses MS/MS spectra and the exact mass of an unknown metabolite to identify metabolites in a reference database that are structurally similar to the unknown metabolites [61]. CSI:FingerID predicts molecular fingerprints based on fragmentation tree trained with machine learning [66]. This fingerprint is then used to search chemical databases, such as PubChem or ChemSpider, and has shown to significantly improve the metabolite identification, according to the 2016 Critical Assessment of Small Molecule Identification (CASMI) competition [67].

CFM-ID is a web server that automatically identifies metabolites by annotating each peak in a MS/MS spectrum for a known chemical structure, predicting the spectra for a given chemical structure, and tentatively identifying the metabolite [62]. The algorithms used in CFM-ID are based on competitive fragmentation modeling, a probabilistic generative model for the MS/MS fragmentation process that uses machine learning techniques to learn its parameters from data. This model estimates the likelihood of any given fragmentation event occurring, thereby predicting those peaks that are most likely to be observed. This freely available web server provides a simple and interactive interface that graphically displays the resulting annotation. The $ALEX^{123}$ framework can be used for lipidomics data to automatically identify and quantify spectral data of lipid species [45]. A key advantage of $ALEX^{123}$ is the storage of lipidome data in a "database table format" which enables robust data processing and visualization. This framework features (1) a database with ionization and fragmentation information for lipid molecules, (2) script for harnessing MS^n (n = 1–3) information in raw mass spectral data files, and (3) auxiliary code for high confidence lipid identification, quantification, and dynamic lipidome visualization. The Global Natural Product Social Molecular Networking (GNPS) is another open-access web platform that can aid in metabolite identification [68]. The GNPS analysis infrastructure allows the fragmentation patterns of each MS/MS to be automatically compared and visualized in form of a network. The information of a known spectra can be used to predict the structure of unknowns by using differences in masses from the MS/MS.

Recent advancement to automate the image generation [69] and metabolite annotation [70] has allowed the MSI community to evaluate their data in greater depth and in less time. METASPACE is a web-based bioinformatics tool that allows for automated database-driven metabolite annotation by screening for metabolites with known sum formulas, an original metabolite-signal match (MSM) score combining spectral and spatial measures, and a target-decoy false discovery rate-estimation approach with a decoy set generated via the use of implausible adducts [70]. The MSM score uses the instrument's resolving power to quantify the likelihood of the presence of a metabolite in the sample by generating its isotopic pattern without MS/MS information.

As demonstrated above, a variety of tools are being used to help with metabolite identification for MSI. Due to the large and complex nature of MSI datasets, statistical methods and imaging software are needed for processing and visualization of mass spectra, statistical analysis, and segmentation and classification of the resulting images. MSiReader is an open source MSI software that allows for a semi-targeted discovery of molecular distributions of interest from MSI data, using an image similarity scoring algorithm to rank images by spatial correlation [71]. This tool enables identification of molecular distributions correlated to some features such as a known region of the sample or the distribution of some known compound such as a disease marker or a drug. Cardinal MSI is an R package that implements statistical tools for analyzing MSI datasets [72]. This open-source software can be used for processing and visualization of mass spectra and for statistical segmentation and classification of resulting images. Commercially available software tools, such as SCiLS Lab (SCiLS), IMAGEREVEAL (Shimadzu), and HDI (Waters), also allow statistical analysis for MSI.

5 Recent Applications

Single-cell resolution, metabolomic-scale MSI exhibits a great potential in the advancement of various scientific disciplines. Not only do these experiments provide a comprehensive picture about the cellular dynamic and its phenotypic fingerprint, but also reveal crucial information about individual cells in a tissue sample that are often unattainable by traditional metabolomics experiments. Here, we summarize some recent applications of cellular and subcellular level tissue MSI in biological, pharmaceutical, and medical sciences.

High-spatial resolution MALDI-MSI was performed on mouse and human pancreatic tissues to study phospholipid and glycolipid distributions in pancreatic islets [73]. In this work, immunofluorescent images were used to accurately co-register and verify islet location, enabling the acquisition of MSI data from selected subregions rather than of the entire tissue section. This demonstrated the importance of both spatial resolution and specificity when it comes to performing molecular measurements of complex heterogeneous tissues. More on this regard, a histology-directed platform used autofluorescence microscopy and MSI data to improve the registration and alignment process [74]. An autofluorescence image was acquired prior to the MSI run in order to align with the microscope image. Then, another autofluorescence image was obtained post MSI to align the matrix burn mark with the corresponding MS spectra. This is advantageous in cellular and subcellular imaging due to the fact that having a microscopy grade view of the tissue structure will be an important aid in localizing the metabolites of interest.

Three-dimensional (3D) MALDI-MSI has also been used to visualize metabolites and lipids at the cellular level in cell cultures [75, 76] and zebrafish embryos [77]. This application can be used in clinical settings to help solve problems, such as understanding how drugs are distributed within the tissue and finding where set metabolites are located. For example, drug penetration into solid tumors is critical for the effectiveness of chemotherapy and cancer chemotherapeutics often fail to reach all diseased cells [78]. To solve this problem, 3D cell cultures can be used as a model system to assess the distribution of anticancer drugs. In a study by the Hummon group, a time-dependent penetration of irinotecan was visualized by tracking the parent drug, as well as some metabolites [75]. This proof-of-principle study demonstrated that spheroids can be used in MALDI-MSI to screen and select drugs in a format that more closely resembles conditions in patients. In another study, MALDI-MSI was applied, for the first time, for 3D chemical imaging of a single cell using newly fertilized individual zebrafish embryos as a model system. MSI was used to map and visualize the 3D spatial distribution of certain lipids, revealing heterogeneous localization of different classes of lipids in the embryo [77].

MALDI-MSI can also enable the exploration of cellular molecular signatures required for many pathology applications [79]. Multivariate data analysis method can be applied to MS imaging data for the automated annotation of tissues. Furthermore, MSI integrates the histology of the sample which allows studying the molecular information in a histopathological context [80]. In a study by the Heeren laboratory, a pixel-wise analysis of MALDI-MSI was used to distinguish between steatotic and nonsteatotic tissue, specifically to study nonalcoholic fatty liver disease. Using this method, they were able to detect subtle changes between the groups and concluded that lipid composition of steatotic and nonsteatotic tissue is highly distinct, implying that spatial context is important for understanding the mechanisms of lipid accumulation in diseases [81].

6 Conclusion and Outlook

High-spatial-resolution MALDI-MSI at the single-cell resolution is essential for detecting chemical signatures of phenotypic heterogeneity at the cellular and subcellular level. Recent advancements in overall analytical workflow and instrumentation have allowed MALDI-MSI to become a unique tool towards cellular or subcellular level imaging at the metabolomic scale. The convergence of spatial resolution at the micrometer scale, the improved sensitivity, and the surge of computational tools available provide exciting new possibilities towards metabolomic-scale imaging at a subcellular level. New insights can be gained about the behavior of individual cells, which can be applied to fields of biology, medicine, and pharmaceutics.

As a technique that is under continuous development, the MSI community still needs to overcome many challenges. These are mainly connected with problems such as management and interpretation of big data, the sensitivity of measurements, reliable methodology for statistical analysis, automated data interpretation, and integration of molecular information provided by MSI with other imaging modalities. The acquired data obtained from MSI are complex and contain features belonging to both known and unknown metabolites. Improvements in software and databases are essential to identify metabolites with high confidence in order to draw biological conclusions. Moreover, advances in quantification methods are essential to differentiate between results that are skewed by matrix effects or ionization efficiency of analytes.

MALDI-MSI coupled with ion mobility separation (IMS) has demonstrated significant utility over the past decade for separation of isobaric species in the gas phase. IMS, a gas phase separation method based on collisional cross-section differences between ions, allows for the molecules to be separated based on charge, size, and shape [82]. MALDI-IMS has not been demonstrated for high-spatial resolution MS imaging yet, but the future of this technique looks promising, especially as multiple commercial instruments have become available. This type of instrument platform will improve separation and identification of metabolites, making it a particularly useful tool in the field for structure determination.

There is still a long way to go before MSI can be implemented in routine metabolomic analysis. Continuous efforts in MSI-based single-cell metabolomics are moving the field towards higher sensitivity, higher throughput, higher reproducibility, and better quantification. Once all of these obstacles are addressed, MSI will revolutionize our understanding of how cells function by revealing unprecedented details of cellular metabolism.

References

1. Gilmore, I. S., Heiles, S., & Pieterse, C. L. (2019). Metabolic imaging at the single-cell scale: Recent advances in mass spectrometry imaging. *Annual Review of Analytical Chemistry, 12*, 201–224.
2. Johnson, R. W., & Talaty, N. (2019). Tissue imaging by mass spectrometry: A practical guide for the medicinal chemist. *ACS Medicinal Chemistry Letters, 10*, 161–167.
3. Fujii, T., Matsuda, S., Tejedor, M. L., Esaki, T., Sakane, I., Mizuno, H., Tsuyama, N., & Masujima, T. (2015). Direct metabolomics for plant cells by live single-cell mass spectrometry. *Nature Protocols, 10*, 1445–1456.
4. Svatoš, A. (2011). Single-cell metabolomics comes of age: New developments in mass spectrometry profiling and imaging. *Analytical Chemistry, 83*, 5037–5044.
5. Zenobi, R. (2013). Single-cell metabolomics: Analytical and biological perspectives. *Science, 342*, 1201.
6. Korte, A., Yandeau-Nelson, M., Nikolau, B., & Lee, Y. (2015a). Subcellular-level resolution MALDI-MS imaging of maize leaf metabolites by MALDI-linear ion trap-Orbitrap mass spectrometer. *Analytical and Bioanalytical Chemistry, 407*, 2301–2309.
7. Lee, Y. J., Perdian, D. C., Song, Z., Yeung, E. S., & Nikolau, B. J. (2012). Use of mass spectrometry for imaging metabolites in plants. *The Plant Journal, 70*, 81–95.
8. Stoeckli, M., Chaurand, P., Hallahan, D. E., & Caprioli, R. M. (2001). Imaging mass spectrometry: A new technology for the analysis of protein expression in mammalian tissues. *Nature Medicine, 7*, 493–496.
9. Cobice, D. F., Goodwin, R. J. A., Andren, P. E., Nilsson, A., Mackay, C. L., & Andrew, R. (2015). Future technology insight: Mass spectrometry imaging as a tool in drug research and development. *British Journal of Pharmacology, 172*, 3266–3283.
10. Nilsson, A., Goodwin, R. J. A., Shariatgorji, M., Vallianatou, T., Webborn, P. J. H., & Andren, P. E. (2015). Mass spectrometry imaging in drug development. *Analytical Chemistry, 87*, 1437–1455.
11. Schwamborn, K., Kriegsmann, M., & Weichert, W. (2017). MALDI imaging mass spectrometry — From bench to bedside. *Biochimica et Biophysica Acta (BBA) – Proteins and Proteomics, 1865*, 776–783.
12. Zhang, A., Sun, H., Wang, P., Han, Y., & Wang, X. (2012). Modern analytical techniques in metabolomics analysis. *Analyst, 137*, 293–300.
13. Baker, T. C., Han, J., & Borchers, C. H. (2017). Recent advancements in matrix-assisted laser desorption/ionization mass spectrometry imaging. *Current Opinion in Biotechnology, 43*, 62–69.
14. Agüi-Gonzalez, P., Jähne, S., & Phan, N. T. N. (2019). SIMS imaging in neurobiology and cell biology. *Journal of Analytical Atomic Spectrometry, 34*, 1355–1368.
15. Nemes, P., & Vertes, A. (2007). Laser ablation electrospray ionization for atmospheric pressure, in vivo, and imaging mass spectrometry. *Analytical Chemistry, 79*, 8098–8106.
16. Swales, J. G., Tucker, J. W., Spreadborough, M. J., Iverson, S. L., Clench, M. R., Webborn, P. J. H., & Goodwin, R. J. A. (2015). Mapping drug distribution in brain tissue using liquid extraction surface analy-

sis mass spectrometry imaging. *Analytical Chemistry, 87*, 10146–10152.

17. Parrot, D., Papazian, S., Foil, D., & Tasdemir, D. (2018). Imaging the unimaginable: Desorption electrospray ionization – Imaging mass spectrometry (DESI-IMS) in natural product research. *Planta Medica, 84*, 584–593.
18. Nguyen, S. N., Liyu, A. V., Chu, R. K., Anderton, C. R., & Laskin, J. (2017). Constant-distance mode Nanospray desorption electrospray ionization mass spectrometry imaging of biological samples with complex topography. *Analytical Chemistry, 89*, 1131–1137.
19. Nguyen, S. N., Sontag, R. L., Carson, J. P., Corley, R. A., Ansong, C., & Laskin, J. (2018). Towards high-resolution tissue imaging using Nanospray desorption electrospray ionization mass spectrometry coupled to shear force microscopy. *Journal of the American Society for Mass Spectrometry, 29*, 316–322.
20. Lamont, L., Baumert, M., Ogrinc Potočnik, N., Allen, M., Vreeken, R., Heeren, R. M. A., & Porta, T. (2017). Integration of ion mobility MSE after fully automated, online, high-resolution liquid extraction surface analysis micro-liquid chromatography. *Analytical Chemistry, 89*, 11143–11150.
21. Feenstra, A. D., Dueñas, M. E., & Lee, Y. J. (2017b). Five Micron high resolution MALDI mass spectrometry imaging with simple, interchangeable, multi-resolution optical system. *Journal of the American Society for Mass Spectrometry, 28*, 434–442.
22. Kompauer, M., Heiles, S., & Spengler, B. (2016). Atmospheric pressure MALDI mass spectrometry imaging of tissues and cells at 1.4-μm lateral resolution. *Nature Methods, 14*, 90.
23. Zavalin, A., Yang, J., & Caprioli, R. (2013). Laser beam filtration for high spatial resolution MALDI imaging mass spectrometry. *Journal of the American Society for Mass Spectrometry, 24*, 1153–1156.
24. Zavalin, A., Yang, J., Haase, A., Holle, A., & Caprioli, R. (2014). Implementation of a Gaussian beam laser and aspheric optics for high spatial resolution MALDI imaging MS. *Journal of the American Society for Mass Spectrometry, 25*, 1079–1082.
25. Jun, J. H., Song, Z., Liu, Z., Nikolau, B. J., Yeung, E. S., & Lee, Y. J. (2010). High-spatial and high-mass resolution imaging of surface metabolites of Arabidopsis thaliana by laser desorption-ionization mass spectrometry using colloidal silver. *Analytical Chemistry, 82*, 3255–3265.
26. Caprioli, R. M., Farmer, T. B., & Gile, J. (1997). Molecular imaging of biological samples: Localization of peptides and proteins using MALDI-TOF MS. *Analytical Chemistry, 69*, 4751–4760.
27. Spengler, B., & Hubert, M. (2002). Scanning microprobe matrix-assisted laser desorption ionization (SMALDI) mass spectrometry: Instrumentation for sub-micrometer resolved LDI and MALDI surface analysis. *Journal of the American Society for Mass Spectrometry, 13*, 735–748.
28. Zavalin, A., Todd, E. M., Rawhouser, P. D., Yang, J., Norris, J. L., & Caprioli, R. M. (2012). Direct imaging of single cells and tissue at subcellular spatial resolution using transmission geometry MALDI MS. *Journal of Mass Spectrometry : JMS, 47*. i–i.
29. Holle, A., Haase, A., Kayser, M., & Höhndorf, J. (2006). Optimizing UV laser focus profiles for improved MALDI performance. *Journal of Mass Spectrometry, 41*, 705–716.
30. Luxembourg, S. L., Mize, T. H., McDonnell, L. A., & Heeren, R. M. A. (2004). High-spatial resolution mass spectrometric imaging of peptide and protein distributions on a surface. *Analytical Chemistry, 76*, 5339–5344.
31. Korte, A. R., Yagnik, G. B., Feenstra, A. D., & Lee, Y. J. (2015b). Multiplex MALDI-MS imaging of plant metabolites using a hybrid MS system. In L. He (Ed.), *Mass spectrometry imaging of small molecules* (pp. 46–62). New York: Springer.
32. Dueñas, M. E., Feenstra, A. D., Korte, A. R., Hinners, P., & Lee, Y. J. (2018). Cellular and subcellular level localization of maize lipids and metabolites using high-spatial resolution MALDI mass spectrometry imaging. In L. M. Lagrimini (Ed.), *Maize: Methods and protocols* (pp. 217–231). New York: Springer New York.
33. Dueñas, M. E., Klein, A. T., Alexander, L. E., Yandeau-Nelson, M. D., Nikolau, B. J., & Lee, Y. J. (2017b). High-spatial resolution mass spectrometry imaging reveals the genetically programmed, developmental modification of the distribution of thylakoid membrane lipids among individual cells of the maize leaf. *The Plant Journal, 89*, 825–838.
34. Feenstra, A. D., Alexander, L. E., Song, Z., Korte, A. R., Yandeau-Nelson, M., Nikolau, B. J., & Lee, Y.-J. (2017a). Spatial mapping and profiling of metabolite distributions during germination. *Plant Physiology, 174*, 2532–2548.
35. Hansen, R. L., Dueñas, M. E., & Lee, Y. J. (2018a). Sputter-coated metal screening for small molecule analysis and high-spatial resolution imaging in laser desorption ionization mass spectrometry. *Journal of the American Society for Mass Spectrometry, 30*, 299–308.
36. Hansen, R. L., Guo, H., Yin, Y., & Lee, Y. J. (2018b). FERONIA mutation induces high levels of chloroplast-localized Arabidopsides which are involved in root growth. *The Plant Journal, 97*, 341–351.
37. Klein, A. T., Yagnik, G. B., Hohenstein, J. D., Ji, Z., Zi, J., Reichert, M. D., MacIntosh, G. C., Yang, B., Peters, R. J., Vela, J., & Lee, Y. J. (2015). Investigation of the chemical Interface in the soybean–aphid and Rice–bacteria interactions using MALDI-mass spectrometry imaging. *Analytical Chemistry, 87*, 5294–5301.
38. Manier, M. L., Spraggins, J. M., Reyzer, M. L., Norris, J. L., & Caprioli, R. M. (2014). A derivatization and validation strategy for determining the spatial localization of endogenous amine metabolites in tissues using MALDI imaging mass spectrometry. *Journal of Mass Spectrometry, 49*, 665–673.
39. Khalil, S. M., Pretzel, J., Becker, K., & Spengler, B. (2017). High-resolution AP-SMALDI mass

spectrometry imaging of Drosophila melanogaster. *International Journal of Mass Spectrometry, 416*, 1–19.
40. Kompauer, M., Heiles, S., & Spengler, B. (2017). Autofocusing MALDI mass spectrometry imaging of tissue sections and 3D chemical topography of nonflat surfaces. *Nature Methods, 14*, 1156.
41. Thiery-Lavenant, G., Zavalin, A. I., & Caprioli, R. M. (2013). Targeted multiplex imaging mass spectrometry in transmission geometry for subcellular spatial resolution. *Journal of the American Society for Mass Spectrometry, 24*, 609–614.
42. Ogrinc Potočnik, N., Porta, T., Becker, M., Heeren, R. M. A., & Ellis, S. R. (2015). Use of advantageous, volatile matrices enabled by next-generation high-speed matrix-assisted laser desorption/ionization time-of-flight imaging employing a scanning laser beam. *Rapid Communications in Mass Spectrometry, 29*, 2195–2203.
43. Perdian, D. C., & Lee, Y. J. (2010). Imaging MS methodology for more chemical information in less data acquisition time utilizing a hybrid linear ion trap–Orbitrap mass spectrometer. *Analytical Chemistry, 82*, 9393–9400.
44. Korte, A., & Lee, Y. (2013). Multiplex mass spectrometric imaging with polarity switching for concurrent Acquisition of Positive and Negative ion Images. *Journal of the American Society for Mass Spectrometry, 24*, 949–955.
45. Husen, P., Tarasov, K., Katafiasz, M., Sokol, E., Vogt, J., Baumgart, J., Nitsch, R., Ekroos, K., & Ejsing, C. S. (2013). Analysis of lipid experiments (ALEX): A software framework for analysis of high-resolution shotgun Lipidomics data. *PLoS One, 8*, e79736.
46. Ellis, S. R., Paine, M. R. L., Eijkel, G. B., Pauling, J. K., Husen, P., Jervelund, M. W., Hermansson, M., Ejsing, C. S., & Heeren, R. M. A. (2018). Automated, parallel mass spectrometry imaging and structural identification of lipids. *Nature Methods, 15*, 515–518.
47. Hansen, R. L., & Lee, Y. J. (2017). Overlapping MALDI-mass spectrometry imaging for in-parallel MS and MS/MS data acquisition without sacrificing spatial resolution. *Journal of the American Society for Mass Spectrometry, 28*, 1910–1918.
48. Feenstra, A. D., Hansen, R. L., & Lee, Y. J. (2015). Multi-matrix, dual polarity, tandem mass spectrometry imaging strategy applied to a germinated maize seed: Toward mass spectrometry imaging of an untargeted metabolome. *Analyst, 140*, 7293–7304.
49. Soltwisch, J., Kettling, H., Vens-Cappell, S., Wiegelmann, M., Müthing, J., & Dreisewerd, K. (2015). Mass spectrometry imaging with laser-induced postionization. *Science, 348*, 211.
50. Shariatgorji, M., Nilsson, A., Källback, P., Karlsson, O., Zhang, X., Svenningsson, P., & Andren, P. E. (2015). Pyrylium salts as reactive matrices for MALDI-MS imaging of biologically active primary amines. *Journal of the American Society for Mass Spectrometry, 26*, 934–939.
51. Toue, S., Sugiura, Y., Kubo, A., Ohmura, M., Karakawa, S., Mizukoshi, T., Yoneda, J., Miyano, H., Noguchi, Y., Kobayashi, T., Kabe, Y., & Suematsu, M. (2014). Microscopic imaging mass spectrometry assisted by on- tissue chemical derivatization for visualizing multiple amino acids in human colon cancer xenografts. *Proteomics, 14*, 810–819.
52. Barré, F. P. Y., Flinders, B., Garcia, J. P., Jansen, I., Huizing, L. R. S., Porta, T., Creemers, L. B., Heeren, R. M. A., & Cillero-Pastor, B. (2016). Derivatization strategies for the detection of triamcinolone Acetonide in cartilage by using matrix-assisted laser desorption/ionization mass spectrometry imaging. *Analytical Chemistry, 88*, 12051–12059.
53. Shimma, S., Kumada, H.-O., Taniguchi, H., Konno, A., Yao, I., Furuta, K., Matsuda, T., & Ito, S. (2016). Microscopic visualization of testosterone in mouse testis by use of imaging mass spectrometry. *Analytical and Bioanalytical Chemistry, 408*, 7607–7615.
54. Wu, Q., Comi, T. J., Li, B., Rubakhin, S. S., & Sweedler, J. V. (2016). On-tissue Derivatization via electrospray deposition for matrix-assisted laser desorption/ionization mass spectrometry imaging of endogenous fatty acids in rat brain tissues. *Analytical Chemistry, 88*, 5988–5995.
55. Dueñas, M. E., Larson, E., & Lee, Y. J. (2019). Towards mass spectrometry imaging in the metabolomics scale: Increasing metabolic coverage through multiple on-tissue chemical modifications. *Frontiers in Plant Science, 10*, 860.
56. Dreisewerd, K., Schürenberg, M., Karas, M., & Hillenkamp, F. (1995). Influence of the laser intensity and spot size on the desorption of molecules and ions in matrix-assisted laser desorption/ionization with a uniform beam profile. *International Journal of Mass Spectrometry and Ion Processes, 141*, 127–148.
57. Knochenmuss, R., & Zhigilei, L. V. (2012). What determines MALDI ion yields? A molecular dynamics study of ion loss mechanisms. *Analytical and Bioanalytical Chemistry, 402*, 2511–2519.
58. Niehaus, M., Soltwisch, J., Below, M., & Dreisewerd, K. (2019). Transmission-mode MALDI-2 mass spectrometry imaging of cells and tissues at subcellular resolution. *Nature Methods, 16*, 925–931.
59. Spivey, E. C., McMillen, J. C., Ryan, D. J., Spraggins, J. M., & Caprioli, R. M. (2019). Combining MALDI-2 and transmission geometry laser optics to achieve high sensitivity for ultra-high spatial resolution surface analysis. *Journal of Mass Spectrometry, 54*, 366–370.
60. Guijas, C., Montenegro-Burke, J. R., Domingo-Almenara, X., Palermo, A., Warth, B., Hermann, G., Koellensperger, G., Huan, T., Uritboonthai, W., Aisporna, A. E., Wolan, D. W., Spilker, M. E., Benton, H. P., & Siuzdak, G. (2018). METLIN: A technology platform for identifying Knowns and unknowns. *Analytical Chemistry, 90*, 3156–3164.
61. Aguilar-Mogas, A., Sales-Pardo, M., Navarro, M., Guimerà, R., & Yanes, O. (2017). iMet: A network-based computational tool to assist in the annotation

of metabolites from tandem mass spectra. *Analytical Chemistry, 89*, 3474–3482.
62. Allen, F., Pon, A., Wilson, M., Greiner, R., & Wishart, D. (2014). CFM-ID: A web server for annotation, spectrum prediction and metabolite identification from tandem mass spectra. *Nucleic Acids Research, 42*, W94–W99.
63. Tsugawa, H., Kind, T., Nakabayashi, R., Yukihira, D., Tanaka, W., Cajka, T., Saito, K., Fiehn, O., & Arita, M. (2016). Hydrogen rearrangement rules: Computational MS/MS fragmentation and structure elucidation using MS-FINDER software. *Analytical Chemistry, 88*, 7946–7958.
64. Wolf, S., Schmidt, S., Müller-Hannemann, M., & Neumann, S. (2010). In silico fragmentation for computer assisted identification of metabolite mass spectra. *BMC Bioinformatics, 11*, 148–148.
65. Ruttkies, C., Schymanski, E. L., Wolf, S., Hollender, J., & Neumann, S. (2016). MetFrag relaunched: Incorporating strategies beyond in silico fragmentation. *Journal of Cheminformatics, 8*, 3.
66. Dührkop, K., Shen, H., Meusel, M., Rousu, J., & Böcker, S. (2015). Searching molecular structure databases with tandem mass spectra using CSI:FingerID. *Proceedings of the National Academy of Sciences, 112*, 12580.
67. Schymanski, E. L., Ruttkies, C., Krauss, M., Brouard, C., Kind, T., Dührkop, K., Allen, F., Vaniya, A., Verdegem, D., Böcker, S., Rousu, J., Shen, H., Tsugawa, H., Sajed, T., Fiehn, O., Ghesquière, B., & Neumann, S. (2017). Critical assessment of small molecule identification 2016: Automated methods. *Journal of Cheminformatics, 9*, 22.
68. Wang, M., Carver, J. J., Phelan, V. V., Sanchez, L. M., Garg, N., Peng, Y., Nguyen, D. D., Watrous, J., Kapono, C. A., Luzzatto-Knaan, T., Porto, C., Bouslimani, A., Melnik, A. V., Meehan, M. J., Liu, W.-T., Crüsemann, M., Boudreau, P. D., Esquenazi, E., Sandoval-Calderón, M., Kersten, R. D., Pace, L. A., Quinn, R. A., Duncan, K. R., Hsu, C.-C., Floros, D. J., Gavilan, R. G., Kleigrewe, K., Northen, T., Dutton, R. J., Parrot, D., Carlson, E. E., Aigle, B., Michelsen, C. F., Jelsbak, L., Sohlenkamp, C., Pevzner, P., Edlund, A., McLean, J., Piel, J., Murphy, B. T., Gerwick, L., Liaw, C.-C., Yang, Y.-L., Humpf, H.-U., Maansson, M., Keyzers, R. A., Sims, A. C., Johnson, A. R., Sidebottom, A. M., Sedio, B. E., Klitgaard, A., Larson, C. B., Boya, C. A., Torres-Mendoza, D., Gonzalez, D. J., Silva, D. B., Marques, L. M., Demarque, D. P., Pociute, E., O'Neill, E. C., Briand, E., Helfrich, E. J. N., Granatosky, E. A., Glukhov, E., Ryffel, F., Houson, H., Mohimani, H., Kharbush, J. J., Zeng, Y., Vorholt, J. A., Kurita, K. L., Charusanti, P., McPhail, K. L., Nielsen, K. F., Vuong, L., Elfeki, M., Traxler, M. F., Engene, N., Koyama, N., Vining, O. B., Baric, R., Silva, R. R., Mascuch, S. J., Tomasi, S., Jenkins, S., Macherla, V., Hoffman, T., Agarwal, V., Williams, P. G., Dai, J., Neupane, R., Gurr, J., Rodríguez, A. M. C., Lamsa, A., Zhang, C., Dorrestein, K., Duggan, B. M., Almaliti, J., Allard, P.-M., Phapale, P., Nothias, L.-F., Alexandrov, T., Litaudon, M., Wolfender, J.-L., Kyle, J. E., Metz, T. O., Peryea, T., Nguyen, D.-T., VanLeer, D., Shinn, P., Jadhav, A., Müller, R., Waters, K. M., Shi, W., Liu, X., Zhang, L., Knight, R., Jensen, P. R., Palsson, B. Ø., Pogliano, K., Linington, R. G., Gutiérrez, M., Lopes, N. P., Gerwick, W. H., Moore, B. S., Dorrestein, P. C., & Bandeira, N. (2016). Sharing and community curation of mass spectrometry data with global natural products social molecular networking. *Nature Biotechnology, 34*, 828.
69. Bokhart, M. T., Nazari, M., Garrard, K. P., & Muddiman, D. C. (2018). MSiReader v1.0: Evolving open-source mass spectrometry imaging software for targeted and untargeted analyses. *Journal of the American Society for Mass Spectrometry, 29*, 8–16.
70. Palmer, A., Phapale, P., Chernyavsky, I., Lavigne, R., Fay, D., Tarasov, A., Kovalev, V., Fuchser, J., Nikolenko, S., Pineau, C., Becker, M., & Alexandrov, T. (2017). FDR-controlled metabolite annotation for high-resolution imaging mass spectrometry. *Nature Methods, 14*, 57–60.
71. Ekelöf, M., Garrard, K. P., Judd, R., Rosen, E. P., Xie, D.-Y., Kashuba, A. D. M., & Muddiman, D. C. (2018). Evaluation of digital image recognition methods for mass spectrometry imaging data analysis. *Journal of the American Society for Mass Spectrometry, 29*, 2467–2470.
72. Bemis, K. D., Harry, A., Eberlin, L. S., Ferreira, C., van de Ven, S. M., Mallick, P., Stolowitz, M., & Vitek, O. (2015). Cardinal: An R package for statistical analysis of mass spectrometry-based imaging experiments. *Bioinformatics, 31*, 2418–2420.
73. Prentice, B. M., Hart, N. J., Phillips, N., Haliyur, R., Judd, A., Armandala, R., Spraggins, J. M., Lowe, C. L., Boyd, K. L., Stein, R. W., Wright, C. V., Norris, J. L., Powers, A. C., Brissova, M., & Caprioli, R. M. (2019). Imaging mass spectrometry enables molecular profiling of mouse and human pancreatic tissue. *Diabetologia, 62*, 1036–1047.
74. Patterson, N. H., Tuck, M., Lewis, A., Kaushansky, A., Norris, J. L., Van de Plas, R., & Caprioli, R. M. (2018). Next generation histology-directed imaging mass spectrometry driven by autofluorescence microscopy. *Analytical Chemistry, 90*, 12404–12413.
75. Liu, X., Weaver, E. M., & Hummon, A. B. (2013). Evaluation of therapeutics in three-dimensional cell culture systems by MALDI imaging mass spectrometry. *Analytical Chemistry, 85*, 6295–6302.
76. Lukowski, J. K., Weaver, E. M., & Hummon, A. B. (2017). Analyzing liposomal drug delivery Systems in Three-Dimensional Cell Culture Models Using MALDI imaging mass spectrometry. *Analytical Chemistry, 89*, 8453–8458.
77. Dueñas, M. E., Essner, J. J., & Lee, Y. J. (2017a). 3D MALDI mass spectrometry imaging of a single cell: Spatial mapping of lipids in the embryonic development of Zebrafish. *Scientific Reports, 7*, 14946.
78. Weaver, E. M., & Hummon, A. B. (2013). Imaging mass spectrometry: From tissue sections to cell

cultures. *Advanced Drug Delivery Reviews, 65*, 1039–1055.

79. Barré, F., Rocha, B., Dewez, F., Towers, M., Murray, P., Claude, E., Cillero-Pastor, B., Heeren, R., & Porta Siegel, T. (2019). Faster raster matrix-assisted laser desorption/ionization mass spectrometry imaging of lipids at high lateral resolution. *International Journal of Mass Spectrometry, 437*, 38–48.
80. Balluff, B., Hanselmann, M., Heeren, R. M. A., Drake, R. R., & McDonnell, L. A. (2017). Chapter Eight – Mass spectrometry imaging for the investigation of intratumor heterogeneity. In *Advances in cancer research* (pp. 201–230). New York: Academic Press.
81. Ščupáková, K., Soons, Z., Ertaylan, G., Pierzchalski, K. A., Eijkel, G. B., Ellis, S. R., Greve, J. W., Driessen, A., Verheij, J., De Kok, T. M., Olde Damink, S. W. M., Rensen, S. S., & Heeren, R. M. A. (2018). Spatial systems Lipidomics reveals nonalcoholic fatty liver disease heterogeneity. *Analytical Chemistry, 90*, 5130–5138.
82. Harvey, S. R., MacPhee, C. E., & Barran, P. E. (2011). Ion mobility mass spectrometry for peptide analysis. *Methods, 54*, 454–461.

Detection of N^6-Methyladenine in Eukaryotes

Baodong Liu and Hailin Wang

1 Introduction

Four bases, adenine, cytosine, guanine, and thymine, constitute the heritable life blueprint. DNA methylation, as part of precision gene expression regulator, usually takes place at the C5 position of cytosine (5mC), N^4 position of cytosine (4mC), and N^6 position of adenine (6mA). In 1973, Gorovsky et al. found 6mA in nuclear DNA of *Tetrahymena pyriformis* using radioactive ^3H labeling technology combined with paper chromatography [1]. In 1981, Pratt et al. detected 6mA in *Tetrahymena pyriformis* by high-performance liquid chromatography with ultraviolet detection (HPLC-UV) and showed that 6mA was rich, but not randomly present in its large nuclear DNA, and further distributed at linker DNA [2]. Based on the restriction endonuclease *Dpn*I recognizing hypermethylated G(6mA)TC site, Harrison et al. confirmed GATC-specific methylation sites at the nuclear DNA of *Tetrahymena pyriformis* [3]. In addition, capillary electrophoresis laser-induced fluorescence (CE-LIF) was also used for 6mA detection [4, 5]. These early 6mA assays have the disadvantages of low detection sensitivity (detection limits of 0.01–0.1% 6mA/dA) and cannot provide structural information for identification of 6mA.

Current 6mA detection methods mainly include UHPLC-MS/MS, 6mA-antibody based assay, and DNA sequencing analysis. In 2015, using the ultrasensitive UHPLC-MS/MS method, we detected 6mA (0.001% ~ 0.07%) in the genome of the model organism *Drosophila* [6]. In order to verify our findings, qualitative examination of "6mA" from fly was performed with 6mA antibody-based assay and HPLC with high-resolution time-of-flight mass spectrometry (TOF MS). The "6mA" from fly and 6mA standard had exact mass of precursor ion, as well as 17 main daughter ions (fragments), and the maximum deviation was less than 4.0 ppm. In addition, the whole 6mA level in genome was analyzed by UHPLC-MS/MS in many species, such as 0.01–0.4% 6mA/dA in *Caenorhabditis elegans* [7], 0.0001–0.0005% in mouse embryonic stem cells [8], 0.00009% 6mA/dA in *Xenopus laevis* [9], and ~ 0.4% in *Chlamydomonas* [10].

6mA antibody-based assays include dot blot, immunofluorescence imaging (IF), enzyme-linked immunosorbent assay (ELISA), and immunoprecipitation (IP). Dot blotting of 6mA [6–9, 11] is a qualitative and semiquantitative method and measures a relative level of 6mA in genomic DNA in vitro. As a visual and in situ 6mA analysis method, IF was performed to show

B. Liu · H. Wang (✉)
State Key Laboratory of Environmental Chemistry and Ecotoxicology, Research Center for Eco-Environmental Sciences, Chinese Academy of Sciences, Beijing, China

University of Chinese Academy of Sciences, Beijing, China
e-mail: hlwang@rcees.ac.cn

S. Hu (ed.), *Cancer Metabolomics*, Advances in Experimental Medicine and Biology 1280,
https://doi.org/10.1007/978-3-030-51652-9_6

6mA dynamic change in early embryonic development of *Drosophila*, *C. elegans*, and zebrafish [6, 7, 11, 12]. ELISA was used to detect 6mA in the genomes of *Mnemiopsis leidyi*, *Beroe abyssicola*, and *Pleurobrachia*, and the abundance of 6mA was 0.02%, 0.01%, and 0.025%, respectively [13]. In addition, immunoprecipitation is an important approach to enrich the DNA fragments containing 6mA, especially for DNA with low 6mA abundance. Then the enriched 6mA containing fragments were sequenced to determine the 6mA-rich region in genome by mapping to the corresponding whole genome sequence. The 6mA antibody-dependent assays require highly specific 6mA antibody.

In addition, photo-crosslinking-exonuclease-assisted method [10, 14, 15] and restriction enzyme method [10] were used to obtain a much higher resolution, even at single-molecule resolution for 6mA analysis. Recently, Hong et al. found that Ag^{+} could effectively cause steady A-C mismatch in polymerase chain reaction, but 6mA-C mismatch was unstable, leading to DNA amplification termination. They demonstrated that in the presence of Ag^{+}, 6mA was discriminated at a single base resolution from dA by rolling circle amplification both at single-strand and double-strand DNA probes [16].

Active DNA cytosine methylation pathway in mammals is well known. It includes writer (DNMT1, DNMT3A/DNMT3B), reader (MBD2, MECP2), and demethylase (TET1/TET2/TET3). Similarly, recent studies have revealed the candidates for writer, reader, and eraser in DNA adenine methylation pathway. We have demonstrated that the TET homologous protein DMAD (DNA N6-methyl adenine demethylase) is a 6mA eraser in fly genome. When DMAD was knocked out in fly, the 6mA level was found to be significantly increased (10–70-fold) at whole genomic level in fly brain and ovary. This result indicates that DMAD may regulate the 6mA demethylation by direct or indirect enzymatic catalysis in vivo. In order to verify DMAD is the direct 6mA demethylase, catalytic domain of DMAD (DMAD-CD) and DMAD-CD^{mut} was purified from 293 T cells and then incubated with adenine methylated calf thymus DNA, respectively [6]. DMAD-CD showed significantly 6mA demethylase activity, but the DMAD-CD^{mut} displayed very poor demethylase activity. Our findings have clearly demonstrated that DMAD is a 6mA demethylase in fly. Greer et al. demonstrated DNA N6-methyl adenine demethylase (NMAD-1) as a 6mA demethylase and DNA N6-methyl methyltransferase (DAMT-1) as a potential 6mA methylase in *Caenorhabditis elegans* [7]. Wu et al. showed that deposition of 6mA in LINE-1 transposons inversely correlated with the evolutionary age, and histone H2A dioxygenase ALKBH1 played the role of 6mA demethylase in vivo and in vitro in mouse embryonic stem cells [8]. Koh et al. demonstrated single-stranded DNA binding protein 1 (SSBP1) as a 6mA reader and mitochondrial ALKBH1 as the eraser in human 293 T cells [15]. In addition, N^{6}-adenine-specific DNA methyltransferase 1 (N6AMT1) and ALKBH1 were reported as the 6mA writer and eraser, respectively, in human [17]. In a word, 6mA has been proposed as a new epigenetic mark in eukaryotes and regulated possibly by several N^{6}-adenine methylases and demethylases. The probable DNA methylation and demethylation pathways of DNA adenine in eukaryotes is shown in Fig. 1.

Cytosine methylation is generally well known as gene suppresser. However, the function of 6mA in gene regulation is much more complicated. In order to obtain the overall relationship between 6mA and gene regulation, the detailed distribution of 6mA in genome was investigated with the RNA-seq data. Using 6mA immunoprecipitation sequencing technique (6mA-DIP-seq), we found that 6mA tended to be enriched in the transposon element region of wild-type *Drosophila* ovary genome, and 6mA was removed from the transposon in $DMAD^{mut}$ *Drosophila* [6]. Global expression profiling analysis showed that transposons with 6mA possessed significantly higher expression level in $DMAD^{mut}$ ovary than those in wild type. Greer et al. found that 6mA was widely distributed in genome of *Caenorhabditis elegans* [7]. Liu et al. demonstrated that 6mA was mainly distributed at the repeat sequence of genome from the early embryo of zebrafish [12]. DNA cytosine modifi-

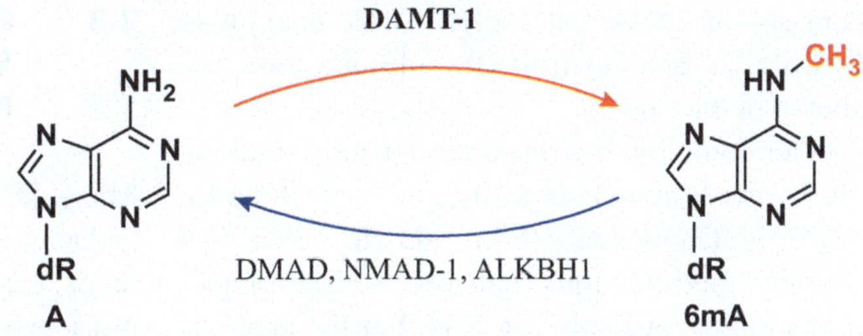

Fig. 1 DNA adenine methylation and demethylation in eukaryotes

cations have been linked to human diseases such as cancer. For instance, studies have shown that global 5-methylcytosine (5mC) contents generally decrease in cancers [18–20]. We found 5-hydroxymethylcytosine (5hmdC) and 5-formylcytosine (5fdC) also declined dramatically in the very early stage of hepatocellular carcinoma [20]. The reduction of 5hmdC and 5fdC was principally due to the decrease of 5mC and was related to hepatitis B virus infection. However, to the best of our knowledge, there is no adequate evidence of the link between 6mA and human diseases.

Next, we will focus on the discussion about the studies of 6mA with analytical methodologies, particularly LC-MS, antibody-based assays, and DNA sequencing technology.

2 LC-MS for Qualitative and Quantitative Analysis of 6mA

HPLC-MS/MS is a hyphenated technique which combines highly efficient chromatographic separation and powerful MS identification. Three forms of DNA methyladenine (1mA, 3mA, and 6mA) can be well differentiated by LC-MS because of their differences in chromatographic behavior and chemical structure. Therefore, LC-MS/MS method has been reliably used for qualitative and quantitative analysis of 6mA.

2.1 MS Analysis of 6mA in Oligos

The in vitro activity of DNA methyltransferase or demethylase is usually verified by incubation with synthetic oligos, and then the 6mA levels in oligos are measured by HPLC-ESI-TOF MS or MALDI-TOF MS. For example, the oxidative demethylation of N6-methyladenosine (m6A) in RNA oligo by alpha-ketoglutarate-dependent dioxygenase (FTO) can be detected by MS. Since producing adenine from methyladenine accompanies with a mass loss of 14 Da, and producing formyladenosine from methyladenine with a mass increase of 14 Da [21], qualitative and quantitative analysis of the 6mA demethylation activity of FTO can be easily attained through the exact mass changes detected by MS.

2.2 Preparation of Mononucleotides by DNA Hydrolysis for LC-MS Analysis

In order to analyze the target DNA modification directly and obtain much higher sensitivity, the DNA from the cells or body fluids was usually digested into mononucleotides for MS analysis. There are two ways of DNA digestion for this purpose. One is robust hydrolysis under strong acidic condition and high temperature (140–170 °C), which produces nucleotide bases and 2′-desoxyribose [22]. This method requires RNA-free DNA, because RNA also contains adenine, cytosine, guanine, and modified bases. For example, RNA m6A, as an abundant modification in RNA, also released N6-methyladenine bases. All the N6-methyladenine base signal will be assigned to 6mA by LC-MS. On one hand, it is time consuming and difficult to achieve pure RNA-free DNA sample. On the other hand, this method, which is based on hot acidic hydrolysis conditions, is not suitable for unstable modified nucleotide analysis. The other approach is DNA hydrolysis by enzymes and the general procedure consists of DNA extraction, DNA enzymatic hydrolysis, and hydrolysate ultrafiltration, as shown in the Fig. 2.

The demethylated products of m6A include N6-hydroxymethyladenosine (hm6A), N6-formyladenosine (f6A), and the other two unstable modifications (half-life, ~3 h) in physiological aqueous solution [21]. For the analysis of the unstable DNA modifications, we have demonstrated two promising DNA hydrolysis strategies. One is mild digestion of DNA by hydrolases, including DNase I, phosphodiesterase, and alkaline phosphatase (ALP) [23], as illustrated in Fig. 3. We found that 1.0 mM Mg^{2+} stimulated the DNase, snake venom phosphodiesterase (SVP), and ALP to digest DNA (~5.0 μg) completely within 2–3 h [24]. It significantly shortens the digestion time than traditionally enzymatic hydrolysis method (6–18 h). In addition, the efficiency of DNase/SVP/ALP set was significantly inhibited by the Na^+ and K^+, which were general components of the phosphate buffered solution. Of note, we observed 2′-deoxycytosine (dC) and 5-methyldeoxycytidine (5mdC) possessed different release rate in the digestion of DNA. Our results suggest that there are differences probably widespread among the release rate of numerous DNA modifications.

The second strategy is that hydrolysis of DNA with immobilized enzyme cascade bioreactors [25, 26]. We constructed a three-enzyme cascade bioreactor, with Benzonase immobilized capillary bioreactor combined with SVP/ALP immobilized capillary bioreactor. Genetic DNA can be fully digested (>99.5%) within 10 min [26]. This three-enzyme cascade bioreactor can be directly combined with LC-MS for DNA modification analysis.

2.3 Enhancement of the MS Signal for Released Nucleosides

Many DNA modifications are essentially polar and tend to be detected by LC-ESI-MS in positive mode. Generally, the pH and additives were optimizable to enhance MS detection of DNA modifications. For example, we found ammonium bicarbonate (NH_4HCO_3) was able to enhance MS signal (1.8–14.3 times) than formic acid for a class of modified nucleosides (5hmdC, 5fdC, acrolein-dG adducts) [27, 28]. To explore the mechanism of the enhancement of MS detection by ammonium bicarbonate, MS2 scan analysis of acrolein-dG was performed. There were abundant $[\text{acrolein-dG} + Na]^+$ and $[\text{acrolein-dG} + K]^+$ relative to $[\text{acrolein-dG} + H]^+$(22.8–72%) under the mobile phase containing HCOOH, $HCOONH_4$, or CH_3COONH_4, but there was only 3.6% to $[\text{acrolein-dG} + H]^+$ at the condition of NH_4HCO_3. This indicated NH_4HCO_3 inhibited the formation of compound acrolein-dG-metallic ions in the process of ionization and then enhanced the portion of acrolein-dG-proton. We speculated NH_4^+ probably formed ionic complexes with acrolein-dG ($[\text{acrolein-dG} + NH_4]^+$), which formed $[\text{acrolein-dG} + H]^+$ with loss of NH_3 by heated gas phase. Meanwhile, the HCO_3^- was liable to be degraded to CO_2 and H_2O. This process was expected to enhance the protonation of acrolein-dG. Also, NH_4HCO_3 was able to enhance chemically labeled nucleoside triphosphates [29]. Of note, ESI negative mode was much more suitable for analysis of 5cadC and 5hmdU.

DNA derivatization is another strategy to enhance the MS detection sensitivity of modified nucleotides. DNA chemical derivatization using 2-bromo-1-(4-dimethylamino-phenyl)-ethanone

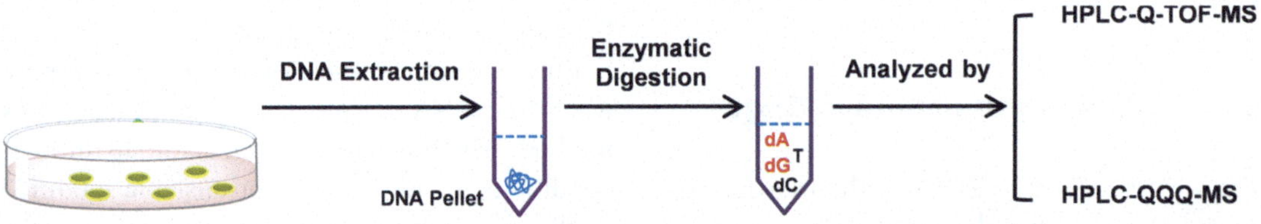

Fig. 2 General procedure of DNA hydrolysis into single nucleotides for HPLC-MS analysis

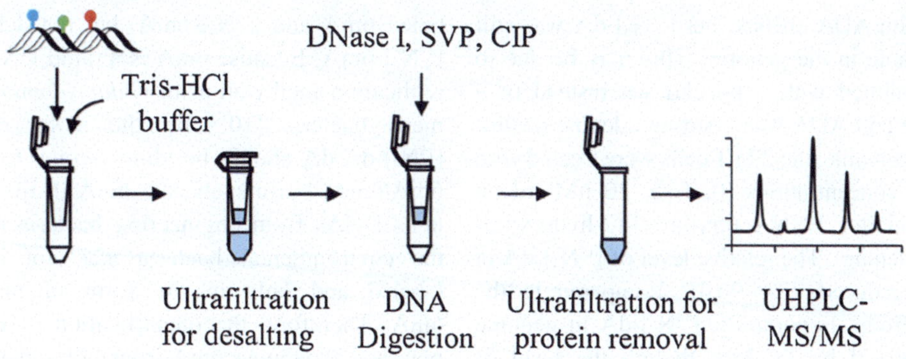

Fig. 3 DNA was desalted and digested with stepwise pretreatment for UHPLC-MS/MS detection [23]. Reprinted with permission from Lai, W., Mo, J., Lyu, C., Wang, H. Anal Chem 110: 173–182. Copyright 2018. American Chemical Society

(BDAPE) [30] and 8-(diazomethyl) quinoline (8-DMQ) [29] was used for enhancing the MS signal of DNA modifications. This method significantly decreased the limits of detection for NTPs from 56- to 137-fold [29]. Enzymatic derivatization of DNA modifications is another promising strategy. For example, 5hmdC can be selectively derivatized by T4 c-glucosyltransferase, into 6-azide-β-glucosyl-5-hydroxymethylcytosine, with an elevated eightfold signal sensitivity by LC-MS [31].

2.4 Stable Isotope Labeling [$^{15}N_5$]-dA Tracing Veritable 6mA

The analysis of 6mA usually faces severe challenge of ubiquitous bacterial contamination [9, 32]. Routine LC-MS and 6mA antibody-based assays are generally not able to distinguish 6mA of different origins. However, the genomic DNA of cultured cells can be labeled by stable isotope labeling nucleotides via the purine salvage pathway, which may be used to distinguish endogenous and exogenous DNA by LC-MS.

2.4.1 Involvement of [$^{15}N_5$]-dA in the Adenine Deamination-Regulated Purine Salvage Pathway

In order to test our approach, 20 μM of [$^{15}N_5$]-dA was added to the culture medium of human 293 T cells. After 24-h treatment, the genomic DNA of 293 T cells was extracted and digested into single nucleotides for UHPLC-TOF MS analysis. Based on the exact mass of labeled and unlabeled dA, we unexpectedly found that [$^{15}N_5$]-dA was almost entirely incorporated into genomic DNA in the form of [$^{15}N_4$]-dA instead of [$^{15}N_5$]-dA in 293 T cells. To determine which ^{15}N atom of [$^{15}N_5$]-dA was replaced with ^{14}N in the transformation in vivo, the co-eluted fraction of dA containing unlabeled dA and [$^{15}N_4$]-dA was collected and analyzed by the Agilent 6530 TOF MS under targeted MS/MS mode. Given a 20-eV collision energy, most of the target precursor ions (dA or [$^{15}N_4$]-dA) were fully dissociated into adenine bases (unlabeled A or [$^{15}N_4$]-A), together with constant neutral loss of 2′-deoxyribose. With a given collision energy of 55 eV, there were 12 and 15 product ions from the unlabeled adenine and [$^{15}N_4$]-adenine, respectively. Based on the reliable dissociative principle of adenine reported in a previous study by Nelson et al. [33], we demonstrated that the exocyclic N atom of [$^{15}N_4$]-dA was unlabeled. It means that the exocyclic N^{6th} ^{15}N of [$^{15}N_5$]-dA undergone certain process of biological deamination in vivo. Adenosine deaminase (ADA) is an important deaminase of adenosine and deoxyadenine [34]. In order to verify the potential role of ADA in the deamination of [$^{15}N_5$]-dA in vivo, ADA expression was knocked down via transfection with ADA siRNA. We found that the relative level of [$^{15}N_4$]-dA/dA in genome significantly decreased ~37.2% after 293 T cells transfected with ADA siRNA, but [$^{15}N_5$]-dA was still undetectable in the genome. This may be due to ADA inhibited with a knockdown instead of a knockout and ADA was a strong adenine deaminase. Meanwhile, the 293 T cells were treated with different concentrations (0, 1, 5, 20 μM) of an ADA inhibitor EHNA (erythro-9-(2-hydroxy-3-nonyl) adenine). The relative level of [$^{15}N_4$]-dA in genome reduced 75%–96.4% compared to the control group. Importantly, [$^{15}N_5$]-dA in genome was observed by LC-MS, though the level of [$^{15}N_5$]-dA/dA was less than 5% under our experimental condition. Our results have demonstrated that [$^{15}N_5$]-dA is overwhelmingly involved in the adenine deamination-regulated purine salvage pathway in 293 T cells (Fig. 4).

2.4.2 Differentiation of the 6mA from Nonproliferative Prokaryotic DNA and Human DNA

We have demonstrated that the incorporation of exogenous nucleoside [$^{15}N_5$]-dA into the genomic DNA was in the form of [$^{15}N_4$]-dA and [$^{15}N_4$]-dG, but not [$^{15}N_5$]-dA itself [35]. After 293 T cells (1×10^5) were treated with 20 μM [$^{15}N_5$]-dA for 24 hrs, the molar ratios of [$^{15}N_4$]-dA/dA and [$^{15}N_4$]-dG/dG were 25.5 ± 0.6% and 29.5 ± 0.2% in the genomic DNA, respectively [35]. Therefore, if 6mA is a chemical modification from dA, there must be two forms of 6mA, unlabeled 6mA and [$^{15}N_4$]-6mA, but not detectable [$^{15}N_5$]-6mA. Because 6mA is a rapid DNA post-replication methylation in *Chlamydomonas* and many bacteria [10, 36], the molar ratio of [$^{15}N_4$]-dA/dA should be almost equal to [$^{15}N_4$]-6mA/6mA. Fortunately, the 6mA in the exogenous DNAs from engineering bacteria or from the environmental bacteria was not isotope-labeled and only in the form of unlabeled 6mA. Therefore, the quantification of endogenous and exogenous 6mA from cultured cells can be straightforward.

2.4.3 Tracing of 6mA Origin by LC-MS with Stable Isotope Labeling

As a common bacterial contaminant of mammalian cell cultures, a plenty of *mycoplasmas* slow the growth of cells by competition for nutrients, but do not cause media turbidity. In order to verify the presence of *mycoplasma*, universal mycoplasma primers and mycoplasma species-specific primers were used in polymerase chain reaction, and the products were separated by 1% agarose gel [35], as shown in Fig. 4. There are two positive strands (strand 1 and 2), corresponding to theoretical products size 425 bp (universal primers) and 334 bp (*Mycoplasma hyorhinis*) [37]. The results demonstrated that the DNA extracted from the 293 T cells with abundance of 6mA contained the bacterial DNA from *Mycoplasma hyorhinis*. This means that the 293 T cells were

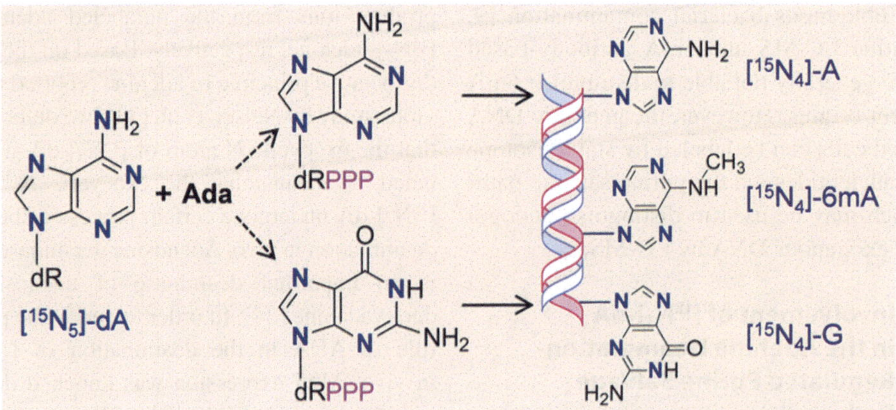

Fig. 4 Incorporation of a metabolically generated code of [$^{15}N_5$]-dA into the genome by adenine deamination-regulated purine salvage pathway in human cells [35]. Reprinted with permission from Liu, B., Liu, X., Lai, W., Wang, H. Anal Chem 89 (11): 6202–6209. Copyright 2017. American Chemical Society

infected with *Mycoplasma hyorhinis* and its bacterial DNA was one source of 6mA (Fig. 5).

We then explored the metabolic difference of ^{15}N-labeled dA between the *Mycoplasma*-positive and *Mycoplasma*-negative 293 T cells by treatment with 20 μM [$^{15}N_5$]-dA for 24 hrs. The DNA was extracted and digested as previously described for UHPLC-MS/MS analysis. The results showed that both [$^{15}N_4$]-dA and [$^{15}N_4$]-dG existed in the two extracted samples. The ratio of [$^{15}N_4$]-dG/dG and [$^{15}N_4$]-dA/dA of *Mycoplasma*-positive genomic DNA was 0.96- and 1.28-fold, respectively, to the *Mycoplasma*-negative DNA (Fig. 6). However, [$^{15}N_5$]-dA, 6mA, and [$^{15}N_5$]-6mA existed only in the *Mycoplasma*-positive 293 T cells, but not in *Mycoplasma*-negative 293 T cells. UHPLC-MS/MS analysis showed that there was about 560 6mA per million dA in the extracted DNA from the 293 T cells. More importantly, the frequency of the three forms of 6mA was unlabeled 6mA (32%), [$^{15}N_4$]-6mA (24%), and [$^{15}N_5$]-6mA (44%) [35]. Of note, [$^{15}N_5$]-6mA was predominated among the three forms of detected 6mA. Consistent with our report, there was ~2% 6mA in the genome of *Mycoplasma hyorhinis* [38] and no detectable ADA activity in *Mycoplasma hyorhinis* [39]. Moreover, *mycoplasma* owned capacity of uptaking nucleotides from both the nucleotide pool of the medium and the host nucleotide pool [40], and there was no detectable 6mA (lower than 0.4 6mdA per million dA) in the *Mycoplasma*-negative cells [35]. Based on these observations, we concluded that the detected 6mA was mainly from mycoplasma, but we could not exclude the possibility of minor 6mA from the host gnomic DNA itself.

It is known that routine LC-MS and antibody-based methods (IF, IP, dot blot) are unable to discriminate the 6mA from different origins, because of their identical exact masses and chemical structures. Due to the high ADA activity in many human or mouse cells [41–43], there should be predominant [$^{15}N_4$]-dA, but not [$^{15}N_5$]-dA after the cells are treated with [$^{15}N_5$]-dA. On one hand, the stable isotope labeling method that we developed was very reliable, rapid, and effective to

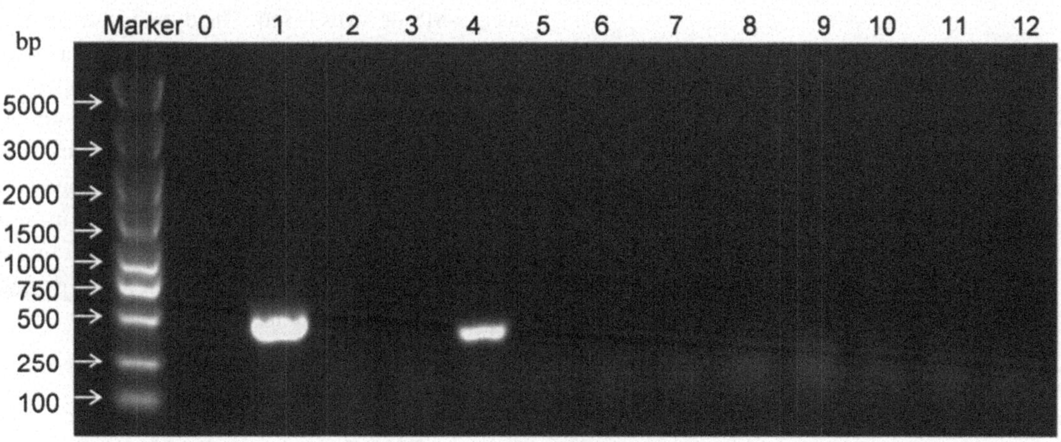

0. Negative Control.
1. Universal
2. *M. arginini*
3. *M. orale*
4. *M. hyorhinis*
5. *M. fermentans*
6. *M. genitalium*
7. *M. laidlawii*
8. *M. hominis*
9. *M. Pirum*
10. *M. pneumoniae*
11. *M. salivarium*
12. *ureaplasma urealyticum*

Fig. 5 Agarose gel electrophoresis (1%) analysis of the PCR products for identification of potential mycoplasma contamination in DNA of infected 293 T cells [35]. Reprinted with permission from Liu, B., Liu, X., Lai, W., Wang, H. Anal Chem 89 (11): 6202–6209. Copyright 2017. American Chemical Society

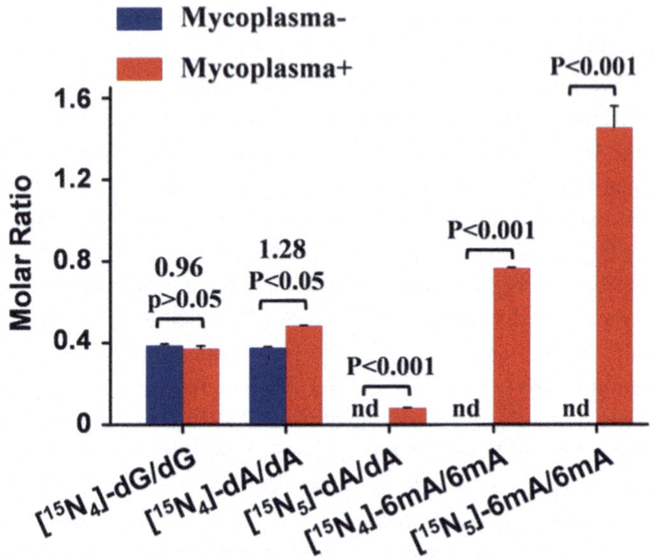

Fig. 6 DNA modification products from metabolism of [$^{15}N_5$]-dA in the genome of *Mycoplasma*-positive or negative 293 T cells treated with [$^{15}N_5$]-dA for 24 h [35]. Reprinted with permission from Liu, B., Liu, X., Lai, W., Wang, H. Anal Chem 89 (11): 6202–6209. Copyright 2017. American Chemical Society

trace 6mA in cultured cells. On the other hand, *Mycoplasma* as a common contamination in cell culture, and other prokaryotes with deficiency in ADA activity [39, 44], can be monitored by the production of [$^{15}N_5$]-6mA and [$^{15}N_5$]-dA with LC-MS.

2.4.4 Undetectable [$^{15}N_4$]-6mA in Mouse Embryonic Stem Cells

The mouse embryonic stem cells (mESCs, 129SvEv) were treated with 20 μM of [$^{15}N_5$]-dA for 5 days and the medium was replaced with the fresh medium with the same concentration of [$^{15}N_5$]-dA every day. The labeling ratio of [$^{15}N_4$]-dA/dA and [$^{15}N_4$]-dG/dG increased from zero to ~0.7 along with the cell growth. Three forms of 6mA were detected, including unlabeled 6mA, [$^{15}N_4$]-6mA, and [$^{15}N_5$]-6mA. The level of unlabeled 6mA was about 4 6mA per 10^7 dA, but [$^{15}N_4$]-6mA and [$^{15}N_5$]-6mA were undetectable (unpublished data). These results indicated there was no detectable N6-adenine methyltransferase activity in the mESCs.

3 Antibody-Based Assays

The 6mA antibody-based assays such as dot blot [6–9, 11], immunofluorescence imaging [6–8, 11], and ELISA [13] have been used for 6mA analysis in many species. Besides a high-quality 6mA antibody, RNA contamination should be completely removed, because of the nonspecific recognition of RNA m6A by 6mA antibody. Therefore, if there is very low abundance of 6mA in a DNA sample, it is essential to verify the actual level of 6mA using other techniques, such as LC-MS or SMRT-Seq. The dynamic change of 6mA in embryonic development [6, 12] has suggested its potential important role in this process. However, it is very difficult to obtain enough number of early mammalian embryonic cells (zygote, 1 cell, and morula, 32 cells) for the 6mA analysis. New analytical methods, e.g., in situ detection, are needed to overcome this sample size issue when analyzing the 6mA levels during embryonic development.

3.1 Enrichment of 6mA-Specific DNA Fragments by Multiple Immunoprecipitation

IP is a common tool for studying the locus-specific DNA methylations and profiling of DNA methylations at a genome-wide level [6, 10]. However, the use of antibodies, microbeads, and protein A/G probably results in nonspecific binding of 6mA-free DNA fragments in 6mA IP. In our previous study [45], prior to 6mA IP, the low methylation Lambda DNA (0.68 6mA modification per 10^4 deoxynucleotides) was fragmented and thermally denatured into single-strand (ss) DNA (~150 nt). Then, five anti-6mA antibodies from different sources (3 μg of each antibody) were incubated with 5 μg ssDNA [45]. The enrichment coefficient of each anti-6mA antibody was determined to be from 5.3-fold to 37-fold. Surprisingly, the ultimate enriched fragments contained 62.7% to 94.6% 6mA-free DNA fragments [45]. The next-generation sequencing (NGS) method could not distinguish the 6mA from dA, which means all the enriched DNA fragments would be read and mapped to the genome as 6mA-rich regions. The oversize false-positive background prevented us from revealing the truth of 6mA distribution in genome (Fig. 7). The single-molecule real-time sequencing was able to distinguish 6mA from dA at single base resolution, but it required large amounts of DNA and was not suitable for sequencing of very low abundant 6mA genome [46].

Based on previous IP results, we speculated the affinities of the 6mA antibodies against 6mA are probably at submicromolar level, in the presence of copious 6mA-free fragments, suggesting that IP is a moderate affinity solid-phase (antibody) extraction. Therefore, the multiple-round 6mA-IP procedure should be very efficient to enrich a high proportion of 6mA-specific fragments in the final pull-down fraction. The first and second round IP enriched 34-fold and 61-fold 6mA fragments, respectively, but 6mA-free fragments remained to be the majority as the 6mA-specific fragments only took up 0.23% and 13.7% of the entire pull-down fraction. Only after the third round IP, 60% 6mA-specific fragments were obtained. Finally, 13.7 ng DNA was enriched and the overall length (2.5×10^{13} nts) was 4700-fold higher than the length of mouse genomes (5.3×10^9 nts). Therefore, the enriched 6mA-specific fragments were enough for construction and sequencing of DNA libraries. The multiple-round 6mA-IP combined with high-throughput sequencing is promising to reveal the authentic genome-wide distribution of low abundance 6mA in multicellular organisms.

4 High-Throughput DNA Sequencing Technology

4.1 Next-Generation Sequence

NGS usually consists of the following steps: library construction, surface attachment and bridge amplification, denaturation and complete amplification, single base extension and sequencing, and data analysis [47]. As a result, PCR-based NGS was not able to directly read the sequence information of DNA modifications, but there are other ways for mapping the DNA modification sequence. For example, bisulfite oxidation deaminizes C to U, but 5mC is invariable in DNA. The U is read as T and 5mC is read as C by the NGS. This so-called BS-Seq method was widely used in genome-wide mapping of 5mC. Similarly, the 6mA and dA are both read as dA by NGS. Unfortunately, as far as we know, there was no sufficiently effective way to convert 6mA to other derivative at genomic level, because of its extreme stability. Of note, 6mA could be demethylated by fly DMAD or

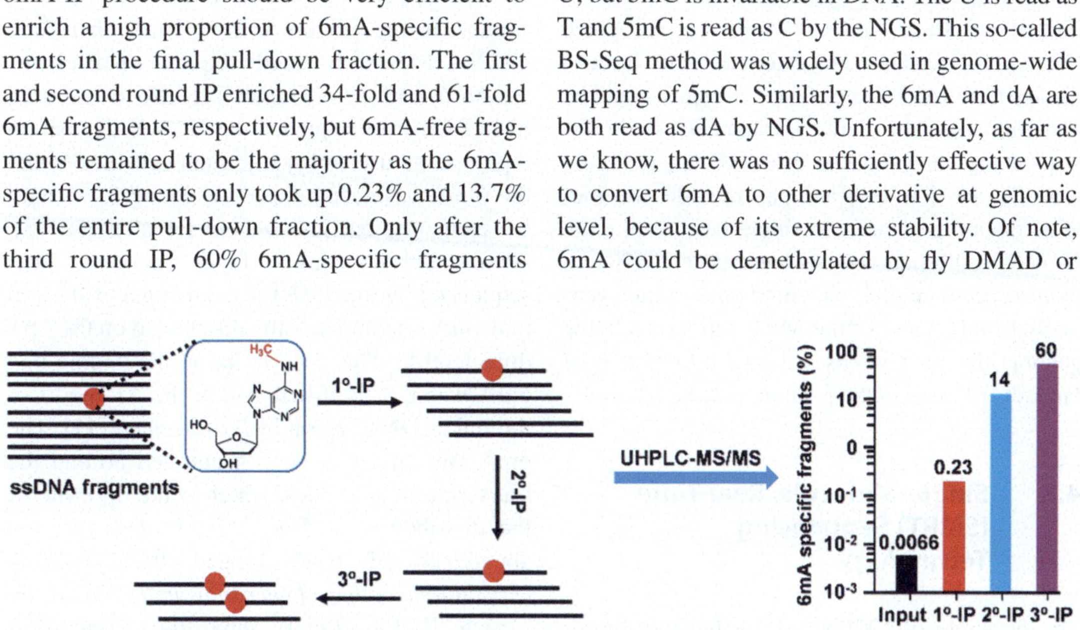

Fig. 7 Multiple-round 6mA-IP significantly enhanced the proportion of 6mA-specific fragments in the total enriched fragments using a genome with very low 6mA abundance [45]. Reprinted with permission from Liu, X., Lai, W., Zhang, N., Wang, H. Anal Chem 90 (9): 5546–5551. Copyright 2018. American Chemical Society

mouse ALKBH1 to potential intermediates such as 6hmA and 6fA. TET2 can stepwise oxidize to 5hmdC and 5fdC [48], and the oxidation may be stalled at 5hmdC by TET2 mutant [49]. Similarly, oxidization of 6mA may be potentially stalled at 6hmA or 6fA by remodeled 6mA demethylases. Derivatization of the hydroxy and formyl groups of the 6hmA and 6fA, which probably are stable under certain conditions, then provides another strategy for the 6mA methylome sequencing.

Sample preparation for sequencing analysis can be carried out with a method combining the use of 6mA antibody with photo-crosslinking and exonuclease digestion. Methylated DNA sample is adequately incubated with 6mA antibody and then photo-crosslinked at UV 254 nm, and the cross-linked DNA was digested by two exonucleases, Lambda exonuclease and RecJf exonuclease for sequencing analysis [10, 15]. With this method, Koh and colleague [15] obtained a single-nucleotide resolution for 6mA analysis, which is different from the previous report (~33 bp 6mA mapping resolution) [10]. This is probably caused by the difference in the degree enzymatic digestion.

Restriction enzyme-based 6mA sequencing (6mA-RE-seq) has also been demonstrated for global-scale 6mA analysis. Luo and colleagues [50] found that *Dpn*I not only can recognize G(6mA)TC in dsDNA but also weakly cut C(6mA) TC and G(6mA) TG sites. The 6mA sites would be at terminal of the derived fragments ready for sequencing analysis. The 6mA-RE-seq is highly sensitive and low cost and can provide genome-wide mapping of 6mA at single base resolution. Of note, restriction endonucleases selectively recognize specific motif containing 6mA, which generally is only a part of the whole 6mA sites in the genome. In other words, a lot of information of 6mA distribution in the genome may be ignored.

4.2 Single-Molecule, Real-Time (SMRT) Sequencing Technology

The principle of SMRT lies in that the fluorophores are cleaved off when dNTPs are incorporated into expanded DNA by the DNA polymerase. A detector detects the fluorescent signal of the nucleotide incorporation, and the base call is made according to the corresponding fluorescence of the dye. SMRT sequencing is antibody independent, without native DNA cloning or amplification, but had an overall lower read accuracy (~87%) [51]. This means much more native DNA is required for SMRT than the NGS method. The read length of SMRT sequencing generally exceed 5 kilobases. The longer read length increases the reliability of mapping genome, decreases the GC bias, and reduces the difficulty of mapping to repetitive elements, paralogous sequences, and phasing alleles in the genome. However, SMRT sequencing consumes more native DNA and the cost is high, which limits its popularity. Generally, to generate a complete human 6mA methylome, no less than 75 runs are required to achieve the minimal ~150× coverage by the SMRT sequencing on the PacBio Sequel System [52].

SMRT sequencing was used to analyze the distribution of 6mA in the *C. elegans* genome, and two methylation-specific sites AGAA and GAGG were verified [7]. Meanwhile, there were no significantly depleted or enriched regions of 6mA in the genome of *C. elegans*. Of note, SMRT cannot distinguish 6mA from 1mA; therefore, UHPLC-MS/MS is usually required to differentiate 6mA and 1mA signals [7]. Wu et al. used SMRT-ChIP to sequence the H2A.X deposition region in mouse embryonic stem cells and found the 6mA was accumulated on young full-length L1 elements, but less on old L1 elements [8]. Also, early-diverging fungi genome was sequenced by the SMRT sequencing and showed that 6mA is symmetrically distributed on the ApT dinucleotide. This was similar to the finding that 6mA was mostly distributed at the AT modif of the linker DNA region in *Tetrahymena* [11]. The 6mA was found to be concentrated around the transcription start sites, which is the opposite of the distribution of 5mC [53]. In *Dikarya*, the abundance of 6mA ranged from 0.048% (*Pucciniomycotina*, *Leucosporidiella creatinivora*) to 0.21% (*Taphrinomycotina*, *Protomyces lactucaedebilis*). The excessively low level of 6mA (0.048%) probably caused the false-positives when using the SMRT sequencing for 6mA mapping [53]. It should be noted that the abundance level of 0.048% (6mA/A) in the genome is generally comparative or higher than the level of 6mA in mammalian somatic cells [8, 17].

References

1. Gorovsky, M. A., Hattman, S., & Pleger, G. L. (1973). (6 N)methyl adenine in the nuclear DNA of a eucaryote, Tetrahymena pyriformis. *The Journal of Cell Biology, 56*(3), 697–701. https://doi.org/10.1083/jcb.56.3.697.
2. Pratt, K., & Hattman, S. (1981). Deoxyribonucleic acid methylation and chromatin organization in Tetrahymena thermophila. *Molecular and Cellular Biology, 1*(7), 600–608. https://doi.org/10.1128/MCB.1.7.600.
3. Harrison, G. S., Findly, R. C., & Karrer, K. (1986). Site-specific methylation of adenine in the nuclear genome of a eucaryote, Tetrahymena thermophila. *Molecular and Cellular Biology, 6*(7), 2364–2370. https://doi.org/10.1128/MCB.6.7.2364.
4. Krais, A. M., Cornelius, M. G., & Schmeiser, H. H. (2010). Genomic N(6)-methyladenine determination by MEKC with LIF. *Electrophoresis, 31*(21), 3548–3551. https://doi.org/10.1002/elps.201000357.
5. Dohno, C., Shibata, T., & Nakatani, K. (2010). Discrimination of N6-methyl adenine in a specific DNA sequence. *Chemical Communications (Cambridge), 46*(30), 5530–5532. https://doi.org/10.1039/c0cc00172d.
6. Zhang, G., Huang, H., Liu, D., Cheng, Y., Liu, X., Zhang, W., Yin, R., Zhang, D., Zhang, P., Liu, J., Li, C., Liu, B., Luo, Y., Zhu, Y., Zhang, N., He, S., He, C., Wang, H., & Chen, D. (2015). N6-methyladenine DNA modification in Drosophila. *Cell, 161*(4), 893–906. https://doi.org/10.1016/j.cell.2015.04.018.
7. Greer, E. L., Blanco, M. A., Gu, L., Sendinc, E., Liu, J., Aristizabal-Corrales, D., Hsu, C. H., Aravind, L., He, C., & Shi, Y. (2015). DNA methylation on N6-adenine in C. elegans. *Cell, 161*(4), 868–878. https://doi.org/10.1016/j.cell.2015.04.005.
8. Wu, T. P., Wang, T., Seetin, M. G., Lai, Y., Zhu, S., Lin, K., Liu, Y., Byrum, S. D., Mackintosh, S. G., Zhong, M., Tackett, A., Wang, G., Hon, L. S., Fang, G., Swenberg, J. A., & Xiao, A. Z. (2016). DNA methylation on N(6)-adenine in mammalian embryonic stem cells. *Nature, 532*(7599), 329–333. https://doi.org/10.1038/nature17640.
9. Koziol, M. J., Bradshaw, C. R., Allen, G. E., Costa, A. S., Frezza, C., & Gurdon, J. B. (2016). Identification of methylated deoxyadenosines in vertebrates reveals diversity in DNA modifications. *Nature Structural & Molecular Biology, 23*(1), 24–30. https://doi.org/10.1038/nsmb.3145.
10. Fu, Y., Luo, G. Z., Chen, K., Deng, X., Yu, M., Han, D., Hao, Z., Liu, J., Lu, X., Dore, L. C., Weng, X., Ji, Q., Mets, L., & He, C. (2015). N6-methyldeoxyadenosine marks active transcription start sites in Chlamydomonas. *Cell, 161*(4), 879–892. https://doi.org/10.1016/j.cell.2015.04.010.
11. Wang, Y., Chen, X., Sheng, Y., Liu, Y., & Gao, S. (2017). N6-adenine DNA methylation is associated with the linker DNA of H2A.Z-containing well-positioned nucleosomes in pol II-transcribed genes in Tetrahymena. *Nucleic Acids Research, 45*(20), 11594–11606. https://doi.org/10.1093/nar/gkx883.
12. Liu, J., Zhu, Y., Luo, G. Z., Wang, X., Yue, Y., Wang, X., Zong, X., Chen, K., Yin, H., Fu, Y., Han, D., Wang, Y., Chen, D., & He, C. (2016). Abundant DNA 6mA methylation during early embryogenesis of zebrafish and pig. *Nature Communications, 7*, 13052. https://doi.org/10.1038/ncomms13052.
13. Dabe, E. C., Sanford, R. S., Kohn, A. B., Bobkova, Y., & Moroz, L. L. (2015). DNA methylation in basal metazoans: Insights from ctenophores. *Integrative and Comparative Biology, 55*(6), 1096–1110. https://doi.org/10.1093/icb/icv086.
14. Chen, K., Lu, Z., Wang, X., Fu, Y., Luo, G. Z., Liu, N., Han, D., Dominissini, D., Dai, Q., Pan, T., & He, C. (2015). High-resolution N(6) -methyladenosine (m(6) A) map using photo-crosslinking-assisted m(6) A sequencing. *Angewandte Chemie (International Ed. in English), 54*(5), 1587–1590. https://doi.org/10.1002/anie.201410647.
15. Koh, C. W. Q., Goh, Y. T., Toh, J. D. W., Neo, S. P., Ng, S. B., Gunaratne, J., Gao, Y. G., Quake, S. R., Burkholder, W. F., & Goh, W. S. S. (2018). Single-nucleotide-resolution sequencing of human N6-methyldeoxyadenosine reveals strand-asymmetric clusters associated with SSBP1 on the mitochondrial genome. *Nucleic Acids Research, 46*(22), 11659–11670. https://doi.org/10.1093/nar/gky1104.
16. Hong, T., Yuan, Y., Wang, T., Ma, J., Yao, Q., Hua, X., Xia, Y., & Zhou, X. (2017). Selective detection of N6-methyladenine in DNA via metal ion-mediated replication and rolling circle amplification. *Chemical Science, 8*(1), 200–205. https://doi.org/10.1039/c6sc02271e.
17. Xiao, C. L., Zhu, S., He, M., Chen, Z. Q., Chen, Y., Yu, G., Liu, J., Xie, S. Q., Luo, F., Liang, Z., Wang, D. P., Bo, X. C., Gu, X. F., Wang, K., & Yan, G. R. (2018). N(6)-methyladenine DNA modification in the human genome. *Molecular Cell, 71*(2), 306–318. e307. https://doi.org/10.1016/j.molcel.2018.06.015.
18. Baylin, S. B. (2005). DNA methylation and gene silencing in cancer. *Nature Clinical Practice. Oncology, 2*(Suppl 1), S4–S11. https://doi.org/10.1038/ncponc0354.
19. Ehrlich, M. (2002). DNA methylation in cancer: Too much, but also too little. *Oncogene, 21*(35), 5400.
20. Liu, J., Jiang, J., Mo, J., Liu, D., Cao, D., Wang, H., He, Y., & Wang, H. (2019). Global DNA 5-hydroxymethylcytosine and 5-formylcytosine contents are decreased in the early stage of hepatocellular car-

cinoma. *Hepatology, 69*(1), 196–208. https://doi.org/10.1002/hep.30146.
21. Fu, Y., Jia, G., Pang, X., Wang, R. N., Wang, X., Li, C. J., Smemo, S., Dai, Q., Bailey, K. A., Nobrega, M. A., Han, K. L., Cui, Q., & He, C. (2013). FTO-mediated formation of N6-hydroxymethyladenosine and N6-formyladenosine in mammalian RNA. *Nature Communications, 4*, 1798. https://doi.org/10.1038/ncomms2822.
22. Yamagata, Y., Szabo, P., Szuts, D., Bacquet, C., Aranyi, T., & Paldi, A. (2012). Rapid turnover of DNA methylation in human cells. *Epigenetics, 7*(2), 141–145. https://doi.org/10.4161/epi.7.2.18906.
23. Lai, W., Mo, J., Yin, J., Lyu, C., & Wang, H. (2019). Profiling of epigenetic DNA modifications by advanced liquid chromatography-mass spectrometry technologies. *TrAC Trends in Analytical Chemistry, 110*, 173–182. https://doi.org/10.1016/j.trac.2018.10.031.
24. Lai, W., Lyu, C., & Wang, H. (2018). Vertical ultrafiltration-facilitated DNA digestion for rapid and sensitive UHPLC-MS/MS detection of DNA modifications. *Analytical Chemistry, 90*(11), 6859–6866. https://doi.org/10.1021/acs.analchem.8b01041.
25. Yin, J., Xu, T., Zhang, N., & Wang, H. (2016). Three-enzyme cascade bioreactor for rapid digestion of genomic DNA into single nucleosides. *Analytical Chemistry, 88*(15), 7730–7737. https://doi.org/10.1021/acs.analchem.6b01682.
26. Yin, J., Chen, S., Zhang, N., & Wang, H. (2018). Multienzyme cascade bioreactor for a 10 min digestion of genomic DNA into single nucleosides and quantitative detection of structural DNA modifications in cellular genomic DNA. *ACS Applied Materials & Interfaces, 10*(26), 21883–21890. https://doi.org/10.1021/acsami.8b05399.
27. Zhang, N., Song, Y., Wu, D., Xu, T., Lu, M., Zhang, W., & Wang, H. (2016). Detection of 1,N(2)-propano-2′-deoxyguanosine adducts in genomic DNA by ultrahigh performance liquid chromatography-electrospray ionization-tandem mass spectrometry in combination with stable isotope dilution. *Journal of Chromatography. A, 1450*, 38–44. https://doi.org/10.1016/j.chroma.2016.04.067.
28. Yin, R., Mo, J., Lu, M., & Wang, H. (2015). Detection of human urinary 5-hydroxymethylcytosine by stable isotope dilution HPLC-MS/MS analysis. *Analytical Chemistry, 87*(3), 1846–1852. https://doi.org/10.1021/ac5038895.
29. Jiang, H. P., Xiong, J., Liu, F. L., Ma, C. J., Tang, X. L., Yuan, B. F., & Feng, Y. Q. (2018). Modified nucleoside triphosphates exist in mammals. *Chemical Science, 9*(17), 4160–4167. https://doi.org/10.1039/c7sc05472f.
30. Tang, Y., Zheng, S. J., Qi, C. B., Feng, Y. Q., & Yuan, B. F. (2015). Sensitive and simultaneous determination of 5-methylcytosine and its oxidation products in genomic DNA by chemical derivatization coupled with liquid chromatography-tandem mass spectrometry analysis. *Analytical Chemistry, 87*(6), 3445–3452. https://doi.org/10.1021/ac504786r.
31. Shahal, T., Koren, O., Shefer, G., Stern, N., & Ebenstein, Y. (2018). Hypersensitive quantification of global 5-hydroxymethylcytosine by chemoenzymatic tagging. *Analytica Chimica Acta, 1038*, 87–96. https://doi.org/10.1016/j.aca.2018.08.035.
32. Luo, G. Z., Blanco, M. A., Greer, E. L., He, C., & Shi, Y. (2015). DNA N(6)-methyladenine: A new epigenetic mark in eukaryotes? *Nature Reviews. Molecular Cell Biology, 16*(12), 705–710. https://doi.org/10.1038/nrm4076.
33. Nelson, C. C., & McCloskey, J. A. (1992). Collision-induced dissociation of adenine. *Journal of the American Chemical Society, 114*(10), 3661–3668.
34. Kaljas, Y., Liu, C., Skaldin, M., Wu, C., Zhou, Q., Lu, Y., Aksentijevich, I., & Zavialov, A. V. (2017). Human adenosine deaminases ADA1 and ADA2 bind to different subsets of immune cells. *Cellular and Molecular Life Sciences, 74*(3), 555–570. https://doi.org/10.1007/s00018-016-2357-0.
35. Liu, B., Liu, X., Lai, W., & Wang, H. (2017). Metabolically generated stable isotope-labeled deoxynucleoside code for tracing DNA N6-methyladenine in human cells. *Analytical Chemistry, 89*(11), 6202–6209. https://doi.org/10.1021/acs.analchem.7b01152.
36. Heyn, H., & Esteller, M. (2015). An adenine code for DNA: A second life for N6-methyladenine. *Cell, 161*(4), 710–713. https://doi.org/10.1016/j.cell.2015.04.021.
37. Molla Kazemiha, V., Shokrgozar, M. A., Arabestani, M. R., Shojaei Moghadam, M., Azari, S., Maleki, S., Amanzadeh, A., Jeddi Tehrani, M., & Shokri, F. (2009). PCR-based detection and eradication of mycoplasmal infections from various mammalian cell lines: A local experience. *Cytotechnology, 61*(3), 117–124. https://doi.org/10.1007/s10616-010-9252-6.
38. Razin, A., & Razin, S. (1980). Methylated bases in mycoplasmal DNA. *Nucleic Acids Research, 8*(6), 1383–1390.
39. Hamet, M., Bonissol, C., & Cartier, P. (1980). Enzymatic activities on purine and pyrimidine metabolism in nine mycoplasma species contaminating cell cultures. *Clinica Chimica Acta, 103*(1), 15–22. https://doi.org/10.1016/0009-8981(80)90225-9.
40. Drexler, H. G., & Uphoff, C. C. (2002). Mycoplasma contamination of cell cultures: Incidence, sources, effects, detection, elimination, prevention. *Cytotechnology, 39*(2), 75–90. https://doi.org/10.1023/A:1022913015916.
41. Traut, T. W. (1994). Physiological concentrations of purines and pyrimidines. *Molecular and Cellular Biochemistry, 140*(1), 1–22.
42. Austin, W. R., Armijo, A. L., Campbell, D. O., Singh, A. S., Hsieh, T., Nathanson, D., Herschman, H. R., Phelps, M. E., Witte, O. N., Czernin, J., & Radu, C. G. (2012). Nucleoside salvage pathway kinases regulate hematopoiesis by linking nucleotide metabolism with replication stress. *The Journal of Experimental Medicine, 209*(12), 2215–2228. https://doi.org/10.1084/jem.20121061.
43. Rebhandl, S., Huemer, M., Greil, R., & Geisberger, R. (2015). AID/APOBEC deaminases and cancer.

Oncoscience, 2(4), 320–333. https://doi.org/10.18632/oncoscience.155.
44. Chang, Z., Nygaard, P., Chinault, A. C., & Kellems, R. E. (1991). Deduced amino acid sequence of Escherichia coli adenosine deaminase reveals evolutionarily conserved amino acid residues: Implications for catalytic function. *Biochemistry, 30*(8), 2273–2280.
45. Liu, X., Lai, W., Zhang, N., & Wang, H. (2018). Predominance of N(6)-methyladenine-specific DNA fragments enriched by multiple immunoprecipitation. *Analytical Chemistry, 90*(9), 5546–5551. https://doi.org/10.1021/acs.analchem.8b01087.
46. Jenjaroenpun, P., Wongsurawat, T., Pereira, R., Patumcharoenpol, P., Ussery, D. W., Nielsen, J., & Nookaew, I. (2018). Complete genomic and transcriptional landscape analysis using third-generation sequencing: A case study of Saccharomyces cerevisiae CEN.PK113-7D. *Nucleic Acids Research, 46*(7), e38. https://doi.org/10.1093/nar/gky014.
47. Shendure, J., & Ji, H. (2008). Next-generation DNA sequencing. *Nature Biotechnology, 26*(10), 1135–1145. https://doi.org/10.1038/nbt1486.
48. Crawford, D. J., Liu, M. Y., Nabel, C. S., Cao, X. J., Garcia, B. A., & Kohli, R. M. (2016). Tet2 catalyzes stepwise 5-methylcytosine oxidation by an iterative and de novo mechanism. *Journal of the American Chemical Society, 138*(3), 730–733. https://doi.org/10.1021/jacs.5b10554.
49. Liu, M. Y., Torabifard, H., Crawford, D. J., DeNizio, J. E., Cao, X. J., Garcia, B. A., Cisneros, G. A., & Kohli, R. M. (2017). Mutations along a TET2 active site scaffold stall oxidation at 5-hydroxymethylcytosine. *Nature Chemical Biology, 13*(2), 181–187. https://doi.org/10.1038/nchembio.2250.
50. Luo, G. Z., Wang, F., Weng, X., Chen, K., Hao, Z., Yu, M., Deng, X., Liu, J., & He, C. (2016). Characterization of eukaryotic DNA N(6)-methyladenine by a highly sensitive restriction enzyme-assisted sequencing. *Nature Communications, 7*, 11301. https://doi.org/10.1038/ncomms11301.
51. Zhou, X., Peris, D., Kominek, J., Kurtzman, C. P., Hittinger, C. T., & Rokas, A. (2016). In silico whole genome sequencer and analyzer (iWGS): A computational pipeline to guide the design and analysis of de novo genome sequencing studies. *G3 (Bethesda), 6*(11), 3655–3662. https://doi.org/10.1534/g3.116.034249.
52. Zhu, S., Beaulaurier, J., Deikus, G., Wu, T. P., Strahl, M., Hao, Z., Luo, G., Gregory, J. A., Chess, A., He, C., Xiao, A., Sebra, R., Schadt, E. E., & Fang, G. (2018). Mapping and characterizing N6-methyladenine in eukaryotic genomes using single-molecule real-time sequencing. *Genome Research, 28*(7), 1067–1078. https://doi.org/10.1101/gr.231068.117.
53. Mondo, S. J., Dannebaum, R. O., Kuo, R. C., Louie, K. B., Bewick, A. J., LaButti, K., Haridas, S., Kuo, A., Salamov, A., Ahrendt, S. R., Lau, R., Bowen, B. P., Lipzen, A., Sullivan, W., Andreopoulos, B. B., Clum, A., Lindquist, E., Daum, C., Northen, T. R., Kunde-Ramamoorthy, G., Schmitz, R. J., Gryganskyi, A., Culley, D., Magnuson, J., James, T. Y., O'Malley, M. A., Stajich, J. E., Spatafora, J. W., Visel, A., & Grigoriev, I. V. (2017). Widespread adenine N6-methylation of active genes in fungi. *Nature Genetics, 49*(6), 964–968. https://doi.org/10.1038/ng.3859.

Microbial Metabolomics: From Methods to Translational Applications

Rui Guo, Xialin Luo, Xu Xin, Lian Liu, Xijun Wang, and Haitao Lu

1 Introduction

Microbes, which are generally divided into five categories, namely, bacteria, viruses, fungi, archaea, and protozoa, are the pathogens responsible for many infectious diseases that remain a leading cause of death worldwide due to the ongoing emergence of new pathogens and resurgence of previous pathogens. For instance, the gut microbiota is a contributing factor to the pathophysiology of obesity. *Escherichia coli* is the major pathogen of urinary tract infection (UTI), which has a high rate of recurrence. Hepatitis C virus (HCV) induces the development of hepatitis C, and some other serious infectious diseases, even cancer, are associated with microbes [1–4].

Conventionally, molecular and cellular biological methods are used to study infections at the gene and protein levels, but these methods cannot be used for precise and direct monitoring of minor changes in biological niches, let alone for pathogenic annotation. As the final downstream event of transcription and translation, metabolism will amplify these changes, which can then be traced back to easily identify the pathogenesis of infectious diseases [5]. To our knowledge, microbial metabolism refers to a series of chemical reactions that occur during the growth, proliferation, and differentiation of microbes and substrate degradation by microbes, including catabolism and anabolism, which are closely associated with pathogenesis and virulence [6]. Therefore, microbial metabolomics provide a new opportunity to study the diagnosis, pathogenesis, and treatment of diverse infections.

Over the past few years, microbial metabolomics, which is designated for global profiling of a large number of small molecules (molecular weight <1000) from a microbiological system,

R. Guo · X. Luo · H. Lu (✉)
Key Laboratory of Systems Biomedicine (Ministry of Education), Shanghai Center for Systems Biomedicine, Shanghai Jiao Tong University, Shanghai, China
e-mail: Haitao.lu@sjtu.edu.cn

X. Xin
Key Laboratory of Systems Biomedicine (Ministry of Education), Shanghai Center for Systems Biomedicine, Shanghai Jiao Tong University, Shanghai, China

National Chinmedomics Research Center, Sino-America Chinmedomics Technology Collaboration Center, National TCM Key Laboratory of Serum Pharmacochemistry, Harbin, China

L. Liu (✉)
School of Biomedical Sciences, Faculty of Health, Queensland University of Technology, Brisbane, Australia

X. Wang
National Chinmedomics Research Center, Sino-America Chinmedomics Technology Collaboration Center, National TCM Key Laboratory of Serum Pharmacochemistry, Harbin, China

S. Hu (ed.), *Cancer Metabolomics*, Advances in Experimental Medicine and Biology 1280,
https://doi.org/10.1007/978-3-030-51652-9_7

has developed rapidly and been introduced into life science research. Owing to the development of techniques such as high-resolution mass spectrometry (MS), methods of sample preparation and biological annotation databases such as the Human Metabolome Database (HMDB), we can precisely target microbiological functions and then apply microbial metabolomics to study the diagnosis, pathogenesis, and treatment of many infections, such as type 1 diabetes (T1D), UTI, and cystic fibrosis (CF) [2].

In this chapter, we attempt to summarize microbial metabolomics from methods to applications in the study of diverse infectious diseases, allowing us to better understand how microbial metabolomics aids the study of the diagnosis, pathogenesis, and treatment of microbe-related infections (Fig. 1).

2 Methods in Microbial Metabolomics

2.1 Key Analytical Tools for Microbial Metabolomics

Microbial metabolomics strives to analyze the metabolomes of microbiological systems and then translates the metabolic differences to phenotypic differences, enhancing our knowledge about the molecular mechanisms of infectious diseases [7]. Accuracy, sensitivity, and high throughput are three basic characteristics that analytical instruments used for microbial metabolomics should possess. However, because the classes and concentrations of metabolites vary greatly and due to the presence of a large number of metabolites in biological samples, it is very challenging for only one analytical tool to meet all three requirements and detect all known and unknown metabolites [8]. Two types of instrumentation platforms based on nuclear magnetic resonance (NMR) and MS are currently preferred, although neither of these platforms can profile all the metabolites present in microbial samples in an unbiased manner.

NMR spectroscopy identifies chemical structures based on the absorption spectra of radio frequency (RF) pulses from the nuclei of atoms in strong magnetic fields. The commonly employed atoms for analysis include ^{1}H, ^{13}C, and ^{31}P, and this technique can analyze metabolites in samples both qualitatively and quantitatively at the same time. The applications of NMR spectroscopy in metabolomics vary widely, with the most common application being qualitative and quantitative analysis of metabolites in body fluid samples. For example, ^{1}H-NMR was applied to

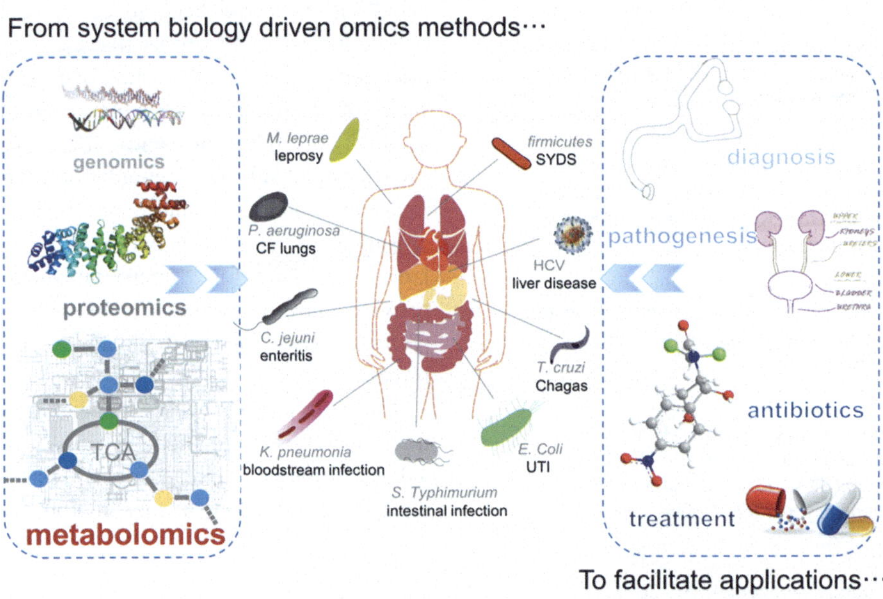

Fig. 1 Applications of metabolomics in the study of microbe-related infectious diseases

compare metabolomes between biofilms, which are associated with many infections, and planktonic cells of *Staphylococcus aureus* [9]. However, due to the complexity of metabolites from microbes and wide range of metabolite concentrations, as well as the relatively low sensitivity and high cost of NMR, the application of NMR in microbial metabolomics has been limited.

To overcome these problems, high-resolution MS has recently become an indispensable tool in metabolomics. Sample preparation techniques such as gas chromatography (GC), liquid chromatography (LC), or capillary electrophoresis (CE) coupled with high-resolution MS methods are broadly employed in microbial metabolomics [7].

GC-MS is a hyphenated technique in which the metabolites of the sample are first separated by GC and then detected and identified by MS [10]. GC-MS only detects volatile and thermally stable compounds, while a majority of microbial metabolites are nonvolatile and thermally labile, such as phosphorylated metabolites, which may degrade when placed at high temperatures in the GC oven. However, this method has been used to analyze microbial metabolites after derivatization due to the advantages of GC, including the ability to efficiently distinguish isomeric compounds, the ease of use, and the low cost compared to other separation tools [8]. For example, a derivatization reaction combined with GC-MS analysis has been used to study numerous microbes, such as *Propionibacterium freudenreichii*, *E. coli*, and *Bacillus subtilis* [7].

LC-MS is another hyphenated technique that offers analyte separation via LC followed by ionization and MS detection. There are two commonly used ionization methods for LC-MS, namely, electrospray ionization (ESI) and atmospheric pressure chemical ionization (APCI), which are both very sensitive. However, ESI is more desirable in microbial metabolomics because ESI-MS preferentially detects polar compounds, while APCI-MS detects nonpolar compounds. In addition, in contrast to GC-MS, LC-MS does not require high temperatures and volatility of analytes, which increases the ease of sample preparation [10]. Furthermore, LC-MS is also highly sensitive with small sample volumes [11]. For example, myxoprincomide, a novel myxobacterial metabolite of *Myxococcus xanthus* DK1622, was discovered by LC coupled with high-resolution MS (LC-HRMS) [12]. Nevertheless, there remain some challenges associated with LC-MS techniques, such as interference by the high salt content in microbial media samples, ionization suppression, and the relatively low resolution of high-performance LC (HPLC). Nevertheless, the emergence of ultrahigh-performance LC (UPLC) has improved chromatographic resolution greatly [10]. For instance, Marcobal and colleagues used an UPLC-MS method to examine the influence of the gut microbiota on the urinary and fecal metabolome of a humanized mouse [13]. CE-MS is another useful tool for metabolomic analysis, the advantages of which include exquisite separation efficiency, very small sample volumes (nL range), and low cost when compared to GC-MS and LC-MS. However, the major shortcoming of CE-MS is the difficulties at the interface between CE and MS [11].

In short, there are several platforms employed in microbial metabolomics (Fig. 2), and each type of instrument has advantages and disadvantages. Researchers should choose the best method or combine the tools to analyze microbial metabolites based on the characteristics of compounds of interest and analytical tools (Fig. 2).

2.2 Sample Preparation and Data Mining of Microbial Metabolomics

Microbial metabolomics focuses on intracellular metabolites that change quickly over time. Therefore, the methods and conditions of sampling and sample preparation, including time, storage condition, and other factors, greatly influence the reproducibility, precision, and accuracy of detection. In addition, the biological variability tends to be larger than analytical variability, which enhances the importance of optimizing sampling and sample preparation methods.

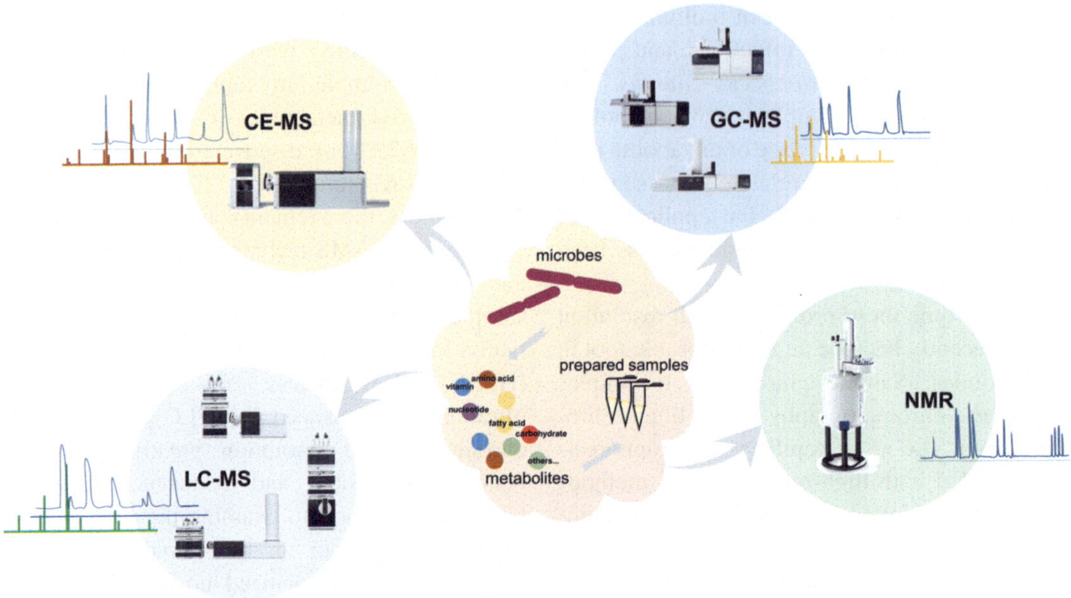

Fig. 2 Platforms used for microbial metabolomics

Some metabolic processes are so rapid (usually less than 2 s) that quick collection of samples from the reactor to stop cell metabolism, especially enzymatic processes, is very crucial. Quick harvesting of metabolites followed by freezing in liquid nitrogen and then storing at −80 °C is commonly used by many researchers. Choosing an effective approach for instant quenching is also rather important for the harvesting of metabolites, and the approach should meet basic requirements such as absence of cell leakage or detection of any leaked metabolites. The use of acidic reagents such as nitric and perchloric acid drastically reduces the number of detected metabolites, and unstable compounds are severely degraded. Hot alcoholic polar (e.g., methanol/water) and nonpolar (e.g., chloroform) extractions are also employed. According to many related studies, prokaryotic microbes such as *E. coli* have a greater tendency to exhibit leakage of intracellular metabolites than eukaryotic microbes such as yeasts when treated with cold methanol, which might be due to the differences in cell wall and membrane structures between the two types of microorganisms. Therefore, cold methanol extraction may be promoted as a common quenching method for extraction of intracellular metabolites from some prokaryotic microbes [14]. A detailed procedure for sampling and sample processing is shown in Fig. 3.

After analyzing the samples via MS-based platform, we obtained the raw data that were very complex. Therefore, data analysis requires the use of appropriate informatics tools for metabolite identification and quantification (Fig. 3). First, pretreatment of raw data to exclude irrelative factors is important and indispensable. Several major processes that involve noise filtering, resolution of overlapping peaks, peak alignment, peak matching, and peak normalization are needed. Current software programs for performing data pretreatment include MetAlign, MET-IDEA, MZmine, Progenesis QI, XCMS, and MSFACTs. The first three can be used to pretreat all LC-MS and GC-MS raw data, while Progenesis QI and XCMS can only process data produced by LC-MS, and MSFACTs is a software for GC-MS data processing. Among the tools mentioned above, MetAlign and MZmine cannot resolve overlapping peaks; MET-IDEA can extract semiquantitative information in addition to resolving overlapping peaks; and XCMS can perform alignment of nonlinear retention times, noise filtering, and other functions. STOCSY (statistical total correlation spectroscopy) is a commonly used method for molecule

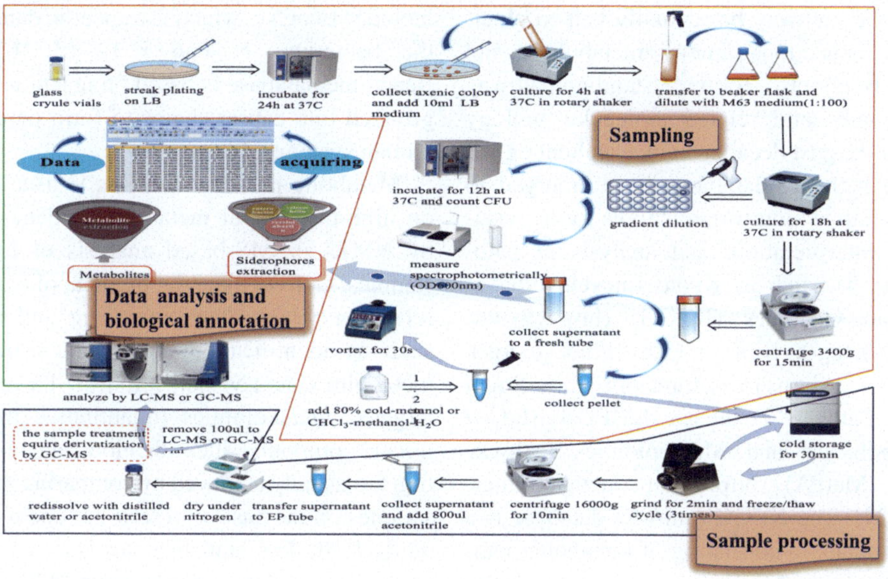

Fig. 3 Sample preparation and data mining of metabolites from *E. coli*

identification in microbial metabolomics based on NMR. It takes advantage of the multicollinearity of the intensity variables in a set of spectra to generate a pseudo-two-dimensional NMR spectrum that displays the correlation among the intensities of the various peaks across the whole sample. This method is not limited to the usual connectivities that are deducible from more standard two-dimensional NMR spectroscopic methods, such as TOCSY. Moreover, two or more molecules involved in the same pathway can also present high intermolecular correlations because of biological covariance or can even be anticorrelated. The combination of STOCSY with supervised pattern recognition and particularly orthogonal projection on latent structure-discriminant analysis (O-PLS-DA) offers a new powerful framework for analysis of metabolomic data. In a first step O-PLS-DA extracts the part of NMR spectra related to discrimination. This information is then cross-combined with the STOCSY results to help identify the molecules responsible for the metabolic variation [15].

In addition to data pretreatment, mining of useful information from a large amount of data and functional annotation of this data is another key challenge in microbial metabolomics. Multivariable data analysis (MVDA) is commonly used to extract information from data sets, including analysis of variables that contribute to classification, identification of biomarkers associated with phenotypes, and annotation of regulatory mechanisms via metabolic pathways. Recently developed MVDA techniques comprise supervised and unsupervised methods as two main types. In microbial metabolomics, supervised methods include clustering analysis (CA) and principal component analysis (PCA), and unsupervised methods include linear discriminant analysis (LDA), partial least squares (PLS) analysis, partial least squares-discriminant analysis (PLS-DA), and artificial neural network (ANN) analysis. Among these analytical methods, PCA and PLS-DA are the most commonly applied methods, yielding classification information via a score plot and revealing metabolites that contribute to the classification as well as the determining the contribution of these metabolites via a loading plot [3, 16, 17].

2.3 Biological Annotation of Differential Metabolic Pathways Characterized by Microbial Metabolomics

After identification of the contributive molecules, the next important step is to identify relevant metabolic pathways that could explain the roles of these molecules in metabolism. Identification of metabolic pathway has actually helped elucidate the connections among metabolites and proven to be effective for understanding pathway genes/enzymes and related molecular biology [18]. Over the past decade, many excellent online metabolic pathway databases have emerged to provide intuitive bioinformatic tools for the visualization, interpretation, and analysis of pathways (Fig. 4), such as Kyoto Encyclopedia of Genes and Genomes (KEGG) (https://www.genome.jp/kegg/), BioCyc (https://biocyc.org/), Reactome (https://reactome.org/), Small Molecule Pathway Database (SMPDB) (http://www.smpdb.ca/), and Metabolomics Pathway Analysis (MetPA) (http://metpa.metabolomics.ca/) [18–24]. The KEGG pathway database is a reference database consisting of metabolic pathway maps with functional significance [25]. BioCyc provides not only a reference for genomes and metabolic pathways but is also a powerful computational analytical tool for prediction of metabolic pathways and operons; BioCyc includes EcoCyc, which is a specific database for the bacterium *E. coli* K-12 MG1655. The Reactome database is based on reactions that are grouped into causal chains to form pathways in human systems [20].

Metabolic pathway analysis is usually based on high-throughput metabolomic data achieved by NMR- or MS-based analysis of biological samples. Correct mapping of metabolic pathways relies on robust data processing and analysis, such as identification and characterization of metabolites, and visualization of the results. In targeted metabolomics (quantitative metabolomics), compound identification and quantification are usually achieved by comparing analytical samples on the basis of a series of chemical standards [26]. For statistical analysis of targeted metabolomic data, openly accessible software/database tools such as MetaboAnalyst (http://www.metaboanalyst.ca/), MeltDB (https://meltdb.cebitec.uni-bielefeld.de/), HMDB, and MeTPA are usually preferred [26–28]. In

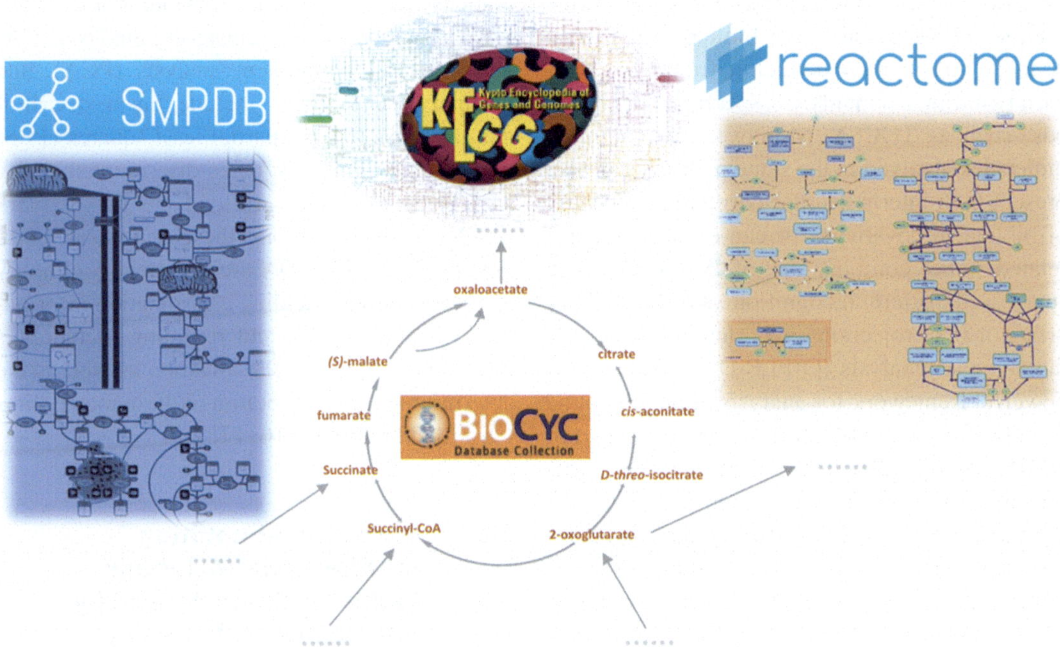

Fig. 4 Online metabolic pathway databases for biological annotation

MetaboAnalyst, detailed and hyperlinked diagrams of pathways can be obtained after uploading a peak list and including information regarding the name and peak intensity of each identified metabolite. MeltDB is similar to MetaboAnalyst to some extent but is only used for MS-based metabolomics data analysis. All the results are linked to the HMDB, which is currently the most comprehensive database of human metabolites and related metabolisms [29]. MetPA is another powerful tool that helps identify the most relevant metabolic pathways and visualizes pathway data.

Metabolic pathway analysis of untargeted metabolomic data is quite challenging because it requires confident identification of a large number of metabolites and building of complex relationships among the identified metabolites. Therefore, comprehensive databases such as the HMDB, METLIN (https://metlin.scripps.edu/), and Madison Metabolomics Consortium Database (MMCD) (http://mmcd.nmrfam.wisc.edu/) [29, 30] are needed to provide the structural properties (e.g., MS/MS spectra) and functional properties of metabolites. Such publicly accessible, web-based databases provide hyperlinks to other databases and share some information in common. HMDB integrates information regarding compound description, chemical structure, and disease associations and reference NMR and MS spectra [29]. METLIN is centered on MS-based data, especially MS/MS data. This database can be used to match metabolites based on MS and MS/MS data. Recently, isoMETLIN, a version for isotope-labeled compounds, has facilitated untargeted global isotope-tracer experiments [30]. The MMCD database supports an extensive search using experimental MS or NMR data, and this database contains information for more than 20,000 biologically relevant small molecules chosen from KEGG, BioCyc, HMDB, and others [31]. These open-source databases allow their content and software infrastructures to be optimized and updated according to user feedback, greatly increasing the convenience and efficiency of metabolic pathway analysis of biological systems.

3 Translational Applications of Microbial Metabolomics

3.1 Diagnosis of Infectious Diseases Caused by Pathogenic Microbes

Many infectious diseases, such as UTI, spleen-yang-deficiency syndrome (SYDS), and CF-associated lung disease, cause serious issues to patients' health. However, diagnosis of these diseases remains highly challenging due to the lack of effective biomarkers. Fortunately, the applications of microbial metabolomics have significantly contributed to the diagnosis of infection diseases. UTI is a serious disease worldwide that mainly affects females, and the most common pathogen is *E. coli* [2]. LC-MS was used to globally profile the metabolites in urine from healthy controls and patients with UTI, and several potential biomarkers were identified successfully (Fig. 5) [32]. Lam et al. applied proton NMR spectroscopy to analyzing 88 urine samples from UTI patients and demonstrated that trimethylamine (TMA) could serve as a human-microbial marker of UTI associated with *E. coli*, and NMR-based urinalysis could aid the etiological diagnosis of this infectious disease [33].

SYDS is a typical syndrome in traditional Chinese medicine (TCM). Patients with SYDS can be distinguished from healthy controls by performing liquid chromatography/quadrupole time-of-flight mass spectrometry (LC-QTOF-MS)-based metabolomics and 16S rRNA sequencing because the number of *Firmicutes* and *Clostridia* bacteria that contribute to energy dysfunction is increased in the gut of SYDS patients. Therefore, *Firmicutes* and *Clostridia* bacteria may become new markers for the diagnosis of SYDS via microbial metabolomics coupled with 16S rRNA sequencing [34]. *Pseudomonas aeruginosa* is one of the most common pathogens and causes CF-associated lung disease. By analyzing the metabolites of CF patients and non-CF patients via LC-MS/MS, sphingolipids were found to be the most abundant molecules in the sputum of CF patients. This study showed that microbial

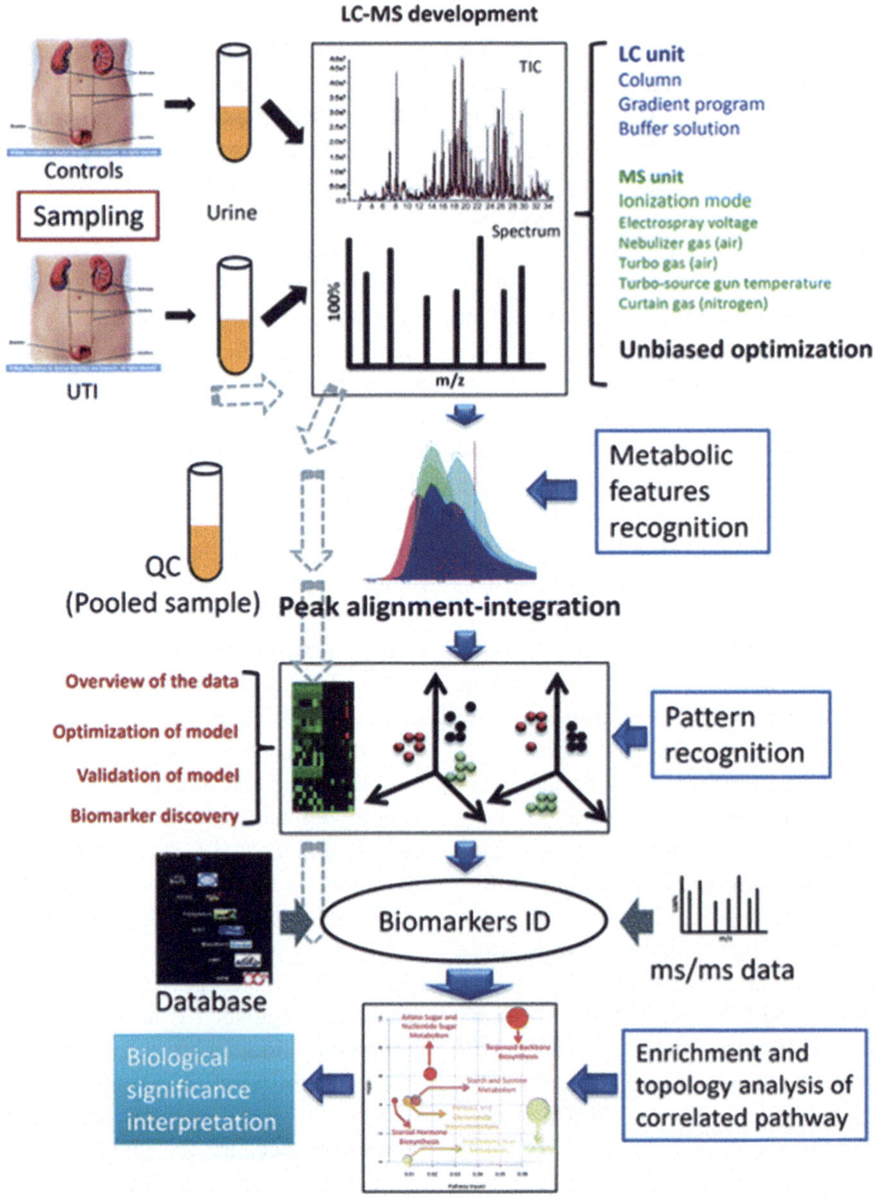

Fig. 5 LC-MS-based global metabolic profiling platform for human urine from healthy controls and patients with UTI

metabolomics could identify specific compounds that are abundant in clinical samples to help diagnose the disease [35].

Microbial metabolomics could also improve the diagnosis of inflammatory bowel disease (IBD), Crohn's disease (CD), and ulcerative colitis (UC) caused by the gut microbiota by identifying the altered metabolite signatures in biological samples [36]. For instance, GC-MS was performed to analyze the fecal samples from 20 UC patients, 22 CD patients, 26 IBS patients, and 19 healthy controls and reveal the increased levels of ester and alcohol derivatives of short chain fatty acids (SCFAs) and indole in the CD group [27]. Based on ^{1}H-NMR analysis, the levels of 3-hydroxybutyrate, β-glucose, α-glucose, and phenylalanine were found to be significantly increased and lipid levels were significantly decreased in the serum samples of UC patients compared to healthy controls [4]. In addition, urinary metabolites, including those originating from the gut microbiota, such as hippurate, acetate, methanol, methylamine and formate, TCA cycle intermediates, creatine, urea, taurine, and trigonelline, were identified as potential biomarkers to distinguish IBD patients from healthy controls [38]. Ahmed et al. reported a comprehensive study of the fecal volatile organic metabolites (VOMs) in the patients with diarrhea-predominant IBS (IBS-D, n = 30), CD (n = 62) or UC (n = 48), and healthy controls (n = 109). Fecal VOMs were extracted by solid-phase microextraction and analyzed by GC-MS. In total, 240 VOMs were identified. Esters of short chain fatty acids, cyclohexanecarboxylic acid, and its ester derivatives were associated with IBS-D, while aldehydes were more abundant in IBD. A predictive model, developed by multivariate analysis, could differentiate IBS-D from active CD, UC, and healthy controls with high sensitivity and specificity [39].

3.2 Pathogenesis Annotation of Microbial Infections

Although many drugs have been developed to treat infections, patients also experience side effects due to the nonspecificity of drug targets. In this regard, microbial metabolomics may be a useful tool to better understand the pathogenesis of infectious diseases and to promote precision treatment. Infections such as T1D, neonatal necrotizing enterocolitis (NEC), and UTI are increasingly prevalent conditions associated with gut microbiota, and the early mechanism of these illnesses remains elusive. By profiling the serum metabolites from transgenic mice with a combined LC-MS and GC-MS approach, decreased levels of lysophosphatidylcholine (LPC) and methionine and accumulation of ceramides were observed, which may facilitate our understanding of early T1D pathogenesis [40]. NEC mainly leads to the mortality of infants with very low birth weight. Metabolomics and next-generation sequencing tools have been used to investigate the contribution of intestinal microbes to NEC pathogenesis. The role of intestinal microbes was redefined and numerous evidences support the supported the hypothesis that NEC is a microbe-mediated disorder [41].

In addition, NMR has been used to determine the relationship between siderophores (secondary metabolites of microorganisms) and the pathogenesis of *E. coli*, the gut microorganism that causes UTI, demonstrating that the molecular interactions between the host and pathogen provide novel insight into pathogenesis (Fig. 6)

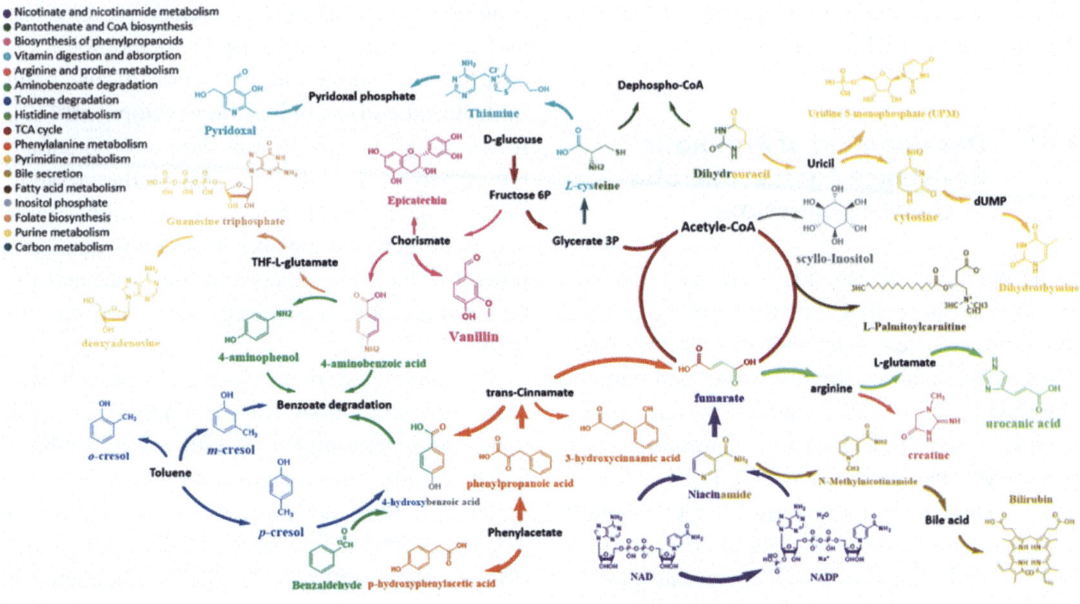

Fig. 6 Urinary metabolites altered by siderophore treatment, as identified via NMR spectroscopy, and related metabolic pathways

[42]. Similarly, GC-MS was employed to explore the relationships among the host, *Salmonella enterica* serovar Typhimurium (*S.* Typhimurium), and the commensal gut bacteria during *S.* Typhimurium-mediated intestinal infection, and the data demonstrated the accumulation of metabolites consumed by commensal microbes. This result offers insights into the molecular interplay among the host, pathogen, and commensal microbes during pathogenesis [43].

Liver disease is a serious illness worldwide, and HCV is the leading cause, but the pathogenesis of HCV is not fully understood. Fortunately, some progress has been made with the help of microbial metabolomics. For instance, Sun and colleagues applied UPLC/ESI-SYNAPT-HDMS to analysis of metabolites of an HCV animal model and identified 38 distinct compounds, such as hypotaurine, glycerophospholipid, and tryptophan, as effective biomarkers for HCV diagnosis and pathogenesis [44]. Another microbe, *Mycobacterium leprae*, causes leprosy, which mainly infects the skin and peripheral nervous system. UPLC-MS was used to investigate the serum samples from the patients with high bacterial indices (BIs) and low BIs, and the levels of arachidonic acid, eicosapentaenoic acid, and docosahexaenoic acid were found to significantly increase, particularly in high-BI patients, which may serve as potential biomarkers and facilitate the study of high-BI pathogenesis [45].

3.3 Development of Antibiotic Resistance Against Microbe-Associated Infections

Penicillin and sulfonamide were the first two effective antimicrobials, and the former has saved thousands of lives. A number of other prevalent antibiotics such as streptomycin, aureomycin, chloramphenicol, and kanamycin were subsequently discovered. However, antibiotic resistance (AR) has emerged with misuse, overuse, and even underuse of antibiotics. In fact, the main reason for the lack of success in AR control is that the wide range of biochemical and physiological mechanisms is poorly understood due to the complexity of the processes that contribute to the emergence and dissemination of resistance [46]. Nonetheless, microbial metabolomics may have potential applications in the control of AR because most AR processes consume cellular energy, which leads to clear downstream changes in microbial metabolism [47].

Biofilms are sessile communities of microbes, usually bacteria or fungi, on surfaces or liquid-air interfaces. Biofilms are closely associated with many health problems, such as UTI, dental caries, chronic osteomyelitis, and CF-associated lung infection. However, these diseases are difficult to treat due to the resistance of biofilms to antibiotics [2]. To overcome the resistance, both MS- and NMR-based metabolomics have recently been used to study biofilms. For instance, Stipetic et al. demonstrated a novel extraction method via bead beating in a chloroform/methanol/water extraction solvent, and the metabolites were then analyzed by LC-MS to detect metabolic alterations between biofilm and planktonic cells of *S. aureus*. Significant changes in arginine biosynthesis were identified [48]. Another study by Hess et al. was performed on a biofilm of *S. aureus* with ^{1}H NMR, and low oxygen concentrations were found to inhibit biofilm formation and regulate the ability of gentamicin and vancomycin. The results showed differential metabolomic profiles between aerobic and anaerobic biofilms and demonstrated that microbial metabolomics is an effective tool for identification of the main molecules involved in biofilm development [49]. In addition, mannoside was shown to potentiate the activity of trimethoprim-sulfamethoxazole in the treatment of UTI [50]. All these studies indicate that microbial metabolomics may serve as a powerful tool to understand the mechanisms underlying the resistance of biofilms to antibiotics.

An untargeted metabolomics approach was used to quantify the short-term metabolic changes that occur in treating *E. coli* with several antibiotics; this study was performed with QTOF-MS to understand the mechanisms of drug action and determine approaches to potentially address AR (Fig. 7). The results revealed that an imbalance of ammonium could improve chloramphenicol tox-

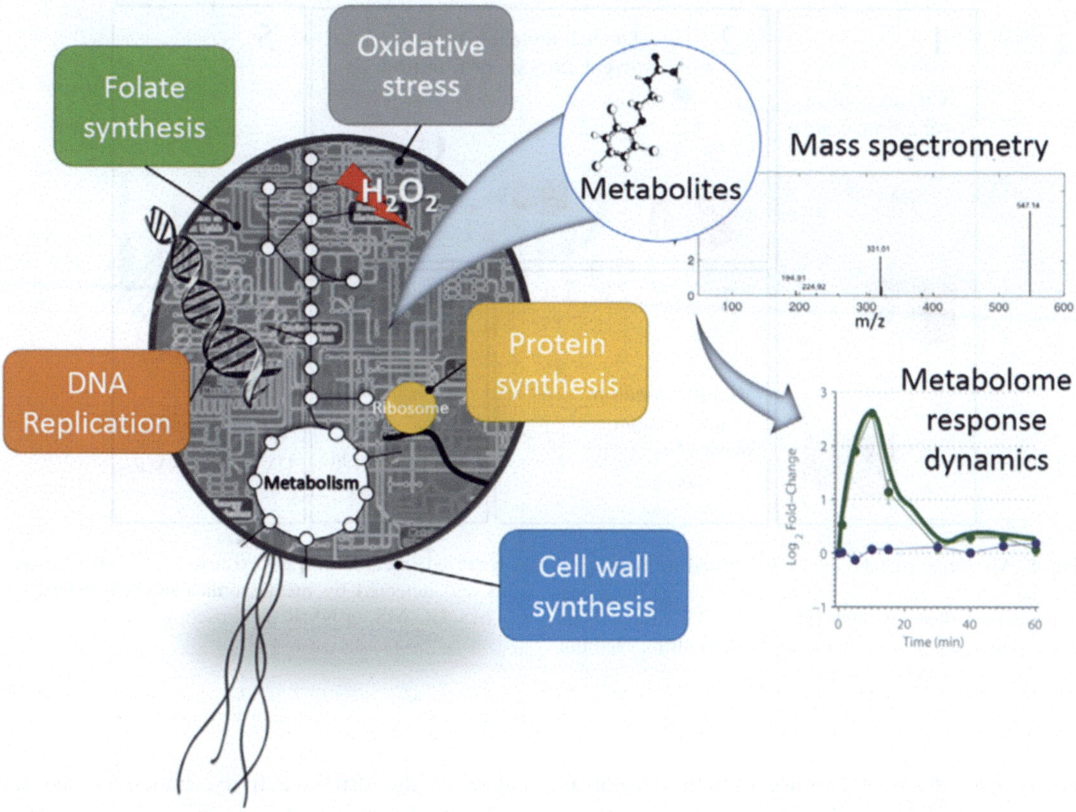

Fig. 7 Monitoring of short-term metabolic changes in *E. coli* after exposure to antibiotics by QTOF-MS

icity and the function of dTDP-rhamnose synthesis in response to quinolone antibiotics [51]. *Klebsiella pneumoniae*, a major pathogen of bloodstream infections, is also an AR-associated strain. Rees and colleagues applied GC × GC-TOFMS to profiling the volatile compounds produced by *K. pneumoniae* in human blood and identified 33 volatile metabolites that are abundant in the pathogenic strain [52]. In addition, *Campylobacter jejuni* (*C. jejuni*), a foodborne microbe, is a great burden on human health due to resistance to antibiotics. UPLC–TOF/MS was used to profile metabolites and discover metabolic signatures associated with chloramphenicol and florfenicol resistance-causing mutations in *C. jejuni*. Up to 41 differential metabolites involved in glycerophospholipid metabolism, sphingolipid metabolism, and fatty acid metabolism were observed in a chloramphenicol-resistant mutant strain of *C. jejuni*. A panel of 40 features was identified in florfenicol-resistant mutants, demonstrating changes in glycerophospholipid metabolism, sphingolipid metabolism, and tryptophan metabolism. This study shows that the UPLC-MS-based metabolomics is a promising and valuable tool to generate new insights into the drug-resistant mechanism of *C. jejuni* [53].

3.4 Treatment of Infectious Diseases Caused by Pathogenic Microbes

Although traditional antibiotics have saved millions of lives and revolutionized the treatment of infectious diseases, side effects associated with the broad use of antibiotics, such as increased

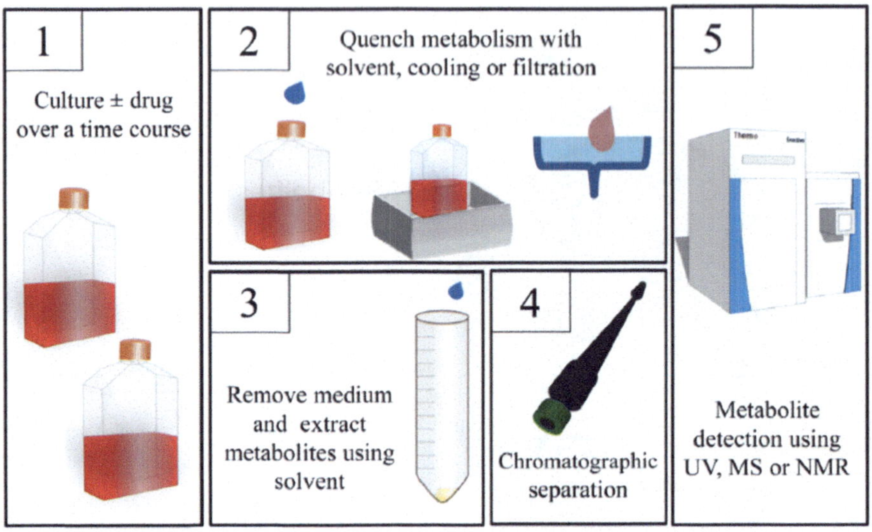

Fig. 8 Microbial metabolomics is applied to investigating the systems actions of antimicrobial drugs involving therapeutic efficiency and toxicology. Microorganisms are grown in the medium with and without drug. Medium is removed; metabolites are extracted from microorganisms and detected by metabolomics methods based on LC-MS, GC-MS, or NMR spectroscopy

emergence of AR and indiscriminate disruption of the beneficial microbiota, have stimulated the need for alternative treatment strategies [54, 55]. One approach is the development of a new generation of antimicrobials that mitigate the spread of AR. Microbial metabolomics could provide the opportunity to understand the biochemistry and pathogenesis of microbial pathogens and facilitate the discovery and development of novel anti-infective drugs [56]. Therefore, investigation of the targets and action modes of drugs via metabolomics can be used to predict the safety and efficacy of a drug (Fig. 8) [57]. For example, a quantitative metabolomics analysis of non-mevalonate isoprenoid synthesis in *Plasmodium falciparum* identified the primary antiparasitic activity of fosmidomycin, and this study will guide future research on the chemical modification of fosmidomycin for treating infections [58]. To investigate the activity of benznidazole, a drug proven to be effective against Chagas disease caused by *Trypanosoma cruzi* (*T. cruzi*), an untargeted LC-MS-based metabolomics approach was developed, and the results revealed that covalent binding of benznidazole with thiols is a primary cause of the drug's activity, which helped us understand the natural variation in *T. cruzi* [59]. A multiomics analysis has facilitated our understanding of the molecular mechanism of eflornithine resistance in African trypanosomes. Metabolic profiling of wild-type *Trypanosoma brucei* (*T. brucei*) and eflornithine-resistant *T. brucei* showed that eflornithine levels were greatly reduced in resistant cells compared to the wild type, and genetic analysis confirmed the role of TbAAT6 (*T. brucei* eflornithine transporter AAT6) in eflornithine action [60]. In addition, triphenylbismuthdichloride (TPBC) has been proven to have toxic effects on many antibiotic-resistant strains, such as methicillin-resistant *Staphylococcus aureus* (*S. aureus*) and vancomycin-resistant enterococci. The use of exometabolomic approaches to monitor metabolic changes in *S. aureus* treated with TPBC showed that this compound has potent antimicrobial activity against many bacterial pathogens, acting by blocking bacterial pyruvate catabolism. Enzymatic studies indicated that TPBC is a highly efficient inhibitor of the bacterial pyruvate dehydrogenase complex [61].

In addition to the development of new antimicrobials, there are alternative approaches for the treatment of infectious diseases, such as photodynamic therapy (PDT), radioimmunotherapy, and bacteriophage treatment. PDT is a technique that combines a nontoxic dye, photosensitizer (PS), and low-intensity visible light in the presence of oxygen to produce cytotoxic species for killing cells [62]. PDT treatment using Green 2 W as the PS has been reported to have a significant effect against *Aspergillus fumigatus* in vitro [63]. Radioimmunotherapy is theoretically useful as an anti-infective therapy against any microbe (including bacteria, fungi, viruses, and parasites) susceptible to radiation. Studies have shown the applicability of radioimmunotherapy to treat *Streptococcus pneumoniae* infections [64]. The efficacy of phages in the treatment of bacterial disease in animal models has been demonstrated, and bacteriophage treatment is a feasible alternative treatment modality for microbe-infected diseases [65]. Nonetheless,

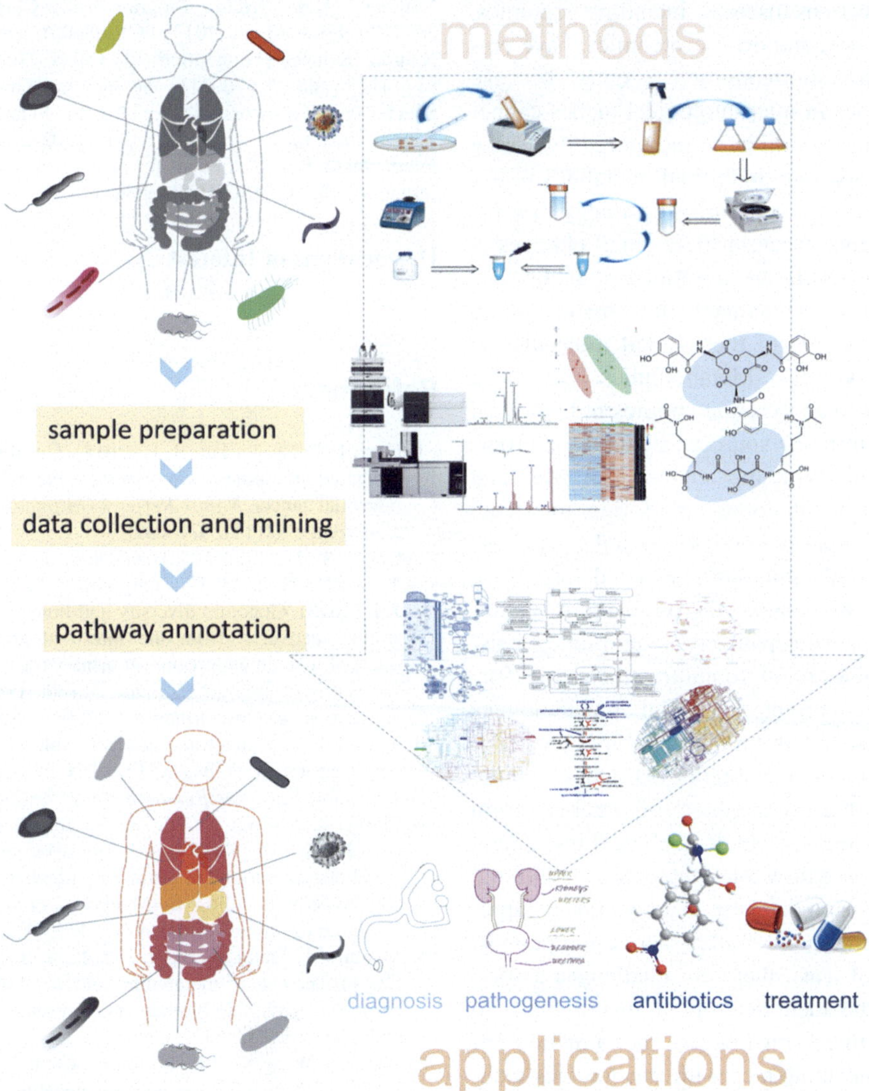

Fig. 9 Overview of microbial metabolomics: from methods to applications

although many therapeutic strategies against infectious diseases have been reported, these strategies remain in the stage of in vitro or animal model experiments.

4 Concluding Remarks and Future Perspective

Microbes contribute to serious infections, such as UTI, CF-associated lung disease, diabetes, and many other diseases, which remain a leading cause of death worldwide. Conventional methods to study infectious diseases, including genomics, transcriptomics, and even proteomics, have presented some shortcomings recently because minor changes in microbiological niches cannot be precisely and directly monitored by these methods. Targeting microbial metabolism has been considered as a promising strategy to solve these problems, because these small changes at gene/protein levels are amplified at metabolite level, which offers valuable information about the functional role of these small molecules in microbial systems. Metabolomics has been widely used to analyze metabolites in biological samples from many sources, including microorganisms [66]. With the advances of MS- and NMR-based metabolomics platforms, microbial metabolomics has been demonstrated as a powerful tool to study microbe-associated infections, particularly the diagnostic biomarkers, pathogenic mechanisms/pathways, antibiotic resistance, and new antimicrobial treatment (Fig. 9).

However, current microbial metabolomics approach has certain limitations. First, the existing methods of metabolite extraction cannot extract all the metabolites of interest from samples. Second, no single analytical instrument alone can perform whole-metabolome profiling. Third, there is no database that contains comprehensive information for all bioactive compounds. Last, but not least, there are challenges associated with the identification of metabolites. To overcome these challenges, combination of microbial metabolomics with other omics technologies, such as genomics, transcriptomics, and proteomics, may become a leading methodology in microbial research.

We hope that this critical review will inspire scientific communities to pay more attention to microbial metabolism from a metabolomics perspective and will significantly advance the discovery and translational applications of microbial metabolomics in clinical diagnosis and pathogenesis, as well as in the discovery of novel therapeutics against a variety of complex infections caused by rapidly expanding microbes.

Acknowledgments This work was supported by the National Key R&D Program of China (No. 2017YFC1308600 and 2017YFC1308605), the National Natural Science Foundation of China Grants (No. 81274175 and 31670031), the Startup Funding for Specialized Professorship Provided by Shanghai Jiao Tong University (No. WF220441502), and the Fundamental Research Funds for the Central Universities (grant no. 106112015CDJZR468808).

Declarations of Interest None.

References

1. Cani, P. D., & Jordan, B. F. (2018). Gut microbiota-mediated inflammation in obesity: A link with gastrointestinal cancer. *Nature Reviews Gastroenterology & Hepatology, 15*(11), 671–682.
2. Chen, S. L., Wu, M., Henderson, J. P., Hooton, T. M., Hibbing, M. E., Hultgren, S. J., & Gordon, J. I. (2013). Genomic diversity and fitness of *E. Coli* strains recovered from the intestinal and urinary tracts of women with recurrent urinary tract infection. *Science Translational Medicine, 5*, 160r–184r.
3. Saccenti, E., & Timmerman, M. E. (2016). Approaches to sample size determination for multivariate data: Applications to PCA and PLS-DA of omics data. *Journal of Proteome Research, 15*, 2379–2393.
4. Zhang, Y., Lin, L., Xu, Y., Lin, Y., Jin, Y., & Zheng, C. (2013). 1h NMR-based spectroscopy detects metabolic alterations in serum of patients with early-stage ulcerative colitis. *Biochemical and Biophysical Research Communications, 433*, 547–551.
5. Mamas, M., Dunn, W. B., Neyses, L., & Goodacre, R. (2011). The role of metabolites and metabolomics in clinically applicable biomarkers of disease. *Archives of Toxicology, 85*, 5–17.
6. Wang, J., Wang, C., Liu, H., Qi, H., Chen, H., & Wen, J. (2018). Metabolomics assisted metabolic network modeling and network wide analysis of metabolites in

microbiology. *Critical Reviews in Biotechnology, 38*, 1–15.
7. Koek, M. M., Muilwijk, B., van der Werf, M. J., & Hankemeier, T. (2006). Microbial metabolomics with gas chromatography/mass spectrometry. *Analytical Chemistry, 78*, 1272–1281.
8. Garcia, D. E., Baidoo, E. E., Benke, P. I., Pingitore, F., Tang, Y. J., Villa, S., & Keasling, J. D. (2008). Separation and mass spectrometry in microbial metabolomics. *Current Opinion in Microbiology, 11*, 233–239.
9. Wu, X., Yu, H., Ba, Z., Chen, J., Sun, H., & Han, B. (2010). Sampling methods for NMR-based metabolomics of *Staphylococcus Aureus*. *Biotechnology Journal, 5*, 75–84.
10. Dunn, W. B., & Ellis, D. I. (2005). Metabolomics: Current analytical platforms and methodologies. *TrAC Trends in Analytical Chemistry, 24*, 285–294.
11. Mashego, M. R., Rumbold, K., De Mey, M., Vandamme, E., Soetaert, W., & Heijnen, J. J. (2007). Microbial metabolomics: Past, present and future methodologies. *Biotechnology Letters, 29*, 1–16.
12. Cortina, N. S., Krug, D., Plaza, A., Revermann, O., & Müller, R. (2012). Myxoprincomide: A natural product from *Myxococcus Xanthus* discovered by comprehensive analysis of the secondary metabolome. *Angewandte Chemie International Edition, 51*, 811–816.
13. Marcobal, A., Kashyap, P. C., Nelson, T. A., Aronov, P. A., Donia, M. S., Spormann, A., Fischbach, M. A., & Sonnenburg, J. L. (2013). A metabolomic view of how the human gut microbiota impacts the host metabolome using humanized and gnotobiotic mice. *The ISME Journal, 7*, 1933–1943.
14. Southam, A. D., Weber, R. J., Engel, J., Jones, M. R., & Viant, M. R. (2016). A complete workflow for high-resolution spectral-stitching nanoelectrospray direct-infusion mass-spectrometry-based metabolomics and lipidomics. *Nature Protocols, 12*, 310–328.
15. Cloarec, O., Dumas, M.-E., Craig, A., Barton, R. H., Trygg, J., Hudson, J., Blancher, C., Gauguier, D., Lindon, J. C., Holmes, E., & Nicholson, J. (2005). Statistical total correlation spectroscopy: An exploratory approach for latent biomarker identification from metabolic 1H NMR data sets. *Analytical Chemistry, 77*(5), 1282–1289.
16. Lv, H. (2013). Mass spectrometry-based metabolomics towards understanding of gene functions with a diversity of biological contexts. *Mass Spectrometry Reviews, 32*, 118–128.
17. Wang, C., Li, M., Jiang, H., Tong, H., Feng, Y., Wang, Y., Pi, X., Guo, L., Nie, M., Feng, H., & Li, E. (2016). Comparative analysis of VOCs in exhaled breath of amyotrophic lateral sclerosis and cervical spondylotic myelopathy patients. *Science Reports-UK, 6*, 26120.
18. Frolkis, A., Knox, C., Lim, E., Jewison, T., Law, V., Hau, D. D., Liu, P., Gautam, B., Ly, S., Guo, A. C., Xia, J., Liang, Y., Shrivastava, S., & Wishart, D. S. (2010). SMPDB: The small molecule pathway database. *Nucleic Acids Research, 38*, D480–D487.
19. Croft, D., O'Kelly, G., Wu, G., Haw, R., Gillespie, M., Matthews, L., Caudy, M., Garapati, P., Gopinath, G., Jassal, B., Jupe, S., Kalatskaya, I., Mahajan, S., May, B., Ndegwa, N., Schmidt, E., Shamovsky, V., Yung, C., Birney, E., Hermjakob, H., D'Eustachio, P., & Stein, L. (2010). Reactome: A database of reactions, pathways and biological processes. *Nucleic Acids Research, 39*, D691–D697.
20. Joshi-Tope, G. (2004). Reactome: A knowledgebase of biological pathways. *Nucleic Acids Research, 33*, D428–D432.
21. Kanehisa, M. (2004). The KEGG resource for deciphering the genome. *Nucleic Acids Research, 32*, 277D–280D.
22. Kanehisa, M., Goto, S., Sato, Y., Kawashima, M., Furumichi, M., & Tanabe, M. (2013). Data, information, knowledge and principle: Back to metabolism in KEGG. *Nucleic Acids Research, 42*, D199–D205.
23. Karp, P. D. (2005). Expansion of the biocyc collection of pathway/genome databases to 160 genomes. *Nucleic Acids Research, 33*, 6083–6089.
24. Xia, J., & Wishart, D. S. (2010). MetPA: A web-based metabolomics tool for pathway analysis and visualization. *Bioinformatics, 26*, 2342–2344.
25. Krummenacker, M., Paley, S., Mueller, L., Yan, T., & Karp, P. D. (2005). Querying and computing with biocyc databases. *Bioinformatics, 21*, 3454–3455.
26. Xia, J., & Wishart, D. S. (2011). Web-based inference of biological patterns, functions and pathways from metabolomic data using MetaboAnalyst. *Nature Protocols, 6*, 743–760.
27. Chong, J., Soufan, O., Li, C., Caraus, I., Li, S., Bourque, G., Wishart, D. S., & Xia, J. (2018). Metaboanalyst 4.0: Towards more transparent and integrative metabolomics analysis. *Nucleic Acids Research, 46*, W486–W494.
28. Neuweger, H., Albaum, S. P., Dondrup, M., Persicke, M., Watt, T., Niehaus, K., Stoye, J., & Goesmann, A. (2008). MeltDB: A software platform for the analysis and integration of metabolomics experiment data. *Bioinformatics, 24*, 2726–2732.
29. Wishart, D. S., Tzur, D., Knox, C., Eisner, R., Guo, A. C., Young, N., Cheng, D., Jewell, K., Arndt, D., Sawhney, S., Fung, C., Nikolai, L., Lewis, M., Coutouly, M. A., Forsythe, I., Tang, P., Shrivastava, S., Jeroncic, K., Stothard, P., Amegbey, G., Block, D., Hau, D. D., Wagner, J., Miniaci, J., Clements, M., Gebremedhin, M., Guo, N., Zhang, Y., Duggan, G. E., MacInnis, G. D., Weljie, A. M., Dowlatabadi, R., Bamforth, F., Clive, D., Greiner, R., Li, L., Marrie, T., Sykes, B. D., Vogel, H. J., & Querengesser, L. (2007). HMDB the human metabolome database. *Nucleic Acids Research, 35*, D521–D526.
30. Guijas, C., Montenegro-Burke, J. R., Domingo-Almenara, X., Palermo, A., Warth, B., Hermann, G., Koellensperger, G., Huan, T., Uritboonthai, W., Aisporna, A. E., Wolan, D. W., Spilker, M. E., Benton,

H. P., & Siuzdak, G. (2018). Metlin: A technology platform for identifying knowns and unknowns. *Analytical Chemistry, 90*, 3156–3164.

31. Cui, Q., Lewis, I. A., Hegeman, A. D., Anderson, M. E., Li, J., Schulte, C. F., Westler, W. M., Eghbalnia, H. R., Sussman, M. R., & Markley, J. L. (2008). Metabolite identification via the Madison metabolomics consortium database. *Nature Biotechnology, 26*, 162–164.
32. Lv, H., Hung, C. S., Chaturvedi, K. S., Hooton, T. M., & Henderson, J. P. (2011). Development of an integrated metabolomic profiling approach for infectious diseases research. *The Analyst, 136*, 4752.
33. Lam, C., Law, C., Sze, K., & To, K. K. (2015). Quantitative metabolomics of urine for rapid etiological diagnosis of urinary tract infection: Evaluation of a microbial-mammalian co-metabolite as a diagnostic biomarker. *Clinica Chimica Acta, 438*, 24–28.
34. Lin, Z., Ye, W., Zu, X., Xie, H., Li, H., Li, Y., & Zhang, W. (2018). Integrative metabolic and microbial profiling on patients with spleen-yang-deficiency syndrome. *Science Reports-UK, 8*, 6619.
35. Quinn, R. A., Phelan, V. V., Whiteson, K. L., Garg, N., Bailey, B. A., Lim, Y. W., Conrad, D. J., Dorrestein, P. C., & Rohwer, F. L. (2016). Microbial, host and xenobiotic diversity in the cystic fibrosis sputum metabolome. *The ISME Journal, 10*, 1483–1498.
36. Preter, V. D., & Verbeke, K. (2013). Metabolomics as a diagnostic tool in gastroenterology. *World Journal of Gastrointestinal Pharmacology and Therapeutics, 4*, 97.
37. Walton, C., Fowler, D. P., Turner, C., Jia, W., Whitehead, R. N., Griffiths, L., Dawson, C., Waring, R. H., Ramsden, D. B., Cole, J. A., Cauchi, M., Bessant, C., & Hunter, J. O. (2013). Analysis of volatile organic compounds of bacterial origin in chronic gastrointestinal diseases. *Inflammatory Bowel Diseases, 19*, 2069–2078.
38. Stephens, N. S., Siffledeen, J., Su, X., Murdoch, T. B., Fedorak, R. N., & Slupsky, C. M. (2013). Urinary NMR metabolomic profiles discriminate inflammatory bowel disease from healthy. *Journal of Crohn's and Colitis, 7*, e42–e48.
39. Ahmed, I., Greenwood, R., Costello, B. L., Ratcliffe, N. M., & Probert, C. S. (2013). An investigation of fecal volatile organic metabolites in irritable bowel syndrome. *PLoS One, 8*, e58204.
40. Overgaard, A. J., Weir, J. M., De Souza, D. P., Tull, D., Haase, C., Meikle, P. J., & Pociot, F. (2016). Lipidomic and metabolomic characterization of a genetically modified mouse model of the early stages of human type 1 diabetes pathogenesis. *Metabolomics, 12*, 13.
41. Morowitz, M. J., Poroyko, V., Caplan, M., Alverdy, J., & Liu, D. C. (2010). Redefining the role of intestinal microbes in the pathogenesis of necrotizing enterocolitis. *Pediatrics, 125*, 777–785.
42. Su, Q., Guan, T., & Lv, H. (2016). Siderophore biosynthesis coordinately modulated the virulence-associated interactive metabolome of uropathogenic *Escherichia Coli* and human urine. *Science Reports-UK, 6*, 24099.
43. Deatherage, K. B., Li, J., Sanford, J. A., Kim, Y. M., Kronewitter, S. R., Jones, M. B., Peterson, C. T., Peterson, S. N., Frank, B. C., Purvine, S. O., Brown, J. N., Metz, T. O., Smith, R. D., Heffron, F., & Adkins, J. N. (2013). A multi-omic view of host-pathogen-commensal interplay in salmonella-mediated intestinal infection. *PLoS One, 8*, e67155.
44. Sun, H., Zhang, A., Yan, G., Piao, C., Li, W., Sun, C., Wu, X., Li, X., Chen, Y., & Wang, X. (2013). Metabolomic analysis of key regulatory metabolites in hepatitis C virus-infected tree shrews. *Molecular & Cellular Proteomics, 12*, 710–719.
45. Al-Mubarak, R., Vander, H. J., Broeckling, C. D., Balagon, M., Brennan, P. J., & Vissa, V. D. (2011). Serum metabolomics reveals higher levels of polyunsaturated fatty acids in lepromatous leprosy: Potential markers for susceptibility and pathogenesis. *PLoS Neglected Tropical Diseases, 5*, e1303.
46. Davies, J., & Davies, D. (2010). Origins and evolution of antibiotic resistance. *Microbiology and Molecular Biology Reviews, 74*, 417–433.
47. Lobritz, M. A., Belenky, P., Porter, C. B. M., Gutierrez, A., Yang, J. H., Schwarz, E. G., Dwyer, D. J., Khalil, A. S., & Collins, J. J. (2015). Antibiotic efficacy is linked to bacterial cellular respiration. *Proceedings of the National Academy of Sciences, 112*, 8173–8180.
48. Stipetic, L. H., Dalby, M. J., Davies, R. L., Morton, F. R., Ramage, G., & Burgess, K. E. V. (2016). A novel metabolomic approach used for the comparison of *Staphylococcus Aureus* planktonic cells and biofilm samples. *Metabolomics, 12*, 1.
49. Hess, D. J., Henry-Stanley, M. J., Lusczek, E. R., Beilman, G. J., & Wells, C. L. (2013). Anoxia inhibits biofilm development and modulates antibiotic activity. *The Journal of Surgical Research, 184*, 488–494.
50. Guiton, P. S., Cusumano, C. K., Kline, K. A., Dodson, K. W., Han, Z., Janetka, J. W., Henderson, J. P., Caparon, M. G., & Hultgren, S. J. (2012). Combinatorial small-molecule therapy prevents uropathogenic *Escherichia Coli* catheter-associated urinary tract infections in mice. *Antimicrobial Agents Chemotherapy, 56*, 4738–4745.
51. Zampieri, M., Zimmermann, M., Claassen, M., & Sauer, U. (2017). Nontargeted metabolomics reveals the multilevel response to antibiotic perturbations. *Cell Reports, 19*, 1214–1228.
52. Rees, C. A., Smolinska, A., & Hill, J. E. (2016). The volatile metabolome of *Klebsiella Pneumoniae* in human blood. *Journal of Breath Research, 10*, 27101.
53. Li, H., Xia, X., Li, X., Naren, G., Fu, Q., Wang, Y., Wu, C., Ding, S., Zhang, S., Jiang, H., Li, J., & Shen, J. (2014). Untargeted metabolomic profiling of amphenicol-resistant campylobacter jejuni by ultra-high-performance liquid chromatography-mass spectrometry. *Journal of Proteome Research, 14*, 1060–1068.
54. Aminov, R. (2017). History of antimicrobial drug discovery: Major classes and health impact. *Biochemical Pharmacology, 133*, 4–19.
55. Dodds, D. R. (2017). Antibiotic resistance: a current epilogue. *Biochemical Pharmacology, 134*, 139–146.

56. de la Fuente-Nunez, C., Torres, M. D., Mojica, F. J., & Lu, T. K. (2017). Next-generation precision antimicrobials: Towards personalized treatment of infectious diseases. *Current Opinion in Microbiology, 37*, 95–102.
57. Vincent, I. M., & Barrett, M. P. (2015). Metabolomic-based strategies for anti-parasite drug discovery. *Journal of Biomolecular Screening, 20*, 44–55.
58. Yoshikawa, T. T. (2002). Antimicrobial resistance and aging: Beginning of the end of the antibiotic era? *Journal of the American Geriatrics Society, 50*, S226–S229.
59. Sajjan, U. S., Tran, L. T., Sole, N., Rovaldi, C., Akiyama, A., Friden, P. M., Forstner, J. F., & Rothstein, D. M. (2001). P-113d, an antimicrobial peptide active against *Pseudomonas Aeruginosa*, retains activity in the presence of sputum from cystic fibrosis patients. *Antimicrobial Agents and Chemotherapy, 45*, 3437–3444.
60. Paton, A. W., Morona, R., & Paton, J. C. (2012). Bioengineered microbes in disease therapy. *Trends in Molecular Medicine, 18*, 417–425.
61. Duan, F., & March, J. C. (2010). Engineered bacterial communication prevents vibrio cholerae virulence in an infant mouse model. *Proceedings of the National Academy of Sciences, 107*, 11260–11264.
62. Hamblin, M. R., & Hasan, T. (2004). Photodynamic therapy: A new antimicrobial approach to infectious disease? *Photochemical & Photobiological Sciences, 3*, 436–450.
63. Friedberg, J. S., Skema, C., Baum, E. D., Burdick, J., Vinogradov, S. A., Wilson, D. F., Horan, A. D., & Nachamkin, I. (2001). In vitro effects of photodynamic therapy on *Aspergillus Fumigatus*. *Journal of Antimicrobial Chemotherapy, 48*, 105–107.
64. Grellier, P., Santus, R., Mouray, E., Agmon, V., Maziere, J. C., Rigomier, D., Dagan, A., Gatt, S., & Schrevel, J. (1997). Photosensitized inactivation of plasmodium falciparum- and babesia divergens-infected erythrocytes in whole blood by lipophilic pheophorbide derivatives. *Vox Sanguinis, 72*, 211–220.
65. Cerveny, K. E., DePaola, A., Duckworth, D. H., & Gulig, P. A. (2002). Phage therapy of local and systemic disease caused by vibrio vulnificus in iron-dextran-treated mice. *Infection and Immunity, 70*, 6251–6262.
66. Yan, L., Nie, W., Parker, T., Upton, Z., & Lu, H. (2013). MS-based metabolomics facilitates the discovery of in vivo functional small molecules with a diversity of biological contexts. *Future Medicinal Chemistry, 5*, 1953–1965.

Tracer-Based Cancer Metabolomic Analysis

Jianzhou Liu, Jing Huang, and Gary Guishan Xiao

1 Introduction

Tumor metabolism is a vast network of metabolic pathways, such as oxidative phosphorylation, glycolysis, the tricarboxylic acid (TCA) cycle, the pentose phosphate pathway (PPP), and the synthesis of nucleotides and lipids. Corresponding functions of these metabolic pathways address the strong biosynthesis needs of rapid growth and reproduction of tumor cells. Otto Warburg first put forward that even with sufficient oxygen supply, tumor cells mainly generate energy (e.g., ATP) by non-oxidative breakdown of glucose (glycolysis). According to his hypothesis (Warburg effect), carcinogenesis stems from the lowering of mitochondrial respiration [1]. Ever since, reports of changes in glucose metabolism of cancer cells have been published extensively. Several signaling pathways contribute to the Warburg effect and other metabolic phenotypes of cancer cells (Fig. 1). For instance, most cancer cells and tissues exhibit high lactate (Lac) secretion rates [2]. There are also strong evidences supporting that tumor cell proliferation can be greatly contributed by the anabolic effects of glutamine [3]. In fact, studies have shown that glycolysis-preferred tumor cells consume more glutamine than normal cells to synthesize proteins, nucleotides, and fatty acids, thereby producing energy to meet the vigorous growth and reproduction needs [4, 5].

In cancer biology, a main bottleneck is to elucidate the cancer metabolism in vivo, which can lead to targets for diagnostics or therapeutics. Metabolomics refers to a global-scale analysis of metabolites in a biological system. In fact, measuring intracellular metabolites is a practical way to record the "snapshots" of biological processes [6]. However, the best method for studying metabolic pathways is to measure flux, which describes the genuine function of specific enzymes or pathways [7]. To this end, the combination of isotope tracers and computational algorithms enable quantitative analysis of intracellular fluxes intensity and relevant confidence intervals in metabolic control systems [8]. The interaction between the central carbon metabolic pathway and other metabolic pathways have been studied with a stable isotope tracer method by using ^{13}C-glucose, ^{15}N-glutamine, ^{13}C-propionate, and other labeled substrates [9]. Stable isotope tracing provides a powerful approach to studying the physiological processes in tumor and its surrounding microenvironment. These methods,

J. Liu · J. Huang
School of Pharmaceutical Science and Technology, Dalian University of Technology, Dalian, China

G. G. Xiao (✉)
School of Pharmaceutical Science and Technology, Dalian University of Technology, Dalian, China

Center of Functional Genomics and Proteomics, Creighton University Medical Center, Omaha, NE, USA
e-mail: gxiao@dlut.edu.cn

S. Hu (ed.), *Cancer Metabolomics*, Advances in Experimental Medicine and Biology 1280,
https://doi.org/10.1007/978-3-030-51652-9_8

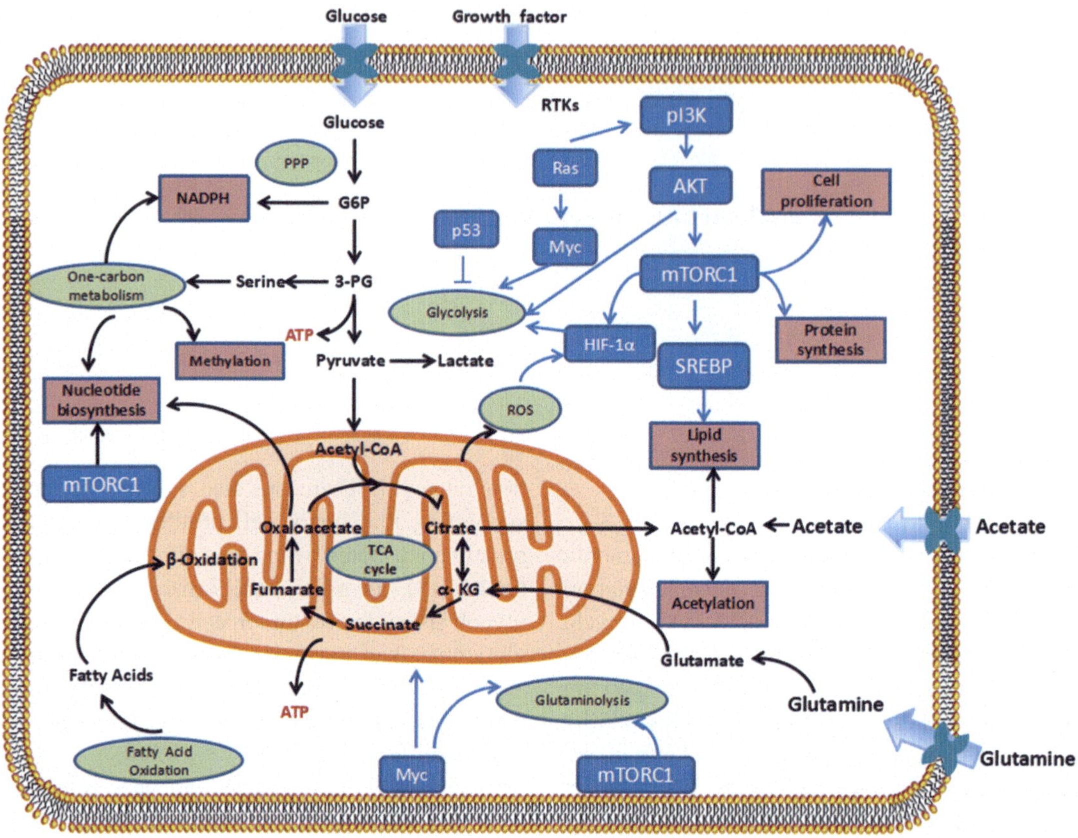

Fig. 1 Signaling pathways that may contribute to the Warburg effect in cancer cells

which usually based on nuclear magnetic resonance spectroscopy (NMR) or mass spectrometry (MS), may find key applications in the study of cancer diseases and advancing personalized medicine for cancer patients in the future [10], and these methodologies can be applied to both in vitro and in vivo studies [6]. In this chapter, we will focus on Stable Isotope Resolution Metabolomics (SIRM) and its applications to studying cancer metabolism.

2 Isotope Analysis of Cancer Metabolism

The isotopic tracer is a compound consisting of one or more tracer atoms. One atom-labeled compound is called a single-labeled tracer whereas a compound with two atoms labeled is called a double-labeled tracer (e.g., $^{2}H_2{}^{18}O$). Tracers can be used to effectively study the unique metabolic pathways of cancer cells. It can also help identifying the complicated interplay among interacting metabolic pathways. Recently, stable isotope-labeled glucose and glutamine have been used as metabolic tracers for cancer metabolism studies. Researchers have used isotopes with a low natural abundance, such as ^{13}C or ^{15}N, as tracer labels and then analyze the ^{13}C and/or ^{15}N distribution within the metabolites to determine the contribution of different metabolic pathways.

2.1 ^{13}C Isotopic Tracer

Since the glycolysis flux significantly increases in cancer cells, ^{13}C-glucose (^{13}C-Glc) tracer can be used to effectively monitor glycolysis. Newly produced ^{13}C-enriched pyruvate equilibrates with lactate and leads to the formation of ^{13}C-enriched lactate, which is distinguishable from the non-enriched counterpart. Due to their fast anabolic processes, cancer cells demand for increased glutamine-derived carbons. Recent reports have shown that reductive carboxylation of α-ketoglutarate (α-KG) by isocitrate dehydrogenase 1 (IDH1) and 2 (IDH2) is a major source of citrate synthesis from glutamine. ^{13}C-Glutamine (^{13}C-Gln) can be used as a tracer to monitor the glutaminolysis flux in cancer cells.

The PPP, which branches from glycolysis at the first committed step of glucose metabolism, is required for the synthesis of ribonucleotides. It is a major source of nicotinamide adenine dinucleotide phosphate (NAPDH), a reducing agent required and consumed during fatty acid synthesis and the scavenging of reactive oxygen species (ROS) [7]. Therefore, the PPP plays an important role in cancer cell metabolism and survival. The involvement of the PPP pathway in overall cellular metabolism can be easily monitored from the analysis of the lactate isotopomer following the administration of [2-^{13}C] Glc [8]. Most of cancer cells have a plethora of oncogene-driven metabolic changes in order to sustain fast growth and proliferation [9]. The use of ^{13}C tracers can clearly detect these metabolic differences between cancer and normal cells.

2.2 ^{15}N Isotopic Tracer

Nucleotides are continually synthesized de novo in cells [10], and glutamine serves as an essential substrate for key enzymes involved in the de novo synthesis of purine and pyrimidine nucleotides. Recently, liquid chromatography mass spectrometry (LC-MS) has been used to quantify glutamine-derived ^{15}N flux into nucleosides and nucleobases (purines and pyrimidines). DNA from bladder cancer cell line is cultured in ^{15}N-labeled glutamine and then enzymatically hydrolyzed by sequential digestion. Subsequently, DNA hydrolysates were separated by LC-MS and selected reaction monitoring (SRM) was employed to identify and quantify the nucleobases and nucleosides. The results indicated that ^{15}N-glutamine flux measurement using LC-MS/MS-SRM can be used for discrimination of aggressive tumors from nonaggressive tumors and may be further adapted for high-throughput analysis of a large set of DNA in a clinical setting [11].

The glutamine and citrulline are indispensable in cell metabolisms and act as fuel source and product, respectively. It has been shown that the administration of ^{15}N-labeled glutamine results in the incorporation of the ^{15}N label into citrulline, but it is not clear which of the three nitrogen groups of citrulline is actually labeled. A rapid LC-MS/MS method was developed to determine the ^{15}N enrichment of the positional isomers of glutamine and citrulline. The method developed provides an additional insight into the metabolism of glutamine and citrulline tracing the precursor-product relationship between these two amino acids [12].

2.3 ^{2}H Isotope Tracer

NADPH is involved in a variety of metabolic reactions, such as the synthesis of lipids, fatty acids, and nucleotides [13]. In order to analyze the dynamic changes in the metabolic substrates converted to NADPH, a D_2-based tracing method has been developed to quantitatively analyze the differences and dynamic changes of NADPH by different metabolic pathways [14]. In cancer cells, the PPP and malic enzyme produce about 30% of NADPH, respectively, while one-carbon metabolism produces about 40% of NADPH. This suggests that one-carbon metabolism plays an important role in cancer cell survival. As metabolism precursors, serine and glycine are used to produce NADPH by one-carbon metabolism. During cell culture, [2,3,3-$^{2}H_3$] serine or [2,2--$^{2}H_2$] glycine can be used for tracing [^{2}H]-NADPH in the cells. As shown in Fig. 2, the conversion of serine to glycine is catalyzed by serine hydroxymethyl transferase 2 to produce NADPH. Similarly, the labeling glycine with ^{2}H reveals that glycine is catalyzed by glycine decarboxylase to produce NADPH.

NADPH is used as an electron carrier for maintaining redox homeostasis and reducing bio-

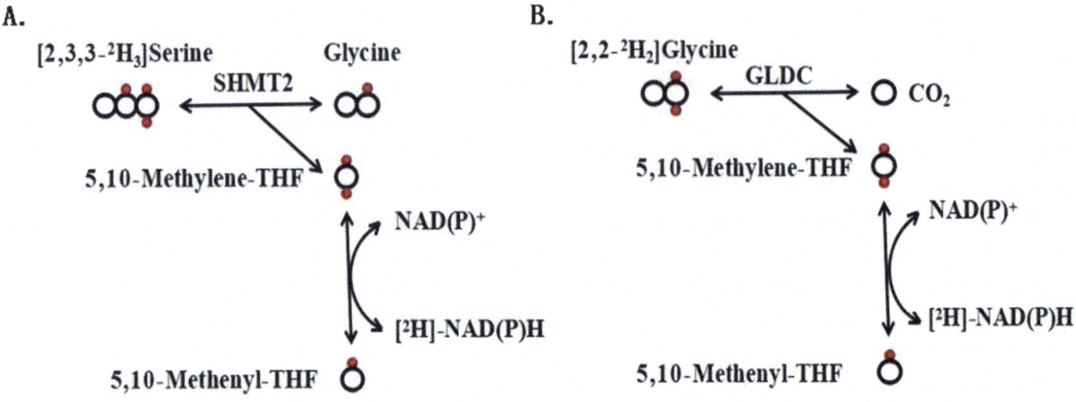

Fig. 2 ^{2}H-labeled amino acid tracers to study one-carbon metabolism in mitochondria [15]. (**a**): Deuterium-labeled serine for NADPH tracing; (**b**): deuterium-labeled glycine for NADPH tracing *SHMT2*, serine hydroxymethyl transferase 2; *GLDC*, glycine decarboxylase; *5,10-methylene-THF*, 5,10-methylene-tetrahydrofolate; *5,10-methenyl-THF*, 5,10-methenyl-tetrahydrofolate

synthesis, wherein individual cytoplasmic and mitochondrial pools provide reducing power at each respective location. This cellular organization of reducing power is critical for many functions, but the use of existing methods complicates metabolic pathway analysis. Theoretically, as much as half of the hydrogen transferred to NADH by GAPDH is derived from glucose. However, exchange with water in the aldolase and triosephosphate isomerase (TPI) reactions reduces the net contribution of the hydrogen atom to NADH (Fig. 3). Lewis et al. [15] cultured A549 and H1299 cells with [4-^{2}H] glucose to trace NADH metabolism. They observed metabolic pathway activity in these distinct cellular compartments and determined the direction of serine/glycine interconversion within the mitochondria and cytosol, highlighting the ability of this approach to resolve compartmentalized reactions in intact cells.

3 Flux Measurement

In order to better understand the metabolic activity as well as the concentration of metabolites, it is also needed to quantify metabolic flux, which is the most direct measurement of enzyme activities in living systems. Kinetic flux profiling is a pioneering method for the quantification of metabolic flux in cultured cells. Briefly, the cells are cultured with identical media that contains isotope-labeled nutrients instead of common media, which will lead to labeling of downstream metabolites. This supplies the information of metabolic flows, even in non-steady-state conditions (e.g., drug treatment and transient nutrient deprivation). Table 1 lists different labeled substrates and related applications to tracing multifaceted metabolism. For instance, ^{13}C-Gln tracing can probe TCA cycle efflux and turning, whereas ^{15}N-Gln tracing can probe the synthetic processes of amino acids and nucleotides. Tracing with these tracers can reveal key changes in particular metabolic pathways in cancer cells and identify the intricate interactions among different metabolic pathways.

3.1 Glycolysis/Lactic Fermentation

Usually, [$^{13}C_6$] Glc is used as the tracer for glycolytic metabolic flux measurement, because it allows each carbon to be labeled to facilitate tracking of the metabolites derived from glycolysis in other metabolic pathways. Recent studies have indicated that the "Warburg effect" can also be found in the non-tumorigenic fast-dividing cells and the tissues that possess a high biosynthetic activity. Glycolysis can be well monitored with the ^{13}C-Glc tracer and can be distinguished

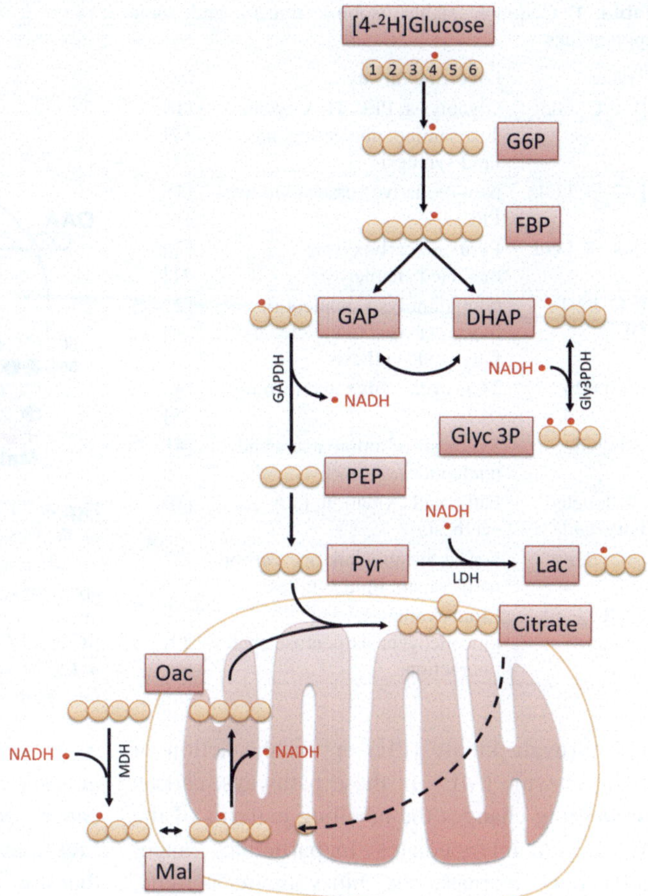

Fig. 3 ^{2}H-labeled tracer to study the NADH metabolic map

by enriched ^{13}C-labeled Lac and pyruvate (Pyr). This distinction can be resolved by 1H-NMR spectroscopy due to direct (^1J HC) and long-range (^2J HC, ^3J HC) 1H-^{13}C scalar-scalar coupling. Therefore, ^{13}C-Lac present in cell culture media is often used as a measure of glycolysis and combined with the disappearance of labeled tracers ([1-^{13}C]-, [U-^{13}C]- or [1,6-$^{13}C_2$]- Glc) to indirectly reflect the contributions of TCA cycle and glycolysis flux to full-scale cellular metabolism.

3.2 Pentose Phosphate Pathway

PPP is an alternative pathway for Glc metabolism, providing a large number of NADPH for the biosynthesis of fatty acids and the breakdown of peroxides while producing 5-phosphate ribose for nucleotide biosynthesis. PPP can be monitored by analyzing the Lac isotopomers after [2-^{13}C]-Glc treatment. Moreover, this tracer results in the appearance of labeling patterns at Lac level, such as [3-^{13}C]- and [1,3-$^{13}C_2$]-Lac. [$^{13}C_6$] Glc can be used to label all carbons of the PPP precursors to detect changes in the PPP of cancer cells with maximum flux. However, the [1,2-$^{13}C_2$] Glc label can distinguish between the oxidized and non-oxidized branches of PPP.

3.3 Pyruvate Cycling

Pyruvate (Pyr) can be carboxylated via the action of pyruvate carboxylase (PC) producing oxaloacetate (OAA); OAA can follow the TCA cycle or be converted back to Pyr via the combination of phosphoenolpyruvate carboxykinase (PEPCK)

Table 1 Common stable isotope tracers and their applications

Tracer	Labeled pathway	Ref.
[U-^{13}C] Glc	Glycolysis, PPP, TCA cycle, hexosamine, nucleotide, and lipid synthesis	[16, 17]
[1,2-^{13}C] Glc	Non-oxidative versus oxidative PPP	[18, 19]
[3,4-^{13}C] Glc	Pyruvate-carboxylase-mediated anaplerosis	[20, 21]
[^{13}C /^{15}N] Glc	Glutaminolysis, nucleotide biosynthesis, TCA cycle, and fatty acid synthesis	[22–24]
[^{13}C] Gln	TCA cycle efflux and turning	[4, 25]
[^{15}N] Gln	Synthesis of amino acids and nucleotides	[4]
^{13}C-labeled fatty acids	Fatty acid oxidation, fatty acid synthesis	[26]
[^{13}C] Ser	Serine metabolism, one-carbon metabolism, lipid synthesis	[27]
[^{13}C] glycerol	Lipid synthesis, gluconeogenesis-pentose cycle interactions	[28, 29]

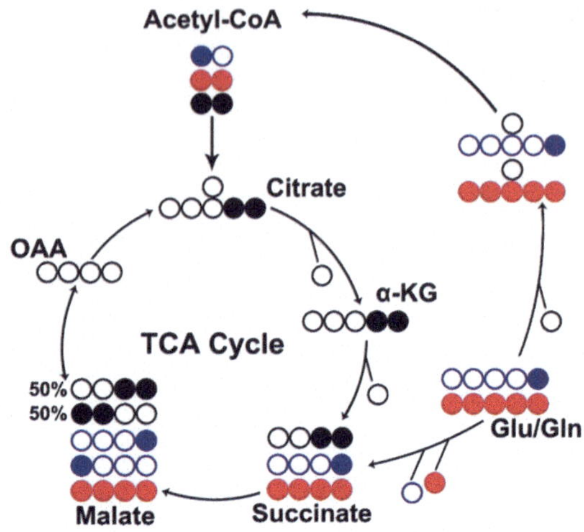

Fig. 4 ^{13}C-labeling patterns via the metabolic pathways of TCA cycle and glutaminolysis. Circles of different colors illustrate the different metabolic pathways. Molecules are represented by their skeletal carbons and depicted as circles. Moreover, the empty and filled circles represent ^{12}C and ^{13}C, respectively
α-KG, α-ketoglutarate; *Acetyl-CoA*, acetyl-coenzyme A; *Gln*, glutamine; *Glu*, glutamate; *OAA*, oxaloacetate

and pyruvate kinase (PK) or via the action of malic enzyme (ME). In these pathways, carbon scrambling changes the labelling patterns of the TCA cycle intermediates. In particular, cancer cells may increase the biosynthetic activity, which involves this Pyr cycling pathway.

3.4 TCA Cycle and Glutaminolysis

The mutations of several enzymes in TCA cycle, such as fumarate hydratase (FH), succinate dehydrogenase (SDH), and isocitrate dehydrogenase (IDH), are associated with tumorigenesis. Briefly, FH and SDH mutations can cause an accumulation and a loss of function of fumarate (Fum) and succinate (Suc), respectively. These changes of metabolite concentrations inhibit prolyl hydroxylases (PHD) that prevents the degradation of the hypoxia inducible factor (HIF) and, finally, results in a pseudohypoxic response and increased glycolysis, which can promote tumorigenesis. Highly abundant metabolites, such as amino acids and ketoacids, are easily transformed into less abundant but also demanded species for protein synthesis or directed toward de novo lipogenesis to account for the higher need of lipids in cancer cells. ^{13}C-enriched anaplerotic metabolites may suffer several carbon rearrangements that are full of information about the interaction between TCA cycle and other major metabolic pathways such as glycolysis, pyruvate cycling, and de novo lipogenesis (Fig. 4).

Cancer cells rely primarily on glycolysis-derived ATP and use the TCA cycle as a metabolic pathway for metabolite interconversion [30].The interaction between glycolysis and TCA cycle can be analyzed with NMR by using ^{13}C-enriched precursors [30]. Acetyl-CoA (AcCoA) should be preferentially labeled in carbon 2 or carbon 1, 2 of the acetyl moiety. That is because the label in carbon 2 of AcCoA produces a label in the various carbons of the TCA cycle intermediate and is sensitive to the level of incorporation of the TCA cycle turnover. For example, after the production of [U-^{13}C] Pyr, [1,2-$^{13}C_2$] AcCoA is produced via the action of pyruvate dehydrogenase (PDH). In the first cycle, oxaloacetate (OAA) carbon 1, 2 or 3, 4 become ^{13}C enriched, followed by condensation with another molecule [1,2-$^{13}C_2$] AcCoA, forming multiple labeled intermediates, i.e., [3,4,5-$^{13}C_3$]- and [2,4,5-$^{13}C_3$]-αKG. In subsequent turns, the enrichment mode is further complicated until the isotope steady state is reached. Due to the balance with the αKG pool, the Glu pool also becomes enriched with ^{13}C. However, special attention must be paid to certain tissue and/or metabolic conditions in which exchange between metabolite pools may be compromised. If Glu pool is not rapidly exchanged with the αKG pool, its labeling mode will not fully reflect the TCA cycle dynamics, and metabolic and isotopic homeostasis must be obtained to derive metabolic conclusions from the isotope data [31, 32].

Gln can be converted to Glu through glutaminase and form other nonessential amino acids via transaminases, which convert amino groups to αKG, thereby producing Glu in quickly reversible reactions. Furthermore, Glu can also be converted to αKG by glutamate dehydrogenase (GLDH), facilitating the carbon entry in the TCA cycle. Compared to any other amino acids, Glu and Gln are always present in higher concentrations. Tumor tissue displays an altered metabolic profile and is usually accompanied with an elevation of Gln uptake. Moreover, the biosynthesis of nucleotide in purines and pyrimidines requires the γ-amido group of Gln and aspartate (Asp). Therefore, the labeled Gln tracer can be used in metabolic flux measurement, and ^{13}C labeling experiments are more important than the ^{15}N labeling experiments. This is because that ^{15}N experiments always need extensive sample preparation and provides less comprehensive data.

3.5 De Novo Lipogenesis

De novo lipogenesis is upregulated in cancer cells to assemble the membranes of dividing cells or organelles. Stable isotope tracers, such as ^2H_2O and ^{13}C-labeled Glc or Gln, can be used to monitor the lipogenic sources. It is possible to obtain the absolute rate of de novo lipogenesis with the ^2H_2O labeling method. Moreover, through the ^{13}C labeling patterns, the contributions of the lipogenic sources and pathways can be obtained at the same time. Briefly, the use of [1,6-$^{13}C_2$]-Glc can produce [2-^{13}C]-AcCoA, and the use of [U-^{13}C]-Gln can produce [1,2-$^{13}C_2$]-AcCoA through the reductive carboxylation via IDH. By using these tracers, we can monitor the prevalence of certain sources or pathways for lipogenesis in cancer cells or tissues by adequately defining the interplay among metabolic pathways.

4 NMR-Based Isotope Tracer Analysis

Isotope tracer analysis using $^{13}C_1$ glucose and NMR was first reported by Ugurbil et al. in 1978 [33]. Under conditions of aerobic and anaerobic, ^{13}C NMR spectra were acquired from *E. coli* cells treated with the tracer for 15 min. Lactate, glutamate, succinate, acetate, valine, alanine Ala, and fructose 1,3-bisphosphate were found to be labeled and labeling positions were identified. In 1988, Malloy et al. investigated the relative activity of anaplerotic and oxidative reactions in the TCA cycle using ^{13}C NMR analysis of the rat hearts perfused with ^{13}C tracers such as $^{13}C_{1,2}$ acetate and $^{13}C_3$ pyruvate [34]. In recent years, more and more studies have been conducted on tracer analysis using NMR isotopes, especially in the field of energy metabolism reprogramming of malignant tumors.

4.1 NMR-Based Isotope Tracing Methodology

In the past 20 years, NMR has become a pivotal technology to study cellular metabolisms, including the metabolic reprogramming of cancer cells. NMR-based isotope analysis can be applied to originate information about the topology and flux analysis of cellular metabolism [35]. NMR and MS are two powerful analytical platforms for cancer metabolism studies. Although the development of MS technology has been more advanced than that of NMR, and more extensively applied to cancer metabolism research, NMR is such a valuable tool for elucidating molecular structures at the atomic level [36]. The unique advantage of NMR lies in its ability to directly detect elements and determine the effect of one element on another by coupling interactions, which together can be used in a large number of isotope-editing experiments to determine specific isotope distributions [37, 38].

In the stable isotope tracer studies, enriched biologically relevant nuclei (e.g., ^{13}C, ^{15}N, or ^{2}H) tracers are introduced into a cell, tissue, or whole organism and incorporated into a variety of metabolites. Isotope labeling is incorporated into specific atomic positions of a given metabolite, depending on the transformation pathway. For example, $^{13}C_2$-glucose can be metabolized into $^{13}C_2$-lactate via glycolysis, and through the PPP $^{13}C_1$-glucose can be metabolized to ribose-5-phosphate. Conversion was determined by metabolite (position isotopomer) and a stable isotope-labeled quantity (mass isotopomer), and the reconstruction can confidently identify the transformation routes. NMR is well suited for positional isomer analysis, while MS is tailored for large-scale isotope analysis. It is worth noting that stable isotope enrichment patterns in metabolites are not only essential for reconstituting metabolic networks, but also the basis for the establishment of flux models, which may require isotope homeostasis or are compatible with dynamic conditions, as necessitated by many studies in vivo [37, 39, 40]. In the early days of metabolomics, one-dimensional proton NMR was commonly used to produce metabolomic profiles. While peaks could be assigned to functional groups (e.g., CH_2 signal from fatty acid tails), most peaks reflected the integrated signals from multiple metabolites. These limitations have been partially resolved by multidimensional NMR [41, 42], and NMR continues to play an important role in metabolomics due to its capacity for structure elucidation and in vivo metabolite measurement [43].

4.2 Applications of NMR-Based Isotope Analysis

An important advantage of the NMR stable isotope tracer method is that the biologically relevant stable isotopes which include ^{13}C, ^{15}N, and ^{2}H can be used to detect the changes of structure and motions in individual sites. ^{13}C and ^{15}N tracers can be easily monitored using a large number of direct and indirect detection by NMR methods. The sensitivity and resolution of NMR analysis, as well as the ability to resolve structures, have been greatly improved. The integrated ^{13}C or ^{15}N labeling pattern for a large number of metabolites can now be ascertained using as little as a sub-milligram quantity of dry cells or tissue biomass or low volumes of biofluids. These advances in NMR, as well as revolutionary progress in MS, have significantly expanded the applications of isotope tracers in metabolomic studies.

Different position-labeled ^{13}C-glucose have been used as tracers for studying different types of cellular metabolisms. For instance, ^{1}H NMR analysis with [1-$^{13}C_1$-], [2-$^{13}C_1$-], or [6-$^{13}C_1$-] Glc tracers was used to track the metabolic progression of ^{13}C-Ala and ^{13}C-Lac in continuously cultured hybridoma cell culture media with a chemostat. Metabolic flux analysis showed that 20% of the consumed glucose was metabolized by the oxidative branch of PPP, and the malic enzyme flux supporting fatty acid biosynthesis was about 10% of the glucose uptake. The biosynthesis rate of cells cultured continuously in the chemostat was found to be higher than that of adherent cells grown in the perfused hollow fiber bioreactor, thereby contributing to the progression of glucose metabolism in mammalian cells [44].

In the SIRM study of mouse models of transgenic tumors, Yuneva and colleagues [45] investigated the metabolic reprogramming caused by the genes C-MYC and MET in liver and lung tumor tissues using NMR and gas chromatography-mass spectrometry (GC-MS) with [U-$^{13}C_6$] Glc and [U-$^{13}C_5$, $^{15}N_2$] Gln tracers. The results indicated that accelerated glycolysis was not always associated with glucose metabolism and the Gln genotype depended not only on oncogenic tumors but also on the tissue environment. Glucose and Gln catabolism were enhanced in MYC-induced liver tumors, and MET-induced liver tumors used glucose to synthesize Gln. These events were associated with decreased levels of glutamine synthetase (GLU1) and the switch from GLS2 to GLS1 glutaminase (reprogrammed expression of glutamine synthetase and glutaminase). In contrast, MYC-induced lung tumors showed enhanced GLU1 and GLS1 expression and accumulated Gln. They further showed that MYC overexpression and Gln catabolism in cancer cells can be inhibited by GLS1 inhibitor. These results suggest that the metabolic profiles of tumors are likely to depend on both the genotype and tissue of origin and have implications regarding the design of synergistic therapies targeting tumor metabolism [37, 45]. The study also showed that SIRM is a powerful tool to elucidate downstream effects of oncogene activation through charactering pivotal metabolic alterations in tumor cells [25, 45].

NMR has the advantage of noninvasiveness and structural resolution capabilities, making it an ideal choice for real-time tracking of metabolic transformation in vivo. NMR can perform detailed kinetic analysis of metabolic pathways using only a single sample, which eliminates the effects of variations between samples while greatly reducing cost and labor. Most importantly, NMR analysis allows the detection of metabolic reactions directly in tissues or whole organisms in a tissue-specific manner, which is a difficult task to achieve with other analytical methods. Technological advances in hyperpolarized NMR methods have further enhanced the utility of ^{13}C NMR in real-time kinetic measurements of specific metabolic reactions in vivo [37].

5 MS-Based Isotope Analysis

In addition to NMR, MS is a commonly used analytical tool for SIRM studies. After isotopically labeling a biological system and extracting its metabolites, the number of heavy atoms (isotopologues) and their positions (isotopomers) can be determined for each metabolite by MS. As ^{13}C has a nominal mass of 1 Da greater than that of ^{12}C, MS can readily determine the number of ^{13}C atoms incorporated. GC and LC methods allow to separate a large number of metabolites, which are often used orthogonally with MS detection. High-resolution MS, such as Orbitrap MS and Fourier transform MS, can well distinguish the metabolites containing ^{13}C, ^{15}N, or ^{2}H, allowing for multiplexed labeling experiments.

5.1 LC-MS-Based Isotope Analysis

LC-MS is a hyphenated analytical technique combining LC separation and MS for detection and identification. LC-MS with stable isotope labeling can be used for isotope tracer analysis and flux measurements in cancer cells (Fig. 5) [46]. Tracing of metabolic pathways can be achieved by analyzing the stable isotope-labeled metabolites using LC-MS with stable isotope tracers such as ^{13}C-Glc and ^{15}N-Gln. Alexander A et al. presented a validated metabolic network model (Cumomer analysis) for the analysis of key pathways in tumor metabolism, including glycolysis, PPP, TCA cycle, and other complementary pathways. To achieve dynamic isotope labeling, they cultured DB-1 melanoma cells for 8 hours in the DMEM medium containing 2 mM [U-$^{13}C_5$, $^{15}N_2$] glutamine and glucose (either 5 or 25 mM), and both culture solutions and cells were lyophilized for LC-MS analysis of isotope-labeled metabolites. The results indicated that melanoma tumors acquired 51% ATP by mitochondrial metabolism and 49% by glycolysis. Although high levels of glutamine uptake were equivalent to about 50% and 100% of TCA circulating flux under hyperglycemic conditions and normal blood glucose conditions, respectively, glutamine flux and its effect on ATP contribution of synthesis was still small [47].

Ying et al. investigated the effects of Kras^{G12D} activity on glucose metabolism using LC-MS and U-$^{13}C_6$-glucose to trace glucose flux. ^{13}C-labeled glucose was added to culture pancreatic cancer cells with high expression of the oncogene K-Ras, and then the cellular metabolites were harvested for LC-MS analysis. They observed that Kras^{G12D} enhanced glycolytic flux but did not affect the glycolytic metabolites entering the TCA cycle [48], and Kras^{G12D} served a vital role in controlling tumor metabolism through stimulation of glucose uptake and channeling of glucose inter-

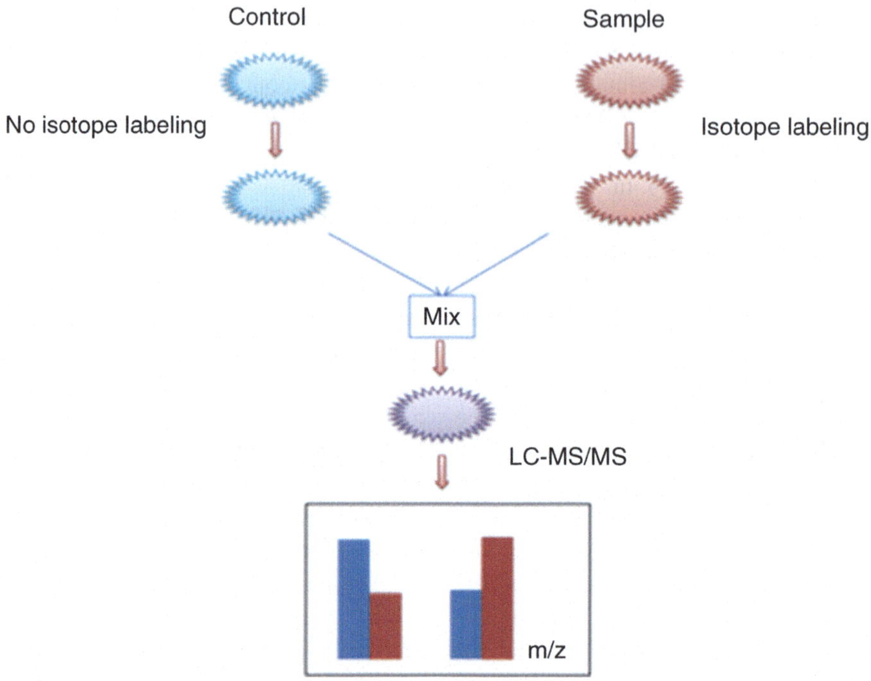

Fig. 5 Isotope tracer analysis by LC-MS/MS with stable isotope labeling. The sample (e.g., cultured cancer cells under treatment) is labeled with a stable isotope whereas the control (untreated, cultured cancer cells) is unlabeled. Metabolites are extracted from both sample and control and mixed for a single LC-MS/MS analysis

mediates into the hexosamine biosynthesis and PPP. This study also revealed that oncogenic Kras promotes ribose biogenesis, and unlike canonical models, KrasG12D drived glycolysis intermediates into the nonoxidative PPP, thereby decoupling ribose biogenesis from NADP/NADPH-mediated redox control. Together, these findings provide in vivo mechanistic insights into how oncogenic Kras promotes metabolic reprogramming in native tumors and illuminates potential metabolic targets that can be exploited for therapeutics in pancreatic cancer. MS-based isotope tracing technology demonstrates unique advantages for quantitative analysis of cellular metabolic dynamics.

5.2 GC-MS-Based Isotope Analysis

In order to maximumly detect and quantify metabolites from biological samples, different analytical platforms such as NMR, LC-MS, and GC-MS may be combined for a more comprehensive analysis [49–53]. Although LC-MS is a very commonly used technique for metabolomic analysis [54, 55], GC-MS is particularly suitable for measuring compounds with low molecular weight (e.g., acetate), high volatility (e.g., alcohols), or not easily ionized by electrospray (e.g., sterols). With chemical derivatization of analytes, GC-MS can also be used to measure medium-sized, charged metabolites (e.g., monophosphates) [56]. Therefore, GC-MS has been commonly used for metabolomic analysis [57]. In addition, GC-MS only requires a very small amount of cellular material for analysis. Therefore, this method can greatly reduce the cost of expensive isotope tracers. So far, isotope labeling and GC-MS have been used to trace metabolites and metabolic flux in a variety of mammalian systems, including hepatocytes [58], cardiac cells [59], and glial cells [60].

Dong et al. investigated the effect of fructose-1,6-biphosphatase (FBP1) on metabolic pathways in MDA-MB231 breast cancer cells using GC-MS and NMR with [U-$^{13}C_6$]-Glc as a tracer.

They found that loss of FBP1 induced glycolysis and resulted in increased glucose uptake, macromolecules biosynthesis, formation of tetrameric PKM2, and maintenance of ATP production under hypoxia. Loss of FBP1 also inhibited oxygen consumption and ROS production by suppressing mitochondrial complex I activity. This study indicates that the loss of FBP1 is a critical oncogenic event in basal-like breast cancer (BLBC) [61].

6 Combined Analysis of NMR and MS Spectra (CANMS)

Although the metabolic pathways are different in mammalian cells, their pathway metabolites sometimes are identical. When using the isotope pattern, this overlap among different pathways complicates subsequent analysis, which requires new model-free approach for data processing. The combination of MS and NMR analyses may provide us a potentially effective approach to solving this issue (Fig. 6). Coupling NMR and ultrahigh-resolution Fourier transform MS (UHR-FTMS) with an atom-resolved metabolic database and tracing tools can lead to robust and unprecedented reconstruction of interconnected pathways and networks [62–65]. When labeled with an isotope such as ^{13}C, information on the mass increments of metabolites can be obtained by MS [66]. However, MS is difficult to distinguish the atomic position of the isotope label, e.g., Ala labeled at C1, 2, or 3 positions [67]. In contrast, NMR can easily identify each position isotope because appropriate NMR techniques yield significant resonances corresponding to each individual ^{13}C position. With the development of two-dimensional NMR methods, more direct and rigorous structural analysis can be achieved, which greatly expands the size range and complexity of molecules that NMR can be applied [68]. In biochemistry, the sources of these carbon atoms are fixed. Through the joint analysis of NMR and MS, we can achieve the quantitative data about the abundance of metabolites labeled by isotopes and the location of the labeled atoms in the metabolites.

Using ^{13}C as a tracer, combined with NMR and GC-MS for SIRM analysis, Fan et al. [69] found that cancer tissues expressed higher levels of many primary metabolites compared with surrounding noncancerous tissues in lung cancer patients. Metabolic changes were investigated by infusing uniformly labeled ^{13}C-glucose into human lung cancer patients, followed by resection and processing of paired noncancerous lung and non-small cell carcinoma tissues. NMR and GC-MS were used for ^{13}C-isotopomer-based metabolomic analysis of the extracts of tissues and blood plasma. Many primary metabolites were consistently found at higher levels in lung cancer tissues than their surrounding noncancerous tissues. ^{13}C enrichment in Lac, Ala, succinate, Glu, Asp, and citrate was also higher in the tumors, suggesting more active glycolysis and TCA cycle in the tumor tissues. Particularly notable were the enhanced production of the Asp isotopomer with three ^{13}C-labeled carbons and the buildup of ^{13}C-2,3-Glu isotopomer in lung tumor tissues. This is consistent with the transformations of glucose into Asp or Glu via glycolysis, anaplerotic pyruvate carboxylation (PC), and the TCA cycle. PC activation in tumor tissues was also shown by an increased level of pyruvate carboxylase mRNA and protein [69].

CANMS allows us to trace the flow of carbon atoms in the metabolic pathways. Figure 7 shows the isotopomer analysis for Lac and Ala by CANMS [70]. Lac and Ala are labeled with [1,2-$^{13}C_2$]-Glc and exhibit typical labeling characteristics. If both are produced by the glycolysis pathway, both C-2,3 Lac and Ala should be labeled and the amount of labeling should be equal. However, due to the presence of the PPP pathway, the C-1 Glc is removed in the first step, and the labeled proportion of C-2,3 Lac and Ala will be different as a result. The labeled Lac obtained from the PPP pathway has three forms [^{13}C-3], [^{13}C-1], and [^{13}C-1,3] [67]. NMR can detect the first isotopomers, but for the isotopomers labeling in C-1, NMR is powerless. Under this situation, only the information of MS can be used to distinguish the two isotopomers. In this analysis, Chong et al.

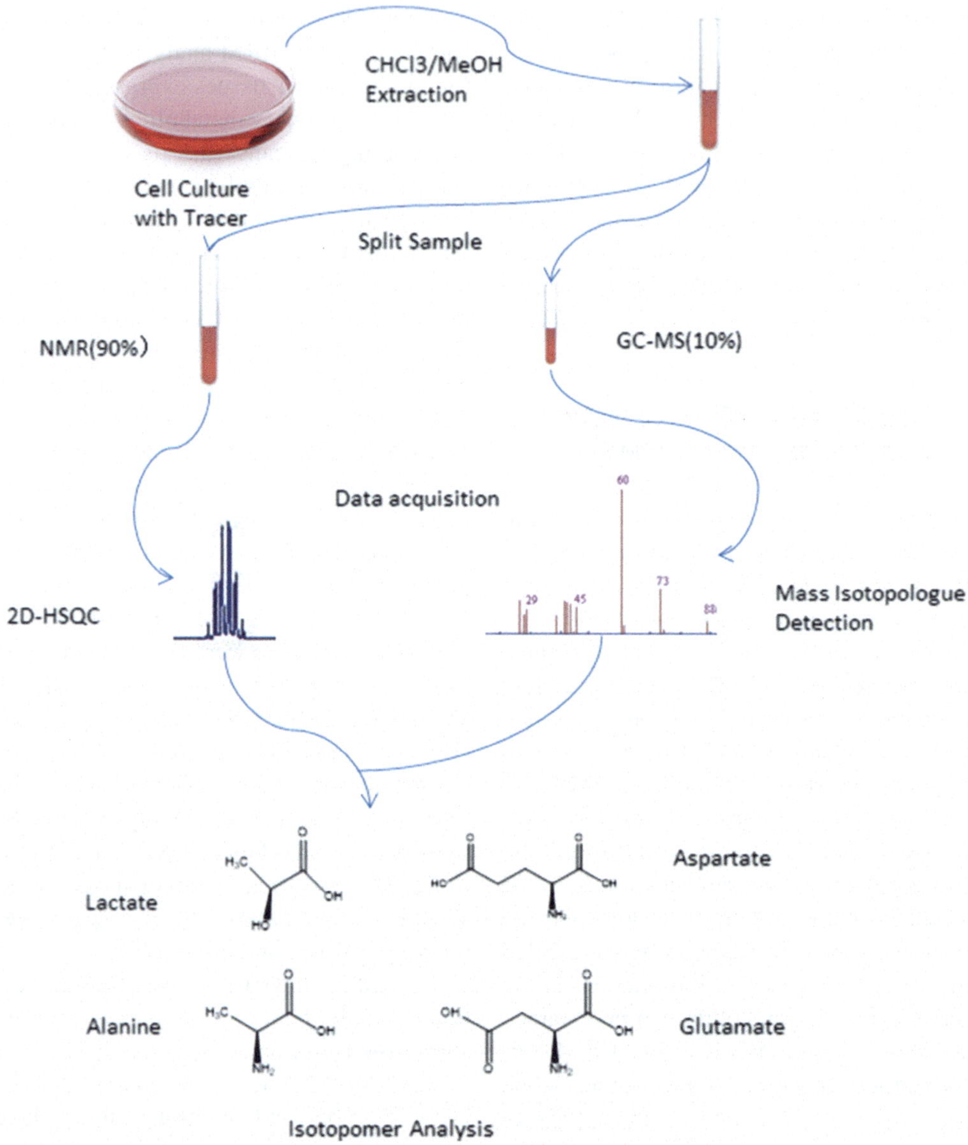

Fig. 6 Schematic representation of model-free isotopomer analysis

observed approximately 3.5% PPP contribution for Lac and Pyr, whereas glycolysis contributes 22.5–23.5% to the label incorporation. Given that the glucose molecule is split into two parts, with one unlabeled for [1,2-^{13}C2]-Glc, this is equivalent to 7% PPP and 45% glycolytic activity, respectively, assuming no Pyr cycling from the TCA cycle [70]. This study demonstrates that CANMS yields highly accurate data about metabolic flux and pathway interactions.

7 Conclusions

Tumor metabolism studies have regained significant attention in recent years. Although the Warburg effect was discovered in the 1920s, our understanding of cancer metabolism remains to be quite limited. While quantification of metabolite concentrations in cancer tissues and cells represents an important aspect of cancer metabolomics, we need to explore how the flow of these metabolites

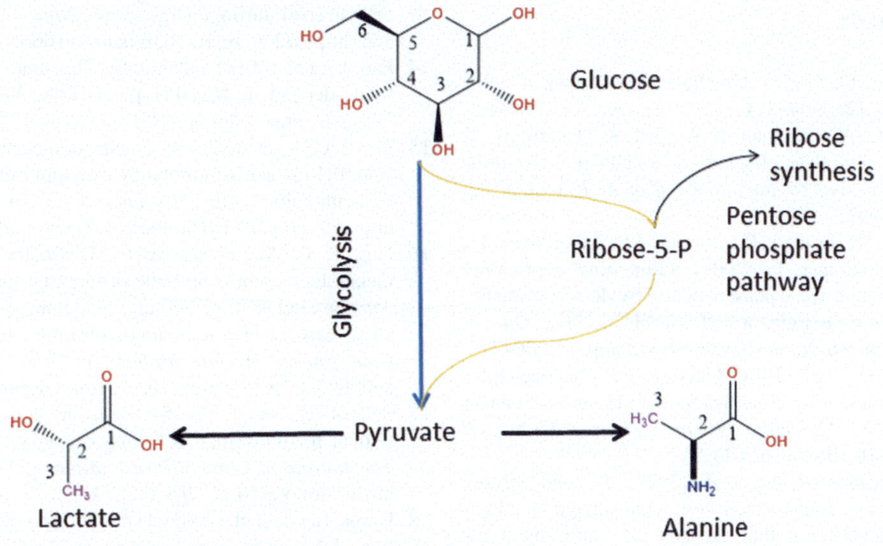

Fig. 7 Tracing central metabolic processes using [1,2-$^{13}C_2$]-Glc

(metabolic flux) per unit time changes in the activated metabolic pathway. In fact, the concentration of metabolites and the flow rate do not always match. For example, when glucose is removed from yeast, glycolytic efflux drops sharply, leading to buildup of lower glycolytic intermediates even though pathway influx is decreased [71].

To identify altered metabolic pathways in cancer cells, SIRM can be used to determine the flow direction and size of the metabolic pathway, so as to accurately determine which metabolic pathways have changed, by measuring the ratio and rate of isotope-labeled metabolic substrate among different pathways [71]. SIRM analysis provides a new global perspective that allows us to better understand the metabolic switch under the regulation of oncogenes or tumor suppressor genes [25]. SIRM can further illustrate the complexity and plasticity of tumor metabolism, which allows tumor cells to better adapt to changes in the microenvironment and utilize more energy. For example, by using tracers and GC-MS or NMR-based metabolomic analyses recent studies have demonstrated the importance of the microenvironment for tumor metabolism through immunoregulation [16] or through direct regulation of stromal cells [72].

SIRM is a useful complement to other omics technologies which are already used in the clinic. It can be combined with genomics and proteomics techniques to greatly promote the development of precision medicine from the perspective of systems biology. Numerous studies have led to the discovery of metabolite biomarkers for early detection of cancer or prediction of anticancer drug responses [73, 74]. A combination of SIRM with genomics and proteomics will lead to the discovery of mechanistic biomarkers for early cancer detection or metabolic targets for therapeutic interventions.

A major challenge in conducting SIRM research is the establishment of data mining and analytical models [71]. Graphical representations of markup patterns and intuitive data interpretation may still be important, but as complexity increases, mathematical modeling may become the core of bio-discovery. This section does not discuss large-scale quantitative flux analysis because the models currently relied on are beyond the capabilities of most wet laboratories. Therefore, developing software that can perform quantitative analysis of flux data is an important task. Nevertheless, it is gratifying to note that many teams in the world are conducting research on tumor metabolic flow calculation algorithms. With the advancement of technology platforms and data analysis models/tools, the applications of SIRM will significantly promote the diagnosis and treatment of cancer diseases.

References

1. Warburg, O. (1956). On the origin of cancer cells. *Science, 123*, 309–314.
2. Sauer, L. A., Stayman, J. W., 3rd, & Dauchy, R. T. (1982). Amino acid, glucose, and lactic acid utilization in vivo by rat tumors. *Cancer Research, 42*, 4090–4097.
3. Gaglio, D., Soldati, C., Vanoni, M., Alberghina, L., & Chiaradonna, F. (2009). Glutamine deprivation induces abortive s-phase rescued by deoxyribonucleotides in k-ras transformed fibroblasts. *PLoS One, 4*, e4715. https://doi.org/10.1371/journal.pone.0004715.
4. Gaglio, D., et al. (2011). Oncogenic K-Ras decouples glucose and glutamine metabolism to support cancer cell growth. *Molecular Systems Biology, 7*, 15. https://doi.org/10.1038/msb.2011.56.
5. DeBerardinis, R. J., et al. (2007). Beyond aerobic glycolysis: Transformed cells can engage in glutamine metabolism that exceeds the requirement for protein and nucleotide synthesis. *Proceedings of the National Academy of Sciences of the United States of America, 104*, 19345–19350. https://doi.org/10.1073/pnas.0709747104.
6. Kurhanewicz, J., et al. (2011). Analysis of cancer metabolism by imaging hyperpolarized nuclei: Prospects for translation to clinical research. *Neoplasia, 13*, 81–97. https://doi.org/10.1593/neo.101102.
7. Patra, K. C., & Hay, N. (2014). The pentose phosphate pathway and cancer. *Trends in Biochemical Sciences, 39*, 347–354. https://doi.org/10.1016/j.tibs.2014.06.005.
8. Delgado, T. C., Castro, M. M., Geraldes, C. F., & Jones, J. G. (2004). Quantitation of erythrocyte pentose pathway flux with [2-13C]glucose and 1H NMR analysis of the lactate methyl signal. *Magnetic Resonance in Medicine, 51*, 1283–1286. https://doi.org/10.1002/mrm.20096.
9. Kroemer, G., & Pouyssegur, J. (2008). Tumor cell metabolism: cancer's Achilles' heel. *Cancer Cell, 13*, 472–482. https://doi.org/10.1016/j.ccr.2008.05.005.
10. Lane, A. N., & Fan, T. W. (2015). Regulation of mammalian nucleotide metabolism and biosynthesis. *Nucleic Acids Research, 43*, 2466–2485. https://doi.org/10.1093/nar/gkv047.
11. Jin, F., et al. (2015). A novel [(15)N] glutamine flux using LC-MS/MS-SRM for determination of nucleosides and nucleobases. *Journal of Analytical & Bioanalytical Techniques, 6*. https://doi.org/10.4172/2155-9872.1000267.
12. Marini, J. C. (2011). Quantitative analysis of 15N-labeled positional isomers of glutamine and citrulline via electrospray ionization tandem mass spectrometry of their dansyl derivatives. *Rapid Communications in Mass Spectrometry: RCM, 25*, 1291–1296. https://doi.org/10.1002/rcm.5007.
13. Jeon, S.-M., Chandel, N. S., & Hay, N. (2012). AMPK regulates NADPH homeostasis to promote tumour cell survival during energy stress. *Nature, 485*, 661–665. https://doi.org/10.1038/nature11066.
14. Fan, J., et al. (2014). Quantitative flux analysis reveals folate-dependent NADPH production. *Nature, 510*, 298–302. https://doi.org/10.1038/nature13236.
15. Lewis, C. A., et al. (2014). Tracing compartmentalized NADPH metabolism in the cytosol and mitochondria of mammalian cells. *Molecular Cell, 55*, 253–263. https://doi.org/10.1016/j.molcel.2014.05.008.
16. Fan, T. W. M., et al. (2016). Distinctly perturbed metabolic networks underlie differential tumor tissue damages induced by immune modulator β-glucan in a two-case ex vivo non-small-cell lung cancer study. *Cold Spring Harbor Molecular Case Studies, 2*, a000893. https://doi.org/10.1101/mcs.a000893.
17. Sellers, K., et al. (2015). Pyruvate carboxylase is critical for non–small-cell lung cancer proliferation. *The Journal of Clinical Investigation, 125*, 687–698. https://doi.org/10.1172/JCI72873.
18. Boros, L. G., et al. (2005). [1,2-13C2]-D-glucose profiles of the serum, liver, pancreas, and DMBA-induced pancreatic tumors of rats. *Pancreas, 31*, 337–343.
19. Lee, W. N., et al. (1998). Mass isotopomer study of the nonoxidative pathways of the pentose cycle with [1,2-13C2]glucose. *The American Journal of Physiology, 274*, E843–E851.
20. Cheng, T., et al. (2011). Pyruvate carboxylase is required for glutamine-independent growth of tumor cells. *Proceedings of the National Academy of Sciences of the United States of America, 108*, 8674–8679. https://doi.org/10.1073/pnas.1016627108.
21. Crown, S. B., Ahn, W. S., & Antoniewicz, M. R. (2012). Rational design of 13C-labeling experiments for metabolic flux analysis in mammalian cells. *BMC Systems Biology, 6*, 43. https://doi.org/10.1186/1752-0509-6-43.
22. Sellers, K., et al. (2015). Pyruvate carboxylase is critical for non-small-cell lung cancer proliferation. *The Journal of Clinical Investigation, 125*, 687–698. https://doi.org/10.1172/jci72873.
23. Xie, H., et al. (2014). Targeting lactate dehydrogenase--A inhibits tumorigenesis and tumor progression in mouse models of lung cancer and impacts tumor-initiating cells. *Cell Metabolism, 19*, 795–809. https://doi.org/10.1016/j.cmet.2014.03.003.
24. Mullen, A. R., et al. (2011). Reductive carboxylation supports growth in tumour cells with defective mitochondria. *Nature, 481*, 385–388. https://doi.org/10.1038/nature10642.
25. Bruntz, R. C., Lane, A. N., Higashi, R. M., & Fan, T. W. (2017). Exploring cancer metabolism using stable isotope-resolved metabolomics (SIRM). *The Journal of Biological Chemistry, 292*, 11601–11609. https://doi.org/10.1074/jbc.R117.776054.
26. Kasumov, T., et al. (2005). Probing peroxisomal beta-oxidation and the labelling of acetyl-CoA proxies with [1-(13C)]octanoate and [3-(13C)]octanoate in the perfused rat liver. *The Biochemical Journal, 389*, 397–401. https://doi.org/10.1042/bj20050144.

27. Cowin, G. J., Willgoss, D. A., Bartley, J., & Endre, Z. H. (1996). Serine isotopmer analysis by 13C-NMR defines glycine-serine interconversion in situ in the renal proximal tubule. *Biochimica et Biophysica Acta, 1310*, 32–40.
28. Qi, J., et al. (2012). The use of stable isotope-labeled glycerol and oleic acid to differentiate the hepatic functions of DGAT1 and -2. *Journal of Lipid Research, 53*, 1106–1116. https://doi.org/10.1194/jlr.M020156.
29. Kurland, I. J., Alcivar, A., Bassilian, S., & Lee, W. N. (2000). Loss of [13C]glycerol carbon via the pentose cycle.Implications for gluconeogenesis measurement by mass isotoper distribution analysis. *Journal of Biological Chemistry, 275*, 36787–36793. https://doi.org/10.1074/jbc.M004739200.
30. Tavares, L. C., Jarak, I., Nogueira, F. N., Oliveira, P. J., & Carvalho, R. A. (2015). Metabolic evaluations of cancer metabolism by NMR-based stable isotope tracer methodologies. *European Journal of Clinical Investigation, 45*, 37–43. https://doi.org/10.1111/eci.12358.
31. Carvalho, R. A., et al. (2001). TCA cycle kinetics in the rat heart by analysis of (13)C isotopomers using indirect (1)H. *American Journal of Physiology. Heart and Circulatory Physiology, 281*, H1413–H1421. https://doi.org/10.1152/ajpheart.2001.281.3.H1413.
32. Weiss, R. G., et al. (1995). Consequences of altered aspartate aminotransferase activity on 13C-glutamate labelling by the tricarboxylic acid cycle in intact rat hearts. *Biochimica et Biophysica Acta, 1243*, 543–548.
33. Ugurbil, K., Brown, T. R., den Hollander, J. A., Glynn, P., & Shulman, R. G. (1978). High-resolution 13C nuclear magnetic resonance studies of glucose metabolism in Escherichia coli. *Proceedings of the National Academy of Sciences of the United States of America, 75*, 3742–3746. https://doi.org/10.1073/pnas.75.8.3742.
34. Malloy, C. R., Sherry, A. D., & Jeffrey, F. M. (1988). Evaluation of carbon flux and substrate selection through alternate pathways involving the citric acid cycle of the heart by 13C NMR spectroscopy. *The Journal of Biological Chemistry, 263*, 6964–6971.
35. Millard, P., Cahoreau, E., Heuillet, M., Portais, J. C., & Lippens, G. (2017). N-15-NMR-based approach for amino acids-based C-13-metabolic flux analysis of metabolism. *Analytical Chemistry, 89*, 2101–2106. https://doi.org/10.1021/acs.analchem.6b04767.
36. Hollinshead, K. E., Williams, D. S., Tennant, D. A., & Ludwig, C. (2016). Probing cancer cell metabolism using NMR spectroscopy. *Advances in Experimental Medicine and Biology, 899*, 89–111. https://doi.org/10.1007/978-3-319-26666-4_6.
37. Fan, T. W. M., & Lane, A. N. (2016). Applications of NMR spectroscopy to systems biochemistry. *Progress in Nuclear Magnetic Resonance Spectroscopy, 92-93*, 18–53. https://doi.org/10.1016/j.pnmrs.2016.01.005.
38. Lane, A. N. (2012). In T. W.-M. Fan, A. N. Lane, & R. M. Higashi (Eds.), *The handbook of metabolomics* (pp. 127–197). Totowa: Humana Press.
39. Fendt, S. M., et al. (2013). Reductive glutamine metabolism is a function of the alpha-ketoglutarate to citrate ratio in cells. *Nature Communications, 4*, 2236. https://doi.org/10.1038/ncomms3236.
40. Mueller, D., & Heinzle, E. (2013). Stable isotope-assisted metabolomics to detect metabolic flux changes in mammalian cell cultures. *Current Opinion in Biotechnology, 24*, 54–59. https://doi.org/10.1016/j.copbio.2012.10.015.
41. Larive, C. K., Barding, G. A., & Dinges, M. M. (2015). NMR spectroscopy for metabolomics and metabolic profiling. *Analytical Chemistry, 87*, 133–146. https://doi.org/10.1021/ac504075g.
42. Markley, J. L., et al. (2017). The future of NMR-based metabolomics. *Current Opinion in Biotechnology, 43*, 34–40. https://doi.org/10.1016/j.copbio.2016.08.001.
43. Mancuso, A., et al. (2004). Real-time detection of 13C NMR labeling kinetics in perfused EMT6 mouse mammary tumor cells and βHC9 mouse insulinomas. *Biotechnology and Bioengineering, 87*, 835–848. https://doi.org/10.1002/bit.20191.
44. Bonarius, H. P., et al. (2001). Metabolic-flux analysis of continuously cultured hybridoma cells using (13)CO(2) mass spectrometry in combination with (13)C-lactate nuclear magnetic resonance spectroscopy and metabolite balancing. *Biotechnology and Bioengineering, 74*, 528–538. https://doi.org/10.1002/bit.1145.
45. Yuneva, M. O., et al. (2012). The metabolic profile of tumors depends on both the responsible genetic lesion and tissue type. *Cell Metabolism, 15*, 157–170. https://doi.org/10.1016/j.cmet.2011.12.015.
46. Fang, Z. Z., & Gonzalez, F. J. (2014). LC-MS-based metabolomics: An update. *Archives of Toxicology, 88*, 1491–1502. https://doi.org/10.1007/s00204-014-1234-6.
47. Shestov, A. A., et al. (2016). (13)C MRS and LC-MS flux analysis of tumor intermediary metabolism. *Frontiers in Oncology, 6*, 135. https://doi.org/10.3389/fonc.2016.00135.
48. Ying, H., et al. (2012). Oncogenic Kras maintains pancreatic tumors through regulation of anabolic glucose metabolism. *Cell, 149*, 656–670. https://doi.org/10.1016/j.cell.2012.01.058.
49. Griffin, J. L., Atherton, H., Shockcor, J., & Atzori, L. (2011). Metabolomics as a tool for cardiac research. *Nature Reviews. Cardiology, 8*, 630–643. https://doi.org/10.1038/nrcardio.2011.138.
50. Griffin, J. L., & Shockcor, J. P. (2004). Metabolic profiles of cancer cells. *Nature Reviews. Cancer, 4*, 551–561. https://doi.org/10.1038/nrc1390.
51. Lu, W., Bennett, B. D., & Rabinowitz, J. D. (2008). Analytical strategies for LC-MS-based targeted metabolomics. Analytical technologies in the biomedical and life sciences. *Journal of Chromatography B, 871*, 236–242. https://doi.org/10.1016/j.jchromb.2008.04.031.

52. Patti, G. J., Yanes, O., & Siuzdak, G. (2012). Metabolomics: The apogee of the omics trilogy. *Nature Reviews. Molecular Cell Biology, 13*, 263. https://doi.org/10.1038/nrm3314.
53. Roberts, L. D., Souza, A. L., Gerszten, R. E., & Clish, C. B. (2012). Targeted metabolomics. *Current Protocols in Molecular Biology, Chapter 30*, Unit 30.32.31–24. https://doi.org/10.1002/0471142727.mb3002s98.
54. Büscher, J. M., Czernik, D., Ewald, J. C., Sauer, U., & Zamboni, N. (2009). Cross-platform comparison of methods for quantitative metabolomics of primary metabolism. *Analytical Chemistry, 81*, 2135–2143. https://doi.org/10.1021/ac8022857.
55. Lu, W., et al. (2010). Metabolomic analysis via reversed-phase ion-pairing liquid chromatography coupled to a stand alone orbitrap mass spectrometer. *Analytical Chemistry, 82*, 3212–3221. https://doi.org/10.1021/ac902837x.
56. Lai, Z., & Fiehn, O. (2018). Mass spectral fragmentation of trimethylsilylated small molecules. *Mass Spectrometry Reviews, 37*, 245–257. https://doi.org/10.1002/mas.21518.
57. Jonsson, P., et al. (2005). High-throughput data analysis for detecting and identifying differences between samples in GC/MS-based metabolomic analyses. *Analytical Chemistry, 77*, 5635–5642. https://doi.org/10.1021/ac050601e.
58. Fiehn, O. (2001). Combining genomics, metabolome analysis, and biochemical modelling to understand metabolic networks. *Comparative and Functional Genomics, 2*, 155–168. https://doi.org/10.1002/cfg.82.
59. Jerby-Arnon, L., et al. (2014). Predicting cancer-specific vulnerability via data-driven detection of synthetic lethality. *Cell, 158*, 1199–1209. https://doi.org/10.1016/j.cell.2014.07.027.
60. Weckwerth, W., & Morgenthal, K. (2005). Metabolomics: From pattern recognition to biological interpretation. *Drug Discovery Today, 10*, 1551–1558. https://doi.org/10.1016/s1359-6446(05)03609-3.
61. Dong, C., et al. (2013). Loss of FBP1 by snail-mediated repression provides metabolic advantages in basal-like breast cancer. *Cancer Cell, 23*, 316–331. https://doi.org/10.1016/j.ccr.2013.01.022.
62. Fan, T. W. M., et al. (2012). Stable isotope-resolved metabolomics and applications for drug development. *Pharmacology & Therapeutics, 133*, 366–391. https://doi.org/10.1016/j.pharmthera.2011.12.007.
63. Higashi, R. M., Fan, T. W., Lorkiewicz, P. K., Moseley, H. N., & Lane, A. N. (2014). Stable isotope-labeled tracers for metabolic pathway elucidation by GC-MS and FT-MS. *Methods in Molecular Biology (Clifton, N.J.), 1198*, 147–167. https://doi.org/10.1007/978-1-4939-1258-2_11.
64. Fan, T. W. M., & Lane, A. N. (2008). Structure-based profiling of metabolites and isotopomers by NMR. *Progress in Nuclear Magnetic Resonance Spectroscopy, 52*, 69–117. https://doi.org/10.1016/j.pnmrs.2007.03.002.
65. Fan, T. W., & Lane, A. N. (2016). Applications of NMR spectroscopy to systems biochemistry. *Progress in Nuclear Magnetic Resonance Spectroscopy, 92–93*, 18–53. https://doi.org/10.1016/j.pnmrs.2016.01.005.
66. Bjarke Christensen, J. N. (1999). Isotopomer analysis using GC-MS. *Metabolic Engineering, 1*, 282–290.
67. Fan, T. W. M., & Lane, A. N. (2011). NMR-based stable isotope resolved metabolomics in systems biochemistry. *Journal of Biomolecular NMR, 49*, 267–280. https://doi.org/10.1007/s10858-011-9484-6.
68. Evans, D. R., & Guy, H. I. (2004). Mammalian pyrimidine biosynthesis: Fresh insights into an ancient pathway. *The Journal of Biological Chemistry, 279*, 33035–33038. https://doi.org/10.1074/jbc.R400007200.
69. Fan, T. W., et al. (2009). Altered regulation of metabolic pathways in human lung cancer discerned by 13C stable isotope-resolved metabolomics (SIRM). *Molecular Cancer, 8*, 41. https://doi.org/10.1186/1476-4598-8-41.
70. Chong, M., et al. (2017). Combined analysis of NMR and MS spectra (CANMS). *Angewandte Chemie (International Ed. in English), 56*, 4140–4144. https://doi.org/10.1002/anie.201611634.
71. Jang, C., Chen, L., & Rabinowitz, D. (2018). *Journal of Metabolomics and Isotope Tracing, 173*, 822.
72. Zhao, H., et al. (2016). Tumor microenvironment derived exosomes pleiotropically modulate cancer cell metabolism. *eLife, 5*, e10250. https://doi.org/10.7554/eLife.10250.
73. Vargas, A. J., & Harris, C. C. (2016). Biomarker development in the precision medicine era: Lung cancer as a case study. *Nature Reviews. Cancer, 16*, 525–537. https://doi.org/10.1038/nrc.2016.56.
74. Hou, Y., et al. (2014). A metabolomics approach for predicting the response to neoadjuvant chemotherapy in cervical cancer patients. *Molecular BioSystems, 10*, 2126–2133. https://doi.org/10.1039/c4mb00054d.

Functional Metabolomics and Chemoproteomics Approaches Reveal Novel Metabolic Targets for Anticancer Therapy

Chang Shao, Wenjie Lu, Haiping Hao, and Hui Ye

1 Introduction

Compared with normal cells, cancer cells feature distinct metabolic phenotypes in order to survive, grow, and proliferate. A growing body of studies has shown that the remodeled metabolic programs of cancer cells are driven by oncogenic signaling and can in return commit more efficient bioenergetics and macromolecule synthesis for the survival and growth of cancer cells [1–3]. Besides modulating the synthesis and degradation of functional metabolites to meet the needs of cancer cells, recent studies have revealed that metabolites and metabolic enzymes can regulate cell fates by affecting a wide range of proteins beyond our previous knowledge, spanning from central players of signaling pathways, such as kinases [4] and transcription factors [5], to highly abundant housekeeping proteins [6].

Based on the metabolic differences between normal and cancer cells, scientists attempted to block abnormal metabolic pathways in order to exert anticancer effects. Some metabolic targets have been successfully adopted in clinics. For example, mutant IDH1 and IDH2 were identified in acute myeloid leukemia (AML) patients (approximately 12% and 8–19%, respectively) [7, 8]. Recently, ivosidenib (mutant IDH1 inhibitor) and enasidenib (mutant IDH2 inhibitor) have been approved by the FDA to treat the AML patients carrying IDH1/2 mutation [9]. In contrast, targeting metabolic enzymes that are essential for both tumor and normal cells have failed in previous clinical trials. For example, 2-deoxy-D-glucose (2-DG) that inhibits glycolysis by binding to hexokinase and subsequently suppresses growth in tumor cells can bring severe side effects such as hypoglycemia to treated subjects [10]. Hence, pressing needs in metabolic target discovery is to examine the metabolic differences between normal and cancer cells and exploit the metabolic differences to develop "precise" anticancer treatments that specifically affect tumor cells.

To accommodate such needs, metabolomics is emerging in the field of cancer metabolism

C. Shao
Pharmacy Department, Shenzhen Luohu People's Hospital, Shenzhen, China

School of Pharmacy, China Pharmaceutical University, Nanjing, China

W. Lu · H. Ye (✉)
Key Laboratory of Drug Metabolism and Pharmacokinetics, State Key Laboratory of Natural Medicines, China Pharmaceutical University, Nanjing, China
e-mail: cpuyehui@cpu.edu.cn

H. Hao (✉)
Key Laboratory of Drug Metabolism and Pharmacokinetics, State Key Laboratory of Natural Medicines, China Pharmaceutical University, Nanjing, China

School of Pharmacy, China Pharmaceutical University, Nanjing, China
e-mail: haipinghao@cpu.edu.cn

S. Hu (ed.), *Cancer Metabolomics*, Advances in Experimental Medicine and Biology 1280,
https://doi.org/10.1007/978-3-030-51652-9_9

research in the past decades due to its capability in delineating the metabolic profiles of cells and tissues on a system level with high sensitivity, speed, and robustness. Its application to biomarker discovery has achieved numerous successes in different types of cancers, such as lung cancer [11], breast cancer [12], and prostate cancer [13]. Nevertheless, the knowledge regarding the pathological causes and consequences of metabolic alterations probed by metabolomics is lacked and awaits to be unraveled by other techniques. To this end, proteomics tools that can analyze the composition, expression, and modification of proteins are complementary to metabolomics. It provides another dimension of biological information and offers valuable insights into the cellular and molecular mechanisms that explain how the abnormal metabolic patterns in cancers are induced and what outcomes the remodeled metabolism may potentially lead to. In turn, the different levels of metabolites can also verify the abundance changes of specific metabolic enzymes detected by proteomics. Hence, the combined use of metabolomics and proteomics can provide a unique and holistic understanding of the abnormal metabolism in cancers and holds potential in discovering metabolic targets of therapeutic value with the aid of biochemical and genetic tools, such as RNAi technology used in vitro and tumor xenograft mice model tested in vivo (See Fig. 1). Therefore, we focused on reviewing the technology advances and diverse applications of metabolomics and proteomics in cancer biomarker discovery and target identification in this chapter.

2 Metabolomics in Anticancer Target Discovery

In contrast to genomics and transcriptomics data that may provide the insights on a pathological process, metabolic profiling of biological samples is instantaneous snapshots of physiological and pathological events that are currently undergoing within bodies and is thus increasingly being utilized to diagnose cancers, predict therapeutic outcomes, understand disease mechanisms, and identify novel targets to develop anticancer therapy.

2.1 Essential Procedures and Advancements of Metabolomics Technologies

2.1.1 Sample Collection and Preparation

Metabolomics relies on the use of cutting-edge analytical techniques to detect and identify metabolites comprehensively from complex biological samples for biomarker or target discovery.

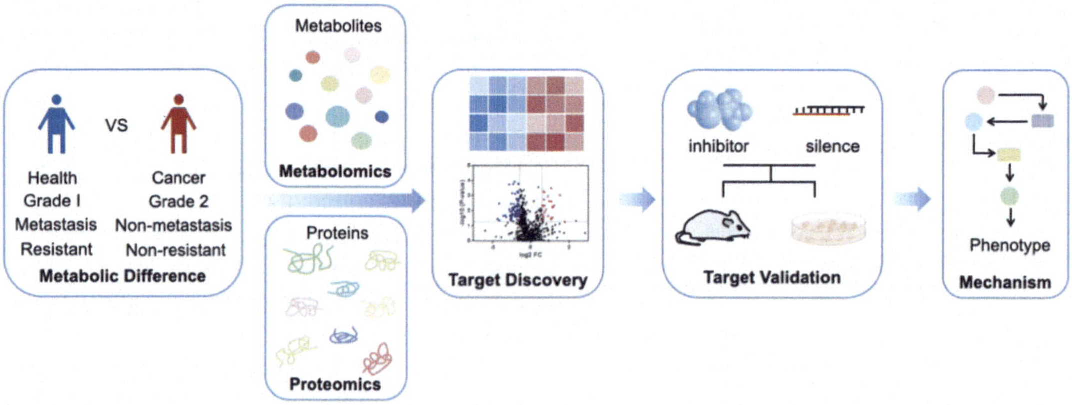

Fig. 1 Schematic workflow of the combined use of metabolomics and proteomics for the discovery of cancer therapeutic targets

Urine, serum, and plasma are easily accessible and contain thousands of metabolites and are thus most frequently used for metabolic biomarker discovery [14]. In addition to this, tissue biopsies and body fluids such as saliva, cerebrospinal fluid, and bile acid have also been used for metabolomic analysis [15].

Nevertheless, metabolites are sensitive and prone to degradation. Hence, reproducible and reliable sample collection and processing protocols are essential for metabolic biomarker discovery. In fact, sample collection and processing steps are of paramount importance. This was demonstrated by studies showing distinct metabolic profiles were obtained due to variances in sample collection and sample preparation. For example, Liu et al. used gas chromatography coupled to mass spectrometry (GC-MS) to analyze the metabolic patterns in serum and plasma from 15 healthy individuals. They found that the incubation of plasma at 4 °C for 2, 3, and 4 h had pronounced influences on detected intensities of plasma metabolites [16]. Therefore, proper collection and storage steps are critical factors to acquire primitive metabolic information from samples. Biological samples subjected to metabolomic analysis are recommended to be stored in liquid nitrogen or − 80 °C and must avoid repeated freezing and thawing.

2.1.2 Metabolomic Acquisition Methods and Data Analysis Tools

Metabolites present in biological samples may possess a wide range of physicochemical properties including polarity, molecular weight, and concentrations [17]. Therefore, it remains a great challenge to comprehensively detect and characterize endogenous metabolites. Nevertheless, advances in state-of-the-art analytical instrumentation and acquisition methods have emerged and posited metabolomics as a current workhorse in bioanalysis. Among different technologies, nuclear magnetic resonance (NMR) and gas/liquid chromatography coupled to mass spectrometry (GC/LC-MS) are most frequently used.

NMR spectroscopy is one of the earliest techniques applied to metabolomic analysis [18]. It uses the energy changes of the nucleus in magnetic field to obtain relevant nuclear information. ^{1}H-NMR, ^{13}C-NMR, ^{15}N-NMR, and ^{31}P-NMR are commonly used with ^{1}H-NMR as the most prevalent technique [19]. Current NMR advances in automation and the capability in unambiguous assignment of molecular identities. Its relatively low sensitivity has been improved by increasing the magnetic field strength and the introduction of cryogenically cooled probes and microprobes [20]. In addition, the unique advantage of NMR in nondestructive analysis is exemplified by a high-resolution magic angle spinning (HRMAS) NMR technology. It is an exciting development that allows to perform metabolic analysis of intact tissues without sample preparation and has been widely applied to probe intact tissues including but not limited to the brain, kidney, and liver [21, 22]. With rapid development in NMR theory and technology, its applications in metabolomics studies have rejuvenated.

Due to their robustness and high sensitivity and throughput, GC/LC-MS has become a core platform for metabolite detection and identification. The coupling of chromatography to MS reduces sample complexity, enabling a comprehensive analysis of metabolome with great coverage. The optimized front end based on separation science thus shines in identification of low-abundance metabolite species and has resulted in successful discovery of a myriad of metabolite biomarkers for various diseases. For instance, Furusho et al. developed a three-dimensional high-performance liquid chromatographic (3D-HPLC) method, which included a reversed-phase column in the first dimension, an anion-exchange column in the second dimension, and an enantioselective column in the third dimension, for metabolite separation. With this setup, they successfully differentiated D-amino acids such as D-alanine, D-serine, D-asparagine, and D-proline from the L-forms in human plasma and found the abundances of D-alanine, D-serine, D-asparagine, and D-proline were significantly increased in the plasma of patients with chronic kidney disease (CKD) compared with those of the healthy donors [23]. Ibáñez et al. combined reversed phase (RP) with hydrophilic interaction chromatography (HILIC) to analyze the cerebrospinal fluids of patients at different stages of Alzheimer's disease (AD) and identified a broader polarity range of metabolites that allows the differentiation of AD developmental stages [24]. Cui and Hu et al. used ion chromatography (IC) as an orthogonal separation method for analysis of charged and polar compounds such as carbohydrates, organic acids, sugar phosphates, and nucleotides from head and neck cancer cells [25] and saliva from gout patients [26], respectively. The outstanding chromatographic resolution of IC even allows differentiation of isobaric and isomeric polar metabolites and thus holds promise for accurate identification of biomarkers for diagnostic and prognostic purposes.

Besides chromatography, cutting-edge technological advances in MS also allow metabolomic analysis with enhanced coverage and accuracy. The development in mass analyzers such as Orbitrap and Q-TOF together with the inclusion of ion mobility cell for gas-phase ion separation has pronouncedly improved the breadth and depth of detected metabolites [27, 28]. For example, Damen et al. combined ion mobility spectrometry and Q-TOF to separate different lipid molecular species and lipid isomers using a charged surface hybrid (CSH) C_{18} column. Compared to conventional MS approach, the combined method delivered a superior performance that can be exemplified by the separation of lipid isomers such as PC 36:3 at *m/z* 784.5851 and PE 36:2 at *m/z* 742.5392 [29].

Although the combination of GC/LC with MS has been successfully implemented for both metabolite identification and biomarker screening, current analytical toolkits are still limited in achieving an in-depth analysis of all metabolites. This limitation could be attributed to multiple factors. First, the most prevalent acquisition method, data-dependent acquisition (DDA), in nontargeted analysis is biased toward the selection of high-abundance ion species for MS/MS fragmentation. A number of biologically significant metabolites may present with relatively low abundance and therefore is limited. To overcome this challenge, data-independent acquisition (DIA) is thus developed as an alternative strategy. Theoretically, DIA methods enable comprehensive fragmentation of all metabolite precursors in a sample run, whereas the data can be repetitively analyzed to re-extract fragment ions for precursors of interest. DIA method has been proven to improve the number of detected endogenous metabolites with better reproducibility through direct comparison with results acquired via the DDA analysis. In addition, quantitative accuracy was improved due to a shortened duty cycle conferred by DIA analysis. A representative example of DIA in metabolomics is that Wang et al. employed sequential windowed acquisition of all theoretical fragment ion (SWATH) MS with variable isolation windows on an ultrahigh-performance liquid chromatography (UPLC)-quadrupole time-of-flight (Q-TOF) to characterize the Standard Reference Material (SRM 1950) in plasma. A total of 1373 unique metabolites was identified, confirming significantly increased coverage compared with DDA [30].

Although the DIA strategy enables acquisition of MS/MS spectra with high quality and efficiency, it is challenging to process the large-scale DIA data. To meet this demand, several approaches have been developed for DIA data analysis. Li et al. developed a program named MetDIA, which identified metabolite by five steps, including peak detection and alignment, targeted chromatogram extractions, generations of peak groups and pseudo MS^2 spectra, metabolite-centric identification, and statistical analysis. Compared with DDA, MetDIA identified five more true positive metabolites in a standard mixture sample containing 30 metabolites. This method was applied to studying the function of Fas-associated protein with death domain (FADD) by comparing metabolome in FADD wild-type and FADD-deficient Jurkat cells. Based on MetDIA, 156 metabolites were identified and 37 metabolites were detected with significant changed abundances [31].

Another factor on metabolome analysis coverage stems from the way the MS/MS fragmentation ions are collected. Normally, a general MS/MS fragmentation parameter is set in the acquisition method that applies to all metabolites. Nevertheless, metabolites are synthesized from different routes and result in production of compounds with distinct molecular structures and physicochemical properties. Therefore, a generalized parameter such as collision energy (CE) is insufficient for all precursors to produce MS/MS spectra of good quality for subsequent structural characterization. Ye et al. have shown that this holds especially true for natural products and developed stepped MS^{All} strategy to produce MS/MS spectra for all detected small molecules by setting pronouncedly wide CE range in each duty cycle [32, 33]. This guarantees precursors are subjected to sufficient MS/MS fragmentation under their optimal settings in a sample run. This application has been further propagated to optimize multiple reaction monitoring (MRM) parameters with automation capability and without the need of a large amount of pure standards for tuning [34, 35]. Another study reported by Luo et al. proposed a pseudotargeted metabolomics approach by generating DIA data from pooled serum metabolites under 20, 40, and 60 eV. Candidate ion pairs for MRM were extracted using a house-developed software MRM-Ion Pair Finder, and 854 transitions were applied to discover metabolites showing abnormal expression levels in sera from hepatocellular carcinoma (HCC) patients [36].

2.1.3 Innovative Metabolomics Data Analysis Approaches

With increasingly more metabolic features being detected, the great challenge lies in how to accurately and specifically identify the detected metabolic features. Conventional approaches rely on searching the acquired *m/z* and fragment ions of metabolites against various online databases including the Encyclopedia of Genes and Genomes (KEGG), METLIN, human metabolome database (HMDB), etc. Matching *m/z* would often result in multiple hits for single precursor query, necessitating the need to match retention time and MS/MS fragmentation ions with those generated from pure standards. This time-consuming task cannot always be accomplished due to limited availability of standards, and this accounts for elusive identities of disease-related metabolic biomarkers in numerous studies.

To solve this dilemma, tremendous efforts have been devoted to structural assignment. Specifically, a recently reported data analysis program termed metabolic pathway extension (MPE) proposed a concept of "submetabolome" and a novel means to infer unknown structures from the pool of metabolites by exploiting the well-classified metabolic reactions normally occurring in biological systems. Firstly, metabolites that displayed abundance changes in response to a drastic intensity change of a "core metabolite" are included as a pool. Then, metabolic reactions are used to connect the metabolites, which leads to the establishment of a network with the core metabolite posited in center. Lastly, metabolites of unknown identities in current databases can be inferred based on its transformation from a known structure within the network. Using the MPE approach, Wang et al. studied the metabolic network of carnitine and validated the assigned molecular structures based on databases. The newly constructed repository of carnitine metabolic network enables identification of more metabolite biomarkers compared to that achieved by database searching in a mice model of fasting. This approach has thus opened up a new window for identification of metabolism-associated compounds (Fig. 2) [35].

Similar to the concept of establishing metabolic network via biotransformations, Shen et al. developed a metabolic reaction network (MRN)-based recursive algorithm (MetDNA), which is based on the assumption that similar MS/MS spectra are produced from seed metabolites and their reaction-paired neighbors due to high structural similarities. Using MetDNA, about 2000 metabolites can be annotated from one dataset, which expands the capability of metabolite annotation and facilitates metabolomics analysis [37]. Another example is Huan et al., who developed a web-based online analytical tool named MyCompoundID.org

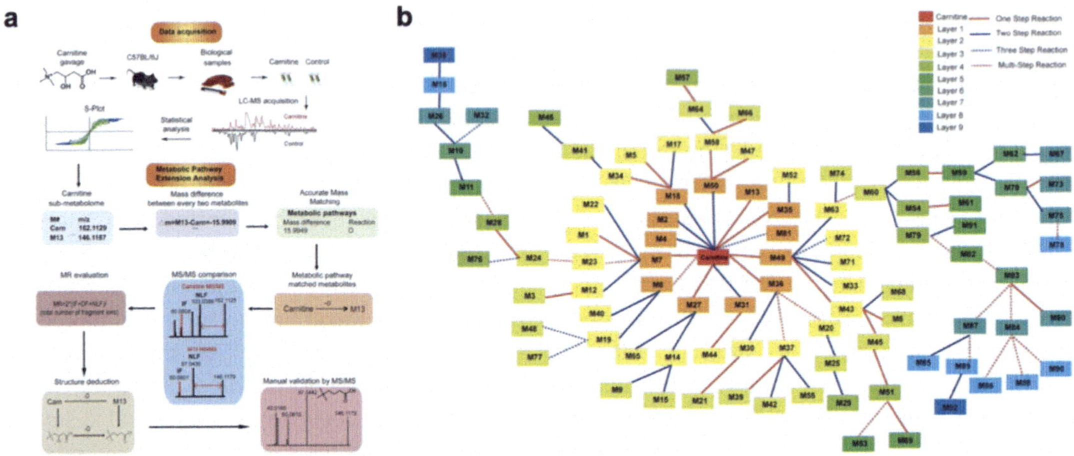

Fig. 2 Metabolic pathway extension (MPE) approach. (**a**) Overall workflow of the MPE approach. Briefly, the carnitine metabolome was first constructed by differential analysis of the plasma samples collected from mice administered with or without the core metabolite, carnitine in this case, by LC-MS. The accurate *m/z* and corresponding MS/MS of the metabolites changed in response to carnitine intake were then extracted from the raw data and imported to a stand-alone program we developed named Metabolic Pathway Extension Analysis (MPEA). The MPEA program used the accurate *m/z* information on the carnitine metabolome to establish the targeted metabolic network of carnitine by calculating the mass differences between any pairs of metabolites within the pool of carnitine metabolome and subsequently matching them against a list of metabolic reactions commonly encountered in biological systems. (**b**) Carnitine metabolome connected by metabolic reactions via the metabolic pathway extension approach. All the metabolites are registered with a number based on *m/z* values, and carnitine is the initial metabolite (highlighted in red). A sequential layer-by-layer characterization strategy enables the connection of the 93 metabolites into the metabolic network of carnitine by one, two, three, or multiple-step metabolic reactions

(MCID). MCID is established by constructing a library of over 383,830 predicted human metabolites by extending the known metabolites with a limited number of biotransformation, which facilitates the identification and validation of novel metabolite structures [38].

2.2 Metabolomics for Biomarker Discovery and Therapeutic Target Identification

Cancer cells purposely reprogram the metabolisms to commit sources to energy production and biosynthesis while maintaining redox balance [39]. These rewired metabolic traits are vital for cancer cell survival, growth, and proliferation. Therefore, the sensitivity, throughput, and robustness offered by metabolomics have made it a powerful tool for profiling the metabolomic alterations between normal and cancerous cells and tissues. The knowledge gained by metabolomics not only enables the discovery of sensitive and specific biomarkers but also provides mechanistic insights regarding the fundamental causes of cancers and therapeutic outcomes. Such information can redefine the targets for anticancer drug discovery and development. In the following sections, successful applications of metabolomics in cancer biomarker discovery and further validation of the key players responsible for mediating the corresponding metabolic changes are reviewed.

2.2.1 Metabolomics in Metabolic Biomarker and Target Discovery

Metabolomics has been frequently used for discovery of cancer diagnostic and prognostic biomarkers as complementary with genomics data and gene risk scores [40]. For instance, lung cancer is the leading cause of cancer-related mortality worldwide [41]. Nevertheless, early diagnosis of lung cancer can increase the survival rate to

85% [42]. Hence, many researchers are striving in exploring the biomarkers for lung cancer diagnosis. Specifically, Mu et al. collected 65 serum samples from nonsmoking female patients with non-small cell lung cancer (NSCLC) and 65 serum samples from healthy donors and examined the metabolomic differences by GC-MS analysis. Cysteine, serine, and 1-monooleoylglycerol were found to significantly decrease in lung cancer patients. These metabolites can be further combined as a biomarker panel for sensitive diagnosis of NSCLC [43]. Rocha et al. employed NMR-based metabolomics to analyze 85 plasma samples collected from primary lung cancer patients and 78 plasma samples from healthy donors as control. They found that several amino acids, including alanine, glutamine and valine, and acetate and formate, were significantly decreased in cancer patients' plasma [44]. Moreover, Ni et al. found glycine, valine, methionine, citrulline, and arginine decreased in sera of 57 lung cancer patients compared with those from the 130 matched healthy control donors. Intriguingly, both studies showed that valine, a branched-chain amino acid (BCAA), was decreased in patients with lung cancer [45]. This finding was supported by a mechanistic study by Mayers et al. showing the BCAA metabolism occurred in NSCLC patients, of which two BCAA transporters, BCAT1 and BCAT2, were both upregulated. These metabolic alterations enabled the tumor cells to adaptively use free BCAAs as a nitrogen source for DNA and macromolecule synthesis. The increased uptake of BCAA into tumor cells explains the reduced BCAAs in NSCLC patients' circulation system. This study suggested the potential of targeting BCAT1 and BCAT2 for therapeutic treatment of NSCLC [46].

Tumor is notorious for its heterogeneity. Heterogeneity leads to different metabolic alterations in specific tissues or variant genetic backgrounds [47–49]. This means metabolic profiles can thus be utilized in tumor classifications. For instance, breast cancer can be classified into luminal A subtype, luminal B subtype, Her-2 positive subtype, basal-like subtype, and triple-negative breast cancer (TNBC) according to the expression level of estrogen receptor (ER), progesterone receptor (PR), and human epidermal growth factor receptor 2 (Her-2) [50, 51]. Cao et al. used high-resolution magic angle spinning magnetic resonance spectroscopy (HR-MAS-MRS) to analyze breast cancer tissue from 75 patients with TNBC or triple-positive breast cancer (TPBC). They found that choline and glutamate were significantly higher in TNBC compared to TPBC tumors. Meanwhile, they also found a significantly lower level of glutamine in TNBC, which indicated an increased glutaminolysis in TNBC [52]. Jin et al. showed that oncogenic receptor tyrosine kinase (RTK) differentially reprogramed the metabolic phenotype in NSCLC cells. Based on metabolomics profiling, they found that NSCLC cells with EGFR mutation were highly dependent on the serine synthesis pathway for nucleotide biosynthesis and redox homeostasis, while NSCLC cells with EGFR amplification utilized lactate as fuel for energy production. The results linked molecular genotype with metabolic dependency and laid the foundation for personalized medical treatment [53]. Combinatorially, these metabolic phenotypes delineated by metabolomics studies demonstrated that signature metabolites may serves as biomarkers for cancer classification. More importantly, these metabolic changes reflect different cell types' need for specific metabolites or metabolic pathways, whereas the metabolic vulnerability can be specifically targeted by selecting tumors that are hypersensitive to these targeted therapies. This information is extremely valuable for cancer types where druggable targets are lacked or expressed at relatively low levels such as diffuse-type gastric cancer [54].

Besides classification of cancer types, metabolomics is used to identify cancer stages as well. Understanding the clinical stages of cancers allows clinicians or surgeons to make righteous treatment decisions. For instance, prostate cancer is the second leading cause of cancer death in men worldwide [13]. According to the American Cancer Society, the 5-year relative survival rates of prostate cancer patients without and with metastasis are 80% and 30%, respectively, whereas the progression-free survival of patients without metastasis was twice that of patients with metastasis [55–57]. Hence, it is necessary to develop biomarkers for the classification of prostate cancer stages. Sreekumar et al. used GC-MS and LC-MS to analyze tissue, blood, and urine samples from 262 clinical subjects classified as prostate cancer and successfully differentiated the benign prostate, clinically localized prostate cancer, and metastatic prostate cancer. One key metabolite, sarcosine, was found to be highly increased when prostate cancer proceeds to the metastatic stage. This accords to a previous study that reported the increase of sarcosine in invasive prostate cancer cell lines such as VCap, DU145, 22RV1, and LNCap compared to benign prostate epithelial cell lines, PeEC and RWPE. Notably, knockdown of a glycine-producing-sarcosine enzyme, glycine-N-methyltransferase, significantly abolished the malignant behaviors of prostate cancer. Taken together, the information gained via integrating clinical and in vitro metabolomics and molecular biology studies indicates that sarcosine plays an important role in the metastasis of prostate cancer cells and can be a potential metabolic biomarker for predicting metastasis. Meanwhile, the sarcosine metabolic pathway also holds potential as a new target for prostate cancer therapy [58]. Recently, Eniu et al. also demonstrated an exemplary application of metabolomics to breast cancer staging. Free amino acids in sera, such as tyrosine, arginine, and alanine, were found to decrease in breast cancer patients, especially during the progression from stage II to stage III [59].

The application of metabolomics in prognostic biomarker discovery has culminated in the finding of oncometabolites such as 2-hydroxyglutarate (2-HG). Wang et al. found that, in 234 cytogenetically normal AML patients, high level of serum 2-HG was associated with poor overall survival and event-free survival. These results suggest that serum 2-HG is a highly valuable prognostic biomarker for AML patients. Besides 2-HG, Chen et al. also found that highly active glycolysis was related to poor overall survival in AML patients. They performed metabolomics analysis of the serum samples from 400 AML patients and 446 healthy controls and identified six serum metabolite biomarkers including lactate, 2-oxoglutarate, pyruvate, 2-HG, glycerol-3-phosphate, and citrate. This panel of six biomarkers could predict the prognostic outcome for AML patients [60]. Mathe et al. analyzed urine samples from 496 patients with lung cancers and 536 healthy controls and found creatine riboside and N-acetylneuraminic acid were significantly elevated in lung cancer patients and associated with poor prognosis [61].

In addition to identifying cancer biomarkers for diagnosis, prognosis, tumor classification, and staging, metabolomics has great potential to deepen our understanding of cancer pathologic mechanisms and thus the discovery of potential therapeutic targets when used in conjugation with biochemical and genetic tools. Huang et al. applied metabolomics to profiling of small cell lung cancer (SCLC) cell lines and identified metabolic heterogeneity and subtype-selective vulnerabilities. Specifically, guanosine nucleotides were found to increase in Achaete-scute homolog-1 (ASCL1) low cells, along with the relatively high expression levels of guanosine synthetic enzymes including inosine monophosphate dehydrogenase-1 and 2 (IMPDH1 and IMPDH2). Inhibition of IMPDH1/2 thwarted the growth of SCLC cells with low ASCL1 expression in both in vitro and in vivo models. These results suggested that IMPDH is a potential therapeutic target for low-ASCL1 expressing SCLC [62]. Wang et al. investigated the metabolomics profiles of the tumor-initiating cells (TICs) from primary NSCLC adenocarcinoma. An increased methionine cycle activity and high S-adenosylmethionine (SAM) consumption were observed in TICs accompanied with elevated transmethylation driven by methionine adenosyltransferase II alpha (MAT2A) that is responsible for SAM synthesis. Consequently, pharmacological inhibition of MAT2A, which leads to the inhibited SAM production, influenced the tumorigenicity of TICs, suggesting that MAT2A holds promise as a potential target for NSCLC therapy [63].

2.2.2 Metabolomics in Cancer Chemotherapy

Metabolomics in predicting and evaluating individual's responses to drug treatment is also widely recognized. The complexity in genetic/protein expressions dictates the need to treat patients with tailored therapy that can mostly benefit them. Drug resistance is one of the main reasons for the failure of cancer therapy [64]. It is reported that cancer cells that gain resistance to therapeutic interventions can remodel their metabolism to adapt and survive from drug treatment [65]. Kominsky et al. used NMR and GC-MS to assess the metabolic differences between chronic myelogenous leukemia (CML) cell lines with different sensitivities to imatinib. They found that, after imatinib treatment, sensitive cells showed decreased glucose uptake and lactate production while resistant cells maintained the highly glycolytic metabolic phenotype. The relatively high glucose uptake and lactate production can thus be used as markers for early detection of imatinib resistance in CML cells [66]. Ruprecht et al. found that the lapatinib-resistant BT-474 cell line showed elevated level of metabolites in glycolysis and increased lactate production after lapatinib treatment compared to the lapatinib-sensitive BT474 cells [67]. Together, these results indicate that metabolomics can be a forecasting method to distinguish patients' sensitivity or resistance to drug intervention [67].

Metabolomics have also been widely applied to profiling of the metabolic alterations after chemotherapy and guide clinical medication therapy. Doxorubicin is the first-line drug in the treatment of breast cancer and has been applied to a wide range of chemotherapy [68, 69]. However, the relatively high dosage of doxorubicin in clinical application could lead to several serious side effects, including myelosuppression and cardiotoxicity [70, 71]. Shao et al. used the breast cancer cell line MCF-7 and administered doxorubicin in a relatively low dosage to establish a metronomic chemotherapy regimen and also in a relatively high dosage to mimic the maximal-tolerated-dose chemotherapy model. Metabolomics and PCR arrays were used to distinguish the metabolic differences between the two dosing regimens. The integral omics data showed that glucose, amino acid, and nucleotide metabolisms were activated in the metronomic chemotherapy group and decreased in the maximal-tolerated-dose chemotherapy group. Pharmacological inhibition of the activated metabolic pathway combined with metronomic chemotherapy exacerbated apoptosis in MCF-7 cells. However, such treatment had no effect on human mammary epithelial MCF-10A cells. These results suggest that disturbing breast cancer cell metabolism with metronomic chemotherapy could selectively kill cancer cells and reduce side effects in normal cells [72].

Metabolomics has significantly facilitated cancer biomarker discovery due to its unique ability in comprehensively profiling metabolic phenotypes and pinpointing metabolic abnormalities. However, the detected metabolic alterations must be linked to causal frameworks, which can then be translated into therapeutic targets for treatment or truly valuable biomarkers for clinical applications. Nevertheless, this cannot be accomplished by metabolomics alone because the underlying metabolic mechanisms need to be answered by other means such as molecular biology methodologies together with metabolomics.

3 Combined Metabolomics and Proteomics in Cancer Metabolic Target Discovery

Although metabolomics provides systematic and sensitive information regarding metabolic alterations induced by cancer occurrence and progression, the causes of these alterations and the underlying mechanisms remain largely elusive. To this regard, proteomics is a complementary methodology that provides insights into the causes and outputs of the observed abnormal metabolism in cancers. Hence, the combined metabolomics and proteomics approach is increasingly being used to deepen the mechanistic understanding of cancer metabolism and identify novel drug targets that modulate such processes.

A representative use of the combined approaches was reported by Celiktas and coauthors. They applied metabolomics and proteomics to investigating lung adenocarcinoma (LADC) with or without liver kinase B1 (LKB1) inactivation. LKB1 is a tumor suppressor and often inactivated in lung cancers, which confers invasive and metastatic properties of cancer cells. Based on quantitative proteomics, they identified carbamoyl phosphate synthetase 1 (CPS1) was elevated in LKB1-inactivated LADC cells compared with LKB1-activated cells. Their metabolomics analysis showed that metabolite intermediates involved in purine/pyrimidine and arginine metabolism pathways were downregulated in CPS1 knockdown H1437 and H1944 cells, indicating that the knockdown of CPS1 could lead to cell growth inhibition. These results suggested that CPS1 is a promising therapeutic target for LADC patients carrying LKB1 mutation [73].

Additionally, Cai et al. used a combined proteomics/metabolomics approach to analyze tissues from patients with gastric cardia cancer (GCC) compared to normal counterparts. They first found that enzymes involved in glycolysis, including fructose-1,6-diphosphate aldolase A (ALDOA), glyceraldehyde-3-phosphate dehydrogenase (GAPDH), and enolase (ENO1) all increased while enzymes involved in TCA cycle, including pyruvate dehydrogenase B (PDHB), aconitate hydratase (ACO2), and fumarate hydratase (FH), were downregulated in cancer tissues via quantitative proteomics. Then, they employed metabolomics tools and revealed that six intermediates involved in glucose metabolism, including fructose-6-phasphate, glyceraldehyde, and pyruvate, were increased during tumorigenesis. These results collectively show activated glycolysis and impaired TCA cycle in GCC cells, whereas channeling the flux from glycolysis to TCA cycle can potentially inhibit growth and migration. Consequently, the inhibition of LDHA and overexpression of PDHB that modulate the metabolic flux are potential therapeutic targets for combating GCC [74].

By using a combined proteomics and metabolomics approach, Dougan et al. found that peroxidasin (PXDN) was elevated in prostate cancer tissues compared to normal tissues and related metabolic pathways. Silencing of PXDN led to decreased cell viability and increased apoptotic rate, and proteomics data showed that PXDN knockdown upregulated multiple proteins that are enriched in biological processes including oxidative stress, mitochondrial dysfunction, and gluconeogenesis. Meanwhile, metabolomic profiling revealed increased metabolites in oxidative stress and decreased metabolites in nucleotide biosynthesis. Therefore, the integral omics data suggested that inhibiting PXDN exerts therapeutic value through increased ROS and inhibited nucleotide synthesis [75].

Besides a handful of cases that successfully integrated these two powerful approaches in developing potential therapeutic targets [76, 77], the integral omics approach can also be used for monitoring cells' responses to chemotherapy and developing anti-resistant therapy in cancer cells. For instance, Wu et al. used metabolomics and proteomics to analyze the metabolism-associated molecular events in senescent and apoptotic cells after doxorubicin treatment. Based on metabolomics, they found that several nucleotides, amino acids, and carbohydrates were elevated in senescent cells while decreased in apoptotic cells. Meanwhile, the proteomics data showed enzymes involved in glycolysis, TCA cycle, pentose phosphate pathway, purine, and pyrimidine biosynthesis were increased in senescent cells yet decreased in apoptotic cells, which in turn supported the metabolic alterations measured by metabolomics (Fig. 3). G6PD, a protein that is responsible for ROS elimination, was significantly upregulated in senescent cells. The coadministration of G6PD inhibitor with Dox managed to induce apoptosis to cancer cells rather than senescence, indicating that senescent cells relied on G6PD to scavenge ROS and repair DNA damage. Therefore, G6PD may serve as a target for treating the chemotherapy-induced resistance [78].

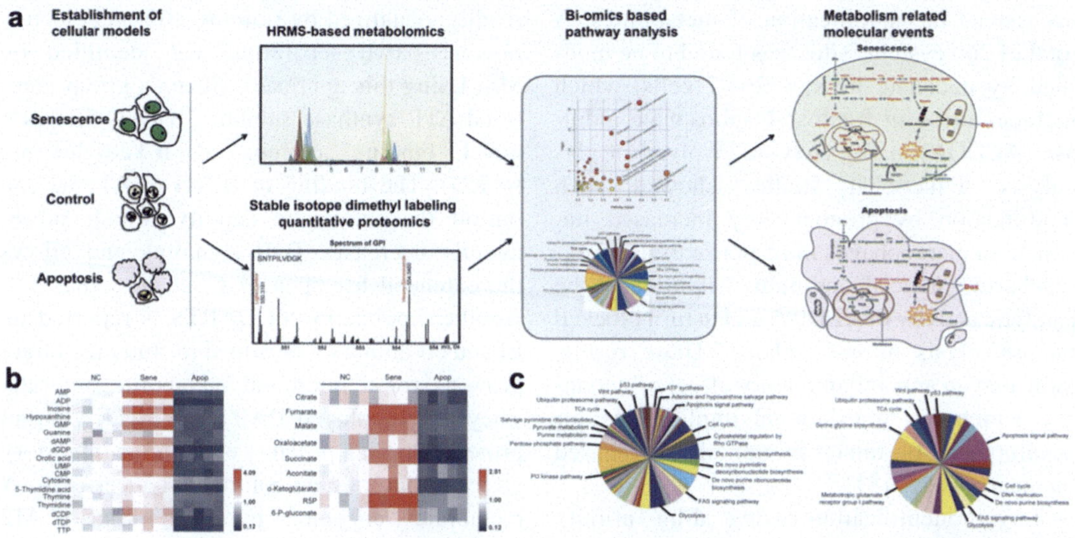

Fig. 3 The combined approach of metabolomics and proteomics was used to analyze the metabolism-associated molecular events in senescent and apoptotic cells after doxorubicin treatment. (**a**) A schematic workflow of the combined approach. (**b**) Heat map of changed metabolites involved in purine and pyrimidine biosynthesis pathway, pentose phosphate pathway, and tricarboxylic acid cycle. (**c**) Gene ontology analysis of proteomic data revealed disturbed pathways in senescent and apoptotic cells

4 Novel Chemoproteomics-Based Approach for Direct Target Identification

Although proteomics can comprehensively record the protein expression changes in diseased states, the measured information is a readout of reprogramed metabolism-induced consequences rather than the direct causes of abnormal metabolism. Therefore, studies have increasingly focused on mapping the direct binding proteome for endogenous functional metabolites in hope that novel functional proteins that exert the biological and pathological functions of altered metabolite abundances can be discovered as therapeutic targets.

Chemoproteomics, an approach that was originally developed to elucidate the target proteins for drugs, has been applied to target identification of endogenous metabolites. For instance, affinity-based protein profiling (AfBPP) is a leading-edge chemical proteomics method that develops probes based on the original structure of targeted small molecules and modifies them with reactive group that allows attachment of the probes to its binding proteins. Fluorophore or other groups for affinity enrichment were devised and incorporated into the probes, which makes subsequent visualization and enrichment for proteomics-based identification accomplishable. Hulce et al. synthesized clickable photoreactive sterol probes in combination with quantitative proteomics and identified 265 cholesterol-binding proteins in HeLa cells. Among the identified proteins, seven proteins have been known to bind to cholesterol [79]. In addition, Moraru et al. synthesized a derivative of methylglyoxal (MGO) that carries a clickable group and identified fatty acid synthase (FASN) as one of the targets of MGO based on AfBPP, imparting a novel druggable target for type 2 diabetes [80]. Furthermore, Qin et al. devised a monosaccharide-based probe, 3,4,6-*O*-Ac_3ManNAz, that competitively labels cysteines with itaconate and applied it to the competitive isotopic tandem orthogonal proteolysis-affinity-based protein profiling (isoTOP-ABPP). The isotope-ABPP does not necessitate the modification of metabolites. A total of 260 cysteine sites was found to be modified by itaconate in Raw 264.7 cells, which includes those in fructose-bisphosphate aldolase (ALDOA), a key enzyme involved in glycolysis. Functional studies showed such modification by pronouncedly increased itaconate in macrophages in response to lipopolysaccharide-induced stimulus inhibited the catalytic activity of ALDOA and in turn blocked the glycolysis of macrophage. These results indicated an anti-inflammatory effect of itaconate, which has translational implications for development of tumor immunotherapy based on macrophages [81].

Target identification using drug affinity responsive target stability (DARTS) is another widely used approach of target discovery for unmodified small molecules of interest. It was originally developed by Lomenick and co-authors. They reasoned that, once the small molecule binds to the target proteins, the interactions would induce conformational change for the bound proteins and confer them greater protease-resistant stability. Therefore, proteins of enhanced stability upon ligand incubation are assigned as binding proteins, which can be readily visualized by staining after gel electrophoresis-based separation and identified by MS. Using this approach, Huang's group identified ATP synthase subunit 5B (ATP5B) as a novel binding protein of α-ketoglutarate (α-KG). The binding of α-KG to ATP5B can inhibit the enzymatic activity, which subsequently decreases TOR signaling and allows the extended life span of *C. elegans* [82, 83]. Another application of DARTS is reported by Li and co-authors who aimed to study the target proteins for a microbial metabolite butyrate. They first employed DARTS to identify target proteins that can possibly explain the inhibitory effect of butyrate on colorectal cancer cells. A metabolic enzyme, pyruvate kinase M2 (PKM2), was identified as the binding protein since butyrate can dose-responsively increased the stability of PKM2 against protease. This finding is validated by metabolomics data showing that pyruvate, the product of PKM2, accumulated after butyrate administration in colorectal cancer cells, suggesting that butyrate might direct bind to and activate PKM2. The biochemical assays also suggested that the activation of PKM2 by butyrate can inhibit the Warburg effect and subsequently suppress the

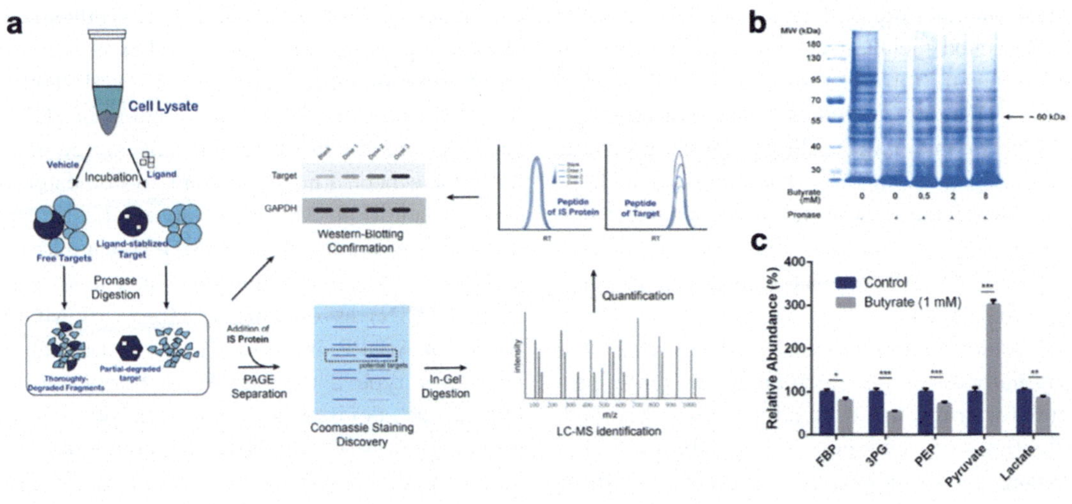

Fig. 4 Target identification for butyrate via the DARTS-based proteomics approach and immunoblotting experiments. (**a**) A schematic workflow. (**b**) SDS-PAGE analysis of pronase-digested cell lysate followed by Coomassie blue staining identified a butyrate-stabilized protein within the ~60 kDa gel band. (**c**) Abundance level changes of representative metabolites suggest modulated PKM2 activity after the 24-h butyrate treatment

proliferation of colorectal cancer cells. Collectively, this study established the first mechanistic link between PKM2-induced metabolic remodeling and the anti-tumorigenic function of butyrate (Fig. 4) [84].

Besides the abovementioned approaches, CETSA (cellular therm mployed to identify proteome-wide binding targets for endogenous metabolites such as 2′,3′-cGAMP in RAW 264.7 cells [85], ATP in K562 cells [86], and arginine in T cells [5]. Noteworthy, proteins of distinct classes and cellular localizations spanning from membrane proteins, transcription factors to cytosol proteins have all been assigned as targets of metabolites, revealing a complex metabolite-protein interaction network heretofore undiscovered [87]. Such information will help elucidate why the deregulated metabolic pathways lead to tumor occurrence, progression, and metastasis through discovering the functionality of the detected metabolite-protein interactions.

5 Conclusion

With the advancement of emerging MS technologies, metabolomics and proteomics have been increasingly used in the discovery of cancer biomarkers and therapeutic targets. The combination of metabolomics and proteomics technology can truly facilitate a better understanding of the pathological causes and biological outcomes of the remodeled cancer metabolism. The integration of metabolomics, proteomics, genomics and reliable bioinformatics tools for omics data analysis are expected to delineate a magnificent landscape of cancer metabolism and facilitate the proteome-wide identification of therapeutic targets to combat cancer.

Acknowledgments This study was financially supported by the National Key R&D Program ofChina (2018YFD0901101), the National Natural Science Foundation of China (grants No. 81872838, 81720108032), the Natural Science Foundation of Jiangsu Province (BK20180079), the Project of State Key Laboratory of Natural Medicines in ChinaPharmaceutical University (SKLNMZZCX201817), the Double First-Rate University project (CPU2018GY09, CPU2018GF09), and the Project for Major New Drugs Innovation and Development (2018ZX09711001-002-003,2018ZX09711002-001-004, 2017ZX09301013).

References

1. Vogelstein, B., & Kinzler, K. W. (2004). Cancer genes and the pathways they control. *Nature Medicine, 10*(8), 789–799.
2. Hanahan, D., & Weinberg, R. A. (2000). The hallmarks of cancer. *Cell, 100*, 57–70.
3. Thompson, C. B. (2011). Rethinking the regulation of cellular metabolism. *Cold Spring Harbor Symposia on Quantitative Biology, 76*, 23–29.
4. Kawaguchi, T., Takenoshita, M., Kabashima, T., & Uyeda, K. (2001). Glucose and cAMP regulate the L-type pyruvate kinase gene by phosphorylation/dephosphorylation of the carbohydrate response element binding protein. *Proceedings of the National Academy of Sciences of the United States of America, 98*(24), 13710–13715.
5. Geiger, R., Rieckmann, J. C., Wolf, T., Basso, C., Feng, Y., Fuhrer, T., Kogadeeva, M., Picotti, P., Meissner, F., Mann, M., Zamboni, N., Sallusto, F., & Lanzavecchia, A. (2016). L-arginine modulates T cell metabolism and enhances survival and anti-tumor activity. *Cell, 167*(3), 829–842.
6. Moellering, R. E., & Cravatt, B. F. (2013). Functional lysine modification by an intrinsically reactive primary glycolytic metabolite. *Science, 341*(6145), 549–553.
7. Parsons, D. W., Jones, S., Zhang, X., Lin, J. C., Leary, R. J., Angenendt, P., Mankoo, P., Carter, H., Siu, I.-M., Gallia, G. L., Olivi, A., McLendon, R., Rasheed, B. A., Keir, S., Nikolskaya, T., Nikolsky, Y., Busam, D. A., Tekleab, H., Diaz, L. A., Hartigan, J., Smith, D. R., Strausberg, R. L., Marie, S. K. N., Shinjo, S. M. O., Yan, H., Riggins, G. J., Bigner, D. D., Karchin, R., Papadopoulos, N., Parmigiani, G., Vogelstein, B., Velculescu, V. E., & Kinzler, K. W. (2008). An integrated genomic analysis of human glioblastoma multiforme. *Science, 321*, 1807–1812.
8. Stein, E. M., DiNardo, C. D., Fathi, A. T., Pollyea, D. A., Stone, R. M., Altman, J. K., Roboz, G. J., Patel, M. R., Collins, R., Flinn, I. W., Sekeres, M. A., Stein, A. S., Kantarjian, H. M., Levine, R. L., Vyas, P., MacBeth, K. J., Tosolini, A., VanOostendorp, J., Xu, Q., Gupta, I., Lila, T., Risueno, A., Yen, K. E., Wu, B., Attar, E. C., Tallman, M. S., & de Botton, S. (2019). Molecular remission and response patterns in patients with mutant-IDH2 acute myeloid leukemia treated with enasidenib. *Blood, 133*(7), 676–687.
9. Mullard, A. (2017). FDA approves first-in-class cancer metabolism drug. *Nature Reviews. Drug Discovery, 16*(9), 593.
10. Dwarakanath, B., Singh, D., Banerji, A. K., Sarin, R., Venkataramana, N., Jalali, R., Vishwanath, P.,

Mohanti, B., Tripathi, R., Kalia, V., & Jain, V. (2009). Clinical studies for improving radiotherapy with 2-deoxy-D-glucose: Present status and future prospects. *Journal of Cancer Research and Therapeutics, 5*(9), 21–26.
11. Jelonek, K., & Widłak, P. (2018). Metabolome-based biomarkers: Their potential role in the early detection of lung cancer. *Contemporary Oncology, 22*(3), 135–140.
12. McCartneya, A., Vignolib, A., Biganzolia, L., Lovec, R., Tenorib, L., Luchinatb, C., & Leoa, A. D. (2018). Metabolomics in breast cancer: A decade in review. *Cancer Treatment Reviews, 67*, 88–96.
13. Kdadra, M., Höckner, S., Leung, H., Kremer, W., & Schiffer, E. (2019). Metabolomics biomarkers of prostate cancer: A systematic review. *Diagnostics, 9*(1), 1–44.
14. Beckonert, O., Keun, H. C., Ebbels, T. M. D., Bundy, J., Holmes, E., Lindon, J. C., & Nicholson, J. K. (2007). Metabolic profiling, metabolomic and metabonomic procedures for NMR spectroscopy of urine, plasma, serum and tissue extracts. *Nature Protocols, 2*(11), 2692–2703.
15. Alvarez-Sanchez, B., Priego-Capote, F., & Castro, L. (2010). Metabolomics analysis I. Selection of biological samples and practical aspects preceding sample preparation. *Trends in Analytical Chemistry, 29*(2), 111–119.
16. Liu, L., Aa, J., Wang, G., Yan, B., Zhang, Y., Wang, X., Zhao, C., Cao, B., Shi, J., Li, M., Zheng, T., Zheng, Y., Hao, G., Zhou, F., Sun, J., & Wu, Z. (2010). Differences in metabolite profile between blood plasma and serum. *Analytical Biochemistry, 406*(2), 105–112.
17. Wishart, D. S., Feunang, Y. D., Marcu, A., Guo, A. C., Liang, K., Vazquez-Fresno, R., Sajed, T., Johnson, D., Li, C., Karu, N., Sayeeda, Z., Lo, E., Assempour, N., Berjanskii, M., Singhal, S., Arndt, D., Liang, Y., Badran, H., Grant, J., Serra-Cayuela, A., Liu, Y., Mandal, R., Neveu, V., Pon, A., Knox, C., Wilson, M., Manach, C., & Scalbert, A. (2018). HMDB 4.0: The human metabolome database for 2018. *Nucleic Acids Research, 46*, D608–D617.
18. Nicholson, J. K., Buckingham, M. J., & Sadler, P. J. (1983). High resolution 1H n.m.r. studies of vertebrate blood and plasma. *The Biochemical Journal, 211*, 605–615.
19. Bothwell, J. H. F., & Griffin, J. L. (2011). An introduction to biological nuclear magnetic resonance spectroscopy. *Biological Reviews, 86*(2), 493–510.
20. Emwas, A.-H. M. (2015). The strengths and weaknesses of NMR spectroscopy and mass spectrometry with particular focus on metabolomics research. *Methods in Molecular Biology, 1277*, 161–193.
21. Au, A., Cheng, K.-K., & Wei, L. K. (2017). Metabolomics, lipidomics and pharmacometabolomics of human hypertension. *Advances in Experimental Medicine and Biology, 956*, 599–613.
22. Beckonert, O., Coen, M., Keun, H. C., Wang, Y., Ebbels, T. M. D., Holmes, E., Lindon, J. C., & Nicholson, J. K. (2010). High-resolution magic-angle-spinning NMR spectroscopy for metabolic profiling of intact tissues. *Nature Protocols, 5*(6), 1019–1032.
23. Furusho, A., Koga, R., Akita, T., Mita, M., Kimura, T., & Hamase, K. (2019). Three-dimensional high-performance liquid chromatographic determination of Asn, Ser, Ala, and Pro enantiomers in the plasma of patients with chronic kidney disease. *Analytical Chemistry, 91*, 11569. https://doi.org/10.1021/acs.analchem.1029b01615.
24. Ibáñez, C., Simó, C., Barupal, D. K., Fiehn, O., Kivipelto, M., Cedazo-Mínguez, A., & Cifuentes, A. (2013). A new metabolomic workflow for early detection of Alzheimer's disease. *Journal of Chromatography A, 1302*, 65–71.
25. Hu, S., Wang, J., Ji, E. H., Christison, T., Lopez, L., & Huang, Y. (2015). Targeted metabolomic analysis of head and neck cancer cells using high performance ion chromatography coupled with a Q exactive HF mass spectrometer. *Analytical Chemistry, 87*(12), 6371–6379.
26. Cui, L., Liu, J., Yan, X., & Hu, S. (2017). Identification of metabolite biomarkers for gout using capillary ion chromatography with mass spectrometry. *Analytical Chemistry, 89*(21), 11737–11743.
27. Wen, C., Lin, F., Huang, B., Zhang, Z., Wang, X., Ma, J., Lin, G., Chen, H., & Hu, L. (2019). Metabolomics analysis in acute paraquat poisoning patients based on UPLC-Q-TOF-MS and machine learning approach. *Chemical Research in Toxicology, 32*(4), 629–637.
28. Hilaire, P. B. S., Hohenester, U. M., Colsch, B., Tabet, J.-C., Junot, C., & Fenaille, F. (2018). Evaluation of the high-field orbitrap fusion for compound annotation in metabolomics. *Analytical Chemistry, 90*(5), 3030–3035.
29. Damen, C. W. N., Isaac, G., Langridge, J., Hankemeier, T., & Vreeken, R. J. (2014). Enhanced lipid isomer separation in human plasma using reversed-phase UPLC with ion-mobility/high-resolution MS detection. *Journal of Lipid Research, 55*(8), 1772–1783.
30. Wang, L., Su, B., Zeng, Z., Li, C., Zhao, X., Lv, W., Xuan, Q., Ouyang, Y., Zhou, L., Yin, P., Peng, X., Lu, X., Lin, X., & Xu, G. (2018). Ion-pair selection method for pseudotargeted metabolomics based on SWATH MS acquisition and its application in differential metabolite discovery of type 2 diabetes. *Analytical Chemistry, 90*(19), 11401–11408.
31. Li, H., Cai, Y., Guo, Y., Chen, F., & Zhu, Z.-J. (2016). MetDIA: Targeted metabolite extraction of multiplexed MS/MS spectra generated by data-independent acquisition. *Analytical Chemistry, 88*(17), 8757–8764.
32. Ye, H., Zhu, L., Sun, D., Luo, X., Lu, G., Wang, H., Wang, J., Cao, G., Xiao, W., Wang, Z., Wang, G., & Hao, H. (2016). Nontargeted diagnostic ion network analysis (NINA): A software to streamline the analytical workflow for untargeted characterization of natural medicines. *Journal of Pharmaceutical and Biomedical Analysis, 131*, 40–47.
33. Ye, H., Wang, L., Zhu, L., Sun, D., Luo, X., Wang, H., Wang, G., & Hao, H. (2016). Stepped colli-

sional energy MS^{All}: An analytical approach for optimal MS/MS acquisition of complex mixture with diverse physicochemical properties. *Journal of Mass Spectrometry, 51*(5), 328–341.
34. Ye, H., Zhu, L., Wang, L., Liu, H., Zhang, J., Wu, M., Wang, G., & Hao, H. (2016). Stepped MS^{All} relied transition (SMART): An approach to rapidly determine optimal multiple reaction monitoring mass spectrometry parameters for small molecules. *Analytica Chimica Acta, 907*, 60–68.
35. Wang, L., Ye, H., Sun, D., Meng, T., Cao, L., Wu, M., Zhao, M., Wang, Y., Chen, B., Xu, X., Wang, G., & Hao, H. (2017). Metabolic pathway extension approach for metabolomic biomarker identification. *Analytical Chemistry, 89*(2), 1229–1237.
36. Luo, P., Dai, W., Yin, P., Zeng, Z., Kong, H., Zhou, L., Wang, X., Chen, S., Lu, X., & Xu, G. (2015). Multiple reaction monitoring-ion pair finder: A systematic approach to transform nontargeted mode to pseudotargeted mode for metabolomics study based on liquid chromatography-mass spectrometry. *Analytical Chemistry, 87*(10), 5050–5055.
37. Shen, X., Wang, R., Xiong, X., Yin, Y., Cai, Y., Ma, Z., Liu, N., & Zhu, Z.-J. (2019). Metabolic reaction network-based recursive metabolite annotation for untargeted metabolomics. *Nature Communications, 10*(1), 1516.
38. Huan, T., Tang, C., Li, R., Shi, Y., Lin, G., & Li, L. (2015). MyCompoundID MS/MS search: Metabolite identification using a library of predicted fragment-ion-spectra of 383,830 possible human metabolites. *Analytical Chemistry, 87*(20), 10619–10626.
39. Kang, S. W., Lee, S., & Lee, E. K. (2015). ROS and energy metabolism in cancer cells: Alliance for fast growth. *Archives of Pharmacal Research, 38*, 338–345.
40. Wishart, D. S. (2016). Emerging applications of metabolomics in drug discovery and precision medicine. *Nature Reviews. Drug Discovery, 15*(7), 473–484.
41. Kumar, N., Shahjaman, M. N. H., Islam, S., & Hoque, A. (2017). Serum and plasma metabolomic biomarkers for lung cancer. *Bioinformation, 13*(6), 202–208.
42. Siegel, R., Ma, J., Zou, Z., & Jemal, A. (2014). Cancer statistics, 2014. *CA: A Cancer Journal for Clinicians, 64*(1), 9–29.
43. Mu, Y., Zhou, Y., Wang, Y., Li, W., Zhou, L., Lu, X., Gao, P., Gao, M., Zhao, Y., Wang, Q., Wang, Y., & Xu, G. (2019). Serum metabolomics study of nonsmoking female patients with non-small cell lung cancer using gas chromatography-mass spectrometry. *Journal of Proteome Research, 18*(5), 2175–2184.
44. Rocha, C. M., Carrola, J., Barros, A. S., Gil, A. M., Goodfellow, B. J., Carreira, I. M., Bernardo, J., Gomes, A., Sousa, V., Carvalho, L., & Duarte, I. F. (2011). Metabolic signatures of lung cancer in biofluids: NMR-based metabonomics of blood plasma. *Journal of Proteome Research, 10*(9), 4314–4324.
45. Ni, J., Xu, L., Li, W., Zheng, C., & Wu, L. (2019). Targeted metabolomics for serum amino acids and acylcarnitines in patients with lung cancer. *Experimental and Therapeutic Medicine, 18*(1), 188–198.
46. Mayers, J. R., Torrence, M. E., Danai, L. V., Papagiannakopoulos, T., Davidson, S. M., Bauer, M. R., Lau, A. N., Ji, B. W., Dixit, P. D., Hosios, A. M., Muir, A., Chin, C. R., Freinkman, E., Jacks, T., Wolpin, B. M., Vitkup, D., & Heiden, M. G. V. (2016). Tissue of origin dictates branched-chain amino acid metabolism in mutant Kras-driven cancers. *Science, 353*(6304), 1161–1165.
47. McGranahan, N., & Swanton, C. (2017). Clonal heterogeneity and tumor evolution: Past, present, and the future. *Cell, 168*(4), 613–628.
48. Cros, J., Raffenne, J., Couvelard, A., & Poté, N. (2018). Tumor heterogeneity in pancreatic adenocarcinoma. *Pathobiology, 85*, 64–71.
49. Marusyk, A., & Polyak, K. (2010). Tumor heterogeneity: Causes and consequences. *Biochimica et Biophysica Acta, 1805*(1), 105–117.
50. Prat, A., & Perou, C. M. (2011). Deconstructing the molecular portraits of breast cancer. *Molecular Oncology, 5*(1), 5–23.
51. Conforti, R., Boulet, T., Tomasic, G., Taranchon, E., Arriagada, R., Spielmann, M., Ducourtieux, M., Soria, J. C., Tursz, T., Delaloge, S., Michiels, S., & Andre, F. (2007). Breast cancer molecular subclassification and estrogen receptor expression to predict efficacy of adjuvant anthracyclines-based chemotherapy: A biomarker study from two randomized trials. *Annals of Oncology, 18*(9), 1477–1483.
52. Cao, M. D., Lamichhane, S., Lundgren, S., Bofin, A., Fjøsne, H., Giskeødegård, G. F., & Bathen, T. F. (2014). Metabolic characterization of triple negative breast cancer. *BMC Cancer, 14*, 941–952.
53. Jin, N., Bi, A., Lan, X., Xu, J., Wang, X., Liu, Y., Wang, T., Tang, S., Zeng, H., Chen, Z., Tan, M., Ai, J., Xie, H., Zhang, T., Liu, D., Huang, R., Song, Y., Leung, E. L.-H., Yao, X., Ding, J., Geng, M., Lin, S.-H., & Huang, M. (2019). Identification of metabolic vulnerabilities of receptor tyrosine kinases-driven cancer. *Nature Communications, 10*(1), 2701.
54. Ge, S., Xia, X., Ding, C., Zhen, B., Zhou, Q., Feng, J., Yuan, J., Chen, R., Li, Y., Ge, Z., Ji, J., Zhang, L., Wang, J., Li, Z., Lai, Y., Hu, Y., Li, Y., Li, Y., Gao, J., Chen, L., Xu, J., Zhang, C., Jung, S. Y., Choi, J. M., Jain, A., Liu, M., Song, L., Liu, W., Guo, G., Gong, T., Huang, Y., Qiu, Y., Huang, W., Shi, T., Zhu, W., Wang, Y., He, F., Shen, L., & Qin, J. (2018). A proteomic landscape of diffuse-type gastric cancer. *Nature Communications, 9*(1), 1–16.
55. Aoun, F., Peltier, A., & van Velthoven, R. (2014). A comprehensive review of contemporary role of local treatment of the primary tumor and/or the metastases in metastatic prostate cancer. *BioMed Research International, 2014*, 1–12.
56. Siegel, R. L., Miller, K. D., & Jemal, A. (2018). Cancer statistics, 2018. *CA: A Cancer Journal for Clinicians, 68*(1), 7–30.

57. Ross, R. W., Xie, W., Regan, M. M., Pomerantz, M., Nakabayashi, M., Daskivich, T. J., Sartor, O., Taplin, M. E., Kantoff, P. W., & Oh, W. K. (2008). Efficacy of androgen deprivation therapy (ADT) in patients with advanced prostate cancer: Association between Gleason score, prostate-specific antigen level, and prior ADT exposure with duration of ADT effect. *Cancer, 112*(6), 1247–1253.
58. Sreekumar, A., Poisson, L. M., Rajendiran, T. M., Khan, A. P., Cao, Q., Yu, J., Laxman, B., Mehra, R., Lonigro, R. J., Li, Y., Nyati, M. K., Ahsan, A., Kalyana-Sundaram, S., Han, B., Cao, X., Byun, J., Omenn, G. S., Ghosh, D., Pennathur, S., Alexander, D. C., Berger, A., Shuster, J. R., Wei, J. T., Varambally, S., Beecher, C., & Chinnaiyan, A. M. (2009). Metabolomic profiles delineate potential role for sarcosine in prostate cancer progression. *Nature, 457*(7231), 910–914.
59. Eniu, D. T., Romanciuc, F., Moraru, C., Goidescu, I., Eniu, D., Staicu, A., Rachieriu, C., Buiga, R., & Socaciu, C. (2019). The decrease of some serum free amino acids can predict breast cancer diagnosis and progression. *Scandinavian Journal of Clinical and Laboratory Investigation, 79*(1–2), 17–24.
60. Wang, J. H., Chen, W. L., Li, J. M., Wu, S. F., Chen, T. L., Zhu, Y. M., Zhang, W. N., Li, Y., Qiu, Y. P., Zhao, A. H., Mi, J. Q., Jin, J., Wang, Y. G., Ma, Q. L., Huang, H., Wu, D. P., Wang, Q. R., Li, Y., Yan, X. J., Yan, J. S., Li, J. Y., Wang, S., Huang, X. J., Wang, B. S., Jia, W., Shen, Y., Chen, Z., & Chen, S. J. (2013). Prognostic significance of 2-hydroxyglutarate levels in acute myeloid leukemia in China. *Proceedings of the National Academy of Sciences of the United States of America, 110*(42), 17017–17022.
61. Mathe, E. A., Patterson, A. D., Haznadar, M., Manna, S. K., Krausz, K. W., Bowman, E. D., Shields, P. G., Idle, J. R., Smith, P. B., Anami, K., Kazandjian, D. G., Hatzakis, E., Gonzalez, F. J., & Harris, C. C. (2014). Noninvasive urinary metabolomic profiling identifies diagnostic and prognostic markers in lung cancer. *Cancer Research, 74*(12), 3259–3270.
62. Huang, F., Ni, M., Chalishazar, M. D., Huffman, K. E., Kim, J., Cai, L., Shi, X., Cai, F., Zacharias, L. G., Ireland, A. S., Li, K., Gu, W., Kaushik, A. K., Liu, X., Gazdar, A. F., Oliver, T. G., Minna, J. D., Hu, Z., & DeBerardinis, R. J. (2018). Inosine monophosphate dehydrogenase dependence in a subset of small cell lung cancers. *Cell Metabolism, 28*(3), 369–382.
63. Wang, Z., Yip, L. Y., Lee, J. H. J., Wu, Z., Chew, H. Y., Chong, P. K. W., Teo, C. C., Ang, H. Y., Peh, K. L. E., Yuan, J., Ma, S., Choo, L. S. K., Basri, N., Jiang, X., Yu, Q., Hillmer, A. M., Lim, W. T., Lim, T. K. H., Takano, A., Tan, E. H., Tan, D. S. W., Ho, Y. S., Lim, B., & Tam, W. L. (2019). Methionine is a metabolic dependency of tumor-initiating cells. *Nature Medicine, 25*(5), 825–837.
64. Yuan, R., Hou, Y., Sun, W., Yu, J., Liu, X., Niu, Y., Lu, J.-J., & Chen, X. (2017). Natural products to prevent drug resistance in cancer chemotherapy: A review. *Annals of the New York Academy of Sciences, 1401*(1), 19–27.
65. Bosc, C., Selak, M. A., & Sarry, J.-E. (2017). Resistance is futile: Targeting mitochondrial energetics and metabolism to overcome drug resistance in cancer treatment. *Cell Metabolism, 26*(5), 705–707.
66. Kominsky, D. J., Klawitter, J., Brown, J. L., Boros, L. G., Melo, J. V., Eckhardt, S. G., & Serkova, N. J. (2009). Abnormalities in glucose uptake and metabolism in imatinib-resistant human BCR-ABL-positive cells. *Clinical Cancer Research, 15*(10), 3442–3450.
67. Ruprecht, B., Zaal, E. A., Zecha, J., Wu, W., Berkers, C. R., Kuster, B., & Lemeer, S. (2017). Lapatinib resistance in breast cancer cells is accompanied by phosphorylation-mediated reprogramming of glycolysis. *Cancer Research, 77*(8), 1842–1853.
68. Tewey, K. M., Rowe, T. C., Yang, L., Halligan, B. D., & Liu, L. F. (1984). Adriamycin-induced DNA damage mediated by mammalian DNA topoisomerase II. *Science, 226*(4673), 3.
69. Cagel, M., Grotz, E., Bernabeu, E., Moretton, M. A., & Chiappetta, D. A. (2017). Doxorubicin: Nanotechnological overviews from bench to bedside. *Drug Discovery Today, 22*(2), 270–281.
70. Chen, T., Shen, H. M., Deng, Z. Y., Yang, Z. Z., Zhao, R. L., Wang, L., Feng, Z. P., Liu, C., Li, W. H., & Liu, Z. J. (2017). A herbal formula, SYKT, reverses doxorubicin-induced myelosuppression and cardiotoxicity by inhibiting ROS-mediated apoptosis. *Molecular Medicine Reports, 15*(4), 2057–2066.
71. Koleini, N., & Kardami, E. (2017). Autophagy and mitophagy in the context of doxorubicin-induced cardiotoxicity. *Oncotarget, 8*(28), 46663–46680.
72. Shao, C., Lu, W., Wan, N., Wu, M., Bao, Q., Tian, Y., Lu, G., Wang, N., Hao, H., & Ye, H. (2019). Integrative omics analysis revealed that metabolic intervention combined with metronomic chemotherapy selectively kills cancer cells. *Journal of Proteome Research, 18*(6), 2643–2653.
73. Celiktas, M., Tanaka, I., Tripathi, S. C., Fahrmann, J. F., Aguilar-Bonavides, C., Villalobos, P., Delgado, O., Dhillon, D., Dennison, J. B., Ostrin, E. J., Wang, H., Behrens, C., Do, K. A., Gazdar, A. F., Hanash, S. M., & Taguchi, A. (2017). Role of CPS1 in cell growth, metabolism and prognosis in LKB1-inactivated lung adenocarcinoma. *Journal of the National Cancer Institute, 109*(3), 1–9.
74. Cai, Z., Zhao, J.-S., Li, J.-J., Peng, D.-N., Wang, X.-Y., Chen, T.-L., Qiu, Y.-P., Chen, P.-P., Li, W.-J., Xu, L.-Y., Li, E.-M., Tam, J. P. M., Qi, R. Z., Jia, W., & Xie, D. (2010). A combined proteomics and metabolomics profiling of gastric cardia cancer reveals characteristic dysregulations in glucose metabolism. *Molecular & Cellular Proteomics, 9*(12), 2617–2628.
75. Dougan, J., Hawsawi, O., Burton, L. J., Edwards, G., Jones, K., Zou, J., Nagappan, P., Wang, G., Zhang, Q., Danaher, A., Bowen, N., Hinton, C., & Odero-Marah, V. A. (2019). Proteomics-metabolomics combined approach identifies peroxidasin as a protector against

metabolic and oxidative stress in prostate cancer. *International Journal of Molecular Sciences, 20*(12), 3046.

76. Wettersten, H. I., Hakimi, A. A., Morin, D., Bianchi, C., Johnstone, M. E., Donohoe, D. R., Trott, J. F., Aboud, O. A., Stirdivant, S., Neri, B., Wolfert, R., Stewart, B., Perego, R., Hsieh, J. J., & Weiss, R. H. (2015). Grade-dependent metabolic reprogramming in kidney cancer revealed by combined proteomics and metabolomics analysis. *Cancer Research, 75*(12), 2541–2552.
77. Shender, V. O., Pavlyukov, M. S., Ziganshin, R. H., Arapidi, G. P., Kovalchuk, S. I., Anikanov, N. A., Altukhov, I. A., Alexeev, D. G., Butenko, I. O., Shavarda, A. L., Khomyakova, E. B., Evtushenko, E., Ashrafyan, L. A., Antonova, I. B., Kuznetcov, I. N., Gorbachev, A. Y., Shakhparonov, M. I., & Govorun, V. M. (2014). Proteome-metabolome profiling of ovarian cancer ascites reveals novel components involved in intercellular communication. *Molecular & Cellular Proteomics, 13*(12), 3558–3571.
78. Wu, M., Ye, H., Shao, C., Zheng, X., Li, Q., Wang, L., Zhao, M., Lu, G., Chen, B., Zhang, J., Wang, Y., Wang, G., & Hao, H. (2017). Metabolomics–proteomics combined approach identifies differential metabolism-associated molecular events between senescence and apoptosis. *Journal of Proteome Research, 16*(6), 2250–2261.
79. Hulce, J. J., Cognetta, A. B., Niphakis, M. J., Tully, S. E., & Cravatt, B. F. (2013). Proteome-wide mapping of cholesterol-interacting proteins in mammalian cells. *Nature Methods, 10*(3), 259–264.
80. Moraru, A., Wiederstein, J., Pfaff, D., Fleming, T., Miller, A. K., Nawroth, P., & Teleman, A. A. (2018). Elevated levels of the reactive metabolite methylglyoxal recapitulate progression of type 2 diabetes. *Cell Metabolism, 27*(4), 926–934.e928.
81. Qin, W., Qin, K., Zhang, Y., Jia, W., Chen, Y., Cheng, B., Peng, L., Chen, N., Liu, Y., Zhou, W., Wang, Y.-L., Chen, X., & Wang, C. (2019). S-glycosylation-based cysteine profiling reveals regulation of glycolysis by itaconate. *Nature Chemical Biology, 15*, 983–991.
82. Fu, X., Chin, R. M., Vergnes, L., Hwang, H., Deng, G., Xing, Y., Pai, M. Y., Li, S., Ta, L., Fazlollahi, F., Chen, C., Prins, R. M., Teitell, M. A., Nathanson, D. A., Lai, A., Faull, K. F., Jiang, M., Clarke, S. G., Cloughesy, T. F., Graeber, T. G., Braas, D., Christofk, H. R., Jung, M. E., Reue, K., & Huang, J. (2015). 2-Hydroxyglutarate inhibits ATP synthase and mTOR signaling. *Cell Metabolism, 22*(3), 508–515.
83. Chin, R. M., Fu, X., Pai, M. Y., Vergnes, L., Hwang, H., Deng, G., Diep, S., Lomenick, B., Meli, V. S., Monsalve, G. C., Hu, E., Whelan, S. A., Wang, J. X., Jung, G., Solis, G. M., Fazlollahi, F., Kaweeteerawat, C., Quach, A., Nili, M., Krall, A. S., Godwin, H. A., Chang, H. R., Faull, K. F., Guo, F., Jiang, M., Trauger, S. A., Saghatelian, A., Braas, D., Christofk, H. R., Clarke, C. F., Teitell, M. A., Petrascheck, M., Reue, K., Jung, M. E., Frand, A. R., & Huang, J. (2014). The metabolite α-ketoglutarate extends lifespan by inhibiting ATP synthase and TOR. *Nature, 510*(7505), 397–401.
84. Li, Q., Cao, L., Tian, Y., Zhang, P., Ding, C., Lu, W., Jia, C., Shao, C., Liu, W., Wang, D., Ye, H., & Hao, H. (2018). Butyrate suppresses the proliferation of colorectal cancer cells via targeting pyruvate kinase M2 and metabolic reprogramming. *Molecular & Cellular Proteomics, 17*(8), 1531–1545.
85. Huber, K. V., Olek, K. M., Muller, A. C., Tan, C. S., Bennett, K. L., Colinge, J., & Superti-Furga, G. (2015). Proteome-wide drug and metabolite interaction mapping by thermal-stability profiling. *Nature Methods, 12*(11), 1055–1057.
86. Reinhard, F. B., Eberhard, D., Werner, T., Franken, H., Childs, D., Doce, C., Savitski, M. F., Huber, W., Bantscheff, M., Savitski, M. M., & Drewes, G. (2015). Thermal proteome profiling monitors ligand interactions with cellular membrane proteins. *Nature Methods, 12*(12), 1129–1131.
87. Diether, M., & Sauer, U. (2017). Towards detecting regulatory protein-metabolite interactions. *Current Opinion in Microbiology, 39*, 16–23.

Ion Chromatography with Mass Spectrometry for Metabolomic Analysis

Eoon Hye Ji, Jason Lee, and Shen Hu

1 Principle of Ion Chromatography

Ion chromatography (IC) or ion-exchange chromatography (IEC) is a form of liquid chromatography (LC) that allows the separation of ions and polar molecules based on their charge. Similar to other forms of LC, IC utilizes a separation column with a stationary phase, a pump that moves the mobile phase and analytes through the column, and a detector that measures the analytes and provides characteristic retention times for them. Prior to separation, the mobile phase is delivered to the system using a high-pressure pump to equilibrate the IC column. The sample is then injected and flows through the ion-exchange column where the ion-exchange separation occurs. Afterward, the analytes are eluted from the column, and the suppressor reduces the conductivity of the eluent and increases the conductivity of the analytes so that they can be sensitively detected with the conductivity detector. Analytical IC is fully automated as the whole system is computer/software controlled, including the sample injection and separation process, data acquisition, and data processing.

E. H. Ji · J. Lee · S. Hu (✉)
School of Dentistry and Jonsson Comprehensive Cancer Center, University of California, Los Angeles, CA, USA
e-mail: shenhu@ucla.edu

Generally speaking, the IEC process consists of four main steps. (1) Equilibration of the stationary phase: When the equilibrium is reached, the functional groups on the stationary phase are associated with exchangeable counterions. (2) Sample injection and wash: Target analytes are retained on the stationary phase via electrostatic interaction with charged functional groups after replacement of the weakly bound counterions. Nonionic sample components are poorly retained and washed out of the column. (3) Elution of retained analytes from the IEC column: This is often carried out by increasing the ionic strength or pH to suppress the interaction between the analytes and stationary phase. (4) Column regeneration: All strongly retained species are removed to restore the full capacity of the IEC column. This step is usually accomplished by changing the eluent pH or buffer composition.

Most charged or ionizable molecules can be separated by IC and the IC stationary phase is derivatized with functional groups which have oppositely charged counterions. There are two types of IC, cation exchange chromatography (CEC) and anion exchange chromatography (AEC), depending on the analytes' surface charge. CEC retains positively charged cations because the stationary phase displays a negatively charged functional group, whereas AEC retains anions using a positively charged functional group. In other words, CEC is used when the analytes of interest are positively charged,

S. Hu (ed.), *Cancer Metabolomics*, Advances in Experimental Medicine and Biology 1280,
https://doi.org/10.1007/978-3-030-51652-9_10

and the separation is based on the interaction between negatively charged stationary phase and positively charged analytes. On the contrary, a positively charged stationary phase is used in AEC for the separation of negatively charged analytes. To elute the retained analytes from the IC column, the concentration of the exchangeable counterions, which competes with the analytes for binding, can be increased or the pH can be changed. A change in pH affects the charge on the particular analytes and, therefore, alters their binding to the stationary phase. The molecules then start eluting out based on their charges. Gradient elution may also be used, in which the concentration of counterions is gradually varied to separate the analytes. Additionally, step elution can be used in which the concentration of counterions is varied step by step.

2 Advantages of IC Separation

One of the primary advantages is only one interaction involved during the IC separation as opposed to other separation techniques. Therefore, IC may have higher matrix tolerance and allows selective analysis of ionic analytes from a complex biological sample. Another advantage of IC lies in its predictability of elution patterns based on the presence of charged groups on the analyte surface. For instance, when CEC is used, positively charged molecules will be eluted out last and the negative charged molecules will be eluted out first and vice versa. In addition, commercial IC columns are highly robust. It is inevitable that over time the injection of crude samples may result in contamination of chromatographic columns, especially with complex matrices. Due to high matrix tolerance, IC columns can be cleaned, regenerated to restore chromatographic resolution with harsh chemical solutions such as KOH and/or H_2SO_4, followed by flush with mobile phase. Lastly, IC columns can be flexible with high or low capacity depending the analytical needs. The use of high capacity columns is necessary to meet the requirement for analysis of complex samples, which contains high concentrations of interfering molecules.

A main limitation of IC techniques is that they are restricted to the separation of ionizable molecules. However, with the use of weak cation and anion exchangers, the coverage of IC separation is quite comprehensive nowadays. In addition, CEC and AEC can be combined to achieve a more in-depth analysis of complex biological samples. Another limitation is that the eluent used in IC may not be compatible with mass spectrometry (MS). This problem can be resolved by using a suppressor [1]. For instance, a suppressor device can be installed after the IC column outlet and before the detector to convert the eluent of high ionic strength (e.g., KOH) to water, which is then compatible with MS detection (Fig. 1).

3 Stationary Phase in IC

An anion exchanger used for IC separation refers to the stationary phase which features positively charged functional groups and attracts anions, whereas a cation exchanger is the stationary phase featuring negatively charged functional groups and attracting cations. A strong ion exchanger can tolerate a wide range of pH buffers and, once the column is equilibrated, does not lose the charge on its matrix. Weak ion exchangers, however, can only maintain their charge within a certain range of pH buffers. If the pH of the buffer goes beyond the capacity range of a weak ion exchanger, the column may lose its charge distribution and the analytes of interest may not be retained on the column during IC separation. Despite the smaller pH range of weak ion exchangers, they are often used due to their high specificity toward certain analyte ions.

The stationary phase of IC columns may contain functional groups such as weak/strong acids or weak/strong bases. There are also special columns that use resins with zwitterionic and amphoteric ion exchangers, where positive and negative charges are located in close proximity. These ion exchangers exhibit alternative ion selectivity to standard anion and cation ion exchangers [2]. Table 1 lists commonly used ion exchangers in IC. Quaternary ammonium (Q)

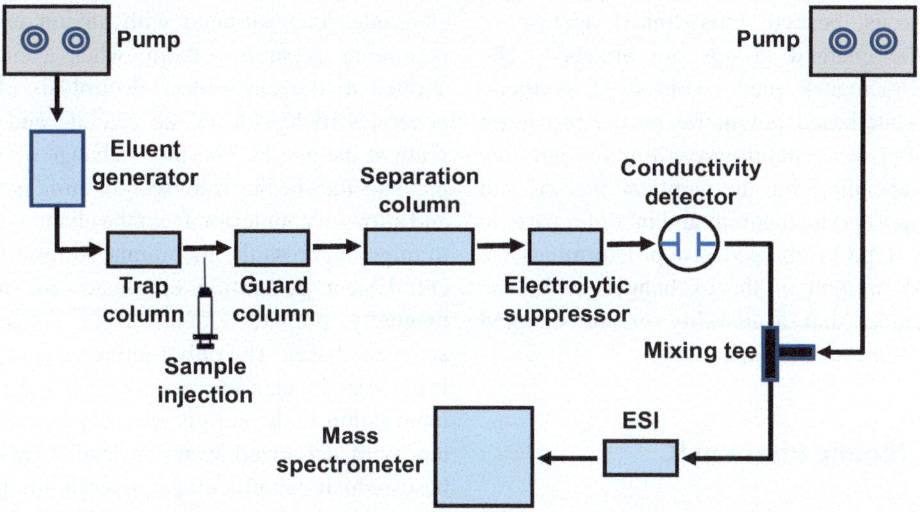

Fig. 1 A schematic diagram of IC-MS instrument for metabolite analysis. Eluent generation allows the automatic production of IC eluent, which eliminates the need to manually prepare an eluent from concentrated acid or base. The trap column is used to remove ionic contaminants from eluents continuously, without the need for offline chemical regeneration. The suppressor in IC is used to remove the eluent and sample counterions and replace them with regenerant ions, thereby converting the eluent to a low conductivity matrix prior to detection. In fact, the electrolytic suppressor operates continuously with a water source as a regenerant, which is compatible with MS detection. Organic desolvation solvent is delivered by using an auxiliary pump, combined with the IC eluent via a mixing tee, before entering the mass spectrometer via the electrospray ionization (ESI) interface

Table 1 Weak and strong ion exchangers used in IC separation

Resin	Functional group	Ion exchanger type	Counter ions[a]	pH range
DEAE Sepharose	Diethylaminoethyl-O-$CH_2CH_2N^+H(CH_2CH_3)_2$	Weak anion	Cl^-	2–9
ANX Sepharose	Diethylaminopropyl-O-$CH_2CHOHCH_2N^+H(CH_2CH_3)_2$	Weak anion	Cl^-	2–9
QAE Sephadex	Quaternary aminoethyl-O-$CH_2CH_2N^+(CH_2CH_3)_2CH_2CH(OH)CH_3$	Strong anion	Cl^-	2–10
Q Sepharose	Quaternary ammonium-$CH_2N^+(CH_3)_3$	Strong anion	Cl^-	2–12
CM Sepharose	Carboxymethyl-O-CH_2COO^-	Weak cation	Na^+	6–10
SP Sepharose	Sulfopropyl-$CH_2CH_2CH_2SO_3^-$	Strong cation	Na^+	4–13
S Sepharose	Methylsulfonate-O-$CH_2CHOHCH_2OCH_2CHOHCH_2SO_3^-$	Strong cation	Na^+	2–12

[a]Many other counterions can be used as well to alter the selectivity for IC separation

and quaternary aminoethyl (QAE) are strong anion exchangers whereas sulfopropyl (SP) and methyl sulfonate (S) are strong cation exchangers. These exchangers can maintain their charge density over a wide pH range. Meanwhile, diethylaminoethyl (DEAE) and diethylaminopropyl (ANX) are weak anion exchangers while carboxymethyl (CM) is a weak cation exchanger. These weak ion exchangers maintain the charge density of the columns over a narrower pH range. Depending on the manufacturers, different resin media may be used for the attachment of functional groups. For instance, Sephadex ion exchangers are produced by introducing functional groups onto Sephadex, a cross-linked dextran matrix. These groups are attached to glucose units in the matrix by stable ether linkages. Sepharose ion exchange media consist of macroporous, beaded, cross-linked agarose to which the charged groups are attached. The Matrix Fractogel® media consist of synthetic methacrylate-based polymeric beads, providing excellent pressure stability resulting in high flow rates. Depending on the application, we can choose appropriate medium and medium particle size. The type of charged group determines the type and strength of the exchanger, while the total number and availability of the charged groups determine the capacity.

4 Mobile Phase in IC

Counterions used in IC separation may include Na^+, K^+, Li^+, and H^+ (cation exchange) and Cl^-, CO_3^{2-}, HCO_3^-, CH_3COO^-, $HCOO^-$, Br^-, I^-, SO_4^{2-}, OH^-, and $CH_3SO_3^-$ (anion exchange). In certain applications, different counterions may improve and even alter the selectivity since they exhibit different elution strength, but it should be noted that using these ions may affect the binding capacity of the medium. Nature and concentration of the counterions and pH of the eluent are the most important factors affecting the elution characteristics of analytes. pH value of eluent can be controlled and adjusted carefully with buffering additives. The buffering compound should not interact with the ion exchanger because it may interfere with the elution. Anionic buffers such as phosphate or MOPS in CEC and cationic buffers such as ethanolamine, Tris, and tricine in AEC may be used. The eluent should be degassed every day to avoid air in the pumps and lower the noise in the detector. This can be performed by purging the eluent bottle with helium while stirring the eluent solution with a stirring bar. In addition, the eluent is usually filtered through a 0.45-μm filter made of chemically inert material such as polyvinylidene difluoride. This prolongs the lifetime of IC separation column and also protects the eluent pump.

Eluent generator allows the automatic production of high purity IC eluents. This is made possible through precise control of the electric current applied to the electrolysis of water to generate hydroxide and hydronium ions. A pair of electrodes is positioned with an ion exchange membrane separating them; when a current is applied to the electrodes, electrolysis of water generates hydroxide at the cathode and hydronium at the anode. The ion exchange membrane prevents the species from recombining into water and allows a counterion from the eluent generator to migrate across the membrane to form the eluent. Eluent generation eliminates the need to manually prepare eluents from concentrated acids and bases. The only routine reagent needed is deionized water. Furthermore, since the instrument pump seals and pistons only come in contact with deionized water instead of acids and bases which can precipitate, overall pump maintenance is significantly reduced. KOH eluent (or NaOH/LiOH) can be generated in situ with this automatic eluent generator for AEC separation. The advantage of using these eluents produced from the eluent generator is that they are extremely stable so the retention times for analytes are highly reproducible [3, 4].

5 Detection Modes in IC

Conductivity detection is widely employed in IC for the measurement of inorganic ions and small organic compounds such as organic acids and amines [5]. It represents a sensitive and quite universal detection mode compared to UV/VIS detection. The sensor of the conductivity detector consists of two electrodes situated into a flow cell. When the eluted analyte ions move into the flow cell, the change in electric current is detected, with a constant voltage imposed between the two electrodes. Conductivity detection is highly susceptible to the effect of temperature fluctuations. A change of 1 °C in mobile phase temperature may cause a change of roughly 2% in electric conductivity. Therefore, a constant temperature flow cell is required to avoid baseline fluctuations of conductivity. The conductivity of IC eluent also has significant effect on the detection, as a high conductivity of an eluent produces a large baseline noise. When the eluent has low conductivity, a non-suppressor method can be applied, although the detection sensitivity is relatively lower. However, if the eluent conductivity is high, it can be reduced after column separation by using a suppressor method, as previously discussed.

Fluorescence detection is highly sensitive and selective. However, there are not many analytes that inherently emit natural fluorescence. Certain analytes such as amino acids or organic amines may be derivatized with fluorescence reagent for fluorescence detection. Amperometry is an alternative detection mode to conductivity and UV/VIS detection, which allows for highly sensitive detection of oxidizable or reducible compounds. Typical applications of amperometric detection include carbohydrates, anions (e.g., cyanide, sulfide, iodide, bromide), cations (e.g., metal ions, amines, aromatic amino acids), and other organic substances such as phenols, catecholamines, and vitamins.

Mass spectrometry (MS) is a highly sensitive and universal detection method that has been well coupled with IC for metabolite analysis. Combining IC with MS takes advantage of the strengths of both techniques. Electrospray ionization (ESI) is typically used to couple IC with MS and introduce the eluted analytes into the mass spectrometer. By using IC with tandem MS followed by database searching against publicly accessible metabolite databases, it is now practical to quantify and identify a large number of metabolites from a metabolomic sample. As discussed earlier, since the IC eluent contains high-level cations or anions, it must be converted to MS-compatible matrix to allow for sensitive detection of metabolites. This is typically accomplished with the installation of an electrolytic eluent suppressor, after the IC column and before the detector, to convert the ionic eluent into water (e.g., convert KOH to water) so that the analytes can be detected with MS. Basically, the IC suppressors are membrane-based devices which are designed to reduce the background conductivity of the eluent from the IC column. It can be used with a conductivity detector to act as a desalting device, thereby removing the interference resulting from the presence of ionic salts in the eluent and enhancing the detection sensitivity. Eluents using ionic gradients and containing organic solvents can be suppressed satisfactorily using either chemical suppression with a micromembrane suppressor or electrolytic suppression using a self-regenerating suppressor. For IC-MS, the electrolytic suppressor is commonly used since it can employ water as the suppressor regenerant and is fully compatible with MS. Because the flow through the suppressor is unobstructed, there is no dispersion and brand broadening that is sometimes observed with packed-bed suppression systems. After the suppressor converts the ionic eluent to water, the only requirement is to introduce an organic solvent using an auxiliary pump and a mixing tee before the eluent enters the electrospray ionization (ESI) source. The organic modifier assists desolvation in the ion source resulting in a significant increase in sensitivity for the analytes (Fig. 1).

6 Application of IC-MS for Metabolomic Analysis

Compared to reversed-phase LC (RP-LC), very few applications demonstrated the use of IC for separation and analysis of metabolites. In earlier studies, IC was used for fractionating a complex metabolite sample prior to LC-MS analysis. For instance, strong cation exchange (SCX) LC was combined with hydrophilic interaction liquid chromatography (HILIC) to further enhance the separation of mostly polar, water-soluble metabolites extracted from *E. coli* and *S. cerevisiae*. Off-line SCX-LC fractions were re-separated with HILIC, followed by tandem MS analysis and identification. This off-line 2-D LC-MS/MS method allowed to detect a total of 141 extracted metabolite species [6]. The use of AEC and CEC also allowed to sub-fractionate the total steroid metabolome, including oxysterols, bile acids, and hormonal steroids, to accomplish a more in-depth analysis [7].

Reversed-phase LC (RPLC) and HILIC are two types of chromatography most commonly coupled with MS for metabolomic analysis [8–10]. HILIC is complementary to RPLC and similar to normal-phase liquid chromatography (NPLC). However, the nonaqueous mobile phase used in NPLC is replaced by an eluent containing organic solvent (e.g., acetonitrile), which means HILIC is well suited for online coupling with ESI-MS [9]. These chromatographic techniques are highly effective for the separation of hydrophobic and polar metabolites, respectively, but there are important classes of metabolites that are poorly resolved or retained using these stationary phases [11]. Burgess et al. demonstrated a capillary flow IC-MS method for metabolomic analysis and compared the technique to HILIC-MS. The capillary flow IC was shown to effectively separate organic acids and sugar di- and triphosphates, many of which are poorly resolved with RPLC or HILIC. Limits of detection for these compounds ranged from 0.01 to 100 pmol on-column. This method was applied to a comparative analysis of energy metabolism in procyclic forms of the parasitic protozoan *Trypanosoma brucei* where cells were grown on glucose or proline as a carbon source. The capillary IC was found to be more effective than HILIC for detection of the organic acids that comprise glucose central metabolism and the tricarboxylic acid (TCA) cycle [11]. Kvitvang et al. also demonstrated a capillary IC (capIC)-negative ESI MS/MS method for quantitative profiling of the phosphometabolome (e.g., sugar phosphates and nucleotides). The metabolite separation was performed with AEC using potassium hydroxide solution as the eluting solvent. The limits of detection (LODs) for these metabolites ranged from 1 to 100 nM, which equal to 5–500 fmol injected onto the column. Metabolite extracts of the human kidney HEK293 cell line were spiked with standards to determine the concentration of each metabolite in the samples, and 44 metabolites were identified and quantified with this method [12]. Si-Hung et al. demonstrated a novel selective cleanup/enrichment method based on metal oxide solid-phase extraction combined with IC-MS for the analysis of phosphorylated metabolites. Metal oxide-based enrichment materials were tested and optimized for both the selective enrichment of 12 phosphorylated compounds from the glycolysis and pentose phosphate pathways and the simultaneous removal of highly abundant matrix components such as organic acids and sugars. The full analytical workflow exhibited a good recovery (>70%) for targeted phosphorylated compounds while many sugars, organic acids, and amino acids were removed. The use of isotopically labeled internal standards added to the samples prior to SPE enables accurate quantification of the metabolites as it compensates for errors introduced during sample pretreatment and LC-MS analysis. This method appears to be effective and selective for the enrichment analysis of intracellular phosphorylated metabolites [13].

A combination of two chromatographic separation techniques is often used to enhance metabolite detection and achieve a more comprehensive metabolomic analysis. Soltow et al. demonstrated a dual chromatography-Fourier transform mass spectrometry (DC-FTMS) method for the study of exposome. For the DC-FTMS, sequential LC-FTMS analyses using RPLC(C18) and AEC were performed, with 10-min run time for each column with gradient elution. In comparison to analysis with the AEC column alone, addition of the second LC-FTMS analysis with the C18 column increased m/z feature detection by 23–36%, yielding a total number of metabolic features up to 7000 for individual samples. DC-FTMS thus provides improved capability for high-performance metabolic profiling of the exposome and maximizes the detection of metabolites characteristics of diseases and environmental exposures in personalized medicine and predictive health [14]. In a separate study, a mixed-mode HILIC/weak anion-exchange LC (HILIC/WAX) method coupled with ESI-MS/MS was demonstrated for the determination of glyphosate and its major metabolite, aminomethylphosphonic acid (AMPA). The best results were obtained when the column was operated under mixed-mode HILIC/WAX elution conditions. An initial 10-min washing step with acetonitrile/water (10:90, v/v) in HILIC mode was used to remove potentially interfering compounds, and then the analytes were eluted in WAX mode with acetonitrile/water containing 0.1 M ammonium hydroxide under gradient elution for the ESI analysis in negative ion mode. The HILIC/WAX-ESI-MS method was an effective way to minimize and compensate for matrix effects and obtain satisfactory quantification of the metabolites [15]. Tharakan et al. demonstrated an integrated platform, which combines microfluidic chip and online SCX separation, for simultaneous metabolomic and peptidomic profiling. The analysis was accomplished by liquid-liquid extraction of peptides and metabolites from tissue samples, online strong cation exchange (SCX) separation, followed by RPLC-MS analysis of peptides and metabolites individually. This easy-to-implement platform was applied to investigating the physiological response to infection in the spleen, showing that the spleen contains an abundance of hemoglobin-derived peptides, which do not appear to change in response to infection, and that there appears to be a large and variable metabolic response to infection [16].

We have demonstrated a highly sensitive capIC-MS method for metabolic profiling of head and neck squamous cell carcinoma (HNSCC) cells. The capIC allowed an excellent separation of anionic polar metabolites, and the sensitivities increased by up to 100-fold compared to RPLC or HILIC. The detection limits for a panel of standard metabolites were between 0.04 and 0.5 nM (0.2 to 3.4 fmol) at a signal-to-noise ratio of 3. This method was applied to an untargeted metabolomic analysis of HNSCC cells and stemlike cancer cells, and isobaric metabolites such as 11 sugar monophosphates were well resolved. Differential metabolomic analysis identified significant changes in energy metabolism pathways such as glycolysis and tricarboxylic acid cycle between cancer stem cells and non-stem cancer cells (Fig. 2). Our study indicates that capIC-MS is a powerful metabolomics tool by providing enhanced separation, reproducibility, and sensitivity for analysis of polar metabolites [3]. Using a similar platform, we profiled the salivary metabolites in eight patients with gout, 15 patients with hyperuricaemia (HUA), and 15 healthy individuals. Forty-nine salivary metabolites were found to be significantly changed between gout patient and healthy control groups, and 26 salivary metabolites were significantly different between gout and HUA patient groups. Three metabolite biomarkers, uric acid, oxalic acid, and l-homocysteic acid (HCA), were selected for validation with enzymatic assays in the saliva samples of 30 patients with gout, 30 patients with HUA, and 30 healthy control subjects. Salivary uric acid and oxalic acid levels were found to be significantly higher in gout patients than healthy controls, whereas salivary HCA level was significantly higher in gout patients than both HUA patients and healthy controls. Our study has demonstrated a new application of IC-MS for the discovery of novel metabolite biomarkers in gout. The validated biomarkers may be used for noninvasive, diagnostic, and prognostic applications in gout [17].

In a separate study, we developed a targeted metabolomics method based on IC-MS and stable isotope-labeled internal standards, for quantitative analysis of metabolites in a specific metabolic pathway in cancer cells. Our method offers great technical advantages for metabolite analysis, including exquisite sensitivity, high speed and reproducibility, and wide dynamic range. We have used this method to quantify pyruvate and TCA cycle metabolites in HNSCC cells and discover distinct metabolic phenotypes between high and low invasive head and neck cancer cells and between CSCs and non-SCCs [4]. Figure 3 presents the IC-MS quantitative analysis of pyruvate and five TCA cycle intermediates between highly invasive UM1 and UMSCC5 and low invasive UM2 and UMSCC6 cancer cells. The expression levels of these metabolites were found to be exceptionally higher in the UMSCC5 cancer cell line, which displays exuberant metabolism, than the other three cancer cell lines. Petucci et al. developed an IC-MS method for targeted metabolomic analysis of 28 organic acids (OAs). The polar nature of these OAs poses a challenge to their measurement with widely used analytical methods. The main advantage of IC is that it separated highly polar OAs that cannot be adequately retained by RPLC. The IC-MS method was used to quantify polar OAs in quadriceps muscle from sedentary mice compared to fatigued mice subjected to either a low intensity, long duration or high intensity, short duration forced treadmill regimen. Among the OAs examined, significant differences

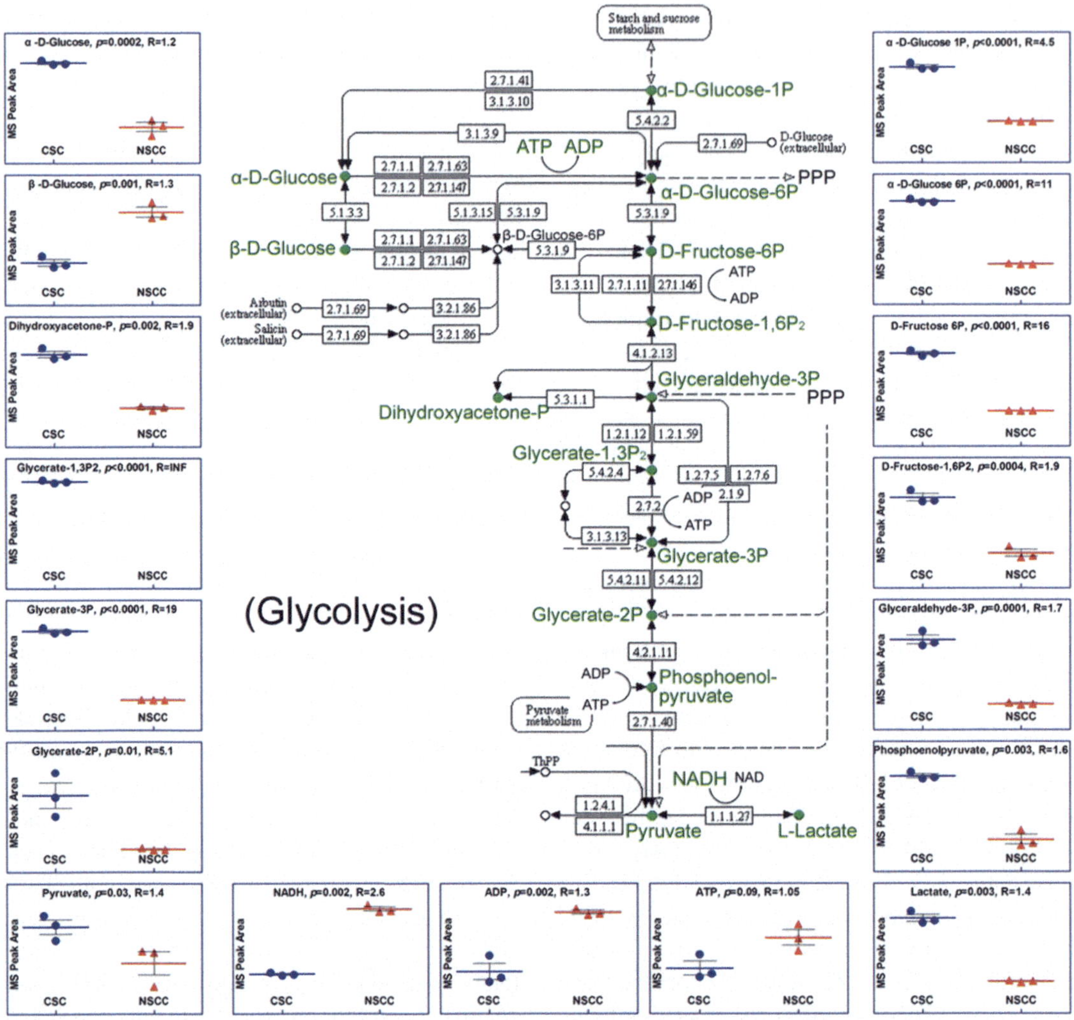

Fig. 2 CapIC-MS analysis revealed differential changes in metabolites of the glycolytic pathway between head and neck cancer stem cells and non-stem cancer cells. Every sample was analyzed in triplicates. *p* p-value, *R* fold change. (Reproduced with permission from Wang et al. [3])

were detected for hippuric acid, malic acid, fumaric acid, and 2-ketoglutaric acid between the sedentary and fatigued mice [18].

Schwaiger et al. developed an IC-MS method for simultaneous targeted and nontargeted metabolite profiling of cancer cells, which is based on AEC for metabolite separation and the use of isotope-labeled internal standards for metabolite quantitation. A list of 45 metabolite standards, including nucleotides and organic acids, were well separated and quantified with the uniformly ^{13}C-labeled *Pichia pastoris* extracts as internal standards. Limits of detection in the low nanomolar range and linear dynamic ranges over 4 orders of magnitude were obtained. Experiments on drug-sensitive versus resistant SW480 cancer cells showed the feasibility of merging analytical tasks into one analytical run and revealed significant differences in distinct metabolic phenotypes between the two cell types. Comparing fingerprinting with and without internal standard proved that the presence of the ^{13}C-labeled internal standards required for absolute quantification was not detrimental to nontargeted data evaluation [19].

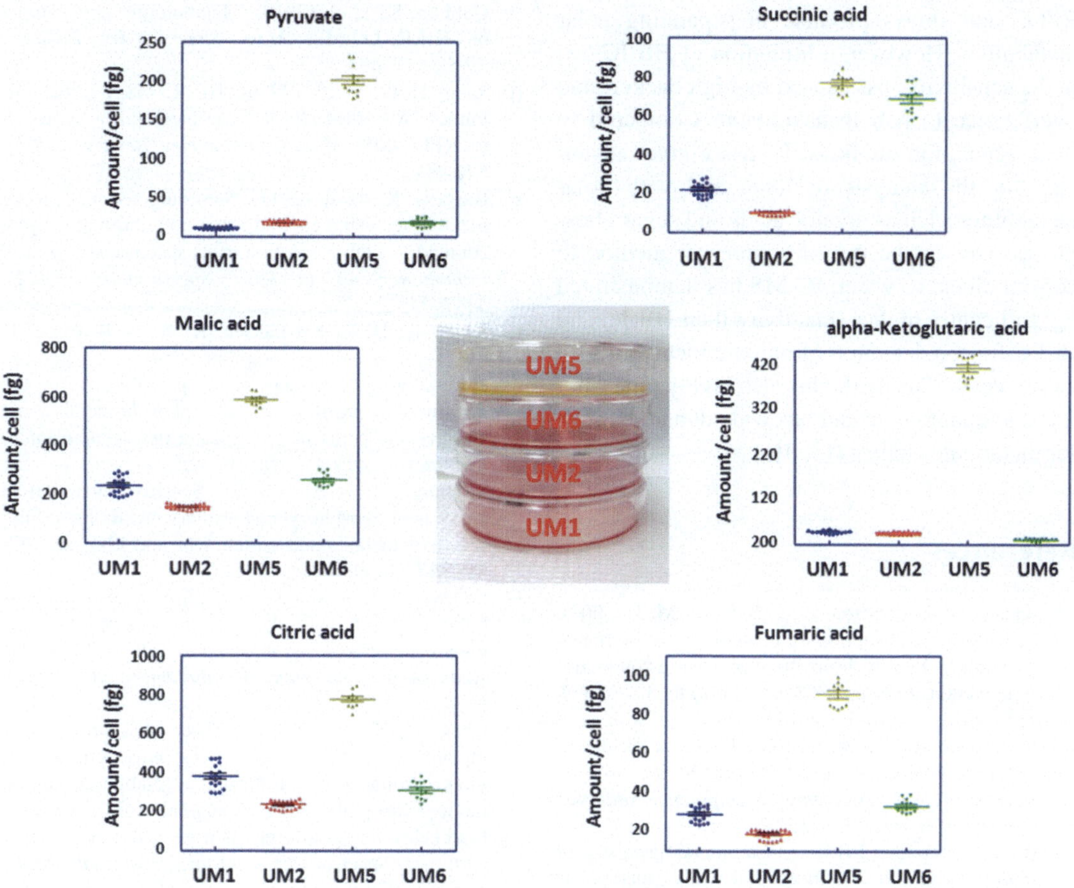

Fig. 3 Quantitative analysis of six targeted metabolites in head and neck cancer cells by IC-MS with isotope-labeled internal standards. The production of these metabolites in UM5 cancer cells is significantly higher than other cell lines. Inserted are the cultures of all four cell lines. Equal number of cells was initially plated and cultured for the same amount of time. (Reproduced with permission from Hu et al. [4])

Casal et al. demonstrated a CEC method with parallel ICP-MS and ESI-MS detection for the study of the metabolomic pattern of selenium in selenium-rich yeast. Ammonium formate gradient in 20% methanol was used as the mobile phase and optimized to obtain efficient separation and sensitive detection. Twenty-seven Se-containing metabolites observed in the CEC-ICP MS chromatogram were identified by ESI-MS based on the Se isotopic pattern, the accurate molecular mass, and the multistage fragmentation patterns. The method, for the first time, allowed the correlation of the differences observed in CEC-ICP MS analysis of Se-rich yeast samples with the identity of the eluted compounds determined by CEC-ESI MS [20].

7 Conclusion

Separation science plays an important role in metabolomics, especially when the separation techniques are coupled with MS for a comprehensive profiling analysis of metabolites. In the past decade, RPLC-MS, HILIC-MS, gas chromatography-MS (GC-MS), and capillary electrophoresis-MS (CE-MS) have been well demonstrated for metabolomic applications [21–24]. However, none of these methods can individually achieve an in-depth, comprehensive metabolome analysis. RPLC is the most commonly used separation technique for metabolomics, but ionic and very polar metabolites may not be retained on RPLC column. HILIC has emerged as an alternative to

RPLC and shows promise in separating polar metabolites. However, a limitation of HILIC lies in the sensitivity loss caused by high background interference to MS measurement. Compared to these separation methods, IC has a great advantage for the analysis of ionic and very polar metabolites such as organic acids and sugar phosphates. Due to the use of suppressor method to convert eluent to water, IC-MS has demonstrated a significantly higher sensitivity than HILIC and RPLC for the detection of anionic metabolites in cancer cells. This method is also highly reproducible and quantitative and has wide dynamic range for metabolite analysis [3, 4].

References

1. Haddad, P. R., Jackson, P. E., & Shaw, M. J. (2003). Developments in suppressor technology for inorganic ion analysis by ion chromatography using conductivity detection. *Journal of Chromatography A, 1000*(1), 725–742.
2. Nesterenko, E. P., Nesterenko, P. N., & Paull, B. (2009). Zwitterionic ion-exchangers in ion chromatography: A review of recent developments. *Analytica Chimica Acta, 652*(1), 3–21.
3. Wang, J., et al. (2014). Metabolomic profiling of anionic metabolites in head and neck cancer cells by capillary ion chromatography with Orbitrap mass spectrometry. *Analytical Chemistry, 86*(10), 5116–5124.
4. Hu, S., et al. (2015). Targeted metabolomic analysis of head and neck cancer cells using high performance ion chromatography coupled with a Q exactive HF mass spectrometer. *Analytical Chemistry, 87*(12), 6371–6379.
5. Buchberger, W. W., & Haddad, P. R. (1997). Advances in detection techniques for ion chromatography. *Journal of Chromatography A, 789*(1), 67–83.
6. Fairchild, J. N., et al. (2010). Two-dimensional liquid chromatography/mass spectrometry/mass spectrometry separation of water-soluble metabolites. *Journal of Chromatography A, 1217*(52), 8161–8166.
7. Griffiths, W. J., & Sjovall, J. (2010). Analytical strategies for characterization of bile acid and oxysterol metabolomes. *Biochemical and Biophysical Research Communications, 396*(1), 80–84.
8. De Vos, R. C. H., et al. (2007). Untargeted large-scale plant metabolomics using liquid chromatography coupled to mass spectrometry. *Nature Protocols, 2*(4), 778–791.
9. Cubbon, S., et al. (2010). Metabolomic applications of HILIC-LC-MS. *Mass Spectrometry Reviews, 29*(5), 671–684.
10. Tang, D.-Q., et al. (2016). HILIC-MS for metabolomics: An attractive and complementary approach to RPLC-MS. *Mass Spectrometry Reviews, 35*(5), 574–600.
11. Burgess, K., et al. (2011). Semi-targeted analysis of metabolites using capillary-flow ion chromatography coupled to high-resolution mass spectrometry. *Rapid Communications in Mass Spectrometry, 25*(22), 3447–3452.
12. Kvitvang, H. F., Kristiansen, K. A., & Bruheim, P. (2014). Assessment of capillary anion exchange ion chromatography tandem mass spectrometry for the quantitative profiling of the phosphometabolome and organic acids in biological extracts. *Journal of Chromatography A, 1370*, 70–79.
13. Si-Hung, L., et al. (2019). Sensitive quantitative analysis of phosphorylated primary metabolites using selective metal oxide enrichment and GC- and IC-MS/MS. *Talanta, 205*, 120147.
14. Soltow, Q. A., et al. (2013). High-performance metabolic profiling with dual chromatography-Fourier-transform mass spectrometry (DC-FTMS) for study of the exposome. *Metabolomics, 9*(1 Suppl), S132–S143.
15. Chen, M. X., et al. (2013). Direct determination of glyphosate and its major metabolite, aminomethylphosphonic acid, in fruits and vegetables by mixed-mode hydrophilic interaction/weak anion-exchange liquid chromatography coupled with electrospray tandem mass spectrometry. *Journal of Chromatography A, 1272*, 90–99.
16. Tharakan, R., et al. (2015). Integrated microfluidic chip and online SCX separation allows untargeted nanoscale metabolomic and peptidomic profiling. *Journal of Proteome Research, 14*(3), 1621–1626.
17. Cui, L., et al. (2017). Identification of metabolite biomarkers for gout using capillary ion chromatography with mass spectrometry. *Analytical Chemistry, 89*(21), 11737–11743.
18. Petucci, C., et al. (2016). Use of ion chromatography/mass spectrometry for targeted metabolite profiling of polar organic acids. *Analytical Chemistry, 88*(23), 11799–11803.
19. Schwaiger, M., et al. (2017). Anion-exchange chromatography coupled to high-resolution mass spectrometry: A powerful tool for merging targeted and non-targeted metabolomics. *Analytical Chemistry, 89*(14), 7667–7674.
20. Casal, S. G., et al. (2010). Study of the Se-containing metabolomes in Se-rich yeast by size-exclusion-cation-exchange HPLC with the parallel ICP MS and electrospray orbital ion trap detection. *Metallomics, 2*(8), 535–548.

21. Shen, Y., et al. (2005). Automated 20 kpsi RPLC-MS and MS/MS with chromatographic peak capacities of 1000–1500 and capabilities in proteomics and metabolomics. *Analytical Chemistry, 77*(10), 3090–3100.
22. Beale, D. J., et al. (2018). Review of recent developments in GC–MS approaches to metabolomics-based research. *Metabolomics, 14*(11), 152.
23. Satoh, K., et al. (2017). Global metabolic reprogramming of colorectal cancer occurs at adenoma stage and is induced by MYC. *Proceedings of the National Academy of Sciences of the United States of America, 114*(37), E7697–E7706.
24. Cui, L., et al. (2019). Predictive metabolomic signatures for safety assessment of metal oxide nanoparticles. *ACS Nano, 13*(11), 13065–13082.

Quantitative Analysis of Oncometabolite 2-Hydroxyglutarate

Bi-Feng Yuan

1 Introduction

The dysregulation of cellular metabolism is considered as an emerging hallmark of cancers [1]. The alterations of endogenous cellular metabolites that are related to cancer-associated metabolic reprogramming have profound impact on gene expression, cellular differentiation, and tumor microenvironment [2, 3]. One of the examples is 2-hydxyglutarate (2HG), a recently identified oncometabolite [4–6].

Gain-of-function mutations of isocitrate dehydrogenase 1 and 2 (IDH1/2) were demonstrated to induce the production and accumulation of 2HG. Mutations of IDH1/2 widely occur in glioma [7–11], acute myeloid leukemia [12–15], chondrosarcoma [16, 17], breast cancer [18], renal cancer [19], biliary cancer [20–23], and giant cell tumor of bone [24]. Normal IDH1/2 are important metabolic enzymes that catalyze the oxidative decarboxylation of isocitrate to generate α-ketoglutarate (α-KG) [25]. Due to the structural similarity between 2HG and α-KG, 2HG has been reported to be a competitor of α-KG and the increased level of 2HG inhibits multiple α-KG-dependent dioxygenases, including approximate 30 histone demethylases and 3 Tet (ten-eleven translocation) proteins [26]. These enzymes are closely linked to diverse cellular processes such as adaptation to hypoxia [27, 28], histone demethylation, and DNA modification [29]. Therefore, the mutations of IDH1/2 are believed to transform cells through modulating the behavior of these specific α-KG-dependent enzymes [5].

2HG carries an asymmetric carbon atom in its carbon backbone and therefore occurs in two distinct enantiomers, D-2-hydroxyglutarate (D-2HG) and L-2-hydroxyglutarate (L-2HG) (Fig. 1) [30]. It is important to note that both D-2HG and L-2HG enantiomers are found in human body [30]. Although D-2HG and L-2HG are similar in their physical and chemical properties, they are different in biochemical properties [30]. Each enantiomer is produced and metabolized in independent biochemical pathway and catalyzed by different enzymes [31]. Cancer-associated IDH1/2 mutants typically convert α-KG to D-2HG (Fig. 2) [7, 32]. The accumulated, excessive D-2HG contributes to elevated risk of malignant tumors due to the inhibition of α-KG-dependent dioxygenases that are critical for regulating the metabolic and epigenetic state of cells (Fig. 2) [33–37]. Increased amount of D-2HG may also cause contractile dysfunction in the heart [38]. L-2HG accumulates in response to cellular reductive stressors like hypoxia [39] and activation of hypoxia-inducible factors [28]. Recently, it was reported L-2HG may also act as

B.-F. Yuan (✉)
Key Laboratory of Analytical Chemistry for Biology and Medicine (Ministry of Education), Department of Chemistry, Wuhan University, Wuhan, China
e-mail: bfyuan@whu.edu.cn

S. Hu (ed.), *Cancer Metabolomics*, Advances in Experimental Medicine and Biology 1280,
https://doi.org/10.1007/978-3-030-51652-9_11

a metabolic signal that coordinates glycolytic flux with epigenetic modifications [40]. In addition, a specific increase of L-2HG was shown to exert similar inhibitory effect as D-2HG on α-KG-dependent dioxygenases in clear cell renal cell carcinoma (Fig. 2) [19]. Therefore, the accurate diagnosis of 2HG-related diseases relies on determining the configuration of the enantiomers, D-2HG or L-2HG, in patients [41, 42]. It is important to investigate the roles of each enantiomer independently in human metabolism and diseases such as malignant tumors.

Routine analytical methods for 2HG include gas chromatography-mass spectrometry (GC-MS), liquid chromatography-mass spectrometry (LC-MS), and magnetic resonance spectroscopy (MRS). However, these methods typically are not able to differentiate the enantiomers of D-2HG and L-2HG, and as a consequence the sum of the two oncometabolites is measured [43, 44]. To address this issue, new methods for determination of these enantiomers have been developed. These analytical strategies for D-2HG and L-2HG mainly include: (1) the use of chiral chromatography medium to facilitate chromatographic separation of enantiomers prior to spectroscopic or mass spectrometric analysis; (2) the use of chiral derivatization reagents to convert the mixture of enantiomers to diastereomers with differential physical and chemical properties that can improve their chromatographic separation; (3) enzymatic assays using enzymes specific for one enantiomeric species or the other. Herein we summarize and discuss the established methods for analysis of total 2HG as well as the determination of the enantiomers of D-2HG and L-2HG (Fig. 3).

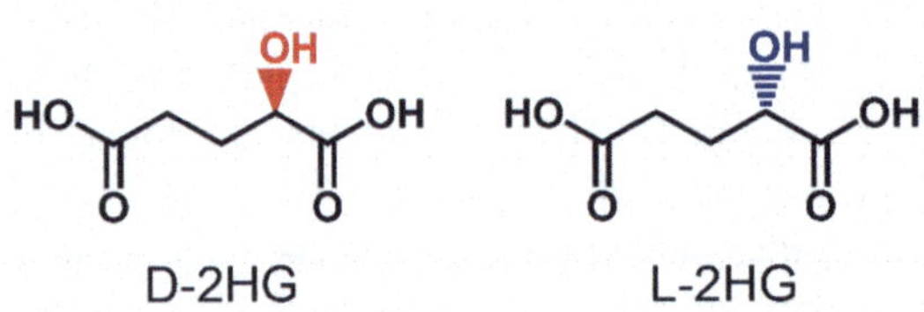

Fig. 1 Chemical structures of D-2HG and L-2HG

2 Methods for Quantitative Analysis of 2HG

2.1 LC-MS-Based Detection of 2HG

LC-MS has been frequently used for the analysis of 2HG [8, 45–50]. Since the enantiomers of D-2HG and L-2HG cannot be effectively separated in normal reversed-phase or hydrophilic interaction LC medium, the measured 2HG generally is the sum of D-2HG and L-2HG. Park et al. [51] recently introduced an analytical method by LC-time-of-flight secondary ion mass spectrometry (LC-TOF-SIMS) for sensitive detection of total 2HG in cancer cells. With this method, 2HG was detectable in 4 × 10^3 cancer

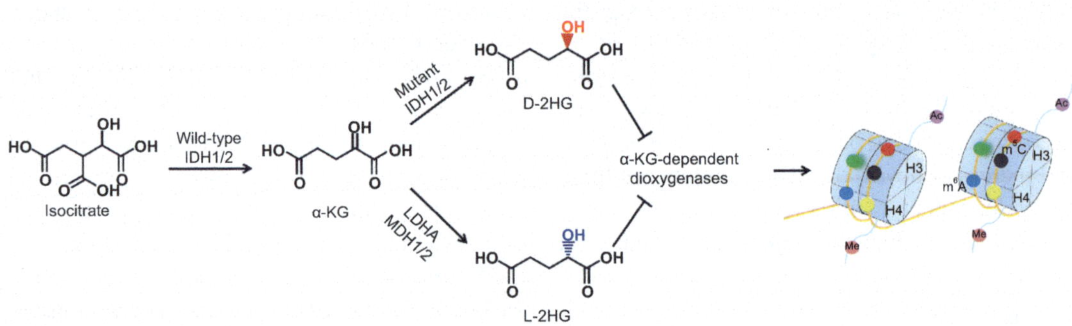

Fig. 2 Somatic mutations in IDH1/2 contribute to the pathogenesis of cancer via the production of D-2HG from α-KG. Enzymatic reduction of α-KG during hypoxia induces the generation of L-2HG by lactate dehydrogenase A (LDHA), with additional contributions from malate dehydrogenase 1 and 2 (MDH1/2). Elevated D-2HG and L-2HG can act as competitive inhibitors of α-KG-dependent enzymes, including Jumonji family histone lysine demethylases and Tet family proteins, which can regulate the epigenetic state of cells

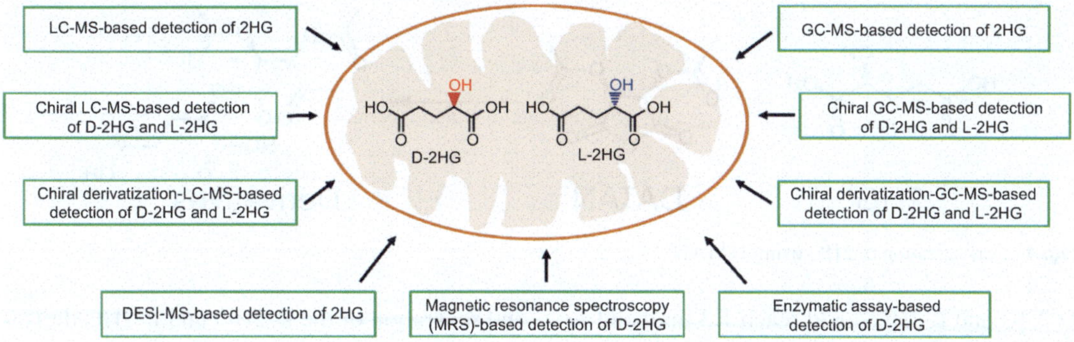

Fig. 3 Summary of the established methods for analysis of total 2HG as well as the determination of the enantiomers of D-2HG and L-2HG

cells. Due to high sensitivity by LC-TOF-SIMS, this method may be applicable to 2HG analysis in chemical screening for drug candidates.

2.2 Chiral LC-MS-Based Detection of D-2HG and L-2HG

Considering that D-2HG and L-2HG enantiomers have identical physical and chemical properties, separation of the enantiomers is challenging. One strategy has been developed to separate and quantify D-2HG and L-2HG by utilizing chiral column combined with MS analysis [52–54]. The enantiomers of D-2HG and L-2HG were satisfactorily separated with baseline resolution. The method is simple, selective, and rapid, although chiral columns are generally expensive. In addition, the detection sensitivity of the method is low due to the poor ionization efficiency of 2HG in MS.

2.3 Chiral Derivatization with LC-MS for the Detection of D-2HG and L-2HG

To differentiate the enantiomers of D-2HG and L-2HG, Struys et al. [55] developed a chiral derivatization strategy by using diacetyl-L-tartaric anhydride (DATAN) to obtain diastereomers, which were then separated on C18 column and detected by MS (Fig. 4). The use of DATAN as a chiral derivatization reagent allowed good separation resolution of the formed diastereomers of D-2HG and L-2HG. The detection limit was 20 pmol for a sample volume of 20 μL. The method was applied to analysis of urinary D-2HG and L-2HG. Recently, Pickard et al. [56] used this method to investigate the intracerebral distribution of D-2HG in mice brain tumors, and they found that D-2HG exited in glioma cells and was present in the interstitial fluid compartment at micromolar concentrations, indicating that inhibition of D-2HG may represent a new strategy to improve tumor immunotherapy. Due to the good performance for the separation of D-2HG and L-2HG by LC upon DATAN derivatization, this chiral derivatization strategy has been widely used for the determination of these two enantiomers [7, 17, 19, 27, 39, 57].

More recently, we developed a new method by using chiral derivatization combined with LC-MS analysis for highly sensitive determination of D-2HG and L-2HG enantiomers. In this strategy, *N*-(p-toluenesulfonyl)-L-phenylalanyl chloride (TSPC) was used for highly efficient labeling of D-2HG and L-2HG under mild reaction conditions (Fig. 5a, b). The results showed that the retention behavior of TSPC-labeled D-2HG and L-2HG enantiomers was greatly improved and they can be well separated in the subsequent LC-MS analysis (Fig. 5c). Moreover, TSPC derivatization greatly enhanced the detection sensitivities of D-2HG and L-2HG by 291 and 346 folds, respectively, due to the introduction of easily ionizable group from TSPC. Upon TSPC derivatization, the limits of detection (LODs) of

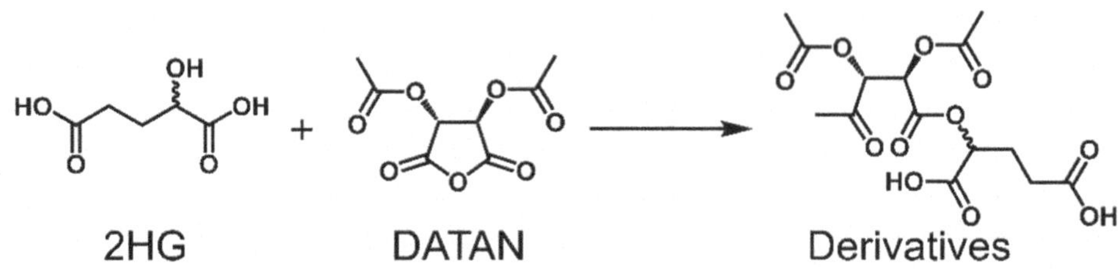

Fig. 4 Derivatization of 2HG using DATAN

D-2HG and L-2HG could reach 1.2 fmol and 1.0 fmol, respectively. Using this method, we achieved a simultaneous quantification of D-2HG and L-2HG in human urines from patients with type 2 diabetes mellitus, lung cancer, colorectal cancer, nasopharyngeal carcinoma, as well as in human clear cell renal cell carcinoma tissues.

2.4 GC-MS-Based Detection of 2HG

GC-MS has often been used for the analysis total 2HG [15, 18, 32, 43, 58–61]. Sahm et al. [58] described a method to detect total 2HG levels in archived, formalin-fixed paraffin-embedded (FFPE) tumor specimens by stable isotope dilution with GC-MS. Samples were derivatized with *N*-methyl-*N*-(trimethylsilyl)heptafluorobutyramide (MSHFBA) for 1 h at 60 °C and analyzed in the selective ion-monitoring mode with electron impact ionization. Gas chromatographic separation was achieved on a capillary column using helium as a carrier gas. Successful detection of 2HG in FFPE specimens allows routinely processed tissue accessible for research on 2HG accumulation and may enable studies on correlation of 2HG levels with clinicopathological data.

2.5 Chiral GC-MS-Based Detection of D-2HG and L-2HG

Neves et al. [62] developed a method for separation of D-2HG and L-2HG by using chiral stationary phase in GC. The esterification of D-2HG and L-2HG was achieved at room temperature by reaction with appropriate alkyl chloroformates, and separation of the D-2HG and L-2HG derivatives was realized by chiral GC-MS. In the study, fused silica capillaries coated with a chiral siloxane copolymer, 1(*R*)-trans-*N*-*N*′-1,2-cyclohexylenebisbenzamideoligodimethyl-siloxane, or with a commercial cyclodextrin were used for separation of the enantiomers. In addition, heptakis(2,3-di-*O*-methyl-6-*O*-tert-butyldimethylsilyl)-β-cyclodextrin was used as a chiral stationary phase in GC-MS for separation and detection of D-2HG and L-2HG [63]. These methods showed highly efficient separation and qualitative determination of D-2HG and L-2HG. However, the preparation of chiral stationary phase for GC-MS generally is time-consuming, which limits the wide use of this method.

2.6 Chiral Derivatization with GC-MS for the Detection of D-2HG and L-2HG

Chiral derivatization of D-2HG and L-2HG by D-2-butanol and acetic anhydride to form their corresponding di-*R*-butyl-*O*-acetyl derivatives was demonstrated for GC separation of D-2HG and L-2HG [64, 65]. These derivatives can be well separated and analyzed by GC-MS. This derivatization strategy was later frequently used for quantitative determination of D-2HG and L-2HG in various studies [40, 66, 67]. Kim et al. [68] also achieved enantiomeric separation of D-2HG and L-2HG after their conversion to *O*-trifluoroacetyl-(−)-menthyl derivatives followed by GC-MS analysis. With this method, D-2HG and L-2HG from urine samples were distinctly identified and quantified.

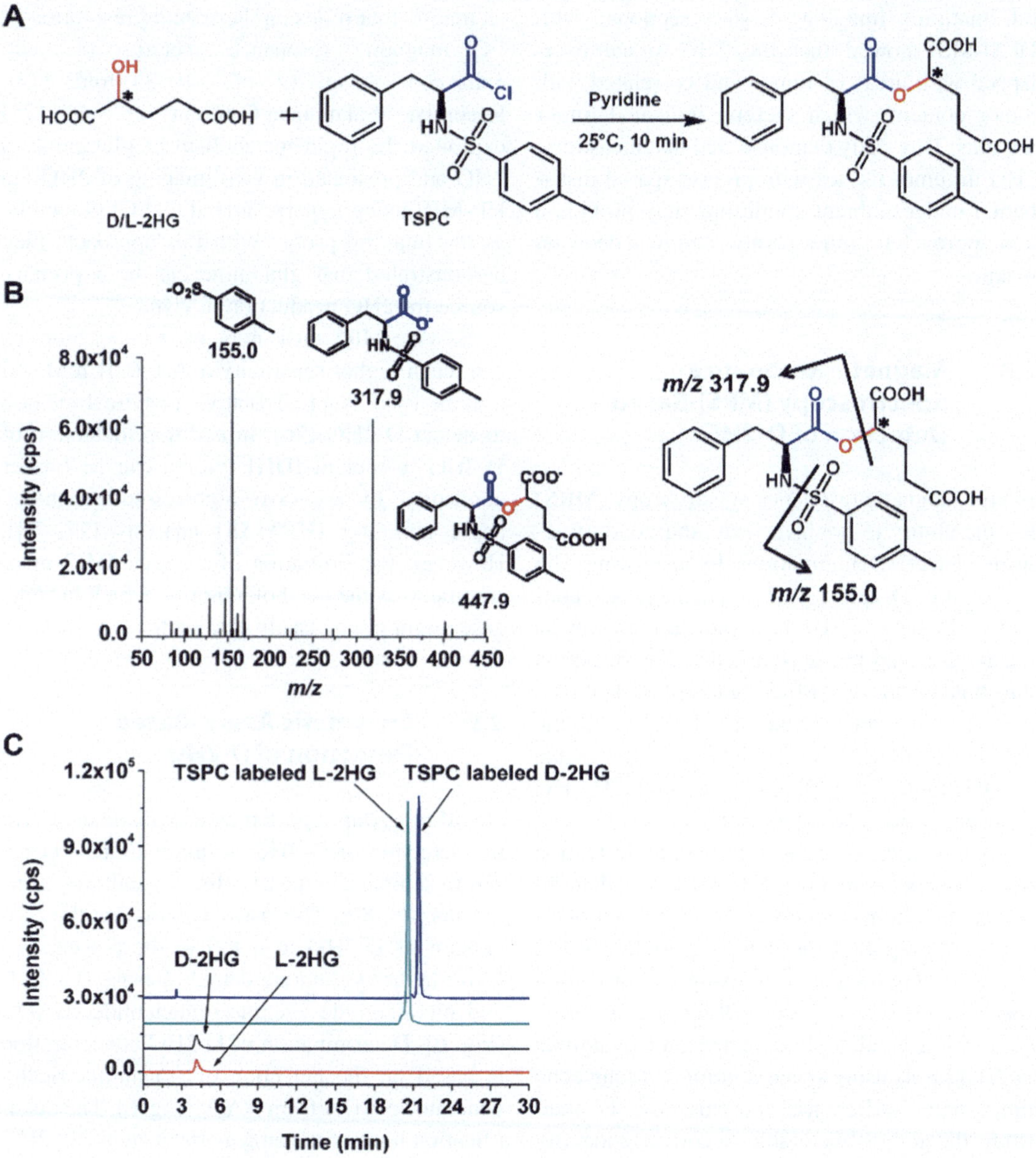

Fig. 5 Determination of D-2HG and L-2HG by chiral TSPC derivatization with LC-MS detection. (**a**) Derivatization of D/L-2HG by TSPC. (**b**) Product ions spectrum of TSPC labeled L-2HG. (**c**) The extracted ion chromatograms of D-2HG and L-2HG before and after TSPC labeling. (Reprinted with permission from *Sci Rep*, 2015, 5, 15217)

2.7 DESI-MS-Based Detection of 2HG

Using desorption electrospray ionization (DESI) MS, Santagata et al. [69] directly detected total 2HG from tissue sections of surgically resected gliomas under ambient conditions without complex tissue preparation. With DESI-MS, the authors identified IDH1 mutant tumors with high sensitivity and specificity, which allows rapid molecular characterization and may provide diagnostic, prognostic, and predictive information. Imaging tissue sections with DESI-MS showed that the 2HG signal overlapped with areas of tumor and correlated with tumor content, which thereby indicated tumor margins. This study demonstrated that measuring 2HG in tumor tissues with precise spatial distribution under ambient conditions may provide a new approach for intraoperative surgical decision making.

2.8 Magnetic Resonance Spectroscopy (MRS)-Based Detection of D-2HG

In vivo magnetic resonance spectroscopy (MRS) has the ability to noninvasively and nondestructively detect IDH mutations by measuring the endogenous D-2HG [70, 71]. The increased content of D-2HG in IDH1 mutant tumors can be readily detected by in vivo MRS. The detection threshold of in vivo MRS generally is approximate 1 mM, which makes D-2HG measurable only in situations where D-2HG accumulates due to IDH1 mutations [70]. On the contrary, D-2HG is not expected to be detectable in tumors without IDH1 mutations or in healthy tissues. Detection of D-2HG with in vivo 1H MRS was demonstrated in glioma patients [72, 73]. Andronesi et al. [72] reported the detection of D-2HG in mutant IDH1 glioma in vivo using 2D correlation spectroscopy (COSY) and J-difference spectroscopy. Choi et al. [73] detected and quantified D-2HG levels using spectral editing at long echo times and J-difference spectroscopy. In their study, the authors were able to correctly identify all patients that have IDH mutations by noninvasively measuring D-2HG.

Although the level of D-2HG is high enough in most tumors to be measured by in vivo MRS, there may be certain tumors in which the levels of D-2HG are below 1 mM detection threshold. Meanwhile, the presence of other abundant metabolites with similar chemical structures to D-2HG makes the detection challenging. Additionally, in vivo MRS cannot assess the carbon sources for D-2HG. Hyperpolarized magnetic resonance imaging (HP-MRI) is an imaging technique that relies on the spectral resolution of ^{13}C magnetic resonance spectroscopy with enhanced sensitivity of >10,000-fold [74]. Recently, Salamanca-Cardona et al. [75] exploited the rapid metabolism of glutamine to 2HG and presented in vivo imaging of 2HG via HP-MRI using hyperpolarized [1-^{13}C] glutamine as the imaging probe. With this approach, they demonstrated that glutamine can be a primary source for 2HG production in vivo.

Ex vivo MRS measurement of intact biopsies can reach higher sensitivity of 0.1–0.01 mM and may be used as an alternative analytical method to detect D-2HG [76]. In addition, detection of D-2HG in mutant IDH1 glioma can be further confirmed by ex vivo high-resolution magic angle spinning (HRMAS) analysis [77, 78]. However, the limitation of ex vivo MRS measurements is the need of a biopsy, which in some case might not be easily obtained.

2.9 Enzymatic Assay–Based Detection of D-2HG

Deimling group reported an enzymatic assay for the detection of D-2HG in tumor tissues, urine/serum samples, cultured cells, and culture supernatants [79, 80]. This assay is based on the conversion of D-2HG to α-KG in the presence of (D)-2-hydroxyglutarate dehydrogenase (HGDH) and nicotinamide adenine dinucleotide (NAD^+) (Fig. 6). Determination of D-2HG concentration is based on the detection of stoichiometrically generated NADH from NAD^+ (Fig. 6). The quantification limit of the enzymatic assay for D-2HG is 0.44 μM in tumor tissue and 2.77 μM in serum, which enables the detection of basal D-2HG levels in human tumor tissues and serum even without IDH mutations. With this method, the levels of D-2HG in frozen and paraffin-embedded tumor tissues containing IDH mutations or in serum from acute myeloid leukemia patients with IDH mutations were found to be significantly higher. The enzymatic assay is considerably less expensive and can be performed on 96-well microtiter plates, which is favorable for the detection of large numbers of clinical samples.

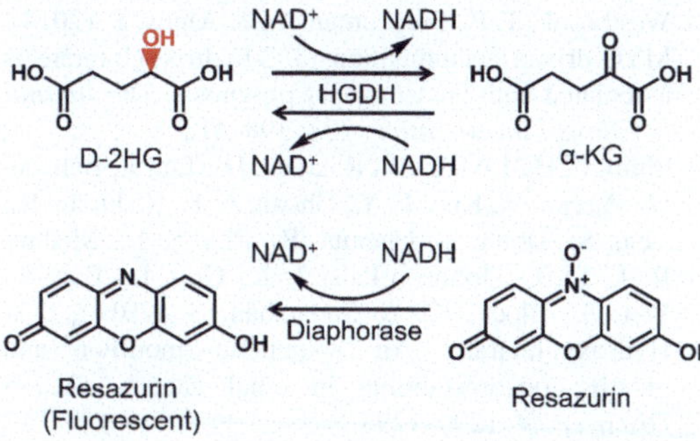

Fig. 6 Scheme for enzymatic assay of D-2HG. (**a**) (D)-2-Hydroxyglutarate dehydrogenase (HGDH) catalyzes the reduction of NAD^+ to NADH by oxidation of D-2HG to α-KG. (**b**) Detection of NADH by diaphorase/resazurin system. Fluorescent product resorufin is exited at 540 nm and detected at 610 nm. (Reprinted with permission from *Acta Neuropathol*, 2012, 124, 883–891)

3 Conclusions

2HG may serve as valuable indicator for tumors with IDH mutations since 2HG is produced as an error product of normal metabolism and generally present at trace levels in cells without IDH mutations. Almost all of the tumors with IDH mutations have increased levels of D-2HG by several orders of magnitude. Hence, quantification of the oncometabolite 2HG may be used to monitor and evaluate the formation and malignant progression of tumors. Furthermore, 2HG levels could also be used to quantify and predict the efficacy of drugs targeting mutant IDH1.

Although it is widely recognized that accumulation of the oncometabolite D-2HG leads to cancer initiation, recently D-2HG has also been demonstrated to have antitumor effects in a subset of tumors by increasing global N^6-methyladenosine RNA modification [81]. The study suggested that 2HG holds therapeutic potential in treating IDH wild-type cancers. Therefore, the biological functions of 2HG may be more complex than we anticipated. While many questions remain regarding the roles of 2HG in tumorigenesis as well as in antitumor effects, in-depth investigations are certainly warranted to uncover new mechanism of 2HG in cancer diseases.

Acknowledgments The authors thank the financial support from the National Natural Science Foundation of China (21672166, 22074110, 21721005).

References

1. Pavlova, N. N., & Thompson, C. B. (2016). The emerging hallmarks of cancer metabolism. *Cell Metabolism, 23*, 27–47.
2. Nielsen, J., & Keasling, J. D. (2016). Engineering cellular metabolism. *Cell, 164*, 1185–1197.
3. Kaelin, W. G., Jr., & McKnight, S. L. (2013). Influence of metabolism on epigenetics and disease. *Cell, 153*, 56–69.
4. Cairns, R. A., & Mak, T. W. (2013). Oncogenic isocitrate dehydrogenase mutations: Mechanisms, models, and clinical opportunities. *Cancer Discovery, 3*, 730–741.
5. Ye, D., Ma, S., Xiong, Y., & Guan, K. L. (2013). R-2-hydroxyglutarate as the key effector of IDH mutations promoting oncogenesis. *Cancer Cell, 23*, 274–276.
6. Rakheja, D., Medeiros, L. J., Bevan, S., & Chen, W. (2013). The emerging role of d-2-hydroxyglutarate as an oncometabolite in hematolymphoid and central nervous system neoplasms. *Frontiers in Oncology, 3*, 169.
7. Dang, L., White, D. W., Gross, S., Bennett, B. D., Bittinger, M. A., Driggers, E. M., Fantin, V. R., Jang, H. G., Jin, S., Keenan, M. C., Marks, K. M., Prins, R. M., Ward, P. S., Yen, K. E., Liau, L. M., Rabinowitz, J. D., Cantley, L. C., Thompson, C. B., Vander Heiden, M. G., & Su, S. M. (2009). Cancer-associated IDH1 mutations produce 2-hydroxyglutarate. *Nature, 462*, 739–744.
8. Jin, G., Reitman, Z. J., Spasojevic, I., Batinic-Haberle, I., Yang, J., Schmidt-Kittler, O., Bigner, D. D., & Yan, H. (2011). 2-hydroxyglutarate production, but not dominant negative function, is conferred by glioma-derived NADP-dependent isocitrate dehydrogenase mutations. *PLoS One, 6*, e16812.
9. Rohle, D., Popovici-Muller, J., Palaskas, N., Turcan, S., Grommes, C., Campos, C., Tsoi, J., Clark, O., Oldrini, B., Komisopoulou, E., Kunii, K., Pedraza, A., Schalm, S., Silverman, L., Miller, A., Wang, F., Yang, H., Chen, Y., Kernytsky, A., Rosenblum, M. K., Liu, W., Biller, S. A., Su, S. M., Brennan, C. W., Chan, T. A., Graeber, T. G., Yen, K. E., & Mellinghoff, I. K. (2013). An inhibitor of mutant IDH1 delays growth and promotes differentiation of glioma cells. *Science, 340*, 626–630.
10. Flavahan, W. A., Drier, Y., Liau, B. B., Gillespie, S. M., Venteicher, A. S., Stemmer-Rachamimov, A. O., Suva, M. L., & Bernstein, B. E. (2016). Insulator dysfunction and oncogene activation in IDH mutant gliomas. *Nature, 529*, 110–114.
11. Mu, L., Long, Y., Yang, C., Jin, L., Tao, H., Ge, H., Chang, Y. E., Karachi, A., Kubilis, P. S., De Leon, G., Qi, J., Sayour, E. J., Mitchell, D. A., Lin, Z., & Huang,

J. (2018). The IDH1 mutation-induced oncometabolite, 2-hydroxyglutarate, may affect DNA methylation and expression of PD-L1 in gliomas. *Frontiers in Molecular Neuroscience, 11*, 82.
12. Wang, F., Travins, J., DeLaBarre, B., Penard-Lacronique, V., Schalm, S., Hansen, E., Straley, K., Kernytsky, A., Liu, W., Gliser, C., Yang, H., Gross, S., Artin, E., Saada, V., Mylonas, E., Quivoron, C., Popovici-Muller, J., Saunders, J. O., Salituro, F. G., Yan, S., Murray, S., Wei, W., Gao, Y., Dang, L., Dorsch, M., Agresta, S., Schenkein, D. P., Biller, S. A., Su, S. M., de Botton, S., & Yen, K. E. (2013). Targeted inhibition of mutant IDH2 in leukemia cells induces cellular differentiation. *Science, 340*, 622–626.
13. Gross, S., Cairns, R. A., Minden, M. D., Driggers, E. M., Bittinger, M. A., Jang, H. G., Sasaki, M., Jin, S., Schenkein, D. P., Su, S. M., Dang, L., Fantin, V. R., & Mak, T. W. (2010). Cancer-associated metabolite 2-hydroxyglutarate accumulates in acute myelogenous leukemia with isocitrate dehydrogenase 1 and 2 mutations. *The Journal of Experimental Medicine, 207*, 339–344.
14. Losman, J. A., Looper, R. E., Koivunen, P., Lee, S., Schneider, R. K., McMahon, C., Cowley, G. S., Root, D. E., Ebert, B. L., & Kaelin, W. G., Jr. (2013). (R)-2-hydroxyglutarate is sufficient to promote leukemogenesis and its effects are reversible. *Science, 339*, 1621–1625.
15. Chan, S. M., Thomas, D., Corces-Zimmerman, M. R., Xavy, S., Rastogi, S., Hong, W. J., Zhao, F., Medeiros, B. C., Tyvoll, D. A., & Majeti, R. (2015). Isocitrate dehydrogenase 1 and 2 mutations induce BCL-2 dependence in acute myeloid leukemia. *Nature Medicine, 21*, 178–184.
16. Amary, M. F., Bacsi, K., Maggiani, F., Damato, S., Halai, D., Berisha, F., Pollock, R., O'Donnell, P., Grigoriadis, A., Diss, T., Eskandarpour, M., Presneau, N., Hogendoorn, P. C. W., Futreal, A., Tirabosco, R., & Flanagan, A. M. (2011). IDH1 and IDH2 mutations are frequent events in central chondrosarcoma and central and periosteal chondromas but not in other mesenchymal tumours. *The Journal of Pathology, 224*, 334–343.
17. Li, L., Paz, A. C., Wilky, B. A., Johnson, B., Galoian, K., Rosenberg, A., Hu, G., Tinoco, G., Bodamer, O., & Trent, J. C. (2015). Treatment with a small molecule mutant IDH1 inhibitor suppresses tumorigenic activity and decreases production of the oncometabolite 2-hydroxyglutarate in human chondrosarcoma cells. *PLoS One, 10*, e0133813.
18. Terunuma, A., Putluri, N., Mishra, P., Mathe, E. A., Dorsey, T. H., Yi, M., Wallace, T. A., Issaq, H. J., Zhou, M., Killian, J. K., Stevenson, H. S., Karoly, E. D., Chan, K., Samanta, S., Prieto, D., Hsu, T. Y., Kurley, S. J., Putluri, V., Sonavane, R., Edelman, D. C., Wulff, J., Starks, A. M., Yang, Y., Kittles, R. A., Yfantis, H. G., Lee, D. H., Ioffe, O. B., Schiff, R., Stephens, R. M., Meltzer, P. S., Veenstra, T. D., Westbrook, T. F., Sreekumar, A., & Ambs, S. (2014). MYC-driven accumulation of 2-hydroxyglutarate is associated with breast cancer prognosis. *The Journal of Clinical Investigation, 124*, 398–412.
19. Shim, E. H., Livi, C. B., Rakheja, D., Tan, J., Benson, D., Parekh, V., Kho, E. Y., Ghosh, A. P., Kirkman, R., Velu, S., Dutta, S., Chenna, B., Rea, S. L., Mishur, R. J., Li, Q., Johnson-Pais, T. L., Guo, L., Bae, S., Wei, S., Block, K., & Sudarshan, S. (2014). L-2-Hydroxyglutarate: An epigenetic modifier and putative oncometabolite in renal cancer. *Cancer Discovery, 4*, 1290–1298.
20. Saha, S. K., Parachoniak, C. A., Ghanta, K. S., Fitamant, J., Ross, K. N., Najem, M. S., Gurumurthy, S., Akbay, E. A., Sia, D., Cornella, H., Miltiadous, O., Walesky, C., Deshpande, V., Zhu, A. X., Hezel, A. F., Yen, K. E., Straley, K. S., Travins, J., Popovici-Muller, J., Gliser, C., Ferrone, C. R., Apte, U., Llovet, J. M., Wong, K. K., Ramaswamy, S., & Bardeesy, N. (2014). Mutant IDH inhibits HNF-4alpha to block hepatocyte differentiation and promote biliary cancer. *Nature, 513*, 110–114.
21. Saha, S. K., Parachoniak, C. A., & Bardeesy, N. (2014). IDH mutations in liver cell plasticity and biliary cancer. *Cell Cycle, 13*, 3176–3182.
22. Kipp, B. R., Voss, J. S., Kerr, S. E., Barr Fritcher, E. G., Graham, R. P., Zhang, L., Highsmith, W. E., Zhang, J., Roberts, L. R., Gores, G. J., & Halling, K. C. (2012). Isocitrate dehydrogenase 1 and 2 mutations in cholangiocarcinoma. *Human Pathology, 43*, 1552–1558.
23. Delahousse, J., Verlingue, L., Broutin, S., Legoupil, C., Touat, M., Doucet, L., Ammari, S., Lacroix, L., Ducreux, M., Scoazec, J. Y., Malka, D., Paci, A., & Hollebecque, A. (2018). Circulating oncometabolite D-2-hydroxyglutarate enantiomer is a surrogate marker of isocitrate dehydrogenase-mutated intrahepatic cholangiocarcinomas. *European Journal of Cancer, 90*, 83–91.
24. Kato, K. M., Liu, X., Oki, H., Ogasawara, S., Nakamura, T., Saidoh, N., Tsujimoto, Y., Matsuyama, Y., Uruno, A., Sugawara, M., Tsuchiya, T., Yamakawa, M., Yamamoto, M., Takagi, M., & Kato, Y. (2014). Isocitrate dehydrogenase mutation is frequently observed in giant cell tumor of bone. *Cancer Science, 105*, 744–748.
25. Dang, L., & Su, S. M. (2017). Isocitrate dehydrogenase mutation and (R)-2-Hydroxyglutarate: From basic discovery to therapeutics development. *Annual Review of Biochemistry, 86*, 305–331.
26. Loenarz, C., & Schofield, C. J. (2011). Physiological and biochemical aspects of hydroxylations and demethylations catalyzed by human 2-oxoglutarate oxygenases. *Trends in Biochemical Sciences, 36*, 7–18.
27. Koivunen, P., Lee, S., Duncan, C. G., Lopez, G., Lu, G., Ramkissoon, S., Losman, J. A., Joensuu, P., Bergmann, U., Gross, S., Travins, J., Weiss, S.,

Looper, R., Ligon, K. L., Verhaak, R. G., Yan, H., & Kaelin, W. G., Jr. (2012). Transformation by the (R)-enantiomer of 2-hydroxyglutarate linked to EGLN activation. *Nature, 483*, 484–488.
28. Intlekofer, A. M., Dematteo, R. G., Venneti, S., Finley, L. W., Lu, C., Judkins, A. R., Rustenburg, A. S., Grinaway, P. B., Chodera, J. D., Cross, J. R., & Thompson, C. B. (2015). Hypoxia induces production of L-2-Hydroxyglutarate. *Cell Metabolism, 22*, 304–311.
29. Wu, X., & Zhang, Y. (2017). TET-mediated active DNA demethylation: Mechanism, function and beyond. *Nature Reviews. Genetics, 18*, 517–534.
30. Struys, E. A. (2013). 2-Hydroxyglutarate is not a metabolite; D-2-hydroxyglutarate and L-2-hydroxyglutarate are! *Proceedings of the National Academy of Sciences of the United States of America, 110*, E4939.
31. Kranendijk, M., Struys, E. A., Salomons, G. S., Van der Knaap, M. S., & Jakobs, C. (2012). Progress in understanding 2-hydroxyglutaric acidurias. *Journal of Inherited Metabolic Disease, 35*, 571–587.
32. Ward, P. S., Patel, J., Wise, D. R., Abdel-Wahab, O., Bennett, B. D., Coller, H. A., Cross, J. R., Fantin, V. R., Hedvat, C. V., Perl, A. E., Rabinowitz, J. D., Carroll, M., Su, S. M., Sharp, K. A., Levine, R. L., & Thompson, C. B. (2010). The common feature of leukemia-associated IDH1 and IDH2 mutations is a neomorphic enzyme activity converting alpha-ketoglutarate to 2-hydroxyglutarate. *Cancer Cell, 17*, 225–234.
33. Reitman, Z. J., Jin, G., Karoly, E. D., Spasojevic, I., Yang, J., Kinzler, K. W., He, Y., Bigner, D. D., Vogelstein, B., & Yan, H. (2011). Profiling the effects of isocitrate dehydrogenase 1 and 2 mutations on the cellular metabolome. *Proceedings of the National Academy of Sciences of the United States of America, 108*, 3270–3275.
34. Xu, W., Yang, H., Liu, Y., Yang, Y., Wang, P., Kim, S. H., Ito, S., Yang, C., Wang, P., Xiao, M. T., Liu, L. X., Jiang, W. Q., Liu, J., Zhang, J. Y., Wang, B., Frye, S., Zhang, Y., Xu, Y. H., Lei, Q. Y., Guan, K. L., Zhao, S. M., & Xiong, Y. (2011). Oncometabolite 2-hydroxyglutarate is a competitive inhibitor of alpha-ketoglutarate-dependent dioxygenases. *Cancer Cell, 19*, 17–30.
35. Lu, C., Ward, P. S., Kapoor, G. S., Rohle, D., Turcan, S., Abdel-Wahab, O., Edwards, C. R., Khanin, R., Figueroa, M. E., Melnick, A., Wellen, K. E., O'Rourke, D. M., Berger, S. L., Chan, T. A., Levine, R. L., Mellinghoff, I. K., & Thompson, C. B. (2012). IDH mutation impairs histone demethylation and results in a block to cell differentiation. *Nature, 483*, 474–U130.
36. Wang, P., Wu, J., Ma, S., Zhang, L., Yao, J., Hoadley, K. A., Wilkerson, M. D., Perou, C. M., Guan, K. L., Ye, D., & Xiong, Y. (2015). Oncometabolite D-2-Hydroxyglutarate inhibits ALKBH DNA repair enzymes and sensitizes IDH mutant cells to alkylating agents. *Cell Reports, 13*, 2353–2361.
37. Janke, R., Iavarone, A. T., & Rine, J. (2017). Oncometabolite D-2-Hydroxyglutarate enhances gene silencing through inhibition of specific H3K36 histone demethylases. *eLife, 6*, e22451.
38. Karlstaedt, A., Zhang, X., Vitrac, H., Harmancey, R., Vasquez, H., Wang, J. H., Goodell, M. A., & Taegtmeyer, H. (2016). Oncometabolite d-2-hydroxyglutarate impairs alpha-ketoglutarate dehydrogenase and contractile function in rodent heart. *Proceedings of the National Academy of Sciences of the United States of America, 113*, 10436–10441.
39. Oldham, W. M., Clish, C. B., Yang, Y., & Loscalzo, J. (2015). Hypoxia-mediated increases in L-2-hydroxyglutarate coordinate the metabolic response to reductive stress. *Cell Metabolism, 22*, 291–303.
40. Li, H., Chawla, G., Hurlburt, A. J., Sterrett, M. C., Zaslaver, O., Cox, J., Karty, J. A., Rosebrock, A. P., Caudy, A. A., & Tennessen, J. M. (2017). Drosophila larvae synthesize the putative oncometabolite L-2-hydroxyglutarate during normal developmental growth. *Proceedings of the National Academy of Sciences of the United States of America, 114*, 1353–1358.
41. Seijo-Martinez, M., Navarro, C., Castro del Rio, M., Vila, O., Puig, M., Ribes, A., & Butron, M. (2005). L-2-hydroxyglutaric aciduria: Clinical, neuroimaging, and neuropathological findings. *Archives of Neurology, 62*, 666–670.
42. Kranendijk, M., Struys, E. A., Gibson, K. M., Wickenhagen, W. V., Abdenur, J. E., Buechner, J., Christensen, E., de Kremer, R. D., Errami, A., Gissen, P., Gradowska, W., Hobson, E., Islam, L., Korman, S. H., Kurczynski, T., Maranda, B., Meli, C., Rizzo, C., Sansaricq, C., Trefz, F. K., Webster, R., Jakobs, C., & Salomons, G. S. (2010). Evidence for genetic heterogeneity in D-2-hydroxyglutaric aciduria. *Human Mutation, 31*, 279–283.
43. Wang, J. H., Chen, W. L., Li, J. M., Wu, S. F., Chen, T. L., Zhu, Y. M., Zhang, W. N., Li, Y., Qiu, Y. P., Zhao, A. H., Mi, J. Q., Jin, J., Wang, Y. G., Ma, Q. L., Huang, H., Wu, D. P., Wang, Q. R., Li, Y., Yan, X. J., Yan, J. S., Li, J. Y., Wang, S., Huang, X. J., Wang, B. S., Jia, W., Shen, Y., Chen, Z., & Chen, S. J. (2013). Prognostic significance of 2-hydroxyglutarate levels in acute myeloid leukemia in China. *Proceedings of the National Academy of Sciences of the United States of America, 110*, 17017–17022.
44. Sellner, L., Capper, D., Meyer, J., Langhans, C. D., Hartog, C. M., Pfeifer, H., Serve, H., Ho, A. D., Okun, J. G., Kramer, A., & Von Deimling, A. (2010). Increased levels of 2-hydroxyglutarate in AML patients with IDH1-R132H and IDH2-R140Q mutations. *European Journal of Haematology, 85*, 457–459.
45. Matsunaga, H., Futakuchi-Tsuchida, A., Takahashi, M., Ishikawa, T., Tsuji, M., & Ando, O. (2012). IDH1

and IDH2 have critical roles in 2-hydroxyglutarate production in D-2-hydroxyglutarate dehydrogenase depleted cells. *Biochemical and Biophysical Research Communications, 423*, 553–556.
46. DiNardo, C. D., Propert, K. J., Loren, A. W., Paietta, E., Sun, Z., Levine, R. L., Straley, K. S., Yen, K., Patel, J. P., Agresta, S., Abdel-Wahab, O., Perl, A. E., Litzow, M. R., Rowe, J. M., Lazarus, H. M., Fernandez, H. F., Margolis, D. J., Tallman, M. S., Luger, S. M., & Carroll, M. (2013). Serum 2-hydroxyglutarate levels predict isocitrate dehydrogenase mutations and clinical outcome in acute myeloid leukemia. *Blood, 121*, 4917–4924.
47. Juratli, T. A., Peitzsch, M., Geiger, K., Schackert, G., Eisenhofer, G., & Krex, D. (2013). Accumulation of 2-hydroxyglutarate is not a biomarker for malignant progression in IDH-mutated low-grade gliomas. *Neuro-Oncology, 15*, 682–690.
48. Akbay, E. A., Moslehi, J., Christensen, C. L., Saha, S., Tchaicha, J. H., Ramkissoon, S. H., Stewart, K. M., Carretero, J., Kikuchi, E., Zhang, H., Cohoon, T. J., Murray, S., Liu, W., Uno, K., Fisch, S., Jones, K., Gurumurthy, S., Gliser, C., Choe, S., Keenan, M., Son, J., Stanley, I., Losman, J. A., Padera, R., Bronson, R. T., Asara, J. M., Abdel-Wahab, O., Amrein, P. C., Fathi, A. T., Danial, N. N., Kimmelman, A. C., Kung, A. L., Ligon, K. L., Yen, K. E., Kaelin, W. G., Jr., Bardeesy, N., & Wong, K. K. (2014). D-2-hydroxyglutarate produced by mutant IDH2 causes cardiomyopathy and neurodegeneration in mice. *Genes & Development, 28*, 479–490.
49. Borger, D. R., Goyal, L., Yau, T., Poon, R. T., Ancukiewicz, M., Deshpande, V., Christiani, D. C., Liebman, H. M., Yang, H., Kim, H., Yen, K., Faris, J. E., Iafrate, A. J., Kwak, E. L., Clark, J. W., Allen, J. N., Blaszkowsky, L. S., Murphy, J. E., Saha, S. K., Hong, T. S., Wo, J. Y., Ferrone, C. R., Tanabe, K. K., Bardeesy, N., Straley, K. S., Agresta, S., Schenkein, D. P., Ellisen, L. W., Ryan, D. P., & Zhu, A. X. (2014). Circulating oncometabolite 2-hydroxyglutarate is a potential surrogate biomarker in patients with isocitrate dehydrogenase-mutant intrahepatic cholangiocarcinoma. *Clinical Cancer Research, 20*, 1884–1890.
50. Walker, O. S., Elsasser, S. J., Mahesh, M., Bachman, M., Balasubramanian, S., & Chin, J. W. (2016). Photoactivation of mutant Isocitrate dehydrogenase 2 reveals rapid Cancer-associated metabolic and epigenetic changes. *Journal of the American Chemical Society, 138*, 718–721.
51. Park, J., Na, H. K., Shon, H. K., Son, H. Y., Huh, Y. M., Lee, S. W., & Lee, T. G. (2018). TOF-SIMS analysis of an isocitrate dehydrogenase 1 mutation-associated oncometabolite in cancer cells. *Biointerphases, 13*, 03B404.
52. Rashed, M. S., AlAmoudi, M., & Aboul-Enein, H. Y. (2000). Chiral liquid chromatography tandem mass spectrometry in the determination of the configuration of 2-hydroxyglutaric acid in urine. *Biomedical Chromatography, 14*, 317–320.
53. Wickenhagen, W. V., Salomons, G. S., Gibson, K. M., Jakobs, C., & Struys, E. A. (2009). Measurement of D: −2-hydroxyglutarate dehydrogenase activity in cell homogenates derived from D: −2-hydroxyglutaric aciduria patients. *Journal of Inherited Metabolic Disease, 32*, 264–268.
54. Kranendijk, M., Salomons, G. S., Gibson, K. M., Aktuglu-Zeybek, C., Bekri, S., Christensen, E., Clarke, J., Hahn, A., Korman, S. H., Mejaski-Bosnjak, V., Superti-Furga, A., Vianey-Saban, C., van der Knaap, M. S., Jakobs, C., & Struys, E. A. (2009). Development and implementation of a novel assay for L-2-hydroxyglutarate dehydrogenase (L-2-HGDH) in cell lysates: L-2-HGDH deficiency in 15 patients with L-2-hydroxyglutaric aciduria. *Journal of Inherited Metabolic Disease, 32*, 713–719.
55. Struys, E. A., Jansen, E. E., Verhoeven, N. M., & Jakobs, C. (2004). Measurement of urinary D- and L-2-hydroxyglutarate enantiomers by stable-isotope-dilution liquid chromatography-tandem mass spectrometry after derivatization with diacetyl-L-tartaric anhydride. *Clinical Chemistry, 50*, 1391–1395.
56. Pickard, A. J., Sohn, A. S., Bartenstein, T. F., He, S., Zhang, Y., & Gallo, J. M. (2016). Intracerebral distribution of the oncometabolite d-2-hydroxyglutarate in mice bearing mutant isocitrate dehydrogenase brain tumors: Implications for tumorigenesis. *Frontiers in Oncology, 6*, 211.
57. Rakheja, D., Mitui, M., Boriack, R. L., & DeBerardinis, R. J. (2011). Isocitrate dehydrogenase 1/2 mutational analyses and 2-hydroxyglutarate measurements in Wilms tumors. *Pediatric Blood & Cancer, 56*, 379–383.
58. Sahm, F., Capper, D., Pusch, S., Balss, J., Koch, A., Langhans, C. D., Okun, J. G., & von Deimling, A. (2012). Detection of 2-hydroxyglutarate in formalin-fixed paraffin-embedded glioma specimens by gas chromatography/mass spectrometry. *Brain Pathology, 22*, 26–31.
59. Luchman, H. A., Stechishin, O. D., Dang, N. H., Blough, M. D., Chesnelong, C., Kelly, J. J., Nguyen, S. A., Chan, J. A., Weljie, A. M., Cairncross, J. G., & Weiss, S. (2012). An in vivo patient-derived model of endogenous IDH1-mutant glioma. *Neuro-Oncology, 14*, 184–191.
60. Ward, P. S., Lu, C., Cross, J. R., Abdel-Wahab, O., Levine, R. L., Schwartz, G. K., & Thompson, C. B. (2013). The potential for isocitrate dehydrogenase mutations to produce 2-hydroxyglutarate depends on allele specificity and subcellular compartmentalization. *The Journal of Biological Chemistry, 288*, 3804–3815.
61. Janin, M., Mylonas, E., Saada, V., Micol, J. B., Renneville, A., Quivoron, C., Koscielny, S., Scourzic, L., Forget, S., Pautas, C., Caillot, D., Preudhomme,

C., Dombret, H., Berthon, C., Barouki, R., Rabier, D., Auger, N., Griscelli, F., Chachaty, E., Leclercq, E., Courtier, M. H., Bennaceur-Griscelli, A., Solary, E., Bernard, O. A., Penard-Lacronique, V., Ottolenghi, C., & de Botton, S. (2014). Serum 2-hydroxyglutarate production in IDH1- and IDH2-mutated de novo acute myeloid leukemia: A study by the acute leukemia French association group. *Journal of Clinical Oncology, 32*, 297–305.
62. dasNeves, H. J. C., Noronha, J. P., & Rufino, H. (1996). New method for the chiral HRGC assay of L-2-hydroxyglutaric acid in urine. *Journal of High Resolution Chromatography, 19*, 161–164.
63. Kaunzinger, A., Rechner, A., Beck, T., Mosandl, A., Sewell, A. C., & Bohles, H. (1996). Chiral compounds as indicators of inherited metabolic disease - simultaneous stereodifferentiation of lactic-, 2-hydroxyglutaric- and glyceric acid by enantioselective cGC. *Enantiomer, 1*, 177–182.
64. Gibson, K. M. B. H. J., Schor, D. S. M., Kok, R. M., Bootsma, A. H., Hoffmann, G. H., & Jakobs, C. (1993). Stable-isotope dilution analysis of D- and L-2-hydroxyglutaric acid: application to the detection and prenatal diagnosis of D- and L-2-hydroxyglutaric acidemias. *Pediatric Research, 34*, 277–280.
65. Chalmers, R. A., Lawson, A. M., Watts, R. W., Tavill, A. S., Kamerling, J. P., Hey, E., & Ogilvie, D. (1980). D-2-hydroxyglutaric aciduria: Case report and biochemical studies. *Journal of Inherited Metabolic Disease, 3*, 11–15.
66. Struys, E. A., Verhoeven, N. M., Roos, B., & Jakobs, C. (2003). Disease-related metabolites in culture medium of fibroblasts from patients with D-2-hydroxyglutaric aciduria, L-2-hydroxyglutaric aciduria, and combined D/L-2-hydroxyglutaric aciduria. *Clinical Chemistry, 49*, 1133–1138.
67. Struys, E. A., Verhoeven, N. M., Brunengraber, H., & Jakobs, C. (2004). Investigations by mass isotopomer analysis of the formation of D-2-hydroxyglutarate by cultured lymphoblasts from two patients with D-2-hydroxyglutaric aciduria. *FEBS Letters, 557*, 115–120.
68. Kim, K. R., Lee, J., Ha, D., Jeon, J., Park, H. G., & Kim, J. H. (2000). Enantiomeric separation and discrimination of 2-hydroxy acids as O-trifluoroacetylated (S)-(+)-3-methyl-2-butyl esters by achiral dual-capillary column gas chromatography. *Journal of Chromatography. A, 874*, 91–100.
69. Santagata, S., Eberlin, L. S., Norton, I., Calligaris, D., Feldman, D. R., Ide, J. L., Liu, X., Wiley, J. S., Vestal, M. L., Ramkissoon, S. H., Orringer, D. A., Gill, K. K., Dunn, I. F., Dias-Santagata, D., Ligon, K. L., Jolesz, F. A., Golby, A. J., Cooks, R. G., & Agar, N. Y. (2014). Intraoperative mass spectrometry mapping of an onco-metabolite to guide brain tumor surgery. *Proceedings of the National Academy of Sciences of the United States of America, 111*, 11121–11126.
70. Andronesi, O. C., Rapalino, O., Gerstner, E., Chi, A., Batchelor, T. T., Cahill, D. P., Sorensen, A. G., & Rosen, B. R. (2013). Detection of oncogenic IDH1 mutations using magnetic resonance spectroscopy of 2-hydroxyglutarate. *The Journal of Clinical Investigation, 123*, 3659–3663.
71. Pope, W. B., Prins, R. M., Albert, T. M., Nagarajan, R., Yen, K. E., Bittinger, M. A., Salamon, N., Chou, A. P., Yong, W. H., Soto, H., Wilson, N., Driggers, E., Jang, H. G., Su, S. M., Schenkein, D. P., Lai, A., Cloughesy, T. F., Kornblum, H. I., Wu, H., Fantin, V. R., & Liau, L. M. (2012). Non-invasive detection of 2-hydroxyglutarate and other metabolites in IDH1 mutant glioma patients using magnetic resonance spectroscopy. *Journal of Neuro-Oncology, 107*, 197–205.
72. Andronesi, O. C., Kim, G. S., Gerstner, E., Batchelor, T., Tzika, A. A., Fantin, V. R., Vander Heiden, M. G., & Sorensen, A. G. (2012). Detection of 2-hydroxyglutarate in IDH-mutated glioma patients by in vivo spectral-editing and 2D correlation magnetic resonance spectroscopy. *Science Translational Medicine, 4*, 116ra114.
73. Choi, C., Ganji, S. K., DeBerardinis, R. J., Hatanpaa, K. J., Rakheja, D., Kovacs, Z., Yang, X. L., Mashimo, T., Raisanen, J. M., Marin-Valencia, I., Pascual, J. M., Madden, C. J., Mickey, B. E., Malloy, C. R., Bachoo, R. M., & Maher, E. A. (2012). 2-hydroxyglutarate detection by magnetic resonance spectroscopy in IDH-mutated patients with gliomas. *Nature Medicine, 18*, 624–629.
74. Salamanca-Cardona, L., & Keshari, K. R. (2015). (13) C-labeled biochemical probes for the study of cancer metabolism with dynamic nuclear polarization-enhanced magnetic resonance imaging. *Cancer & Metabolism, 3*, 9.
75. Salamanca-Cardona, L., Shah, H., Poot, A. J., Correa, F. M., Di Gialleonardo, V., Lui, H., Miloushev, V. Z., Granlund, K. L., Tee, S. S., Cross, J. R., Thompson, C. B., & Keshari, K. R. (2017). In vivo imaging of glutamine metabolism to the oncometabolite 2-hydroxyglutarate in IDH1/2 mutant tumors. *Cell Metabolism, 26*(830–841), e833.
76. Beckonert, O., Coen, M., Keun, H. C., Wang, Y., Ebbels, T. M., Holmes, E., Lindon, J. C., & Nicholson, J. K. (2010). High-resolution magic-angle-spinning NMR spectroscopy for metabolic profiling of intact tissues. *Nature Protocols, 5*, 1019–1032.
77. Elkhaled, A., Jalbert, L. E., Phillips, J. J., Yoshihara, H. A. I., Parvataneni, R., Srinivasan, R., Bourne, G., Berger, M. S., Chang, S. M., Cha, S., & Nelson, S. J. (2012). Magnetic resonance of 2-hydroxyglutarate in IDH1-mutated low-grade gliomas. *Science Translational Medicine, 4*, 116ra115.
78. Kalinina, J., Carroll, A., Wang, L., Yu, Q., Mancheno, D. E., Wu, S., Liu, F., Ahn, J., He, M., Mao, H., & Van Meir, E. G. (2012). Detection of "oncometabo-

lite" 2-hydroxyglutarate by magnetic resonance analysis as a biomarker of IDH1/2 mutations in glioma. *Journal of Molecular Medicine (Berlin, Germany), 90*, 1161–1171.

79. Balss, J., Pusch, S., Beck, A. C., Herold-Mende, C., Kramer, A., Thiede, C., Buckel, W., Langhans, C. D., Okun, J. G., & von Deimling, A. (2012). Enzymatic assay for quantitative analysis of (D)-2-hydroxyglutarate. *Acta Neuropathologica, 124*, 883–891.

80. Pusch, S., Schweizer, L., Beck, A. C., Lehmler, J. M., Weissert, S., Balss, J., Miller, A. K., & von Deimling, A. (2014). D-2-Hydroxyglutarate producing neo-enzymatic activity inversely correlates with frequency of the type of isocitrate dehydrogenase 1 mutations found in glioma. *Acta Neuropathologica Communications, 2*, 19.

81. Su, R., Dong, L., Li, C., Nachtergaele, S., Wunderlich, M., Qing, Y., Deng, X., Wang, Y., Weng, X., Hu, C., Yu, M., Skibbe, J., Dai, Q., Zou, D., Wu, T., Yu, K., Weng, H., Huang, H., Ferchen, K., Qin, X., Zhang, B., Qi, J., Sasaki, A. T., Plas, D. R., Bradner, J. E., Wei, M., Marcucci, G., Jiang, X., Mulloy, J. C., Jin, J., He, C., & Chen, J. (2018). R-2HG exhibits anti-tumor activity by targeting FTO/m(6)A/MYC/CEBPA signaling. *Cell, 172*, 90–105 e123.

Methods of Lipidomic Analysis: Extraction, Derivatization, Separation, and Identification of Lipids

Ya Xie, Zongyuan Wu, Zuojian Qin, Bangfu Wu, Xin Lv, Fang Wei, and Hong Chen

1 Sample Collection and Extraction

1.1 Sample Collection

The first step in lipidomics studies involves the collection of analytical samples from plants, animals, or microbes. These samples can be solid in nature (e.g., tissues [1], cells [2], solid fecal material [3], seeds [4], leaves [5], or root hairs [6]) or comprise highly complex fluids (e.g., plasma [7, 8], serum [9], urine [10], synovial fluid [11], milk [12], or oils [13]). A typical procedure begins when samples are frozen quickly in liquid nitrogen before they are stored at very low temperatures (e.g., −80 °C). This initial step helps to inhibit enzymatic activity and reduce the rate of oxidation, peroxidation, and hydrolytic degradation of lipids containing unsaturated bonds [14]. To ensure that the profile of the extracted lipids is a good representative of the entire sample, the next step of the protocol involves sample homogenization, and then appropriate extraction buffers are used to extract lipids from the homogenate. In contrast, with the focus solely on optimizing the extraction efficiencies of lipid classes of interest using different solvent systems, the sample preparation protocol for fluids tends to be more straightforward. Following lipid extraction, the stability of lipid species in the extraction solvent is also an important consideration, particularly if the samples are subjected to multiple freeze-thaw cycles. As described above, lipid molecules containing unsaturated double bonds may be subjected to oxidation and are also susceptible to hydrolysis in the presence of water. To minimize the breakdown of unsaturated bonds on these molecules, aliquots of lipid extracts into smaller volumes can be considered, which will reduce the number of freeze-thaw cycles.

1.2 Sample Extraction

In general, the application of lipidomics requires sample extraction methods that are highly efficient, reproducible, and able to cover a wide range of analytes with different polarities. The extraction protocol also needs to take into account that a limited amount of sample may be available for lipidomic analysis. With the goal of improving overall lipid coverage, liquid–liquid extraction (LLE), solid-phase extraction (SPE), solid-phase microextraction (SPME), and other emerging techniques have been applied to lipid extraction.

Y. Xie · Z. Wu · Z. Qin · B. Wu · X. Lv · F. Wei
H. Chen (✉)
Oil Crops Research Institute of the Chinese Academy of Agricultural Sciences, Key Laboratory of Biology and Genetic Improvement of Oil Crops, Ministry of Agriculture, Wuhan, People's Republic of China

Hubei Key Laboratory of Lipid Chemistry and Nutrition, Wuhan, China
e-mail: Chenhong@oilcrops.cn

S. Hu (ed.), *Cancer Metabolomics*, Advances in Experimental Medicine and Biology 1280,
https://doi.org/10.1007/978-3-030-51652-9_12

1.2.1 Liquid–Liquid Extraction (LLE)

LLE is the most predominant extraction technique for lipids. In order to achieve exhaustive and comprehensive extraction of key lipid classes, LLE involves the use of two immiscible organic solvents – most commonly a mixture of chloroform and methanol with water, introduced more than 70 years ago by Folch et al. [15] (chloroform/methanol/water ratio 8:4:3 v/v/v) and subsequently modified by Bligh and Dyer [16] (chloroform/methanol/water ratio 1:2:0.8 v/v/v). Most lipidomics studies still rely on these general extraction procedures, often in modified versions. Due to its lower toxicity, dichloromethane has been used as a substitute for chloroform [17].

The high chance of contamination of the samples is a pitfall of two-phase extraction method, because of the need of retrieving lipids from the lower chloroform-rich layer. In 2008, Matyash et al. [18] demonstrated a new sample extraction procedure employing methyl tert-butyl ether (MTBE). The method involves addition of MeOH and MTBE (1.5:5, v/v) to the sample and phase separation is induced by adding water. Compared to conventional two-phase chloroform-containing solvent systems, this extraction method utilizes the low density of the lipid-containing organic phase to form the upper layer during phase separation. This greatly simplified sample collection and minimized dripping losses. Furthermore, compared to chloroform, MTBE is nontoxic and noncarcinogenic, which reduces potential health risks for exposed personnel. While the method has the advantage over conventional chloroform-containing solvents, unsatisfactory recovery for more polar lipid classes has been observed [19].

One-phase lipid extraction has recently been demonstrated, which is an "all-in-one-tube" approach eliminating the need for phase separation. This is achieved by using solvents such as butanol/methanol (3:1, v/v) [20] or MMC solvent mixture (MeOH/MTBE/$CHCl_3$, 1.33:1:1, v/v/v) [21] to denature proteins that are later removed by centrifugation. With an untargeted lipidomics approach, Andres et al. [21] explored the differences/similarities between the most commonly used two-phase extraction methods (Folch, Bligh and Dyer, and MTBE) and one-phase extraction method based on the MMC solvent mixture. The four extraction methods were evaluated and thoroughly compared against a pooled extract that qualitatively and quantitatively represents the average of the combined extracts. The results showed that the lipid profile obtained with the MMC system displayed the highest similarity to the pooled extract, indicating that it was most representative of the lipidome in the original sample. Furthermore, it had better extraction efficiencies for moderate and highly polar lipid species in comparison with the Folch, Bligh and Dyer, and MTBE extraction systems.

1.2.2 Solid-Phase Extraction (SPE)

While LLE represents a somewhat universal extraction method in lipidomic analysis, SPE could well enrich lipids of extremely low endogenous abundance via minimizing background matrix and ensure satisfactory detection upon mass spectrometric (MS) analysis. SPE is a well-established sample preparation method, which utilizes a solid (stationary) phase and a liquid (mobile) phase to capture selectively specific classes of molecules with similar properties [22]. Selective retention of specific molecules of interest on the solid phase can be achieved through the differential interaction of analytes between the two phases.

The most commonly used SPE-column chemistries for lipid extraction include normal-phase silica, reversed-phase (C8 and C18), and ion-exchange columns (packed with aminopropyl) [23]. Silica and aminopropyl columns are often used for separation and sub-fractionation of neutral and polar lipids, which can be achieved by changing the eluent solvents [24, 25], while C8 and C18 columns have been used to isolate PC, cerebrosides, gangliosides, and fatty acids from polar compounds in water based samples [26]. HybridSPE phospholipid (HybridSPE-PL, zirconia-coated silica stationary phase) has been successfully used to remove PL interferences of biological samples based on the Lewis acid-base interaction between zirconia and the phosphate moiety of PLs. Therefore, HybridSPE-PL is also an ideal choice for the isolation and enrichment of all kinds of PLs from complex biological samples. HybridSPE-PL instead of LLE was used to rapidly enrich and recover PL molecular species from human plasma by Wei et al [8].

1.2.3 Solid-Phase Microextraction (SPME)

SPME has also been introduced as a rapid equilibrium-based sample preparation technique, for which a small amount of extraction phase is coated, typically on a solid support, and then used to remove a small portion of analyte from the sample. This technique is commonly used in conjunction with gas chromatography (GC) or GC-MS analysis, as the headspace available in a SPME cartridge enables the enrichment of volatile analytes typically monitored by GC.

SPME has been used successfully together with GC-MS for the extraction of fatty acids and fatty acid esters from solid samples, such as lung tissue [27] and hair [28], and biofluids, such as sputum [29]. This approach can be useful when the sample amount is very limited (e.g., synovial fluid or cyst fluid) or when targeted compounds of interest are expressed at low concentrations. Due to the small sample sizes and extraction volumes required for SPME, sample cleanup tends to be highly efficient, resulting in fewer matrix effects, such as ion suppression or enhancement, in subsequent MS-based analysis [30].

1.2.4 Emerging Techniques for Lipid Extraction

In addition to these established lipid extraction techniques, there are alternative methods, which may have shorter extraction time and lower solvent requirements. These techniques include supercritical fluid extraction (SFE) and ultrasound-assisted extraction (UAE), which are more commonly used for the extraction of metabolites from biological samples such as plant and food materials.

The principle of SFE is based on an increase in solvation power of a supercritical fluid when its pressure and temperature are raised above critical values. This increase in solvation power, coupled with the relatively low viscosity and high diffusivity of such fluids, allows to extract and separate effectively different compound classes (including oils, fats, and vitamins) in a sample [31]. SFE has been used for lipid extraction in plant, animal tissues [32], and, more interestingly, dried human-plasma spot samples [33]. Uchikata et al. [33] compared the extraction of PLs by SFE with a traditional LLE method (Bligh and Dyer) and concluded that SFE was more effective, as it resulted in higher levels of selected PL species, including PC, lysoPC, PE, and SM.

UAE) is an efficient and reproducible extraction technique. It helps improve the yield and quality of the lipid extract and does not raise the temperature of the system. This makes it attractive to extraction of heat-unstable lipids. In addition, UAE can be combined with conventional LLE methods to improve the extraction efficiency of lipid species present in biological samples. For example, Liu et al. successfully developed a combined UAE and LLE protocol for human serum samples, which led to a 5–60% increase in the levels of fatty acids compared to the conventional LLE method [34]. A similar approach was adopted by Pizarro et al. [35] for human blood plasma samples, of which the use of MTBE with UAE resulted in the detection of 30% more lipid species when compared to a conventional MTBE-based LLE method. The MTBE-UAE technique also showed high reproducibility, with relative standard deviation values of less than 6% and lipid-component recoveries of more than 70%.

2 Derivatization

2.1 Advantages of Derivatization

Many trace level compounds in complex matrices which have essential biological functions cannot be well detected by MS-based methods, especially if they are difficult to ionize or to fragment. Derivatization is a specific chemical reaction, which aims to modify the structure of the target compounds and, as a consequence, the chemical and physical properties. The advantages of combining derivatization with MS analysis include: (1) improvement of selectivity and sensitivity [36, 37], (2) enhancement of ionization efficiency [8], (3) improvement of structural elucidation [38], (4) increase accuracy for quantification [1], and (5) facilitation of isomer separation [39].

2.2 Lipid Analysis After Derivatization

Certain lipids, including fatty acyls, glyceride (GLs), glycerophospholipids (GPs), sphingolipids (SPs), sulfatides (STs), phenolic lipids, saccharolipids, and polyketides, contain functional groups, such as carbonyl, hydroxyl (alcohol or phenol), and amine group, and they are suitable for introducing a fragmentable moiety by chemical derivatization. There are challenges when performing derivatization reaction, including formation of by-products, nonquantitative reaction, requirement for harsh reaction conditions, long reaction time, and product degradation. To achieve an effective derivatization-based MS analysis, the derivatization reaction should be fast, efficient, and specific and form relatively stable products.

Fatty acids (FAs), a basic element of all lipids, contain at least one carboxyl group and a long aliphatic chain. Yang et al. developed a LC-MS method for the identification and quantification of FAs through derivatization with 2-bromo-1-methylpyridinium iodide and 3-carbinol-1-methylpyridinium iodide, forming 3-acyloxymethyl-1-methylpyridinium iodide (AMMP) [40]. This derivatization reaction attached a quaternary amine to analytes and enabled electrospray ionization (ESI)-MS analysis with the positive ionization mode. Detection sensitivity was generally 2500-fold higher than in the negative mode of ionization used for underivatized FAs. The main derivatives for FAs and modified FAs are quaternary amine derivatives [41, 42], tertiary amine derivatives [43], piperazine-pyrimidine derivatives [44], benzofuran derivatives [45], and other derivatives [46] for enhancing the assay sensitivity or accuracy of quantification. Kloos D et al. [47] reviewed the most recent trends in analysis of FAs by chromatography and MS employing derivatization techniques. Derivatization has also been applied to analysis of PLs [1, 8], glyceride [48, 49], and steroids [50, 51]. In addition, there are a number of derivatization strategies for determining the location of double bonds in lipids, such as derivatization of C=C bond with acetone [52], N-(4-aminomethylphenyl)-pyridinium [53], ozonolysis [54], ozone-induced dissociation, or olefin cross-metathesis [53].

3 Chromatographic Methods

3.1 Thin-Layer Chromatography (TLC)

TLC is not commonly applied for lipidomic analysis but shows great potential for the separation of lipids by class. The separated analyte species can be acquired from the spots on the TLC plate and extracted with chloroform and methanol. The lipids can then be analyzed by matrix-assisted laser desorption/ionization (MALDI)-MS, ESI-MS, or GC-MS. TLC-MALDI-MS has been demonstrated for analysis of PLs in bronchoalveolar lavage (BAL) fluids, and the study showed a prospective for direct MALDI-MS measurements on the TLC plates in the mass spectrometer [55].

3.2 GC Separation of Lipids

Because of their nonvolatile property, the use of GC for direct analysis of global lipids is impossible. Most early methods relied on hydrolysis of PLs by phospholipase C to diacylglycerols, which is followed by methyl transesterification, producing fatty acid methyl esters that are subsequently analyzed by GC [56].

The first application of GC for FAs can be traced back to the 1950s [57]. There are two methods available to quantify FAs. The first method is through simple peak integration. It may provide uncertain results if peaks are not fully recognized, which is often the case for molecules with similar structures, such as PLs that may only distinguish by a single double bond [58]. The second method is to use a flame ionization detector (FID), which combusts the sample into fragments that are ionized by an electrode. The charged ions will flow to the electrode in the detector, yielding a current. FID is a very sensitive detector; however the disadvantage of using FID is that it destroys the sample [59].

3.3 LC Separation of Lipids

LC separates different classes of analytes according to their physicochemical properties. Reversed-phase LC (RPLC), normal-phase LC (NPLC), and hydrophilic interaction LC (HILIC) are commonly used for lipidomic analysis. The mechanism of action by RPLC for lipids lies in the basic of lipophilicity, which is regulated by the carbon chain length and the number of double bonds. Thus, lipid species containing longer acyl chains are eluted from the column later than shorter chain lipids, and saturated acyl structures are eluted later than polyunsaturated analogs. However, NPLC and HILIC typically separated lipid species based on their hydrophilicity. Therefore, lipids are separated according to their representative polar head group classes [60]. Other LC methods used for lipid separation include nonaqueous RPLC [61], silver-ion RPLC [62], chiral LC [63], and supercritical fluid chromatography (SFC) [64].

3.3.1 RPLC

RPLC utilizes a mobile phase that is more polar than the stationary phase, which permits complex lipidomes to be separated prior to MS analysis. The lipids are separated based on lipophilicity owing to the combined chain length and number of double bonds present in the fatty acid side chains [65].

Due to the hydrophobic property of lipids, the most common separation method for LC-MS-based lipidomics is RPLC with a C18 column. Lipids are adsorbed to the stationary phase and eluted based on the relative affinity, and the gradient allows for controlled elution of lipids over a wide range of polarities [66]. The mobile phase composition can be changed throughout the separation process, increasing the hydrophobicity of mobile phase and hence increasing the elution effect. By contrast, greater separation of lipid classes can be achieved if the mobile phase composition is held constant [67]. However, this amelioration in separation is only available for a narrow range of polarities and can result in long retention times.

3.3.2 NPLC and HILIC

Compared to RPLC, NPLC and HILIC utilize polar stationary phases, therefore more strongly retaining polar analytes. Retention of lipid classes on a RP column is influenced by acyl and alkyl chain length and desaturation; however, the retention on HILIC columns largely relies on the polarity of the lipid head groups [68, 69]. This allows efficient separation of lipid classes, which is not observed with RPLC.

In fact, HILIC and RPLC are highly orthogonal, leading to different elution profiling [70]. As neither method is capable of fully analyzing all lipid compounds in complex matrix, it is possible to couple the two modes of separation using two-dimensional LC (2D-LC). In this configuration, the co-eluting lipid species from the first-dimensional RPLC are loaded onto the second-dimensional HILIC for further separation [71]. However, challenges exist in the development of 2D-LC systems. First, the mobile phase composition for HILIC has a high elution strength in RP. Second, it is difficult to have the second dimension keep up with the sampling frequency of the first dimension. To overcome some of these challenges, trapping columns have been placed between the first and second dimensions to retain analytes while the second dimension is resolved. Alternatively, widely different column sizes and flow rates may be used between the first and second dimensions, generally requiring mobile phase splitters to reduce flow rate into the ion source [71].

3.3.3 SFC

Recently, SFC has emerged as a viable alternative to LC for lipidomic analysis [72]. The most common supercritical fluid used in SFC is CO_2 as it is cheap and easy to achieve and has a low polarity, similar to hexane. The requirement to use mobile phase modifiers, such as methanol, to adjust polarity is important [73]. SFC has been demonstrated for fast separations of lipid classes [74]. Supercritical fluid has higher diffusivity and lower viscosity than a common liquid, thereby facilitating higher-throughput analysis as compared with LC [75]. In addition, supercritical CO_2 used as a mobile phase has almost the same polarity as hexane, and its polarity can be adjusted by adding a modifier such as methanol. These advantages make SFC eminently suitable for simultaneous analysis of lipids with a wide range of polarities. Studies have reported a higher detection sensitivity for carotenoids in SFC than LC, and structural isomers were successfully separated using SFC but not resolved by LC [64, 76].

4 MS Analysis of Lipids

4.1 Ionization Methods

The ionization mode used in MS detection plays an important role in lipidomic analysis. One ionization method may not work for all types of lipid classes, since some lipids are better ionized with one ionization mode while other lipids are ionized more evidently with another mode [77, 78]. Ionization efficiency can be enhanced by the additives present in the mobile phase leading to the formation of different type of adducts. ESI in positive mode (ESI+) is the most common mode in LC-MS because it can effectively ionize a wide range of lipids, while negative ionization mode (ESI−) provides superior results for certain lipid classes, such as PI, PS, and PA [79]. Atmospheric pressure chemical ionization (APCI) has been applied to lipidomic analysis and is preferred for more nonpolar lipids (e.g., triacylglycerols).

When using RPLC for lipid separation, 53% of the studies were performed with both ESI+ and ESI− modes and 38% with ESI+ mode only, while 45% of NPLC/HILIC studies were performed with both ionization modes and 41% with ESI− only [80]. The reason for these differences lies in that NPLC/HILIC methods are often used for analysis of PLs, in which ESI− allows effective ionization of these lipids, while RPLC well separates the lipids that can be effectively ionized with ESI (+), such as cholesteryl esters.

4.2 MS Detection

After lipid compounds are ionized and enter a mass spectrometer, the ions are then measured with a mass analyzer. Depending on the type of mass spectrometer, ions can be filtered by m/z using a quadrupole, accelerated along a flight path to measure their m/z, or orbited around an electrode to measure m/z ratios [81]. Quadrupole mass analyzers often act as mass filters by only allowing ions within a small m/z window to pass through and by contrast, time-of-flight, Orbitrap, and cyclotron-based mass analyzers acquire a mass spectrum in a single scan [82, 83]. Time-of-flight mass analyzers measure the time of flight of an ion in the flight tube, which is then converted to the m/z. Orbitrap, same as cyclotron mass analyzers, traps ions in an orbital motion. The image current from the trapped ions is detected and converted to a mass spectrum using the Fourier transform of the frequency signal [84]. These mass analyzers differ significantly in terms of mass resolution [81]. Compared to quadrupole and time-of-flight mass analyzers, Orbitrap and cyclotron mass analyzers in general have higher resolution and therefore superior resolving power [85]. However, due to the narrow peak widths generated with UHPLC and the long scan times for high-resolution mass spectra, operating these instruments at the highest mass resolution is only commonly used by direct infusion [86, 87].

In tandem MS (MS/MS) , two or more mass analyzers, e.g., triple quadrupole, quadrupole time-of-flight, and linear ion trap-Orbitrap, are coupled together using an additional reaction step to increase their abilities to analyze and identify biomolecules. In these configurations, quadrupoles can form mass filters or collision cells, whereby ions undergo collision-induced dissociation with an inert gas, causing fragmentation of the molecules [80]. Fragmentation can also be accomplished within an ion trap which can supply complementary fragment ions to quadrupole-based fragmentation [88]. Ions entering the mass spectrometer from the ion source are referred to as precursor ions, while ions produced following fragmentation are referred to as product ions and fragmentation products can provide structural information about the precursor ions.

5 Quality Control

During large-scale lipidomics studies, drifts in LC peak shape and retention time may happen due to sample residue or column aging, and signal intensity attenuation may occur in direct infusion MS due to the contamination of ion source components of the mass analyzer. It appears difficult to maintain repeatability and stability during large dataset acquisition over the time. A potential solution is to utilize a standard quality control sample (QC sample) for real-time monitoring the stability of the MS system [89]. This is due to the following reasons: First, the analytical platform needs to be tested with QC sample to ensure that data are reproducible before vital samples are analyzed. Observed peak drift or signal attenuation prior to analyzing vital samples is not acceptable [90]. Second, QC samples analysis can be used as a quality assurance (QA) tool [91]. Third, data produced from QC samples can be used to correct signals between analytical runs and mine in-depth information within the data from different analytical batches [92]. Finally, standards are required for normalization if using community QC samples [93].

The matrix composition of QC samples should be theoretically similar to that of experimental samples. Four types of QC samples are commonly used: (i) internal standards (ISs) were often employed to evaluate the stability of the instrument in the past. However, the limited number of available ISs was not enough to estimate all the lipid features [94]; (ii) batch QC was formed from the small aliquots of each sample to be studied in a batch; (iii) pooled QC was prepared independent by pooling the related samples from laboratory's bank [95]; this type of QC, together with batch QC, is easily prepared and can monitor each lipid features to minimize the variations of intra- and inter-batch. Luo [94] compared the differences between the two QC samples; no significant differences were observed. However, pooled QC samples are more suitable to monitor the data of long-term lipidomics study to increase their comparability; (iv) Standard Reference Material (SRM) may be available as a QC sample in lipidomics studies. For instance, the "SRM 1950 Metabolites in Frozen Human Plasma" is intended primarily for validation of methods for determining metabolites such as fatty acids, hormones, and amino acids in human plasma and similar materials [96]. It may be used for data comparisons among different laboratories.

Regarding how to use QC samples in the analytical runs during lipidomic profiling analysis, the following setup may be considered: (i) before analysis of actual sequence of samples, five and ten QC samples are recommended to be run in order to equilibrate the shotgun-MS and LC-MS system, respectively [97]; (ii) the injection frequency of QC samples has been assessed in relation to the accuracy and robustness during signal correction process, 3–25 injections of samples between each QC injection were reported [98, 99]. Kamleh [95] evaluated the effect of the injection frequency of QC samples, and the signal drift correction procedure always represented better for the most frequency of injections. Considering the balance between the analysis time and the quality of the data acquisition, at least one QC sample should be injected for every ten sample injections; (iii) the NIST SRM 1950 should be injected during the analytical sequence if there is a need to compare the experimental data between laboratories [100]; (iv) in order to monitor possible sample contamination (e.g., contamination caused by extraction) and check the quality of mobile phases, every series of sample analysis are supposed to contain blank samples [95]; (v) randomizing the sample sequence is vital to ensure that there is no correlation among extraneous factors (e.g., preparation or analysis order) and no bias from the analyst [96, 101].

6 Data Processing and Analysis

6.1 Spectral Data Processing

Spectral data processing for MS-based lipidomic analysis may include spectral filtering, peak detection, alignment, and baseline correction. For peak picking from the features of the chromatographic data, a variety of algorithms [102–104] have been proposed. A widely recognized method is to cut the LC/MS data into slices a fraction of a mass unit (0.1 m/z) wide and then operate on those individual slices in the chromatographic time domain. The peak detection algorithm thus handles low-resolution, high-resolution, and centroided data in a flexible and robust manner.

According to Brown and colleagues [77], most of the methods [105–107] commonly used for retention time alignment are based, in some manner, on the correlation between spectra. Since the retention times in lipidomic analysis are well constrained within individual classes by the observed retention times of internal standards, species of interest are bracketed by the standards in time. This information is often used to effectively time-shift spectra within the time-m/z domain of each class without complex spectral computations. The required alignment shifts can then be chosen to maximize the correlation of time-lag-shifted spectrum against one arbitrarily chosen sample from that session of MS analysis.

The correction of the background contribution to the peak intensities of a mass spectrum is important for peak detection and accurate quantification of each analyte, particularly when the species is at low abundance. Accurate baseline correction could reduce the complications faced by uncertainty about the intercept of the standard calibration curve in LC-MS analysis and thus remove reliance on any latent subtraction of noise through the intercept term. Most of identification and noise reduction are typically based on filtering or smoothing functions of LC-MS data analysis tools. However, applying such kind of filtering tools, which implies a model of the noise and/or the peak shapes present in the original data, may lead to distortion of peak identification. According to the study by Smith et al. [105], group methods from LC/MS data, background subtraction may add more noise than it eliminates. Instead, the problem can be reduced to simply finding the appropriate retention time window boundaries for a given m/z.

6.2 Annotation of Lipid Species

Two metabolomic databases, Metlin [108] and HMDB (human metabolome database) [109], are commonly used for database search to identify metabolites including lipids. High-resolution LC-MS, combined with database searching, has been used for lipidomic profiling of human and animal model samples [110]. Derivatization and stable isotope labeling are usually used for the analysis of fatty acids of lipid species in LC-MS-based lipidomic analysis [111]. For instance, fatty acids can be derivatized with 2-bromo-1-methylpyridinium iodide and 3-carbinol-1-methylpyridinium iodide, forming 3-acyloxymethyl-1-methylpyridinium iodide (AMMP). AMMP derivatives have unique tandem mass spectra characterized by common ions at m/z 107.0, 124.0, and 178.0, and individual fatty acids also display unique fingerprint regions that allowed the identification of their carbon skeleton number, number of double bonds, and double bond position.

6.3 Bioinformatics Tools for Lipidomic Data Processing

To simplify the work of processing complex LC-MS data, software tools have been developed to perform multiple data processing steps, including spectral filtering, peak detection, alignment, normalization, and exploratory data analysis and visualization. Here we briefly discuss several software tools that are commonly used in lipidomic analysis. MZmine mainly focuses on LC-MS data analysis [106]. The functionality includes the identification of peaks using online databases, MS^n data support, improved isotope pattern support, scatter plot visualization, and a new method for peak list alignment based on the random sample consensus algorithm. The current version of MZmine 2 is suitable for processing large batches of data and has been applied to both targeted and nontargeted lipidomic analyses. OpenMS 2.0 is an updated version of cross-platform software [112], which provides a set of 185 tools and ready-made workflows for common MS data processing tasks. It also provides implementations to address the most common tasks in quantitative proteomics and metabolomics, including quantification, identification, and visualization, as well as algorithms for isotopic deconvolution, chromatographic peak picking, and so on. The only challenge is to build your custom workflows which can be time-consuming. XCMS2 allows to automatically search MS/MS data against high-quality experimental MS/MS data from known metabolites contained in a reference library [113]. It features the same functions such as peak picking, peak alignment, and statistical analysis of features but with the added capability of automatic searching of MS/MS spectra against the METLIN database. MS-DIAL is a data processing pipeline for untargeted lipidomics applicable to either data-independent or data-dependent fragmentation methods [114]. Identification is achieved through analyses of retention time, mass accuracy, and isotope ratio along with MS/MS similarity matching to libraries from publicly available databases. Other software tools for shotgun lipidomics data analysis include LipidXplorer [115], LipidProfiler [116], AMDMS-SL [117], and so on. These software packages are very useful for identifying and quantifying individual lipid species from the data obtained with MS-based lipidomic analysis.

6.4 Biostatistical Analysis and Data Visualization

After qualitative and quantitative results are obtained from analysis of lipidomic data, the next step is to perform statistical analysis of the data to determine significant lipid species and reveal the biological interpretation. In a simplest setting, the descriptive data analysis can be carried out with statistical methods such as two-sample Student's t-test, Wilcoxon test, Wilcoxon signed-rank test, and Mann-Whitney U test. Analysis variance (ANOVA) may be used to compare the means of two or more groups assuming that sampled population are normally distributed. Correlational analysis can be performed to determine the degree of relationship between two variables, which is measured using a correlation coefficient. Statistical methods are also in place for analysis of multivariate data. Principal component analysis (PCA) is a useful statistical technique for multivariate analysis of correlated variables. It is mostly used as a tool in exploratory data analysis and for making predictive models. Hierarchical clustering analysis (HCA) is widely used for multivariate data analysis, displaying cluster analysis results with heat maps. Partial least square-based discriminant analysis (PLS-DA) is a widely used, supervised classification algorithm when dimensionality reduction is needed, and discrimination is sought in multivariate analysis. Multivariate analysis of variance (MANOVA) is a statistical test procedure for comparing multivariate (population) means of several groups, which uses the variance/covariance between variables in testing the statistical significance of the mean differences. Many of the abovementioned tools are available from commercial software (e.g., SAS, NCSS, IBM SPSS, SIMCA-P). Graphic display is often used for data visualization and presentation in lipidomic analysis. Many software tools such as MetaboAnalyst 2.0, Prism, Origin, and R package can be useful for graphic display of lipidomic data.

References

1. Wang, X., Wei, F., Xu, J. Q., Lv, X., Dong, X. Y., Han, X., et al. (2016). Profiling and relative quantification of phosphatidylethanolamine based on acetone stable isotope derivatization. *Analytica Chimica Acta, 902*, 142–153. https://doi.org/10.1016/j.aca.2015.11.003.
2. Ivanisevic, J., Zhu, Z. J., Plate, L., Tautenhahn, R., Chen, S., O'Brien, P. J., et al. (2013). Toward 'omic scale metabolite profiling: A dual separation – Mass spectrometry approach for coverage of lipids and central carbon metabolism. *Analytical Chemistry, 85*(14), 6876–6884.

3. Camera, E., Ludovici, M., Galante, M., Sinagra, J. L., & Picardo, M. (2010). Comprehensive analysis of the major lipid classes in sebum by rapid resolution high-performance liquid chromatography and electrospray mass spectrometry. *Journal of Lipid Research, 51*(11), 3377.
4. Li, M., Baughman, E., Roth, M. R., Han, X., Welti, R., & Wang, X. (2014). Quantitative profiling and pattern analysis of triacylglycerol species in Arabidopsis seeds by electrospray ionization mass spectrometry. *The Plant Journal, 77*(1), 160–172. https://doi.org/10.1111/tpj.12365.
5. Vu, H. S., Shiva, S., Roth, M. R., Tamura, P., Zheng, L., Li, M., et al. (2014). Lipid changes after leaf wounding in Arabidopsis thaliana: Expanded lipidomic data form the basis for lipid co-occurrence analysis. *The Plant Journal, 80*(4), 728–743. https://doi.org/10.1111/tpj.12659.
6. Wei, F., Fanella, B., Guo, L., & Wang, X. (2016). Membrane glycerolipidome of soybean root hairs and its response to nitrogen and phosphate availability. *Scientific Reports, 6*, 36172. https://doi.org/10.1038/srep36172.
7. Jong Min, C., Tae-Eun, K., Joo-Youn, C., Hwa Jeong, L., & Byung, H. J. (2014). Development of lipidomic platform and phosphatidylcholine retention time index for lipid profiling of rosuvastatin treated human plasma. *Journal of Chromatography B, 944*, 157–165.
8. Wei, F., Wang, X., Ma, H. F., Lv, X., Dong, X. Y., & Chen, H. (2018). Rapid profiling and quantification of phospholipid molecular species in human plasma based on chemical derivatization coupled with electrospray ionization tandem mass spectrometry. *Analytica Chimica Acta, 1024*, 101.
9. Cui, L., Lee, Y. H., Kumar, Y., Xu, F., Lu, K., Ooi, E. E., et al. (2013). Serum metabolome and lipidome changes in adult patients with primary dengue infection. *PLoS Neglected Tropical Diseases, 7*(8), e2373.
10. Min, H. K., Lim, S., Chung, B. C., & Moon, M. H. (2011). Shotgun lipidomics for candidate biomarkers of urinary phospholipids in prostate cancer. *Analytical and Bioanalytical Chemistry, 399*(2), 823–830.
11. Giera, M., Ioan-Facsinay, A., Toes, R., Gao, F., Dalli, J., Deelder, A. M., et al. (2012). Lipid and lipid mediator profiling of human synovial fluid in rheumatoid arthritis patients by means of LC-MS/MS. *BBA – Molecular and Cell Biology of Lipids, 1821*(11), 1415–1424.
12. Dugo, P., Fawzy, N., Cichello, F., Cacciola, F., Donato, P., & Mondello, L. (2013). Stop-flow comprehensive two-dimensional liquid chromatography combined with mass spectrometric detection for phospholipid analysis. *Journal of Chromatography A, 1278*(4), 46–53.
13. Wei, F., Hu, N., Lv, X., Dong, X. Y., & Chen, H. (2015). Quantitation of triacylglycerols in edible oils by off-line comprehensive two-dimensional liquid chromatography–atmospheric pressure chemical ionization mass spectrometry using a single column. *Journal of Chromatography A, 1404*, 60–71.
14. Christie, W. W. (2012). Preparation of lipid extracts from tissues. *Advances in Lipid Methodology*.
15. Folch, J. L. M., & Sloane Stanley, G. H. (1957). A simple method for the isolation and purification of total lipides from animal tissues. *The Journal of Biological Chemistry, 226*(1), 497–509. Epub 509.
16. Bligh, E. L. G., & Dyer, W. J. A. (1959). A rapid method of total lipid extraction and purification. *Canadian Journal of Biochemistry and Physiology, 37*(8), 911–917.
17. Carlson, L. A. (1985). Extraction of lipids from human whole serum and lipoproteins and from rat liver tissue with methylene chloride-methanol: A comparison with extraction with chloroform-methanol. *Clinica Chimica Acta, 149*(1), 89–93.
18. Matyash, V., Liebisch, G., Kurzchalia, T. V., Shevchenko, A., & Schwudke, D. (2008). Lipid extraction by methyl-tert-butyl ether for high-throughput lipidomics. *Journal of Lipid Research, 49*(5), 1137–1146.
19. Löfgren, L., Ståhlman, M., Forsberg, G. B., Saarinen, S., Nilsson, R., & Hansson, G. I. (2012). The BUME method: A novel automated chloroform-free 96-well total lipid extraction method for blood plasma. *Journal of Lipid Research, 53*(8), 1690–1700.
20. Löfgren, L., Forsberg, G. B., & Ståhlman, M. (2016). The BUME method: A new rapid and simple chloroform-free method for total lipid extraction of animal tissue. *Scientific Reports, 6*, 27688.
21. Gil, A., Zhang, W., Wolters, J. C., Permentier, H., Boer, T., Horvatovich, P., et al. (2018). One- vs two-phase extraction: Re-evaluation of sample preparation procedures for untargeted lipidomics in plasma samples. *Analytical and Bioanalytical Chemistry, 410*(23), 5859–5870. https://doi.org/10.1007/s00216-018-1200-x.
22. Callesen, A. K., Madsen, J. S., Vach, W., Kruse, T. A., Mogensen, O., & Jensen, O. N. (2010). Serum protein profiling by solid phase extraction and mass spectrometry: A future diagnostics tool? *Proteomics, 9*(6), 1428–1441.
23. Panagiotopoulou, P. M., & Tsimidou, M. (2002). Solid phase extraction: Applications to the chromatographic analysis of vegetable oils and fats. *Grasas y Aceites, 53*(1), 84–95.
24. Kim, H. Y., & Salem, N., Jr. (1990). Separation of lipid classes by solid phase extraction. *Journal of Lipid Research, 31*(12), 2285–2289.
25. Hamilton, J. G., & Comai, K. (1988). Rapid separation of neutral lipids, free fatty acids and polar lipids using prepacked silica Sep-Pak columns. *Lipids, 23*(12), 1146–1149.
26. Bodennec, J., & Portoukalian, J. (2005). Lipid classes: Purification by solid-phase extraction. *Encylopedia of Chromatography, 2*, 970–972.
27. Cha, D., Liu, M., Zeng, Z., Cheng, D. E., & Zhan, G. (2006). Analysis of fatty acids in lung tissues using gas chromatography–mass spectrometry preceded

by derivatization-solid-phase microextraction with a novel fiber. *Analytica Chimica Acta, 572*(1), 47–54.
28. Pragst, F., Rothe, M., Moench, B., Hastedt, M., Herre, S., & Simmert, D. (2010). Combined use of fatty acid ethyl esters and ethyl glucuronide in hair for diagnosis of alcohol abuse: Interpretation and advantages. *Forensic Science International, 196*(1), 101–110.
29. Cha, D., Cheng, D. E., Liu, M., Zeng, Z., Hu, X., & Guan, W. (2009). Analysis of fatty acids in sputum from patients with pulmonary tuberculosis using gas chromatography–mass spectrometry preceded by solid-phase microextraction and post-derivatization on the fiber. *Journal of Chromatography A, 1216*(9), 1450–1457.
30. Vuckovic, D., Zhang, X., Cudjoe, E., & Pawliszyn, J. (2010). Solid-phase microextraction in bioanalysis: New devices and directions. *Journal of Chromatography A, 1217*(25), 4041–4060.
31. Izhyk, A., Novik, G., & Dey, E. S. (2012). Extraction of polar lipids from bifidobacteria by supercritical carbon dioxide (scCO2). *Journal of Supercritical Fluids, 62*(2), 149–154.
32. Liu, X., Wang, F., Liu, X., Chen, Y., & Wang, L. (2011). Fatty acid composition and physicochemical properties of ostrich fat extracted by supercritical fluid extraction. *European Journal of Lipid Science and Technology, 113*(6), 775–779.
33. Uchikata, T., Matsubara, A., Fukusaki, E., & Bamba, T. (2012). High-throughput phospholipid profiling system based on supercritical fluid extraction-supercritical fluid chromatography/mass spectrometry for dried plasma spot analysis. *Journal of Chromatography A, 1250*(15), 69–75.
34. Liu, Y., Chen, T., Qiu, Y., Cheng, Y., Cao, Y., Zhao, A., et al. (2011). An ultrasonication-assisted extraction and derivatization protocol for GC/TOFMS-based metabolite profiling. *Analytical and Bioanalytical Chemistry, 400*(5), 1405–1417.
35. Pizarro, C., Arenzanarámila, I., Pérezdelnotario, N., Pérezmatute, P., & Gonzálezsáiz, J. M. (2013). Plasma lipidomic profiling method based on ultrasound extraction and liquid chromatography mass spectrometry. *Analytical Chemistry, 85*(24), 12085–12092.
36. Liu, M., Wei, F., Lv, X., Dong, X. Y., & Chen, H. (2017). Rapid and sensitive detection of free fatty acids in edible oils based on chemical derivatization coupled with electrospray ionization tandem mass spectrometry. *Food Chemistry, 242*, 338.
37. Todoroki, K., Hashimoto, H., Machida, K., Itoyama, M., Hayama, T., Yoshida, H., et al. (2013). Fully automated reagent peak-free liquid chromatography fluorescence analysis of highly polar carboxylic acids using a column-switching system and fluorous scavenging derivatization. *Journal of Separation Science, 36*(2), 232–238.
38. Wang, M., Han, R. H., & Han, X. (2013). Fatty acidomics: Global analysis of lipid species containing a carboxyl group with a charge-remote fragmentation-assisted approach. *Analytical Chemistry, 85*(19), 9312–9320.
39. Wang, M., Palavicini, J. P., Cseresznye, A., & Han, X. (2017). Strategy for quantitative analysis of isomeric bis(monoacylglycero)phosphate and phosphatidylglycerol species by shotgun lipidomics after one-step methylation. *Analytical Chemistry, 89*(16), 8490–8495. https://doi.org/10.1021/acs.analchem.7b02058.
40. Yang, W. C., Jiri Adamec, A., & Regnier, F. E. (2007). Enhancement of the LC/MS analysis of fatty acids through derivatization and stable isotope coding. *Analytical Chemistry, 79*(14), 5150–5157.
41. Welham, K. J., Domin, M. A., Johnson, K., Jones, L., & Ashton, D. S. (2000). Characterization of fungal spores by laser desorption/ionization time-of-flight mass spectrometry. *Rapid Communications in Mass Spectrometry, 14*(5), 307–310.
42. Johnson, D. W., Trinh, M. U., & Oe, T. (2003). Measurement of plasma pristanic, phytanic and very long chain fatty acids by liquid chromatography-electrospray tandem mass spectrometry for the diagnosis of peroxisomal disorders. *Journal of Chromatography B, 798*(1), 159–162.
43. Liu, M., Wei, F., Lv, X., Dong, X. Y., & Chen, H. (2018). Rapid and sensitive detection of free fatty acids in edible oils based on chemical derivatization coupled with electrospray ionization tandem mass spectrometry. *Food Chemistry, 242*, 338–344. https://doi.org/10.1016/j.foodchem.2017.09.069.
44. Fan, R. J., Guan, Q., Zhang, F., Leng, J. P., Sun, T. Q., & Guo, Y. L. (2016). Benzylic rearrangement stable isotope labeling for quantitation of guanidino and ureido compounds in thyroid tissues by liquid chromatography-electrospray ionization mass spectrometry. *Analytica Chimica Acta, 908*, 132–140.
45. Tsukamoto, Y., Santa, T., Saimaru, H., Imai, K., & Funatsu, T. (2010). Synthesis of benzofurazan derivatization reagents for carboxylic acids and its application to analysis of fatty acids in rat plasma by high-performance liquid chromatography-electrospray ionization mass spectrometry. *Biomedical Chromatography, 19*(10), 802–808.
46. Dupuy, A., Faouder, P. L., Vigor, C., Galano, J. M., Dray, C., Lee, C. Y., et al. (2016). Simultaneous quantitative profiling of 20 isoprostanoids from omega-3 and omega-6 polyunsaturated fatty acids by LC-MS/MS in various biological samples. *Analytica Chimica Acta, 921*, 46–58.
47. Kloos, D., Lingeman, H., Mayboroda, O. A., Deelder, A. M., Niessen, W. M. A., & Giera, M. (2014). Analysis of biologically-active, endogenous carboxylic acids based on chromatography-mass spectrometry. *Trends in Analytical Chemistry, 61*(2), 17–28.
48. Wang, M., Hayakawa, J., Yang, K., & Han, X. (2014). Characterization and quantification of diacylglycerol species in biological extracts after one-step derivatization: A shotgun lipidomics approach.

Analytical Chemistry, 86(4), 2146–2155. https://doi.org/10.1021/ac403798q.

49. Leiker, T. J., Barkley, R. M., & Murphy, R. C. (2011). Analysis of diacylglycerol molecular species in cellular lipid extracts by normal-phase LC-electrospray mass spectrometry. *International Journal of Mass Spectrometry, 305*(2–3), 103–109. https://doi.org/10.1016/j.ijms.2010.09.008.
50. Xu, X., Veenstra, T. D., Fox, S. D., Roman, J. M., Issaq, H. J., Falk, R., et al. (2005). Measuring fifteen endogenous estrogens simultaneously in human urine by high-performance liquid chromatography-mass spectrometry. *Analytical Chemistry, 77*(20), 6646–6654.
51. Bussy, U., Chungdavidson, Y. W., Buchinger, T. J., Li, K., & Li, W. (2017). High-sensitivity determination of estrogens in fish plasma using chemical derivatization upstream UHPLC-MSMS. *Steroids, 123*, 13.
52. Xiaoxiao, M., & Yu, X. (2014). Pinpointing double bonds in lipids by Paternò-Büchi reactions and mass spectrometry. *Angewandte Chemie, 126*(10), 2630–2634.
53. Kwon, Y., Lee, S., Oh, D. C., & Kim, S. (2011). Simple determination of double-bond positions in long-chain olefins by cross-metathesis. *Angewandte Chemie, 123*(36), 8425–8428.
54. Ren, J., Franklin, E. T., & Yu, X. (2017). Uncovering structural diversity of unsaturated fatty acyls in cholesteryl esters via photochemical reaction and tandem mass spectrometry. *Journal of the American Society for Mass Spectrometry, 28*(7), 1432–1441.
55. Sommerer, D., Suss, R., Hammerschmidt, S., Wirtz, H., Arnold, K., & Schiller, J. (2004). Analysis of the phospholipid composition of bronchoalveolar lavage (BAL) fluid from man and minipig by MALDI-TOF mass spectrometry in combination with TLC. *Journal of Pharmaceutical and Biomedical Analysis, 35*(1), 199–206. https://doi.org/10.1016/j.jpba.2003.12.016.
56. Tserng, K.-Y., & Griffin, R. (2003). Quantitation and molecular species determination of diacylglycerols, phosphatidylcholines, ceramides, and sphingomyelins with gas chromatography. *Analytical Biochemistry, 323*(1), 84–93. https://doi.org/10.1016/j.ab.2003.08.026.
57. Bondia-Pons, I., Castellote, A. I., & Lopez-Sabater, M. C. (2004). Comparison of conventional and fast gas chromatography in human plasma fatty acid determination. *Journal of Chromatography B, 809*(2), 339–344. https://doi.org/10.1016/j.jchromb.2004.07.002.
58. Peterson, B. L., & Cummings, B. S. (2006). A review of chromatographic methods for the assessment of phospholipids in biological samples. *Biomedical Chromatography, 20*(3), 227–243. https://doi.org/10.1002/bmc.563.
59. Lima, E. S., & Abdalla, D. S. P. (2002). High-performance liquid chromatography of fatty acids in biological samples. *Analytica Chimica Acta, 465*(1–2), 81–91.
60. Sandra, K., & Sandra, P. (2013). Lipidomics from an analytical perspective. *Current Opinion in Chemical Biology, 17*(5), 847–853. https://doi.org/10.1016/j.cbpa.2013.06.010.
61. Lisa, M., Netusilova, K., Franek, L., Dvorakova, H., Vrkoslav, V., & Holcapek, M. (2011). Characterization of fatty acid and triacylglycerol composition in animal fats using silver-ion and non-aqueous reversed-phase high-performance liquid chromatography/mass spectrometry and gas chromatography/flame ionization detection. *Journal of Chromatography A, 1218*(42), 7499–7510. https://doi.org/10.1016/j.chroma.2011.07.032.
62. Nikolova-Damyanova, B. (2009). Retention of lipids in silver ion high-performance liquid chromatography: Facts and assumptions. *Journal of Chromatography A, 1216*(10), 1815–1824. https://doi.org/10.1016/j.chroma.2008.10.097.
63. Mesaros, C., Lee, S. H., & Blair, I. A. (2009). Targeted quantitative analysis of eicosanoid lipids in biological samples using liquid chromatography-tandem mass spectrometry. *Journal of Chromatography B, 877*(26), 2736–2745. https://doi.org/10.1016/j.jchromb.2009.03.011.
64. Bamba, T., Lee, J. W., Matsubara, A., & Fukusaki, E. (2012). Metabolic profiling of lipids by supercritical fluid chromatography/mass spectrometry. *Journal of Chromatography A, 1250*, 212–219. https://doi.org/10.1016/j.chroma.2012.05.068.
65. Perona, J. S., & Ruiz-Gutierrez, V. (2003). Simultaneous determination of molecular species of monoacylglycerols, diacylglycerols and triacylglycerols in human very-low-density lipoproteins by reversed-phase liquid chromatography. *Journal of Chromatography B, 785*(1), 89–99.
66. Cajka, T., & Fiehn, O. (2016). Increasing lipidomic coverage by selecting optimal mobile-phase modifiers in LC–MS of blood plasma. *Metabolomics, 12*(2). https://doi.org/10.1007/s11306-015-0929-x.
67. Weir, J. M., Wong, G., & Barlow, C. K. (2013). Plasma lipid profiling in a large population based cohort. *Journal of Lipid Research*. (jlr):P035808.
68. Tang, D. Q., Zou, L., Yin, X. X., & Ong, C. N. (2016). HILIC-MS for metabolomics: An attractive and complementary approach to RPLC-MS. *Mass Spectrometry Reviews, 35*(5), 574–600. https://doi.org/10.1002/mas.21445.
69. Hines, K. M., Herron, J., & Xu, L. (2017). Assessment of altered lipid homeostasis by HILIC-ion mobility-mass spectrometry-based lipidomics. *Journal of Lipid Research*. jlr.D074724.
70. Buszewski, B., & Noga, S. (2012). Hydrophilic interaction liquid chromatography (HILIC)–a powerful separation technique. *Analytical and Bioanalytical Chemistry, 402*(1), 231–247. https://doi.org/10.1007/s00216-011-5308-5.
71. Holcapek, M., Ovcacikova, M., Lisa, M., Cifkova, E., & Hajek, T. (2015). Continuous comprehensive two-

dimensional liquid chromatography-electrospray ionization mass spectrometry of complex lipidomic samples. *Analytical and Bioanalytical Chemistry, 407*(17), 5033–5043. https://doi.org/10.1007/s00216-015-8528-2.

72. Laboureur, L., Ollero, M., & Touboul, D. (2015). Lipidomics by supercritical fluid chromatography. *International Journal of Molecular Sciences, 16*(6), 13868–13884. https://doi.org/10.3390/ijms160613868.
73. Al Hamimi, S., Sandahl, M., Armeni, M., Turner, C., & Spegel, P. (2018). Screening of stationary phase selectivities for global lipid profiling by ultrahigh performance supercritical fluid chromatography. *Journal of Chromatography A, 1548*, 76–82. https://doi.org/10.1016/j.chroma.2018.03.024.
74. Lisa, M., Cifkova, E., Khalikova, M., Ovcacikova, M., & Holcapek, M. (2017). Lipidomic analysis of biological samples: Comparison of liquid chromatography, supercritical fluid chromatography and direct infusion mass spectrometry methods. *Journal of Chromatography A, 1525*, 96–108. https://doi.org/10.1016/j.chroma.2017.10.022.
75. Yamada, T., Uchikata, T., Sakamoto, S., Yokoi, Y., Nishiumi, S., Yoshida, M., et al. (2013). Supercritical fluid chromatography/Orbitrap mass spectrometry based lipidomics platform coupled with automated lipid identification software for accurate lipid profiling. *Journal of Chromatography A, 1301*, 237–242. https://doi.org/10.1016/j.chroma.2013.05.057.
76. Lee, J. W., Uchikata, T., Matsubara, A., Nakamura, T., Fukusaki, E., & Bamba, T. (2012). Application of supercritical fluid chromatography/mass spectrometry to lipid profiling of soybean. *Journal of Bioscience and Bioengineering, 113*(2), 262–268. https://doi.org/10.1016/j.jbiosc.2011.10.e009.
77. Myers, D. S., Ivanova, P. T., Milne, S. B., & Brown, H. A. (2011). Quantitative analysis of glycerophospholipids by LC-MS: Acquisition, data handling, and interpretation. *Biochimica et Biophysica Acta, 1811*(11), 748–757. https://doi.org/10.1016/j.bbalip.2011.05.015.
78. Bird, S. S., Marur, V. R., Sniatynski, M. J., Greenberg, H. K., & Kristal, B. S. (2011). Serum lipidomics profiling using LC-MS and high-energy collisional dissociation fragmentation: Focus on triglyceride detection and characterization. *Analytical Chemistry, 83*(17), 6648–6657. https://doi.org/10.1021/ac201195d.
79. Seppanen-Laakso, T., & Oresic, M. (2009). How to study lipidomes. *Journal of Molecular Endocrinology, 42*(3), 185–190. https://doi.org/10.1677/JME-08-0150.
80. Cajka, T., & Fiehn, O. (2014). Comprehensive analysis of lipids in biological systems by liquid chromatography-mass spectrometry. *Trends in Analytical Chemistry, 61*, 192–206. https://doi.org/10.1016/j.trac.2014.04.017.
81. Kofeler, H. C., Fauland, A., Rechberger, G. N., & Trotzmuller, M. (2012). Mass spectrometry based lipidomics: An overview of technological platforms. *Metabolites, 2*(1), 19–38. https://doi.org/10.3390/metabo2010019.
82. Hager, J. W., & Le Blanc, J. C. Y. (2003). High-performance liquid chromatography–tandem mass spectrometry with a new quadrupole/linear ion trap instrument. *Journal of Chromatography A, 1020*(1), 3–9. https://doi.org/10.1016/s0021-9673(03)00426-6.
83. Michalski, A., Damoc, E., & Hauschild, J. P. (2011). Mass spectrometry-based proteomics using Q Exactive, a high-performance benchtop quadrupole Orbitrap mass spectrometer. *Molecular & Cellular Proteomics*. mcp. M111. 011015.
84. Hu, Q., Noll, R. J., Li, H., Makarov, A., Hardman, M., & Graham, C. R. (2005). The Orbitrap: A new mass spectrometer. *Journal of Mass Spectrometry, 40*(4), 430–443. https://doi.org/10.1002/jms.856.
85. Schuhmann, K., Almeida, R., Baumert, M., Herzog, R., Bornstein, S. R., & Shevchenko, A. (2012). Shotgun lipidomics on a LTQ Orbitrap mass spectrometer by successive switching between acquisition polarity modes. *Journal of Mass Spectrometry, 47*(1), 96–104. https://doi.org/10.1002/jms.2031.
86. Fhaner, C. J., Liu, S., Ji, H., Simpson, R. J., & Reid, G. E. (2012). Comprehensive lipidome profiling of isogenic primary and metastatic colon adenocarcinoma cell lines. *Analytical Chemistry, 84*(21), 8917–8926. https://doi.org/10.1021/ac302154g.
87. Ghaste, M., Mistrik, R., & Shulaev, V. (2016). Applications of Fourier Transform Ion Cyclotron Resonance (FT-ICR) and Orbitrap based high resolution mass spectrometry in metabolomics and lipidomics. *International Journal of Molecular Sciences, 17*(6). https://doi.org/10.3390/ijms17060816.
88. Almeida, R., Pauling, J. K., Sokol, E., Hannibal-Bach, H. K., & Ejsing, C. S. (2015). Comprehensive lipidome analysis by shotgun lipidomics on a hybrid quadrupole-orbitrap-linear ion trap mass spectrometer. *Journal of the American Society for Mass Spectrometry, 26*(1), 133–148. https://doi.org/10.1007/s13361-014-1013-x.
89. Xie, Y., Ma, H., Wei, F., Lyu, X., Wu, Z., Wu, B., Xu, S., Dong, X., Chen, H., & Huang, F. (2017). Importance of quality control in lipidomics profiling based on mass spectrometry. *Oil Crop Science, 2*(4), 217.
90. Michopoulos, F., Lai, L., Gika, H., Theodoridis, G., & Wilson, I. (2009). UPLC-MS-based analysis of human plasma for metabonomics using solvent precipitation or solid phase extraction. *Journal of Proteome Research, 8*(4), 2114–2121.
91. Zhu, C., Dane, A., Spijksma, G., Wang, M., Van der Greef, J., Luo, G., et al. (2012). An efficient hydrophilic interaction liquid chromatography separation of 7 phospholipid classes based on a diol column. *Journal of Chromatography A, 1220*(1), 26–34.
92. Fm, V. D. K., Bobeldijk, I., Verheij, E. R., & Jellema, R. H. (2009). Analytical error reduction using single point calibration for accurate and precise metabo-

lomic phenotyping. *Journal of Proteome Research, 8*(11), 5132–5141.
93. Quehenberger, O., Armando, A. M., Brown, A. H., Milne, S. B., Myers, D. S., Merrill, A. H., et al. (2010). Lipidomics reveals a remarkable diversity of lipids in human plasma. *Journal of Lipid Research, 51*(11), 3299–3305.
94. Luo, P., Yin, P., Zhang, W., Zhou, L., Lu, X., Lin, X., et al. (2016). Optimization of large-scale pseudotargeted metabolomics method based on liquid chromatography-mass spectrometry. *Journal of Chromatography A, 1437*, 127–136.
95. Kamleh, M. A., Ebbels, T. M. D., Spagou, K., Masson, P., & Want, E. J. (2012). Optimizing the use of quality control samples for signal drift correction in large-scale urine metabolic profiling studies. *Analytical Chemistry, 84*(6), 2670.
96. Dunn, W. B., Broadhurst, D., Begley, P., Zelena, E., Francismcintyre, S., Anderson, N., et al. (2011). Procedures for large-scale metabolic profiling of serum and plasma using gas chromatography and liquid chromatography coupled to mass spectrometry. *Nature Protocols, 6*(7), 1060–1083.
97. Zelena, E., Dunn, W. B., Broadhurst, D., Francis-Mcintyre, S., Carroll, K. M., Begley, P., et al. (2009). Development of a robust and repeatable UPLC-MS method for the long-term metabolomic study of human serum. *Analytical Chemistry, 81*(4), 1357–1364.
98. Weir, J. M., Wong, G., Barlow, C. K., Greeve, M. A., Kowalczyk, A., Almasy, L., et al. (2013). Plasma lipid profiling in a large population-based cohort. *Journal of Lipid Research, 54*(10), 2898–2908.
99. Meikle, P. J., Wong, G., Tsorotes, D., Barlow, C. K., Weir, J. M., Christopher, M. J., et al. (2011). Plasma lipidomic analysis of stable and unstable coronary artery disease. *Arteriosclerosis, Thrombosis, and Vascular Biology, 11*(2), 2723–2732.
100. Ulmer, C. Z., Ragland, J. M., Koelmel, J. P., Heckert, A., Jones, C. M., Garrett, T., et al. (2017). LipidQC: Method validation tool for visual comparison to SRM 1950 using NIST interlaboratory comparison exercise lipid consensus mean estimate values. *Analytical Chemistry, 89*(24).
101. Dunn, W. B., Wilson, I. D., Nicholls, A. W., & Broadhurst, D. (2012). The importance of experimental design and QC samples in large-scale and MS-driven untargeted metabolomic studies of humans. *Bioanalysis, 4*(18), 2249–2264.
102. Windig, W., Phalp, J. M., & Payne, A. W. (1997). A noise and background reduction method for component detection in liquid chromatography/mass spectrometry. *Analytical Chemistry*.
103. Andreev, V. P., Rejtar, T., Chen, H.-S., & Moskovets, E. V. (2003). A universal denoising and peak picking algorithm for LC–MS based on matched filtration in the chromatographic time domain. *Analytical Chemistry, 75*(22), 6314–6326.
104. Fredriksson, M. J., Petersson, P., Axelsson, B. O., & Bylund, D. (2009). An automatic peak finding method for LC-MS data using Gaussian second derivative filtering. *Journal of Separation Science, 32*(22), 3906–3918. https://doi.org/10.1002/jssc.200900395.
105. Smith, C. A., Want, E. J., O'Maille, G., Abagyan, R., & Siuzdak, G. (2006). XCMS: Processing mass spectrometry data for metabolite profiling using nonlinear peak alignment, matching, and identification. *Analytical Chemistry, 78*(3), 779–787.
106. Pluskal, T., Castillo, S., Villar-Briones, A., & Oresic, M. (2010). MZmine 2: Modular framework for processing, visualizing, and analyzing mass spectrometry-based molecular profile data. *BMC Bioinformatics, 11*, 395. https://doi.org/10.1186/1471-2105-11-395.
107. Katajamaa, M., & Oresic, M. (2007). Data processing for mass spectrometry-based metabolomics. *Journal of Chromatography A, 1158*(1–2), 318–328. https://doi.org/10.1016/j.chroma.2007.04.021.
108. Sana, T. R., Roark, J. C., Li, X., Waddell, K., & Fischer, S. M. (2008). Molecular formula and METLIN Personal Metabolite Database matching applied to the identification of compounds generated by LC_TOF-MS. *Journal of Biomolecular Techniques, 19*(4), 258.
109. Wishart, D. S., Tzur, D., Knox, C., Eisner, R., Guo, A. C., Young, N., et al. (2007). HMDB: The human metabolome database. *Nucleic Acids Research, 35*(Database issue), D521–D526. https://doi.org/10.1093/nar/gkl923.
110. Bird, S. S., Marur, V. R., Sniatynski, M. J., Greenberg, H. K., & Kristal, B. S. (2011). Lipidomics profiling by high-resolution LC-MS and high-energy collisional dissociation fragmentation: Focus on characterization of mitochondrial cardiolipins and monolysocardiolipins. *Analytical Chemistry, 83*(3), 940–949. https://doi.org/10.1021/ac102598u.
111. Yang, W.-C., Adamec, J., & Regnier, F. E. (2007). Enhancement of the LCMS analysis of fatty acids through derivatization and stable isotope coding. *Analytical Chemistry, 79*(14), 5150–5157.
112. Sturm, M., Bertsch, A., Gropl, C., Hildebrandt, A., Hussong, R., Lange, E., et al. (2008). OpenMS – An open-source software framework for mass spectrometry. *BMC Bioinformatics, 9*, 163. https://doi.org/10.1186/1471-2105-9-163.
113. Benton, H. P., Wong, D. M., Trauger, S. A., & Siuzdak, G. (2008). XCMS2: Processing tandem mass spectrometry data for metabolite identification and structural characterization. *Analytical Chemistry, 80*(16), 6382–6389. https://doi.org/10.1021/ac800795f.
114. Tsugawa, H., Cajka, T., Kind, T., Ma, Y., Higgins, B., Ikeda, K., et al. (2015). MS-DIAL: Data-independent MS/MS deconvolution for comprehensive metabolome analysis. *Nature Methods, 12*(6), 523–526. https://doi.org/10.1038/nmeth.3393.
115. Herzog, R., Schuhmann, K., Schwudke, D., Sampaio, J. L., Bornstein, S. R., Schroeder, M., et al. (2012). LipidXplorer: A software for consensual

cross-platform lipidomics. *PLoS One, 7*(1), e29851. https://doi.org/10.1371/journal.pone.0029851.

116. Ejsing, C. S., Duchoslav, E., Sampaio, J., Simons, K., Bonner, R., Thiele, C., Ekroos, K., & Shevchenko, A. (2006). Automated identification and quantification of glycerophospholipid molecular species by multiple precursor ion scanning. *Analytical Chemistry, 78*(17), 6202–6214.

117. Yang, K., Cheng, H., Gross, R. W., & Han, X. (2009). Automated lipid identification and quantification by multidimensional mass spectrometry-based shotgun lipidomics. https://doi.org/10.1016/j.jchromb.2008.1012.1043.

Capillary Electrophoresis-Mass Spectrometry for Cancer Metabolomics

Xiangdong Xu

1 Introduction

Metabolomics is an analytical toolbox to profile the whole low-molecular-weight metabolites in a biological system, such as cells, tissues, urine, serum, and plasma. Metabolomic analysis is a promising omics approach to not only investigating the altered metabolic regulation in cancer cells but also identifying biomarkers for early cancer detection and prediction of treatment response in cancer patients. Untargeted metabolomics can be performed to gain a comprehensive metabolite profile of a biological sample. Targeted metabolomics may also be applied to quantitative analysis of preselected metabolites and related metabolic pathway. The goal of a metabolomics study is to obtain an answer to a specific biological or clinical question [1]. While genomic and proteomic analyses may not tell the whole story of what might be happening in a cell, metabolic profiling can give an instantaneous snapshot of the physiology of that cell. To accomplish a comprehensive metabolomic analysis of complex biological samples, there is a high demand for the analytical techniques used in metabolomics due to the large variations in physicochemistry properties and expression levels of metabolites. Currently, advanced analytical techniques, such as NMR spectroscopy, gas chromatography with mass spectrometry (GC-MS), and liquid chromatography with mass spectrometry (LC-MS), have become well-established tools for metabolomics studies [2, 3]. A comprehensive overview of the possibilities of these techniques for metabolomics studies can be found in recent reviews [3, 4]. Despite significant developments in LC column technology and methodology, such as hydrophilic interaction liquid chromatography, the selective and efficient analysis of highly polar and charged metabolites is still challenging.

Capillary electrophoresis (CE) is a powerful separation technique but still underused for complex sample analysis. CE-MS has shown considerable potential for profiling of polar ionogenic compounds in metabolomics. However, relatively speaking, there have been not many papers published on CE-MS-based metabolomic analysis. Hyphenation of CE with MS is generally performed via a sheath-liquid interface. However, the electrophoretic effluent is significantly diluted in this configuration, thereby limiting the utility of this method for highly sensitive metabolomic analysis. Moreover, in this setup the intrinsically low-flow property of CE is not effectively utilized in combination with electrospray ionization (ESI). In this chapter, we will discuss the CE-MS fundamentals, methodologies and interfacing, as well as its applications in cancer metabolomics.

X. Xu (✉)
School of Public Health and Key Laboratory of Environment and Human Health, Hebei Medical University, Shijiazhuang, China
e-mail: xuxd@hebmu.edu.cn

S. Hu (ed.), *Cancer Metabolomics*, Advances in Experimental Medicine and Biology 1280,
https://doi.org/10.1007/978-3-030-51652-9_13

2 Capillary Electrophoresis with Mass Spectrometry

2.1 Separation Modes of Capillary Electrophoresis

CE is a general term for a range of separation techniques based on different separation principles, including capillary zone electrophoresis (CZE), micellar electrokinetic capillary chromatography (MECC or MEKC), nonaqueous capillary electrophoresis (NACE), capillary gel electrophoresis (CGE), capillary isoelectric focusing (CIEF), capillary electrochromatography (CEC), and capillary isotachophoresis (CITP). Depending on the complexity of the sample and the nature of the present analytes, each of these techniques will provide various advantages for the separation and detection of different substances.

2.1.1 Capillary Zone Electrophoresis

CZE is a main separation mode used with MS because volatile buffers can be employed. It separates the analytes first in CZE based on their charge-to-size ratios and then in the MS on the basis of their mass-to-charge ratio (m/z). Prior to analysis, CE running buffer is flushed through the capillary by pressure. Afterward, the sample is injected and high voltage is applied for the separation (Fig. 1). Since CE separates analytes based on the differences in charge-to-size ratio, relatively small and highly charged analytes have high electrophoretic mobility, whereas relatively large and poorly charged compounds exhibit low electrophoretic mobility. Obviously, neutral compounds will not be separated because their charge-to-size ratio is zero. The CZE-MS method used for global metabolomic profiling in biological samples was demonstrated by Soga et al. [5]. The coupling to MS is important in untargeted metabolomic analysis although it limits the buffer additives to those that can be made volatile [6].

2.1.2 Micellar Electrokinetic Chromatography

The classic CZE method is not suited for the separation of neutral molecules, which migrate toward the detector with the same velocity as the EOF (Fig. 1). MEKC is a commonly used electrophoretic technique developed in the early 1990s that extended the applicability of CE to analysis of neutral analytes. It is based on the differential partitioning of an analyte between the two-phase system: the mobile aqueous phase and micellar pseudostationary phase. In MEKC, surfactants are added to the buffer solution in concentration above their critical micellar concentrations; consequently micelles are formed. These micelles have a nonpolar inside, and a polar (or charged) surface, and undergo electrophoretic migration like any other charged particle under high electric field. Analytes are

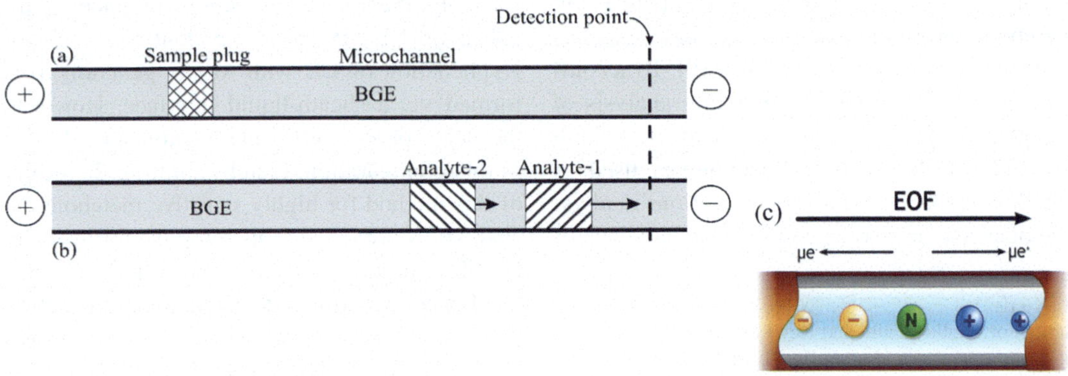

Fig. 1 The principle of capillary zone electrophoresis (CZE). Sample is injected into the separation capillary (**a**) and the analytes are electrophoretically separated by the applied high voltage. The velocity of migration of an analyte in CE also depends on the rate of electroosmotic flow (EOF) of the background electrolytes (BGE) (**c**)

partitioned between the micelles and the buffer solution, dependable on the affinity to the micelles, and separated with the applied high voltage [7].

2.1.3 Nonaqueous Capillary Electrophoresis

With NACE, analytes that are insoluble in water are separated, mainly depending on the use of organic solvents. The viscosity and dielectric constants of organic solvents affect both ion mobility of analytes and the rate of EOF. Recently, NACE was applied as a multiplexed separation platform for analysis of more than 20 nonesterified fatty acids in human serum or plasma samples [8]. Following a simple methyl-tert-butyl ether extraction, seven serum extracts were analyzed directly by multisegment injection-NACE-MS within a single run (<4 min/sample) under negative ion mode detection that incorporates stringent measures for quality control, including batch correction adjustment. Overall, excellent technical variance (RSD = 10%) and mutually agreed results for the measurement of the fatty acids in 50 serum samples were achieved by MSI-NACE-MS and GC/MS within the same laboratory (mean bias = 24%, n = 600).

2.1.4 Capillary Gel Electrophoresis

CGE is carried out with using a gel matrix inside the capillary for size-based separation of biomolecules. Small molecules migrate faster than large molecules under the CGE separation mode. Therefore, CGE is frequently employed for separation of proteins and DNA fragments.

2.1.5 Capillary Isoelectric Focusing

When a pH gradient is formed across the separation capillary, and a high voltage is applied from low pH region (positive) to high pH (negative), analytes would migrate to the pH value that equals their pI value. At lower pH, the analytes are positively charged, whereas at higher pH the analytes are negatively charged. In this separation mode, all the analytes are separated according to their pI. CIEF is commonly used to separate proteins, particularly useful for resolving protein isoforms.

2.1.6 Capillary Electrochromatography

With CEC separation, a capillary is packed with silica-based particles as a stationary phase. When high voltage is applied across the capillary, the buffer starts to migrate due to the present EOF. Similar to HPLC, the analytes are separated based on their interaction with the stationary phase. The difference between HPLC and CEC is that HPLC utilizes a high-pressure pump to mobilize the mobile phase whereas, in CEC, a high voltage is applied to drive the EOF. CEC is capable of separating both neutral and charged molecules. However, CEC has bubble formation issue caused by Joule heating during experiments, which may lead to column dryout and current disruption. Therefore, pressure-assisted CEC (pCEC), with EOF combined with supplemental pressurized flow as its driving force, has been used to overcome this problem. pCEC has been demonstrated for metabolomic profiling of urine samples from lung cancer patients and healthy controls [9].

2.1.7 Capillary Isotachophoresis

A discontinuous buffer system is used in CITP. The sample is introduced between a zone of fast leading electrolyte (LE) and a zone of slow terminating electrolytes (TE). The analytes of interest have intermediate ionic mobility between LE and TE. Under the high voltage applied, a low electrical field is formed in the LE zone whereas a high electrical field is formed in the TE zone. If an analyte is situated in the TE zone, it will be under a higher electric field, giving it a higher speed. Meanwhile, if an analyte is situated in the LE zone, it would be under a lower electric field and migrate slower; the result is that the analytes are focused at the LE/TE interface. For this reason, CITP is often used to concentrate large-volume injections, and low concentration samples are strongly concentrated into very narrow zones.

It was reported that the integration of transient-isotachophoresis (t-ITP) as an in-capillary preconcentration procedure with sheathless CE-MS resulted in subnanomolar limits of detection for metabolites, and more than 1300 metabolic features were detected in urine.

Compared to the classical CE-MS approaches, the integration of t-ITP combined with the use of a sheathless interface provides up to 2 orders of magnitude sensitivity improvement [10]. It was also reported that the use of t-ITP and pH-mediated stacking, coupled with FT-ICR MS, improved the overall detection of cationic metabolites in bacterium [11].

2.2 CE Interface with MS

ESI is a commonly used ionization mode in CE-MS. ESI enables molecules in the liquid phase to be converted directly into ions in the gas phase. It can be easily adapted for online coupling of MS with CE. CE separates mostly charged compounds and ESI is appropriate for ionization of polar and ionic compounds. The interface to MS is a little more complicated in CE than in HPLC owing to a low flow rate of the effluent from the capillary and incompatible electrolytes used in the running buffer. Most commercial LC-MS systems can be adapted for CE-MS with modification in the interface.

2.2.1 Sheath-Flow Interface

A CE-ESI-MS system has to complete the electrical circuit for analyte separation while simultaneously providing an electrical potential to the spray tip. This is generally accomplished using a sheath-flow or sheathless interface [12, 13]. Sheath-flow interfaces have been popular since the early years of CE-MS applications. In this configuration, the separation capillary is inserted coaxially into a stainless-steel tube with a slightly larger diameter, and a sheath liquid is mixed with the BGE at the capillary outlet. The nebulizing gas is supplied via a third coaxial tube, and this assists with stable spray formation and desolvation [14]. Dovichi's group developed a highly robust electrokinetically pumped sheath-flow nanospray interface for coupling CZE with MS, which has been commercialized by the Agent Technologies (Fig. 2). They demonstrated the system for high-throughput proteomic analysis, and 27,000 peptide and nearly 4400 protein identifications were achieved with single-shot CZE-MS [15–18]. A mixture of an aqueous volatile acid (formic acid or acetic acid) and an organic solvent (methanol, propanol, or acetonitrile) is often used as the sheath liquid. The sheath liquid composition and flow rate and the nebulizing gas flow rate, therefore, need to be optimized to create a stable electrospray and maintain separation efficiency and detection sensitivity [19, 20]. Sarver et al. modified the sheath-flow nanospray interface developed by Dovichi's group [21] in order to perform ESI in negative ionization mode [22]. They obtained stable spray conditions by using 10 mM ammonium acetate in 70% methanol as sheath liquid and coating of the emitter with 3-aminopropyltrimethoxysilane to reverse the EOF in the used glass emitter. However, recent calculations and measurements indicate that the EOF is not the driving force in this type of interface and rather the sheath liquid is important to obtain stable spray conditions [23].

Fang et al. designed a nano-flow sheath liquid interface with an extendable tip, featuring a so-called surface flow [24]. The separation capillary with a 20 μm id is chemically etched to reduce the od to 30 μm and is introduced into a tapered sheath flow capillary made of glass with 35 μm id and 40 μm od (Fig. 3). After optimization, the separation capillary protrudes by approximately 200 μm from the outer capillary and serves as the electrospray emitter. The sheath liquid is driven by a syringe pump and flows on the surface of the separation capillary and mixes with the separation effluent inside the Taylor cone with a volume of 4 pL, under a flow rate of 200 nL/min. Extension of the tip showed improved sensitivity when compared to the assembly with retracted tip. The interface was applied to the analysis of a peptide mixture, showing good repeatability for peak intensity and spray stability. While this interface might offer great sensitivity due to its small dimensions with minimum dead volume and low sheath liquid flows, it might be difficult to manufacture.

2.2.2 Sheathless Interface

Sheathless interface benefits from the absence of additional liquid diluting the capillary effluent by

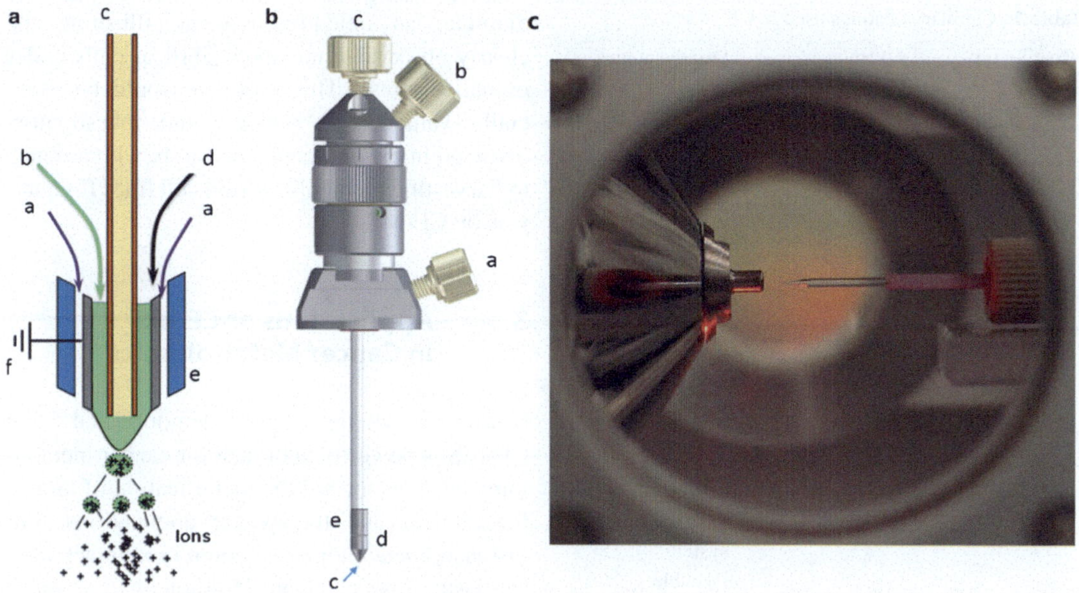

Fig. 2 (**a**) Pictorial representation of Agilent coaxial sheath-liquid CE-MS interface: a, nebulizing gas, b, sheath liquid, c, CE-capillary with BGE, d, stainless steel spray needle 0.4 mm i.d., 0.5 mm o.d., e, outer tube, f, ground connection. (**b**) Engineered sketch of the coaxial sheath-liquid CE-MS interface (graphics courtesy from the Agilent Technologies). (**c**) Electrokinetically pumped sheath-flow nanospray interface developed by Dovichi's group (https://dovichilab.weebly.com/). Reproduced with permission [21]

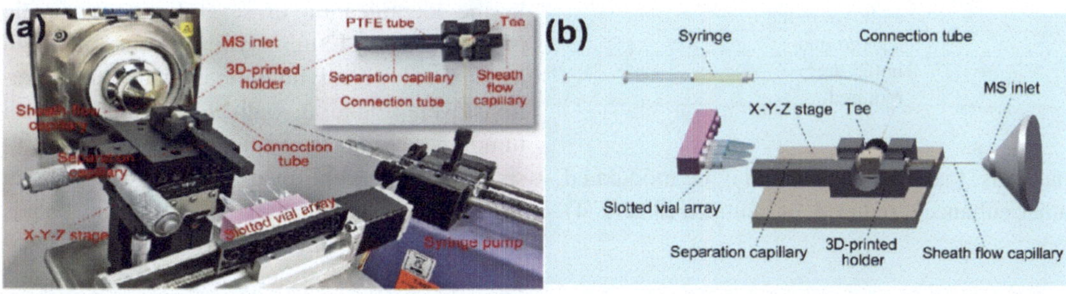

Fig. 3 Image (**a**) and schematic diagram (**b**) of the extendable sheath-flow interface. The inset in (**a**) shows the image of the whole interface. Reproduced with permission [24]

spraying the BGE directly, resulting in high ionization efficiency. However, the lack of supporting liquid can compromise separation and electrospray conditions, since pH value, EOF, capillary coating, organic solvent, or inlet pressure need to be considered to achieve an effective spray. CE-MS with commercial sheathless interfaces have been demonstrated for metabolic profiling of glioblastoma cells and colon and stomach cancer tissues [25, 26].

2.3 Capillary Coating

In CE-MS, capillary coatings are used to prevent analyte adsorption and to provide appropriate conditions for CE-MS interfacing. It can enhance the performance and stability of a CE-MS system, producing accurate and reproducible analytical results. Table 1 shows different types of capillary coatings and their advantages/disadvantages. Depending the charge states of the coating

Table 1 Capillary coatings used in CE

Coating type	Advantages	Disadvantages
Covalent	High reusability (in the order of months)	Complex synthesis procedures
	No further additives in the background buffer are required	Lower reproducibility
Dynamic	Higher repeatability and reproducibility	Require the presence of reagents in the background buffer
	Faster and simpler preparation and optimization	Possible compatibility problems with the detection system
		Possible background buffer heating
Semipermanent	Faster and simpler preparation, optimization, and regeneration	Low reusability (in the order of a few runs)
	No further additives in the background buffer are required	

materials, the EOF direction may be modulated, either enhanced, reduced, or neutralized (Fig. 4).

2.4 Sample Preparation in CE-MS-Based Metabolomic Analysis

Preparation of uniform samples for CE-MS-based metabolomic analysis is a critical issue that remains to be addressed. Maruyama et al. presented an easy protocol for extracting aqueous metabolites from cultured adherent cells for metabolomic analysis using CE-MS [27]. Aqueous metabolites from cultured cells are analyzed by culturing and washing cells, treating cells with methanol, extracting metabolites, and removing proteins and macromolecules with spin columns for CE-MS analysis. Representative results using lung cancer cell lines treated with diamide, an oxidative reagent, illustrate the clearly observable metabolic shift of cells under oxidative stress. This protocol would be especially valuable to students and investigators involved in metabolomics research, who are new to harvesting metabolites from cell lines for analysis by CE-MS.

3 Applications of CE-MS in Cancer Metabolomics

Numerous studies have demonstrated that CE-MS is powerful approach for cancer metabolome analysis toward the identification of targets for clinical and therapeutic applications. For instance, metabolomes of colon or stomach cancer tissues obtained from 16 colon or 12 stomach cancer patients were profiled with CE-MS [28]. Quantification of 94 metabolites in colon cancer tissues and 95 metabolites in stomach cancer tissues involved in glycolysis, the pentose phosphate pathway, the TCA and urea cycles, and amino acid and nucleotide metabolisms resulted in the identification of several cancer-specific metabolic traits. Extremely low glucose and high lactate and glycolytic intermediate concentrations were found in both colon and stomach tumor tissues, which indicated enhanced glycolysis and thus confirmed the Warburg effect. Significant accumulation of all amino acids except glutamine in the tumors implied autophagic degradation of proteins and active glutamine breakdown for energy production, i.e., glutaminolysis. In addition, significant organ-specific differences were found in the levels of TCA cycle intermediates, which reflected the dependency of each tissue on aerobic respiration according to oxygen availability. A similar research was accomplished by Chen et al. [29] by using CE-MS for metabolomic analysis of urine sample from colorectal cancer patients and healthy adults. The results indicated that the urine metabolomes of colorectal cancer patients had significant alterations when compared to those of normal controls, and there were also differences in the metabolomes between early stage and advanced colorectal cancer patients. Compared

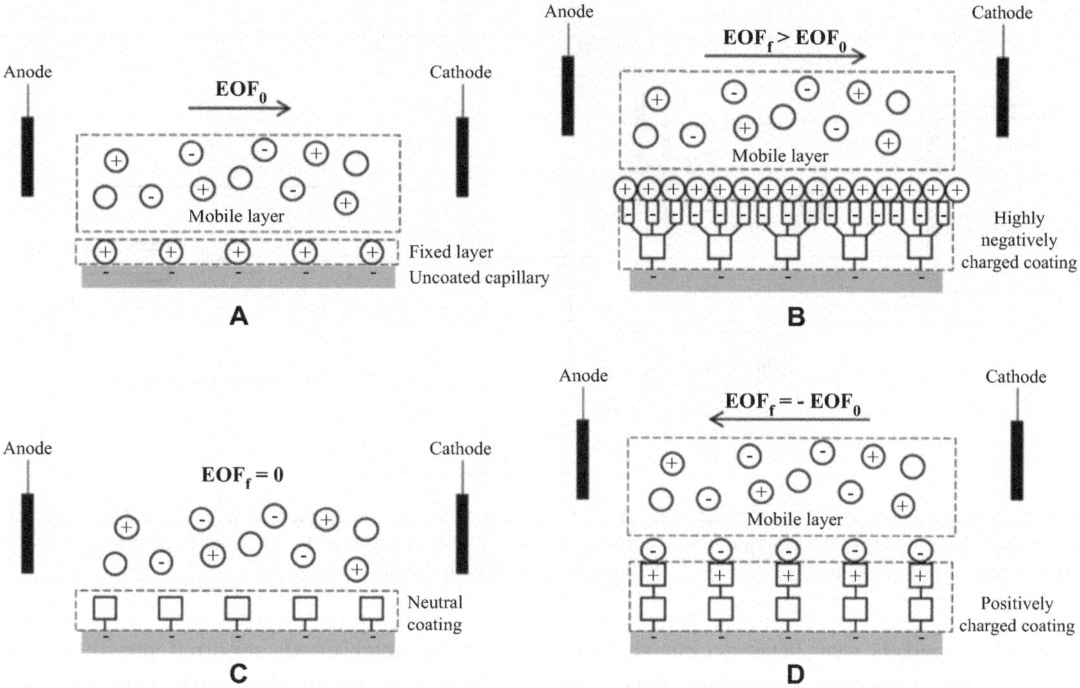

Fig. 4 Schematic representation of the modulation of EOF by capillary coating. (**a**) EOF in an untreated capillary. (**b**) EOF enhancement by formation of a highly negatively charged coating. (**c**) EOF suppression by formation of a neutral coating. (**d**) EOF inversion by formation of a positively charged coating [7]

with the control group, the levels of isoleucine, valine, arginine, lactate acid, and leucine significantly increased, but those of histidine, methionine, serine, aspartic acid, citric acid, succinate, and malic acid significantly decreased in urine samples from colorectal cancer. The levels of isoleucine and valine were lower in the urine samples of patients with advanced colorectal cancer than those in early stage colorectal cancer. Further validation of these urinary markers may lead to a noninvasive method for the early diagnosis of colorectal cancer.

Wu et al. introduced a pCEC method coupled with Q-TOF-MS for metabolomic analysis (Fig. 5) [9]. Three interfaces were compared in this study and a sheathless interface was selected, and the method was applied to lung cancer metabolomic analysis under the optimized conditions. The hyphenated pCEC-Q-TOF-MS system was investigated with mixed standards and pooled urine samples to evaluate its precision, repeatability, linearity, sensitivity, and selectivity. Multivariate data analysis was subsequently performed and used to distinguish lung cancer patients from healthy controls successfully. In a similar approach, Hirayama et al. fabricated a sheathless interface by making a small crack approximately 2 cm from the end of a capillary column and then covering the crack with a dialysis membrane to prevent metabolite loss during separation. CE-MS with the sheathless interface was applied for nontargeted metabolome analysis of human cancer cells and the number of peaks detected was about 2.5 times higher than the standard coaxial sheath liquid interface [30].

The incidence and recurrence rate of bladder cancer is high, especially in developed countries; however, current methods for diagnosis are limited to detecting high-grade tumors using often invasive methods. By using LC-MS and CE-MS, Alberice et al. revealed a total of 27 metabolites that were significantly different among different patient groups, some of which were specific to the stage/grade of cancer or tumor recurrence. The identified

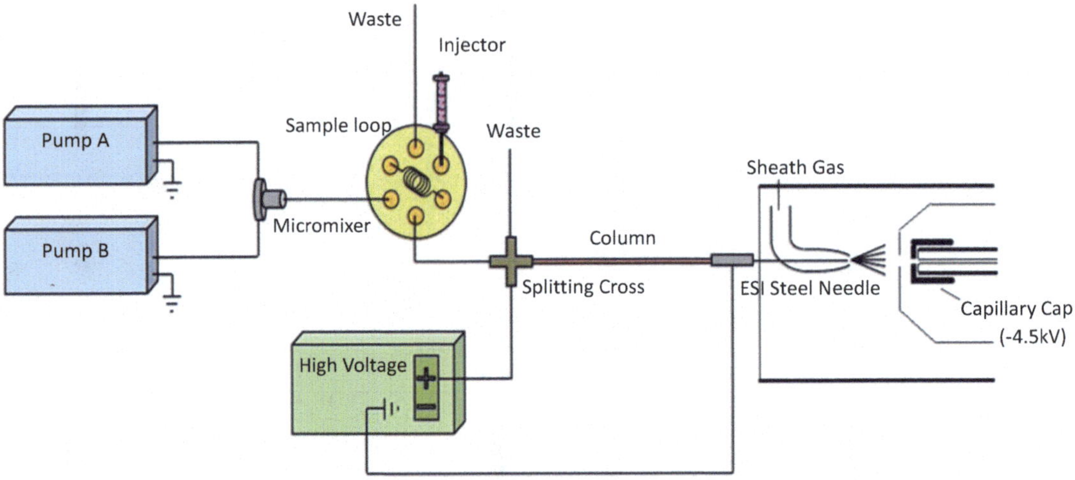

Fig. 5 Schematic overview of pCEC coupled to QTOF-MS. Chromatographic separation was performed on a reversed-phase column of 25 cm (25 cm was packed) × 150 μm id packed with 5 μm C18 particles using a TriSep-2100 pCEC system. (Reproduced from [9] with permission)

potential biomarkers were betaine, cysteine, histidine, tyrosine, carnosine, decanoylcarnitine, and uric acid, where the former four were associated with high risk and the latter three with low risk. Potential biomarkers associated with recurrence were Nε, Nε, Nε-trimethyllysine, N-acetyltryptophan, dopaquinone, leucine, and hypoxanthine, where the former two coincided with high risk and the latter three with low risk [31].

In general, metabolomic analyses lead to the detection of the total amount of all covered metabolites. This is currently a major limitation with respect to metabolites showing high turnover rates, but no changes in their concentration. A stable isotope tracing CE-MS metabolomic approach was developed by Zeng et al., to cover both polar metabolites and isotopologues in a nontargeted way [32]. An in-house developed software enables high-throughput processing of complex multidimensional data. The method was used for analyzing [U-^{13}C]-glucose exposed prostate cancer and non-cancer cells. This CE-MS-based analytical methodology complements polar metabolite profiles through isotopologue labeling patterns, thereby improving not only the metabolomic coverage but also the understanding of metabolism.

Schönemeier et al. reported possible biomarkers in saliva to distinguish between pancreatic cancer and chronic pancreatitis [33]. Salivary samples were collected from patients with pancreatic cancer (PC, n = 39), those with chronic pancreatitis (CP, n = 14), and healthy controls (C, n = 26). Polyamines, such as spermine, N1-acetylspermidine, and N1-acetylspermine, showed a significant difference between patients with PC and healthy controls, and the combination of four metabolites including N1-acetylspermidine showed high accuracy in discriminating PC from the other two groups. These data show the potential of using salivary biomarkers for screening test of PC.

A sheathless CE-MS method has been developed to anionic metabolomic profiling of glioblastoma cells [26]. The BGE, i.e., 10% acetic acid (pH 2.2), previously used for cationic metabolic profiling was assessed for anionic metabolic profiling by using MS detection in negative ion mode. For test compounds, RSDs for migration times and peak areas were below 2 and 11%, respectively, and plate numbers ranged from 60,000 to 40,0000. Critical metabolites with low or no retention on reversed-phase LC were efficiently separated and analyzed by the sheathless CE-MS method. An injection volume of only circa 20 nL resulted in LODs between 10 and 200 nM (corresponding to an amount of 0.4–4 fmol), which was an at least tenfold improvement as compared to LODs obtained by conventional CE-MS approaches for these analytes. The method can also be used for cationic metabolic profiling studies by only switching the MS detection and separation voltage polarity (Table 2).

Table 2 A partial list of CE-MS applications in cancer metabolomics

Analytes	Sample matrix	BGE	Sample pretreatment	MS analyzer	Refs.
Cationic metabolites	Urines from patients diagnosed of lung cancer	Binary solvents of A (0.1% FA in 2% ACN, v/v) and B (1% FA in ACN-methanol-water 49:49:2, v/v/v) were used in gradient elution	Mixed into chlorophenylalanine, vortexed for 1 min, and then centrifuged	TOF	[9]
Cationic metabolites	Colorectal cancer cells	10% acetic acid (pH 2.2)	Homogenization, centrifugation	TOF	[34]
Cationic metabolites	Colon cancer cells	1 M formic acid (pH 1.8)	Ultrafiltration, methanol precipitation, and two SPE procedures evaluated	TOF	[35]
Cationic metabolites	Colon cancer cells	1 M formic acid (pH 1.8)	Methanol purification; cytosolic fraction centrifugated with 3 kDa filter	TOF	[36]
Cationic and anionic metabolites	Colon and stomach cancer tissues	For cation, 1 mol/L formic acid; for anion, cationic-polymer-coated SMILE(+) capillary (Nacalai Tesque) filled with 50 mmol/L ammonium acetate solution (pH 8.5)		TOF	[28]
Cationic metabolites	Urine from patients diagnosed of urothelial bladder cancer	0.8 ml L − 1 formic acid (pH 1.9) and 10% methanol (v/v)	Diluted with Milli-Q water (1/5 v/v), centrifuged, and transferred to vials for analysis	TOF	[31]
Cationic and anionic metabolites	Prostate cancer and non-cancer cells	For cation, 1 mol/L formic acid; for anion, ammonium acetate solution (50 mmol/L; pH 8.5)	Centrifugally filtered	TOF	[32]
Anionic metabolites	Glioblastoma cell line extracts	10% acetic acid (pH 2.2)	Ultrafiltration	TOF	[26]
Cationic and anionic metabolites	Saliva of pancreatic cancer	For cation, 1 mol/L formic acid; for anion, ammonium acetate solution (50 mmol/L; pH 8.5)	Centrifuged, add 2 mM of methionine sulfone, 2-[N-morpholino]-ethanesulfonic acid (MES), D-Camphol-10-sulfonic acid, sodium salt, 3-aminopyrrolidine, and trimesate	TOF	[33]
Cationic and anionic metabolites	Saliva and tissue of oral cancer	For cation, 1 mol/L formic acid; for anion, ammonium acetate solution (50 mmol/L; pH 8.5)	Saliva: the same as tissue. Homogenized, centrifuged, and filtered	TOF	[37]

4 Conclusion and Perspective

Over the past decade, the applicability of CE-MS for targeted and nontargeted cancer metabolomics studies was well demonstrated. CE-MS represents a high efficiency microscale separation and identification platform for profiling of polar/ionic metabolites that is ideal for volume-restricted biological specimens with minimal sample workup. Compared to other analytical techniques employed for metabolomics studies, the application of CE-MS in this field remains rather limited, which might be due to the issues with concentration sensitivity and reproducibility However, significant progress has been made in the development of robust interfaces for coupling CE with MS over the past decade. In this context, the sheathless porous tip sprayer and the flow-through microvial interface offered new perspectives for highly sensitive metabolic profiling of biological samples [38–42], as both interfaces allowed to perform CE-MS analyses at low flow rate conditions. Moreover, the use of in-capillary preconcentration techniques, such as dynamic pH junction and transient isotachophoresis, could improve the concentration sensitivity of CE-MS for metabolomic analysis as they allowed the injection of large sample volumes. Chromatographic preconcentration techniques, using SPE, can also be used for improving the concentration sensitivity.

In order to increase the applicability of CE-MS for (clinical) metabolomics studies, the utility of CE-MS needs to be demonstrated for the analysis of large cohorts of samples. In this regard, reproducibility of migration times and peak areas is of utmost importance for a reliable comparison of metabolic profiles and to observe small changes in large sample cohorts. A promising approach to achieve reproducible CE-MS methods for metabolomic profiling of body fluids is the use of non-covalently coated capillaries. Small-volume sample consumption is another important aspect of CE-MS. Scaling down LC-MS approaches is still a challenging process, while CE, on the other hand, is a "nanoscale technique" by its nature. Therefore, the analysis of volume-limited samples remains to be an important advantage of CE-MS in the field of metabolomics. In fact, CE-MS has great potential for metabolomic analysis of individual cells [43]. To improve the sensitivity of CE-MS for single cell metabolomic analysis, an efficient ionization emitter, named as a "nanoCESI" emitter, was recently demonstrated, which had a thin-walled (~10 μm) and tapered (5–10 μm) end. The thin conductive wall enabled sheathless ionization and minimized the flow rate of ionizing sample, and the tapered end efficiently ionized analytes via ESI, providing up to 3.5-fold increase in sensitivity compared with a conventional sheathless emitter. CE-MS with such nanoCESI emitter achieved a limit of detection of 170 pM (850 zmol). Meanwhile, a sample enrichment method, large-volume dual preconcentration by isotachophoresis and stacking (LDIS), was combined with nanoCESI to achieve up to 800-fold increase of sensitivity in total when compared to normal sheathless CE-MS. By using this method for metabolome analyses of single HeLa cells, 20 amino acids were successfully quantified and 40 metabolites were identified with quadrupole-time-of-flight MS [44]. Such CE-MS-based system may have great potential to study the heterogeneity of cancer cell metabolism and cancer microenvironment.

References

1. Srivastava, A., & Creek, D. J. (2019). Discovery and validation of clinical biomarkers of cancer: A review combining metabolomics and proteomics. *Proteomics, 19*(10), e1700448.
2. Hoang, G., Udupa, S., & Le, A. (2019). Application of metabolomics technologies toward cancer prognosis and therapy. *International Review of Cell and Molecular Biology, 347*, 191–223.
3. Belinato, J. R., et al. (2018). Opportunities for green microextractions in comprehensive two-dimensional gas chromatography/mass spectrometry-based metabolomics – A review. *Analytica Chimica Acta, 1040*, 1–18.
4. Liu, W. J., et al. (2019). Advanced liquid chromatography-mass spectrometry enables merging widely targeted metabolomics and proteomics. *Analytica Chimica Acta, 1069*, 89–97.
5. Soga, T., et al. (2002). Simultaneous determination of anionic intermediates for Bacillus subtilis metabolic pathways by capillary electrophoresis electrospray

ionization mass spectrometry. *Analytical Chemistry, 74*(10), 2233–2239.
6. Garcia, A., et al. (2017). Capillary electrophoresis mass spectrometry as a tool for untargeted metabolomics. *Bioanalysis, 9*(1), 99–130.
7. Ramos-Payan, M., et al. (2018). Recent trends in capillary electrophoresis for complex samples analysis: A review. *Electrophoresis, 39*(1), 111–125.
8. Azab, S., Ly, R., & Britz-McKibbin, P. (2019). Robust method for high-throughput screening of fatty acids by multisegment injection-nonaqueous capillary electrophoresis-mass spectrometry with stringent quality control. *Analytical Chemistry, 91*(3), 2329–2336.
9. Wu, Q., et al. (2014). Pressurized CEC coupled with QTOF-MS for urinary metabolomics. *Electrophoresis, 35*(17), 2470–2478.
10. Ramautar, R., et al. (2012). Enhancing the coverage of the urinary metabolome by sheathless capillary electrophoresis-mass spectrometry. *Analytical Chemistry, 84*(2), 885–892.
11. Baidoo, E. E., et al. (2008). Capillary electrophoresis-fourier transform ion cyclotron resonance mass spectrometry for the identification of cationic metabolites via a pH-mediated stacking-transient isotachophoretic method. *Analytical Chemistry, 80*(9), 3112–3122.
12. Hirayama, A., Wakayama, M., & Soga, T. (2014). Metabolome analysis based on capillary electrophoresis-mass spectrometry. *Trac-Trends in Analytical Chemistry, 61*, 215–222.
13. Liu, C. S., et al. (1998). On-line nonaqueous capillary electrophoresis and electrospray mass spectrometry of tricyclic antidepressants and metabolic profiling of amitriptyline by Cunninghamella elegans. *Electrophoresis, 19*(18), 3183–3189.
14. Britz-McKibbin, P. (2011). Capillary Electrophoresis-Electrospray Ionization-Mass Spectrometry (CE-ESI-MS)-based metabolomics. *Metabolic Profiling: Methods and Protocols, 708*, 229–246.
15. Sun, L., et al. (2014). Over 10,000 peptide identifications from the HeLa proteome by using single-shot capillary zone electrophoresis combined with tandem mass spectrometry. *Angewandte Chemie (International Ed. in English), 53*(50), 13931–13933.
16. Amenson-Lamar, E. A., et al. (2019). Detection of 1zmol injection of angiotensin using capillary zone electrophoresis coupled to a Q-Exactive HF mass spectrometer with an electrokinetically pumped sheath-flow electrospray interface. *Talanta, 204*, 70–73.
17. Zhang, Z., et al. (2018). Production of over 27 000 peptide and nearly 4400 protein identifications by single-shot capillary-zone electrophoresis-mass spectrometry via combination of a very-low-electroosmosis coated capillary, a third-generation electrokinetically-pumped SHEATH-flow nanospray interface, an orbitrap fusion lumos tribrid mass spectrometer, and an advanced-peak-determination algorithm. *Analytical Chemistry, 90*(20), 12090–12093.
18. Liu, C. C., Zhang, J., & Dovichi, N. J. (2005). A sheath-flow nanospray interface for capillary electrophoresis/mass spectrometry. *Rapid Communications in Mass Spectrometry, 19*(2), 187–192.
19. Timischl, B., et al. (2008). Development of a quantitative, validated capillary electrophoresis-time of flight-mass spectrometry method with integrated high-confidence analyte identification for metabolomics. *Electrophoresis, 29*(10), 2203–2214.
20. Kato, M., et al. (2009). A capillary electrochromatography-electron spray ionization-mass spectrometry method for simultaneous analysis of charged and neutral constituents of a hepatocarcinoma cell metabolome. *Journal of Chromatography A, 1216*(47), 8277–8282.
21. Sun, L., et al. (2015). Third-generation electrokinetically pumped sheath-flow nanospray interface with improved stability and sensitivity for automated capillary zone electrophoresis-mass spectrometry analysis of complex proteome digests. *Journal of Proteome Research, 14*(5), 2312–2321.
22. Sarver, S. A., et al. (2017). Capillary electrophoresis coupled to negative mode electrospray ionization-mass spectrometry using an electrokinetically-pumped nanospray interface with primary amines grafted to the interior of a glass emitter. *Talanta, 165*, 522–525.
23. Hocker, O., Montealegre, C., & Neususs, C. (2018). Characterization of a nanoflow sheath liquid interface and comparison to a sheath liquid and a sheathless porous-tip interface for CE-ESI-MS in positive and negative ionization. *Analytical and Bioanalytical Chemistry, 410*(21), 5265–5275.
24. Fang, P., Pan, J. Z., & Fang, Q. (2018). A robust and extendable sheath flow interface with minimal dead volume for coupling CE with ESI-MS. *Talanta, 180*, 376–382.
25. Moini, M. (2007). Simplifying CE-MS operation. 2. Interfacing low-flow separation techniques to mass spectrometry using a porous tip. *Analytical Chemistry, 79*(11), 4241–4246.
26. Gulersonmez, M. C., et al. (2016). Sheathless capillary electrophoresis-mass spectrometry for anionic metabolic profiling. *Electrophoresis, 37*(7–8), 1007–1014.
27. Maruyama, A., et al. (2019). Extraction of aqueous metabolites from cultured adherent cells for metabolomic analysis by capillary electrophoresis-mass spectrometry. *Jove-Journal of Visualized Experiments, 148*.
28. Hirayama, A., et al. (2009). Quantitative metabolome profiling of colon and stomach cancer microenvironment by capillary electrophoresis time-of-flight mass spectrometry. *Cancer Research, 69*(11), 4918–4925.
29. Chen, J.-L., et al. (2012). Urine metabolite profiling of human colorectal cancer by capillary electrophoresis mass spectrometry based on MRB. *Gastroenterology Research and Practice, 2012*, 125890–125890.
30. Hirayama, A., Tomita, M., & Soga, T. (2012). Sheathless capillary electrophoresis-mass

spectrometry with a high-sensitivity porous sprayer for cationic metabolome analysis. *The Analyst, 137*(21), 5026–5033.

31. Alberice, J. V., et al. (2013). Searching for urine biomarkers of bladder cancer recurrence using a liquid chromatography-mass spectrometry and capillary electrophoresis-mass spectrometry metabolomics approach. *Journal of Chromatography A, 1318*, 163–170.
32. Zeng, J., et al. (2019). Comprehensive profiling by non-targeted stable isotope tracing capillary electrophoresis-mass spectrometry: A new tool complementing metabolomic analyses of polar metabolites. *Chemistry, 25*(21), 5427–5432.
33. Asai, Y., et al. (2018). Elevated polyamines in saliva of pancreatic cancer. *Cancers (Basel), 10*(2).
34. Hirayama, A., et al. (2018). Development of a sheathless CE-ESI-MS interface. *Electrophoresis, 39*(11), 1382–1389.
35. Simo, C., et al. (2011). Is metabolomics reachable? Different purification strategies of human colon cancer cells provide different CE-MS metabolite profiles. *Electrophoresis, 32*(13), 1765–1777.
36. Ibanez, C., et al. (2012). CE/LC-MS multiplatform for broad metabolomic analysis of dietary polyphenols effect on colon cancer cells proliferation. *Electrophoresis, 33*(15), 2328–2336.
37. Ishikawa, S., et al. (2016). Identification of salivary metabolomic biomarkers for oral cancer screening. *Scientific Reports, 6*, 31520.
38. Tokunaga, M., et al. (2018). Metabolome analysis of esophageal cancer tissues using capillary electrophoresis-time-of-flight mass spectrometry. *International Journal of Oncology, 52*(6), 1947–1958.
39. MacLennan, M. S., et al. (2018). Capillary electrophoresis-mass spectrometry for targeted and untargeted analysis of the sub-5 kDa urine metabolome of patients with prostate or bladder cancer: A feasibility study. *Journal of Chromatography B-Analytical Technologies in the Biomedical and Life Sciences, 1074*, 79–85.
40. Gao, P., et al. (2017). Capillary electrophoresis – Mass spectrometry metabolomics analysis revealed enrichment of hypotaurine in rat glioma tissues. *Analytical Biochemistry, 537*, 1–7.
41. Ibanez, C., et al. (2015). Metabolomics of adherent mammalian cells by capillary electrophoresis-mass spectrometry: HT-29 cells as case study. *Journal of Pharmaceutical and Biomedical Analysis, 110*, 83–92.
42. Zeng, J., et al. (2014). Metabolomics study of hepatocellular carcinoma: Discovery and validation of serum potential biomarkers by using capillary electrophoresis-mass spectrometry. *Journal of Proteome Research, 13*(7), 3420–3431.
43. Lapainis, T., Rubakhin, S. S., & Sweedler, J. V. (2009). Capillary electrophoresis with electrospray ionization mass spectrometric detection for single-cell metabolomics. *Analytical Chemistry, 81*(14), 5858–5864.
44. Kawai, T., et al. (2019). Ultrasensitive single cell metabolomics by capillary electrophoresis–mass spectrometry with a thin-walled tapered emitter and large-volume dual sample preconcentration. *Analytical Chemistry, 91*(16), 10564–10572.

NMR-Based Metabolomics in Cancer Research

Rui Hu, Tao Li, Yunhuang Yang, Yuan Tian, and Limin Zhang

1 Introduction

Cancer is a disease when abnormal cells rapidly grow and divide in an uncontrolled way and eventually invade or spread into other tissues/organs of the body. According to the World Health Organization (WHO) reports, cancer has becoming the second leading cause of death globally, causing about 9.6 million deaths in 2018 and the number will increase by 70% over the next 20 years. Lung, prostate, colorectal, stomach, and liver cancers are the most common types of cancer in men, while breast, colorectal, lung, cervix, and thyroid cancers are the most common among women (https://www.who.int/cancer/en/). Despite the advances in surgery, radiotherapy, chemotherapy, and immunotherapy, the survival rates for many solid malignancies have not significantly improved because many patients were diagnosed at late stage. Therefore, early diagnosis and correct staging of cancer diseases are critical for treatment decision making and therefore reducing the mortality rate of cancer patients. Although cancer is traditionally considered as a genetic disease, many cancer biologists now believe it is a metabolic disorder. In 1920, Otto Heinrich Warburg unveiled a link between cancer and cell metabolism [1]. It was found, under aerobic conditions, tumor tissues metabolize approximately tenfold more glucose to lactate in a given time than normal tissues, a phenomenon known as the "Warburg effect" (Fig. 1) [2]. Since then, a vast number of investigations have been focused on elucidating the cancer metabolism and understanding the metabolic reprogramming in cancer cells at different progression stages.

R. Hu · Y. Yang · L. Zhang
State Key Laboratory of Magnetic Resonance and Atomic Molecular Physics, Key Laboratory of Magnetic Resonance in Biological Systems, National Center for Magnetic Resonance in Wuhan, Wuhan National Laboratory for Optoelectronics, Wuhan Institute of Physics and Mathematics, Chinese Academy of Sciences,
Wuhan, China

T. Li
State Key Laboratory of Magnetic Resonance and Atomic Molecular Physics, Key Laboratory of Magnetic Resonance in Biological Systems, National Center for Magnetic Resonance in Wuhan, Wuhan National Laboratory for Optoelectronics, Wuhan Institute of Physics and Mathematics, Chinese Academy of Sciences, Wuhan, China

University of Chinese Academy of Sciences,
Beijing, China

Y. Tian (✉)
State Key Laboratory of Magnetic Resonance and Atomic Molecular Physics, Key Laboratory of Magnetic Resonance in Biological Systems, National Center for Magnetic Resonance in Wuhan, Wuhan National Laboratory for Optoelectronics, Wuhan Institute of Physics and Mathematics, Chinese Academy of Sciences, Wuhan, China

Department of Veterinary and Biomedical Sciences, Pennsylvania State University,
University Park, PA, USA
e-mail: yzt11@psu.edu

S. Hu (ed.), *Cancer Metabolomics*, Advances in Experimental Medicine and Biology 1280,
https://doi.org/10.1007/978-3-030-51652-9_14

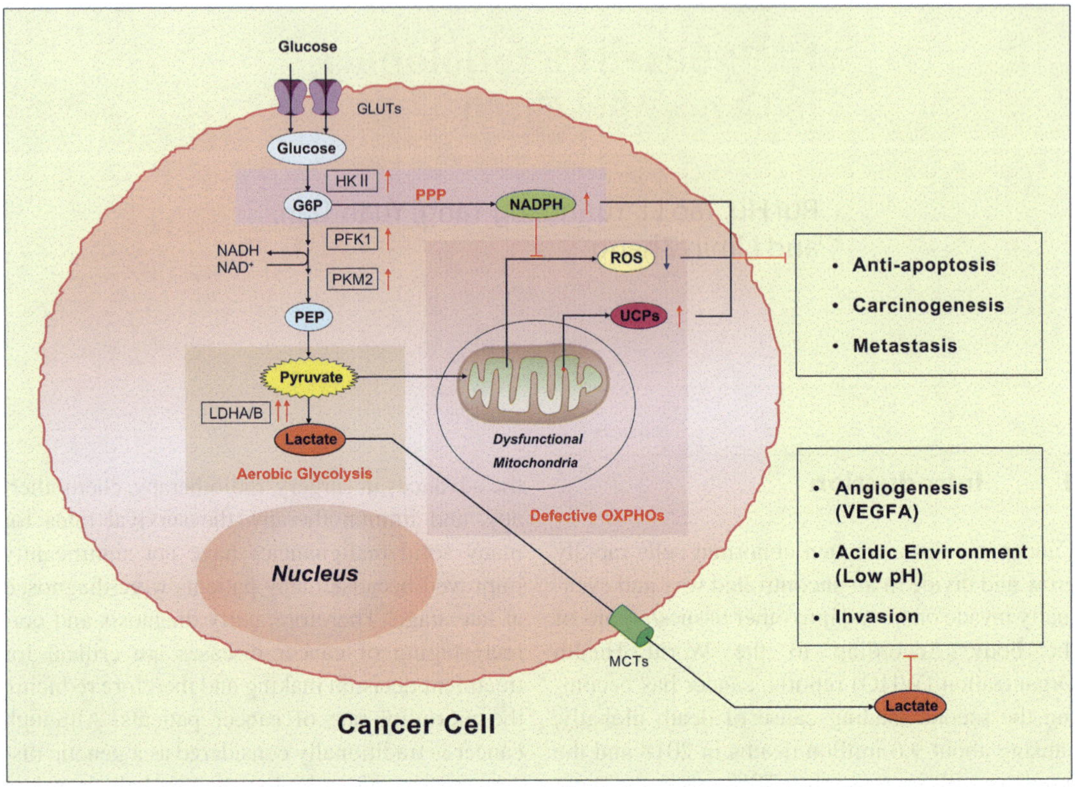

Fig. 1 The Warburg effect in cancer cells [2], reproduced with permission. As shown in this diagram, the Warburg effect is mainly induced by mitochondrial dysfunction. *NADPH*, nicotinamide adenine dinucleotide phosphate; *ROS*, reactive oxygen species; *UCPs*, uncoupling proteins; *PEP*, phosphoenolpyruvate; *GLUTs*, glucose transporters; *HK*, hexokinase; *G6P*, glucose 6 phosphate; *MCTs*, monocarboxylate transporters; *PPP*, pentose phosphate pathway; *PFK1*, phosphofructokinase-1; *LDHA/B*, lactate dehydrogenase A/B

Metabolomics, one of the omics disciplines in systems biology, is the global analysis and identification of endogenous small-molecule biochemicals (metabolites) within a biologic system. Metabolomic analysis of biofluids [3–5], tissues [6–9], and cell line models [10–12] can yield insights into the impact caused by diseases, aging [13], or external stimuli [14–18]. The two leading analytical technologies for metabolomics are mass spectrometry (MS) and nuclear magnetic resonance spectroscopy (NMR). As one of the mainstream metabolomic platforms, NMR is widely used in metabolomic analysis to identify and quantify metabolites because of its ability for quantification and nondestructive measurement of a variety of structurally different metabolites. Since in vivo NMR can be applied in high field NMR spectrometers, NMR analyses have a proven track record of translating in vitro findings into in vivo clinical applications. Moreover, NMR is highly reproducible, quantitative over a wide dynamic range, unmatched for determining unknown structures, and require minimal sample preparation in comparison with MS.

Since the first fully transistorized NMR instrument was constructed in 1960s by German physicist Gunther Laukien, NMR has been continually advanced and applied to cancer research. In 2015, ^{1}H high-resolution magic angle spinning NMR (^{1}H HRMAS NMR) spectroscopy was used to analyze the metabolic profiles of intact breast tumor tissues in comparison with intact nontumor breast tissues obtained from patients, and the results revealed phosphocholine as a biomarker of breast cancer malignant transformation

[19]. Similarly, ^{1}H-NMR-based metabolomic approach was used to profile fecal metabolites of 68 colorectal cancer (CRC) patients (stage I/II = 20, stage III = 25, and stage IV = 23) and 32 healthy controls (HC). Statistical results based on orthogonal partial least squares-discriminant analysis (OPLS-DA) indicated that each stage of CRC could be clearly distinguished from HC based on their NMR-based metabolomic profiles [20]. In 2016, typical NMR methods such as homonuclear total correlations spectroscopy (^{1}H-^{1}H TOCSY) and heteronuclear single quantum coherence spectroscopy (^{1}H-^{13}C HSQC) were used to confirm chemical shift assignment of serum metabolite signatures in lung cancer patients, and the metabolite profiles reflected the temporal discrimination between patient samples before, during, and after receiving therapy [21]. In addition, urinary ^{1}H NMR metabolomic signatures were found to serve as a suitable and noninvasive tool for prostate cancer detection [22]. According to these studies, appropriate NMR methods should be selected to optimize the metabolomic analysis of respective samples from different types of cancers.

Although MS-based approaches are more commonly used in metabolomic studies, MS and NMR offer unique strengths and can be used synergistically for a more comprehensive metabolomic analysis [23]. Despite its relatively lower sensitivity, NMR spectroscopy offers several unparalleled advantages over MS [24, 25]. NMR provides a practical means for identifying and quantifying relatively abundant compounds present in biological fluids, cells, and tissues without the need for elaborate sample preparation or fractionation. NMR can analyze the compounds that are difficult to ionize or require derivatization in MS analysis and is currently the primary method for determining the structure of an unknown compound. In addition, NMR allows to measure isotopic distributions in metabolites. By means of stable isotopic labeling, NMR can be used to elucidate the kinetics and mechanisms of metabolite conversion and to explore the localization of metabolic pathways. Finally, site-specific NMR imaging and spectroscopy provide an important method for metabolomics studies in vivo.

2 NMR-Based Metabolomic Approach

Figure 2 shows an overview of NMR-based metabolomic analysis workflow. The main steps in NMR-based metabolomic analysis are experi-

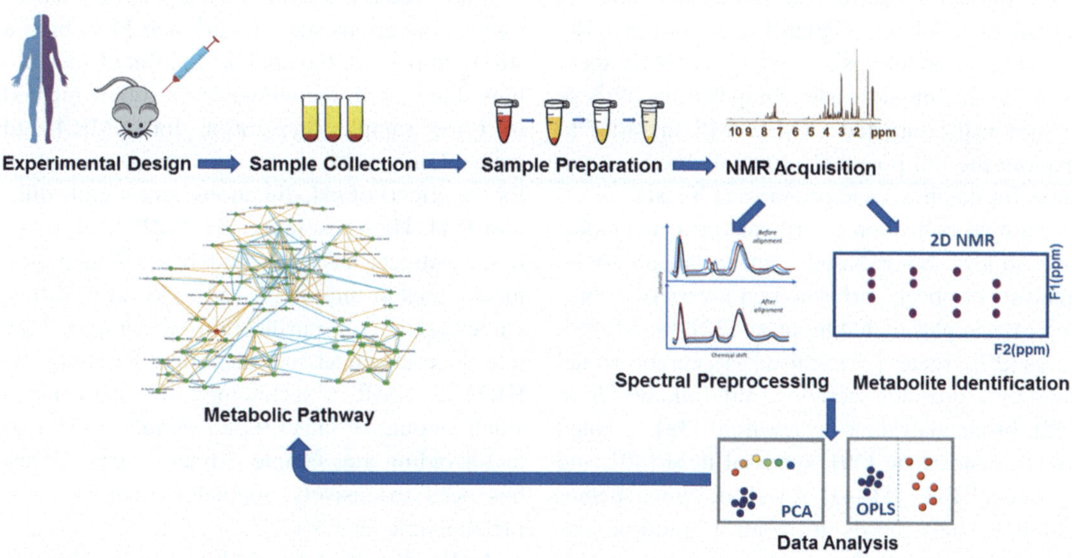

Fig. 2 The basic workflow of NMR-based metabolomics

mental design, NMR sample collection and preparation, spectra acquisition and processing, metabolite identification and statistical data analysis, and data interpretation including a search for biomarkers or pathways associated with a specific disease. Since multiple options exist for each step in the workflow, it is essential to choose appropriate protocol for each metabolomic analysis in order to obtain most robust and valid results.

2.1 Experimental Design and Sample Collection

The ultimate goal of most metabolomic analysis in cancer research is to discover cancer-specific diagnostic, prognostic, or predictive biomarkers. Metabolomics approaches can be categorized as either targeted or untargeted. Untargeted metabolomics studies, as a hypothesis generation strategy, aim to profile the greatest number of metabolites and trace both known and unknown metabolic changes [26, 27]. Targeted approaches focus on one or more metabolites of known or interest, in order to investigate specific metabolic pathways or to validate identified biomarkers [28, 29]. The combination of targeted and untargeted analyses can also be applied to obtaining a more comprehensive and accurate metabolome profiling. For instance, Tian et al. analyzed the global metabolomic signatures of human CRC and thyroid nodule tissues using ^{1}H NMR spectroscopy and the fatty acid compositions of these tissues using targeted GC-FID/MS in order to explore the full potential of metabolomic signatures for diagnosis and prognosis [30, 31].

Sample collection is critical for a metabolomic study. NMR-based cancer metabolomic analysis has been performed on a variety of biological samples including urine [32], blood [33], feces [20], tissues [31], saliva [34], cerebrospinal fluid [35], prostatic secretion [36], follicular fluid [37], bronchoalveolar lavage fluid [38], exhaled breath condensate [39], synovial fluid [40], and cancer cell lines [41–43]. A well-designed metabolomics study needs to control multiple cofounding factors such as gender, age, diet, fasting state, and lifestyle, which may introduce variations or possibly systematic bias into the results. Moreover, the collection and storage of samples should have minimal or no effect on the metabolome of the sample being studied. Notably, these biological samples, especially tissues, should be rapidly quenched when the metabolic pathways with a high metabolic flux in cancer cells are studied (e.g., the glycol tic and TCA pathways).

2.2 Sample Preparation and Data Acquisition

Sample preparation for a metabolomic experiment depends on the study goals. Urine and blood are typical biofluids used for cancer clinical metabolomics studies [44–47]. For metabolite profiling of serum or plasma samples, how to alleviate the interference from the massive amount of serum/plasma proteins is a major challenge. Traditionally, a water-presaturated Carr-Purcell-Meiboom-Gill (CPMG) pulse sequence by adjusting the spin-spin relaxation delays ($2n\tau$ ~100 ms) is used for macromolecule signal suppression in blood samples [47–49]. Recent studies suggested a new protein precipitation approach for blood metabolite quantitation using ^{1}H NMR analysis and enabled the identification of 67 blood metabolites, of which ~ one third are new compared with those reported previously [50]. For the urine samples, the pH and concentrations of cations such as Ca^{2+} and Mg^{2+} have a strong impact on the chemical shifts of metabolites. Jiang et al. recommended a robust method of urine sample preparation for NMR-based metabolomic analysis taking into consideration for the effects of pH, di-cations, and sample dilution [51]. High-resolution ^{1}H NMR analysis of tissue extracts has been widely used to profile metabolites in tumors [52–54]. However, different extraction or purification of samples may introduce chemical modifications. Recently, ^{1}H HRMAS NMR, a technology for analyzing a small amount of intact tissue samples (~15 mg) and avoiding any sample extraction procedures, has been extensively applied to cancer tissue metabolomic analysis [27, 30, 31].

NMR signals of metabolites can be obtained by different NMR pulse sequences. The majority of NMR-based metabolomics analyses are conducted using two 1D pulse sequences, Nuclear Overhauser Enhancement Spectroscopy (NOESY) and CPMG.1D NOESY with presaturation, which have been applied to biological samples including blood [50], urine [51], feces [55], cells [43], and tissues [31], due to its ability to greatly suppress the water peak without intensity losses for most of the other peaks. As mentioned above, CPMG with presaturation by adjusting the spin-spin relaxation delays is usually used to remove the broad protein signals for blood samples [47–49]. Correspondingly, the diffusion-edited spectra have been applied to acquire the information from macromolecules such as lipids, lipoproteins, and long-chain fatty acids according to their diffusion coefficient [56, 57]. Furthermore, the stable isotope tracer methods, such as ^{13}C NMR [58], ^{15}N NMR [59], and ^{31}P NMR [60], have also been widely applied to track metabolic flux analysis in cancer research.

2.3 Metabolite Assignment and Data Analysis

Metabolite assignment is another crucial step in metabolomics study. A great deal of useful information can be derived from 1D ^1H NMR spectra including chemical shifts, spin-spin coupling, the half bandwidth, and the signal intensities. However, too many overlapping peaks represent a major problem for ^1H NMR analysis of biological samples due to its narrow spectral width. To overcome the signal overlap, 2D NMR methods have been developed to improve metabolite assignment based on the atomic connectivity. Among them, 2D ^1H J-resolved NMR spectroscopy (JRES), ^1H-^1H correlation spectroscopy (COSY), ^1H-^1H total correlation spectroscopy (TOCSY), ^1H-^{13}C heteronuclear single quantum correlation (HSQC), and ^1H-^{13}C heteronuclear multiple bond correlation (HMBC) experiments are commonly applied to metabolite identification [61, 62]. Various databases including the Human Metabolome Database (HMDB) [63], the Madison Metabolomics Consortium Database (MMCD) [64], the Biological Magnetic Resonance Bank (BMRB) [65], and the Birmingham Metabolite Library (BML) [66] provide thousands of standard NMR spectra of endogenous metabolites as references. Moreover, some commercial software packages, such as the Chenomx NMR Suite, also offer library database [67].

The data processing steps for NMR spectra are as follows: phase correction, baseline correction, peak alignment, chemical shift calibration, binning, data normalization, and scaling [68]. After spectra and data preprocessing, the multivariate data analysis is performed to extract variables that may be informative about the metabolic differences between groups. Principal component analysis (PCA), an unsupervised method, is initially applied to show intergroup differences and the possible presence of outliers [69]. Subsequently, supervised data analysis methods including projection to latent structure discriminant analysis (PLS-DA) and orthogonal projection to latent structure discriminant analysis (OPLS-DA) are used for further data mining in the search for biomarkers [70]. Recently, Duan et al. developed a useful high-throughput analysis method based on multiple univariate data (MUDA) to extract statistically significant findings on metabolites [71, 72], which is particularly useful when only limited variables (metabolites) are significant. Moreover, receiver operating characteristic (ROC) curve analysis has often been applied to evaluating the sensitivity, specificity, and accuracy of a diagnostic test (e.g., a panel of metabolite biomarkers), particularly in cancer studies [30, 31].

2.4 Interpretation and Validation

Data visualization is a new challenge for analysis of omics data, particularly metabolomics data. Software tools, including R package [73], MATLAB [48, 55], and MetaboAnalyst [74, 75], are available for comprehensive NMR-based metabolomic data analysis, interpretation, and integration with other omics data. In 1993, Merchant et al. developed a correlation coefficient loading plot generated from the OPLS-DA models, which were color-coded with the

Pearson linear correlation coefficients of variables using an in house-written script with MATLAB. In these loading plots, the warm-colored variables meant more significant contributions to intergroup differentiations than cool-colored ones [60].

Once potential diagnostic or prognostic biomarkers are identified, the target needs to be validated: (i) Validation should include repeating the same findings among at least one independent cohort of samples. (ii) Validation could also be performed with cell line or animal models or on human samples to achieve full mechanistic understanding of the disease and the altered metabolic pathways. (iii) In certain cases, validation studies could be performed using stable isotope tracer method to verify the metabolic flux through specific metabolic pathways. For example, ^{13}C-labeled glucose have been evaluated in cancer cell lines including liver cancer [76], colorectal cancer [77], and breast cancer [78] to monitor glucose pathways during interventions.

3 NMR-Based Cancer Metabolomics

The metabolic characteristics of cancer cells refer to the alterations in cellular metabolism and related pathways when compared to normal cells. Typical alterations in cancer cells include: (i) deregulated uptake of glucose and amino acids, (ii) use of opportunistic modes of nutrient acquisition, (iii) use of glycolysis/TCA cycle intermediates for biosynthesis and NADPH production, (iv) increased demand for nitrogen, (v) alterations in metabolite-driven gene regulation, and (vi) metabolic interactions with the microenvironment [79]. Accumulating evidence suggests that the metabolic reprogramming characteristics can be used as a clinical tool for cancer diagnostics, prognostics, and intervention monitoring [30, 31, 47, 72]. Here, an overview of NMR-based cancer metabolomics applications is presented according to the biological matrices used for metabolomic analysis (Figs. 3 and 4).

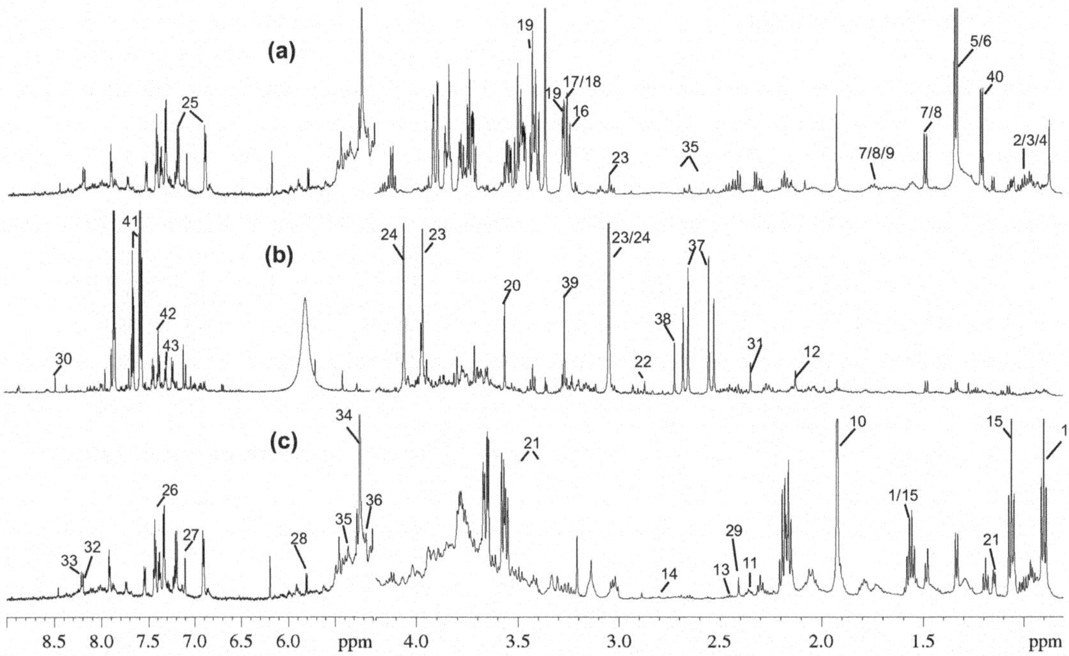

Fig. 3 Representative 600 MHz ^1H NMR spectra of (**a**) serum, (**b**) urine, and (**c**) stool originating from the same CRC cancer patient. Identities: 1, butyrate; 2, isoleucine; 3, leucine; 4, valine; 5, lactate; 6, threonine; 7, alanine; 8, lysine; 9, arginine; 10, acetate; 11, glutamate; 12, methionine; 13, glutamine; 14, aspartate; 15, propionate; 16, choline; 17, phosphocholine (PC); 18, glycerophosphocholine (GPC); 19, taurine; 20, glycine; 21, α-ketoisovalerate; 22, trimethylamine (TMA); 23, creatine; 24, creatinine; 25, tyrosine; 26, phenylalanine; 27, histidine; 28, uracil; 29, succinate; 30, formate; 31, pyruvate; 32, adenine; 33, inosine; 34, glucose; 35, galactose; 36, fucose; 37, citrate; 38, dimethylamine (DMA); 39, trimethylamine-N-oxide (TMAO); 40, 3-hydroxybutyrate; 41, hippurate; 42, indoxyl sulfate; 43, phenylacetylglycine

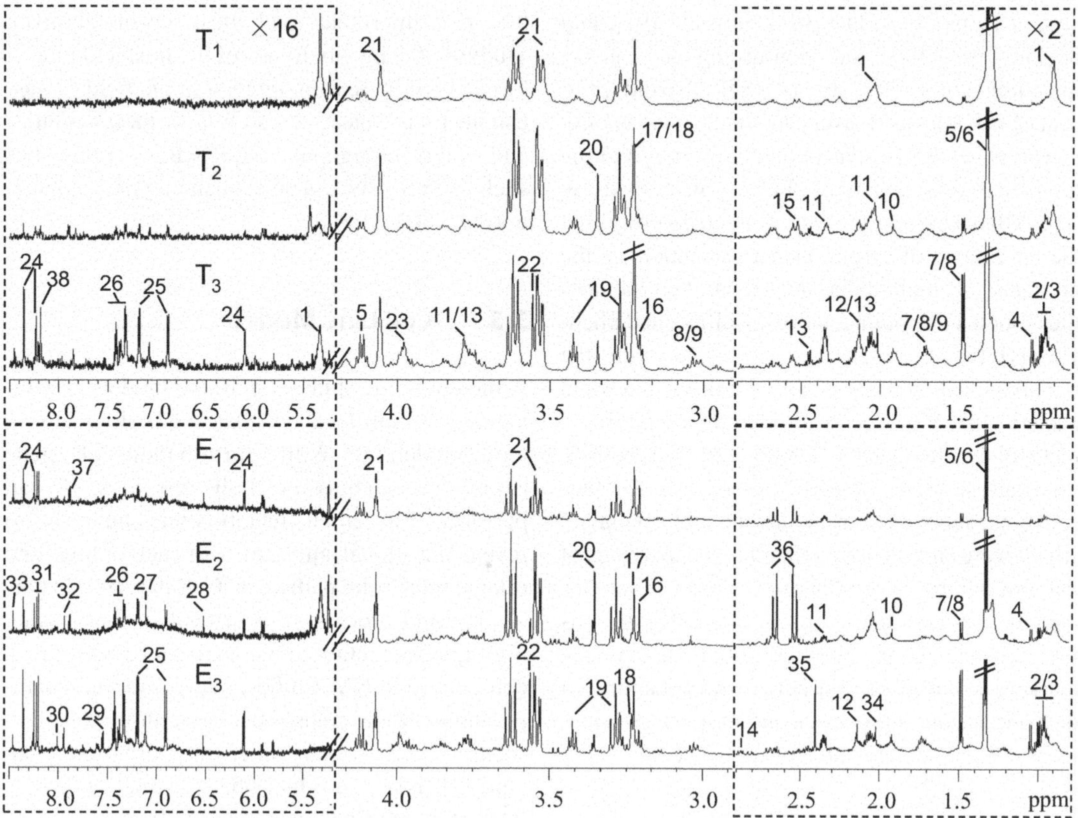

Fig. 4 Representative 600 MHz ^{1}H spectra of intact thyroid tissue (T) and tissue aqueous extracts (E) originating from healthy adjacent thyroid tissue (T1, E1), benign thyroid lesion (T2, E2), and malignant thyroid lesion (T3, E3). Identities: 1, lipid; 2, isoleucine; 3, leucine; 4, valine; 5, lactate; 6, threonine; 7, alanine; 8, lysine; 9, arginine; 10, acetate; 11, glutamate; 12, methionine; 13, glutamine; 14, aspartate; 15, glutathione (GSH); 16, choline; 17, phosphocholine (PC); 18, glycerophosphocholine (GPC); 19, taurine; 20, *scyllo*-inositol; 21, *myo*-inositol; 22, glycine; 23, phosphoethanolamine (PE); 24, inosine; 25, tyrosine; 26, phenylalanine; 27, histidine; 28, fumarate; 29, uracil; 30, guanosine; 31, hypoxanthine; 32, xanthine; 33, formate; 34, acetamide; 35, succinate; 36, citrate; 37, uridine; 38, U1. (Reproduced with permission from Yuan Tian 2015 [30])

3.1 Biofluids

Blood and urine are typical biofluids used in cancer metabolomic analysis due to simple and noninvasive sample collection. NMR-based metabolomic analysis of blood samples has been successfully applied to identifying metabolite signatures associated with cancer risk, detection, and prognosis in various cancer studies including lung cancer [80–82], CRC [83, 84], breast cancer [85], pancreatic cancer [86], thyroid cancer [87], prostate cancer [88], and head and neck cancer [89]. For example, Rocha et al. summarized a systemic serum metabolic signatures for lung cancer including enhanced glycolysis, glutaminolysis, and gluconeogenesis, together with suppressed TCA cycle and reduced lipid catabolism, which were presented at initial disease stages and could be related to known cancer biochemical hallmarks [81]. Fan et al. used [U-^{13}C]-glucose as a tracer for ^{13}C isotopomer-based metabolomic analysis of lung cancer by NMR and gas chromatography-mass spectrometry (GC-MS). The results revealed accelerated glycolysis and altered capacity of the TCA cycle and anaplerotic pyruvate carboxylation pathways in tumor tissues [90].

Due to its nature of noninvasiveness, low cost, and minimal time demand, measurement of urinary biomarkers using NMR has been demonstrated for the detection of cancers of urological system including kidney [91], prostate [92], and bladder [93, 94] and non-urological cancers including colon [32], breast [85], thyroid [87], ovary [95], lung [85], liver [96], and pancreas [53]. Srivastava et al. demonstrated that urinary taurine is a potential biomarker of bladder cancer by using ^{1}H NMR spectroscopy [97]. It is noteworthy that the alterations of certain urinary metabolites, the products of mammalian-microbial "co-metabolites" such as hippurate, indoxyl sulfate, and phenylacetylglycine, might be associated with the modulation of activity or population of intestinal bacteria [48, 98]. Lee et al. identified 25 urinary metabolites involved in amino acid metabolism, especially aromatic or sulfur amino acids, and bioactive nutrients, such as isoflavone and riboflavin, which were significantly related to the activities of gut microflora by comparing pseudo germ-free rats to conventionally raised rats [99]. In this regard, focusing on those potential urinary biomarkers would lead to a better understanding of host and bacterial processes aiding in the development of therapeutic treatment for cancers.

3.2 Stool Samples

Metabolomic analysis of stool samples has been applied to a wide range of diseases, especially for CRC cancer [100, 20, 101]. In one of the first fecal metabolomic studies of CRC, Bezabeh et al. analyzed the metabolomes of stool samples from 500 CRC patients using ^{1}H NMR coupled with statistical classification strategy and demonstrated that ^{1}H NMR-based stool metabolomic analysis has the potential to be used as an effective screening tool in aiding diagnosis for CRC [100]. Lin et al. used ^{1}H NMR-based metabolomics to analyze fecal metabolites from CRC patients and identified distinct metabolites involved in the disruption of normal bacterial ecology, malabsorption of nutrients, and increased glycolysis and glutaminolysis [20]. The fecal metabolic profiles of healthy controls can be distinguished from CRC patients, even in the early stage (stage I/II), highlighting the potential utility of NMR-based fecal metabolomic fingerprints as predictors for early diagnosis of CRC [20]. Notably, stool metabolomic analysis could provide a wide array of information that reflects the gut microbial and host co-metabolism. Studying the metabolomes of the host and microbiome is of increasing interest in the field of gastrointestinal cancer research with metabolomics and high-throughput sequencing approaches such as 16S rRNA gene sequencing and metagenomics [101–103].

3.3 Cell Line Models

A metabolomic study of cell line models is valuable for system-level analysis and biological system modeling. With perturbation of gene expression, such as metabolic enzymes, we can perform differential metabolomic analysis to reveal the global alterations in metabolites and related metabolic pathways. Cellular sample harvesting and processing is critical for harnessing high-quality metabolomic analysis results. From cell culture to NMR tubes, many important sample preparation steps, such as culture medium washing, cell scraping, quenching in liquid nitrogen, cell lysis, and dual phase extraction procedure of metabolites are required [104].

Nittoli et al. studied the effects of alpha-zearalenol (α-zol) on the metabolomic profiles of an estrogen-positive breast cancer cell line, MCF-7, and estrogen-negative breast cancer cell line, MDA-MB-231. They evaluated cell cycle progression, levels of reactive oxygen species (ROS), and metabolomic profiling of MCF-7 and MDA-MB-231 cells before and after 72-h treatment using ^{1}H-NMR techniques. The results showed that α-zol was able to increase the protein biosynthesis as well as lipid metabolism in MCF-7 cells and, hence, to induce estrogen-positive breast cancer progression [105]. Ilaria et al. reported the analysis of the endo-metabolomes of human colon cancer cells (HCT116) by NMR and investigated DNA G-quadruplex ligands as novel anticancer drugs. The study demonstrated an optimized protocol for NMR-based metabolomic analysis of adherent mammalian cell lines and its application to validate anticancer treatment [106]. The study of cell lines by NMR-based metabolomics represents a powerful tool for understanding how local metabolism and biochemical pathways are influenced by external or internal stimuli.

3.4 Cancer Tissues

Cancer tissue metabolomics is a useful tool for studying the abnormal metabolism of human malignancies including CRC [31], thyroid cancer [30], liver cancer [27], breast cancer [85], prostate cancer [107], bone cancer [108], gastric cancer [109], brain cancer [109], and lung cancer [52]. There are different methods for metabolite determination in cancer tissues by NMR. The main ones include in vivo magnetic resonance spectroscopy, liquid high-resolution proton NMR spectroscopy, and high-resolution magic angle spinning (HRMAS ^{1}H-NMR). Each of the above methods has its own advantages and disadvantages and complements each other. The combined use of these methods allows a more comprehensive understanding of the various physiological and biochemical pathways involved in cancer initiation and progression.

Schmahl et al. systematically analyzed NMR-based metabolic profiles of urine, serum, feces, and pancreatic tissues from mice with pancreatic tumors and identified the potential biomarkers including decreased 3-indoxylsulfate, benzoate, and citrate in urine; decreased glucose, choline, and lactate in blood; and decreased phenylalanine and benzoate and increased acetoin in fecal extracts [53]. Recently, HRMAS ^{1}H-NMR analysis of intact tissue metabolic profiles ex vivo has shown great potential for cancer research due to the nondestructive nature of this technique [27, 30, 31]. Tian et al. analyzed the metabolomic signatures of 50 human CRC tissues and their adjacent noninvolved tissues (ANIT) using HRMAS ^{1}H-NMR spectroscopy and demonstrated that tissue metabolic phenotypes not only discriminated CRC from ANIT but also distinguished low-grade tumors (stages I–II) from high-grade ones (stages III–IV) with high sensitivity and specificity [31]. Moreover, Tian et al. used ^{1}H NMR to analyze the metabolic profiles of thyroid tissues and their extracts from thyroid lesion patients. The findings showed that thyroid lesions are accompanied with disturbances of multiple metabolic pathways, including alterations in energy metabolism (glycolysis, lipid, and TCA cycle), protein turnover, nucleotide biosynthesis, as well as phosphatidylcholine biosynthesis [30].

4 Challenge and Innovation

NMR-based metabolomics has shown its strengths and played an important role in cancer research. However, several aspects of NMR-based metabolomic analysis remain to be improved, including sample preparation, data processing and analysis, and detection sensitivity. Innovative methods are being developed to address these challenges to achieve a more comprehensive metabolomic analysis.

4.1 Sample Preparation

Conventional NMR sample tubes have certain limitation for metabolomic analysis of trace amounts of samples, as these tubes are generally 5 mm in diameter and their sample size requirement is at least 500 μl. For small volume of clinical samples, NMR detection may not be feasible while diluted samples might not reach the NMR detection limit. Even if a nuclear magnetic tube with diameters of 3 and 1.7 mm is used, the cost is high, and sample recovery and NMR tube cleaning are difficult. In addition, for samples with high salt concentration or viscosity, the use of existing conventional nuclear magnetic tubes directly affects NMR signal collection, affecting the accuracy of NMR analysis. Therefore, a variety of NMR tubes were developed and dedicated to microscale samples to ensure NMR analysis of biological samples without sample dilution [110].

4.2 High-Resolution Microcoil NMR

For scarce samples of natural products, impurities or degradants of pharmaceuticals, or disease tissues, conventional 5 mm probes are not well suited for the task of acquiring NMR data [111]. The use of microcoil probes is an effective means to increase NMR sensitivity of particularly mass or volume-limited samples. Based on the principle of reciprocity, described by Hoult and Richards [112], it has been shown that the sensitivity of an NMR coil is inversely proportional to its diameter for a constant length-to-diameter ratio [113]. As shown in Eq. 1 [114], ω_0 is the

Larmor frequency, B_1 is the magnitude of the oscillation magnetic field produced by the radio frequency pulse per unit of current i, V_s is the sample volume, and V_{noise} is the noise of the receiver coil and associated circuits. The term B_1/i is referred to as the quality of an NMR probe.

$$S/N = \eta \frac{\omega_0^{\,2} \frac{B_1}{i} V_s}{V_{\text{noise}}} \qquad (1)$$

For a solenoidal coil, the term $B1/i$ from Eq. 1 can also be defined as below:

$$\frac{B_1}{i} = \frac{\mu_0 n}{d\sqrt{1+\left[h/d\right]^2}} \qquad (2)$$

As shown in Eq. 2, μ_0 is the permeability of free space, n is the number of turns in the solenoid coil, h is the coil length, and d is the coil diameter. From Eq. 2 [115], it can be concluded that, for a constant h/d ratio, the coil sensitivity increases as diameter decreases. This is the fundamental premise that has driven the development of solenoidal microcoil NMR probes for improving sensitivity in measurements of mass or volume-limited samples, which indicates that when the detection coli is sufficiently miniaturized, the sample volume can even be reduced to nanoliters.

Another improvement in the signal-to-noise ratio (*S/N*) level has been achieved by cooling the coil, producing cryogenic coils. As shown in Eqs. 3 and 4 [116], the most important factor in determining the *S/N* or the sensitivity of an NMR experiment in an NMR probe, insofar as the hardware itself is concerned, is the coil temperature, T_c [111]. Temperature control is a major contributor to V_{noise} reduction. These equations show the inversely proportional relationship of sensitivity and temperature.

$$V_{\text{noise}} = \sqrt{4k_b T_c R_{\text{noise}} \Delta f} \qquad (3)$$

$$R_{\text{noise}} = \frac{1}{p}\sqrt{\frac{\mu\mu_0\omega_0\rho(T_c)}{2}} \qquad (4)$$

The parameters and experimental results are summarized for different probes in Table 1 [117]. For a conventional room temperature (RT) probe, a 3 mm probe will result in a 40% increase in mass sensitivity compared with a 5 mm conventional probe, while a 1.7 mm microcoil probe demonstrates a twofold increased sensitivity over a 5 mm probe and a 1 mm probe by fourfold increased sensitivity. In addition, a 5 mm cryoprobe shows a fivefold enhancement over its conventional counterpart and a 1.7 mm cryoprobe shows a mass sensitivity almost 20-fold higher than a 5 mm RT probe. The development of microcoil and cryoprobes will significantly promote the applications of NMR-based metabolomics [111].

4.3 LC with NMR

Improved NMR detection efficiency on a small amount of sample can be achieved by the online combination of liquid separation techniques with NMR. For example, solid-phase extraction (SPE), capillary electrophoresis (CE), liquid chromatography (LC), and capil-

Table 1 Comparison of the detection sensitivity of various probes [117]

Probe type[a]	Total volume[b] (mL)	Relative volume (%)	Typical SNR[c] at 500 MHz	Scaled SNR[d] SNR/vol.	Relative SNR (%)
5.0 mm RT	0.55	100.0	900	900.0	100.0
3.0 mm RT	0.19	34.5	430	1244.7	138.3
1.7 mm RT	0.03	5.4	100	1833.3	203.7
1.0 mm	0.005	0.9	34	3740.0	415.5
5.0 mm cryo	0.55	100.0	4500	4500.0	500.0
1.7 mm cryo	0.035	6.4	900	14142.9	1571.4

[a]*RT* room temperature
[b]Total volume refers to the optimal filling volume of samples
[c]SNR values shown are typical performances of such probes and do not represent specifications
[d]Scaled SNR represents the mass sensitivity of a probe

lary electrochromatography (CEC) can be combined for metabolomic analysis of small amounts of samples. In fact, LC-NMR originated in the 1980s [118], but LC-NMR is far less popular than LC-MS. LC-NMR requires to overcome two major difficulties. First is the low detection sensitivity of NMR and the second is that LC elution solvent causes serious interference in NMR detection. A schematic diagram of an LC-NMR system is shown in Fig. 5 [119]. After decades of development of NMR instruments and experimental methods, higher field strength NMR instruments have emerged, with more advanced NMR probes designed, and more sophisticated pulse sequence technology developed. These advances have largely solved the problems of low detection sensitivity and solvent compatibility with detection in LC-NMR, which has led to the rapid increase in LC-NMR applications. LC-NMR can be used for the identification of drug metabolites, including polar or unstable metabolites. Spraul et al. lyophilized the urine samples of an experimenter taking the anti-inflammatory drug ibuprofen and then identified its metabolites using HPLC-NMR [120]. Later, the same method has been used to analyze the second-stage metabolites of ibuprofen in animal urine. Akira et al. have used LC-NMR to identify a tauric acid metabolite in a hereditary hypertensive rat and found that this hypotensive-related taurine metabolite was more abundant in the urine of hereditary hypertensive rats than normal rats [121].

4.4 Optimization of Data Processing

Despite the fact that high field strength and microcoil probes are effective to improve NMR analysis, data processing is also critical for obtaining meaningful results with NRM-based metabolomic analysis. In NMR spectra, baseline correction is used to remove low-frequency artifacts or altera-

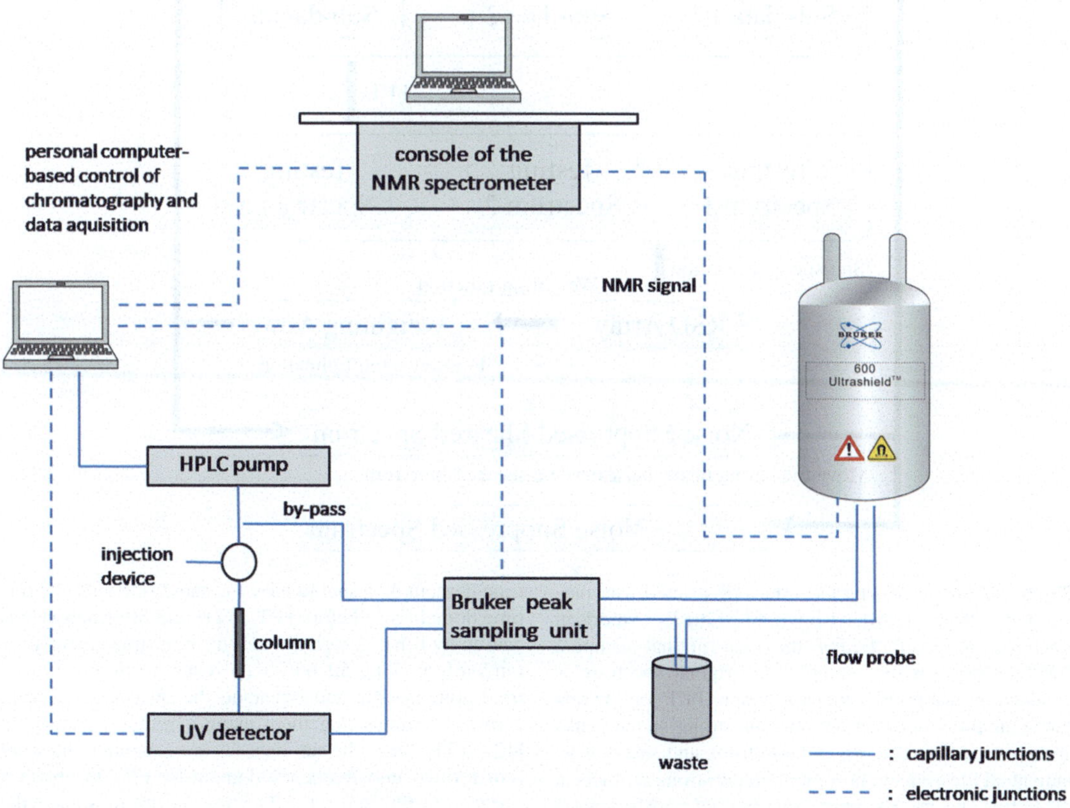

Fig. 5 Instrument configuration for analytical LC-NMR analysis

tions caused by experimental and instrumental variation [122–124]. After baseline correction, the application of high-frequency filters may be necessary to remove electronic noise present in the data that is generated by the measurement equipment [125]. In 2013, Bin Jiang et al. developed an effective approach for simultaneous noise and artifact suppression in NMR spectroscopy [126]. This is called NASR (noise and artifact suppression using resampling), based on resampling, a category of statistical learning methods that uses subsets to derive robust estimates of statistical parameters [127]. NASR is an effective approach for suppressing both noise and nonuniform sampling artifacts and for enhancing the S/N ratio in 1D and 2D-NMR spectroscopy [126] (Fig. 6).

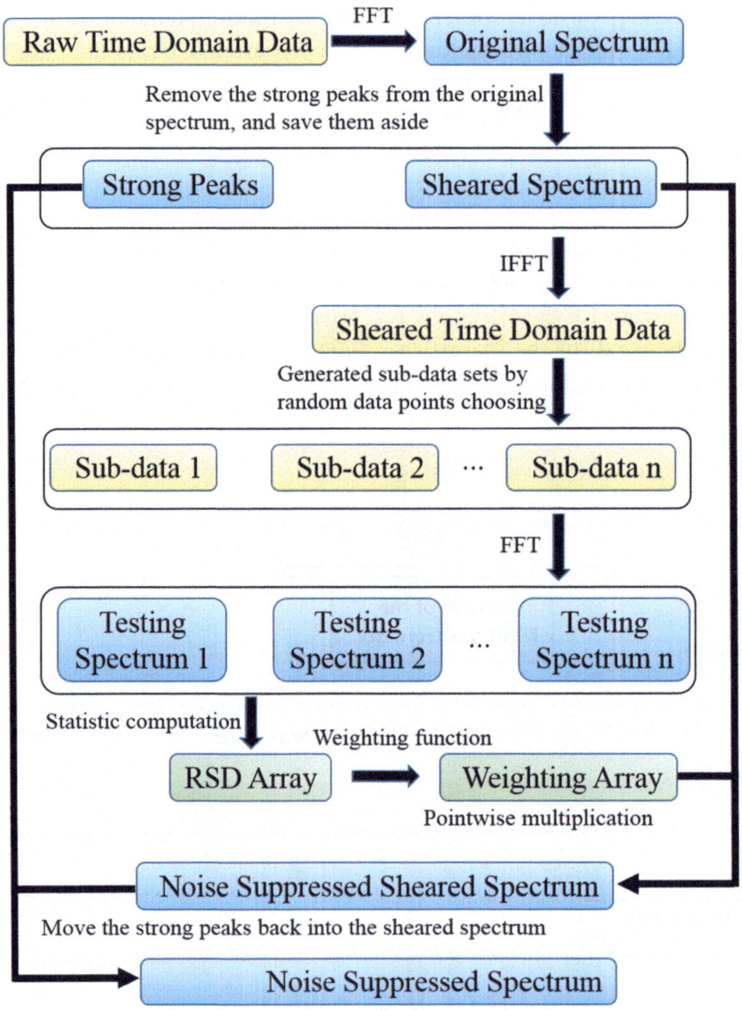

Fig. 6 NASR processing procedure (Reprinted with permissions from [126]. Copyright (2013) American Chemical Society). Taking the conventional sampled NMR experiment for example, an original spectrum is obtained by fast Fourier transformation (FFT) on the raw time domain data. Then the obvious strong signal peaks are removed from the original spectrum, and saved as an individual file aside, to prevent inducing strong artifacts in the testing spectra. By inverse fast Fourier transformation (IFFT), the sheared spectrum is transformed into time domain, called sheared time domain data. The sheared time domain data should have the same size with the raw time domain data before FFT, to prevent information loss caused by IFFT. A series of sub-datasets are generated by randomly picking 50–65% data points from the sheared time domain data and replacing the missing ones with zero or compensating them using a gridding algorithm [132, 133]. Once the sub-datasets are generated, they are transformed into frequency domain by FFT to obtain a series of testing spectra. All testing spectra must have the same size with the original spectrum

In addition, NMR spectra of biofluids contain many background signals that could be noisy and overlapped, due to the existence of hundreds of metabolites [128]. Under these circumstances, the identification and quantification of certain metabolites is a complicated task. Therefore, precise data processing and statistical analysis are required to obtain useful and reliable information from these metabolic profiles. Nowadays, there are many software programs available for statistical analysis of the metabolomic NMR datasets. In 2009, MetaboAnalyst was first released, which is a very popular interface for processing NMR data [75]. The same authors also developed another data analysis software called MetaboMiner to identify metabolites in 2D-NMR spectra [129]. In 2011, MetaboLab was developed to facilitate NMR data processing by providing automated algorithms for the processing a series of spectra in a reproducible fashion [130]. In addition, MetaboHunter is a Web server application aimed at identifying metabolites in 1H-NMR spectra in an automated manner [131]. These powerful analytical tools have greatly promoted the applications of NMR-based metabolomics.

5 Conclusion

In comparison with MS, conventional NMR suffers from relatively low sensitivity. However, the new advances, including high field instruments, microcoil and cryoprobes, LC-NMR, and data analysis tools, have been made to improve NMR sensitivity for metabolomic analysis. NMR is user independent, highly reproducible, nonselective, and nondestructive and allows to analyze metabolite structure, concentration, and even metabolic flux, particularly the identification and quantification of unknown metabolites. Owing to the complexity of biological and clinical samples, a combination of NMR and MS may be required for a more comprehensive metabolomic analysis, facilitating our in-depth understanding of the metabolic reprogramming in cancers.

References

1. Warburg, O. (1920). The reduction of salpeter acid in green cells. *Naturwissenschaften, 8*, 594–596.
2. Fu, Y., Liu, S., Yin, S., et al. (2017). The reverse Warburg effect is likely to be an Achilles' heel of cancer that can be exploited for cancer therapy. *Oncotarget, 8*(34), 57813.
3. Barton, R. H., Nicholson, J. K., Elliott, P., et al. (2008). High-throughput 1H NMR-based metabolic analysis of human serum and urine for large-scale epidemiological studies: Validation study. *International Journal of Epidemiology, 37*(Suppl 1), i31–i40.
4. Fonville, J. M., Maher, A. D., Coen, M., et al. (2010). Evaluation of full-resolution J-resolved 1H NMR projections of biofluids for metabonomics information retrieval and biomarker identification. *Analytical Chemistry, 82*(5), 1811–1821.
5. Schicho, R., Nazyrova, A., Shaykhutdinov, R., et al. (2010). Quantitative metabolomic profiling of serum and urine in DSS-induced ulcerative colitis of mice by (1)H NMR spectroscopy. *Journal of Proteome Research, 9*(12), 6265–6273.
6. Beckonert, O., Coen, M., Keun, H. C., et al. (2010). High-resolution magic-angle-spinning NMR spectroscopy for metabolic profiling of intact tissues. *Nature Protocols, 5*(6), 1019–1032.
7. Cheng, L. L., Burns, M. A., Taylor, J. L., et al. (2005). Metabolic characterization of human prostate cancer with tissue magnetic resonance spectroscopy. *Cancer Research, 65*(8), 3030–3034.
8. Somashekar, B. S., Kamarajan, P., Danciu, T., et al. (2011). Magic angle spinning NMR-based metabolic profiling of head and neck squamous cell carcinoma tissues. *Journal of Proteome Research, 10*(11), 5232–5241.
9. Want, E. J., Masson, P., Michopoulos, F., et al. (2013). Global metabolic profiling of animal and human tissues via UPLC-MS. *Nature Protocols, 8*(1), 17–32.
10. Ackerstaff, E., Pflug, B. R., Nelson, J. B., et al. (2001). Detection of increased choline compounds with proton nuclear magnetic resonance spectroscopy subsequent to malignant transformation of human prostatic epithelial cells. *Cancer Research, 61*(9), 3599–3603.
11. Martineau, E., Tea, I., Loaec, G., et al. (2011). Strategy for choosing extraction procedures for NMR-based metabolomic analysis of mammalian cells. *Analytical and Bioanalytical Chemistry, 401*(7), 2133–2142.
12. Sellick, C. A., Hansen, R., Stephens, G. M., et al. (2011). Metabolite extraction from suspension-cultured mammalian cells for global metabolite profiling. *Nature Protocols, 6*(8), 1241–1249.
13. Gu, H. W., Pan, Z. Z., Xi, B. W., et al. (2009). H-1 NMR metabolomics study of age profiling in children. *NMR in Biomedicine, 22*(8), 826–833.

14. Assfalg, M., Bertini, I., Colangiuli, D., et al. (2008). Evidence of different metabolic phenotypes in humans. *Proceedings of the National Academy of Sciences of the United States of America, 105*(5), 1420–1424.
15. Lindon, J. C., Holmes, E., & Nicholson, J. K. (2004). Metabonomics and its role in drug development and disease diagnosis. *Expert Review of Molecular Diagnostics, 4*(2), 189–199.
16. Martin, F. P., Sprenger, N., Montoliu, I., et al. (2010). Dietary modulation of gut functional ecology studied by fecal metabonomics. *Journal of Proteome Research, 9*(10), 5284–5295.
17. Yap, I. K., Li, J. V., Saric, J., et al. (2008). Metabonomic and microbiological analysis of the dynamic effect of vancomycin-induced gut microbiota modification in the mouse. *Journal of Proteome Research, 7*(9), 3718–3728.
18. Zhao, L., Nicholson, J. K., Lu, A., et al. (2012). Targeting the human genome-microbiome axis for drug discovery: Inspirations from global systems biology and traditional Chinese medicine. *Journal of Proteome Research, 11*(7), 3509–3519.
19. Maria, R. M., Altei, W. F., Andricopulo, A. D., et al. (2015). Characterization of metabolic profile of intact non-tumor and tumor breast cells by high-resolution magic angle spinning nuclear magnetic resonance spectroscopy. *Analytical Biochemistry, 488*, 14–18.
20. Lin, Y., Ma, C. C., Liu, C. K., et al. (2016). NMR-based fecal metabolomics fingerprinting as predictors of earlier diagnosis in patients with colorectal cancer. *Oncotarget, 7*(20), 29454–29464.
21. Hao, D., Sarfaraz, M. O., Farshidfar, F., et al. (2016). Temporal characterization of serum metabolite signatures in lung cancer patients undergoing treatment. *Metabolomics: Official Journal of the Metabolomic Society, 12*, 58.
22. Capati, A., Ijare, O. B., & Bezabeh, T. (2017). Diagnostic applications of nuclear magnetic resonance-based urinary metabolomics. *Magnetic Resonance Insights, 10*. 1178623X17694346.
23. Markley, J. L., Bruschweiler, R., Edison, A. S., et al. (2017). The future of NMR-based metabolomics. *Current Opinion in Biotechnology, 43*, 34–40.
24. Fan, T. W. M., & Lane, A. N. (2016). Applications of NMR spectroscopy to systems biochemistry. *Progress in Nuclear Magnetic Resonance Spectroscopy, 92–93*, 18–53.
25. Nagana Gowda, G. A., & Raftery, D. (2015). Can NMR solve some significant challenges in metabolomics? *Journal of Magnetic Resonance (San Diego, Calif: 1997), 260*, 144–160.
26. Jayaraman, A., Kumar, P., Marin, S., et al. (2018). Untargeted metabolomics reveals distinct metabolic reprogramming in endothelial cells co-cultured with CSC and non-CSC prostate cancer cell subpopulations. *PLoS One, 13*(2).
27. Yang, Y. X., Li, C. L., Nie, X., et al. (2007). Metabonomic studies of human hepatocellular carcinoma using high-resolution magic-angle spinning H-1 NMR spectroscopy in conjunction with multivariate data analysis. *Journal of Proteome Research, 6*(7), 2605–2614.
28. Mpanga, A. Y., Siluk, D., Jacyna, J., et al. (2018). Targeted metabolomics in bladder cancer: From analytical methods development and validation towards application to clinical samples. *Analytica Chimica Acta, 1037*, 188–199.
29. Wang, W. C., Yang, J., Edin, M. L., et al. (2019). Targeted metabolomics identifies the cytochrome P450 monooxygenase eicosanoid pathway as a novel therapeutic target of Colon tumorigenesis. *Cancer Research, 79*(8), 1822–1830.
30. Tian, Y., Nie, X., Xu, S., et al. (2015). Integrative metabonomics as potential method for diagnosis of thyroid malignancy. *Scientific Reports, 5*.
31. Tian, Y., Xu, T. P., Huang, J., et al. (2016). Tissue metabonomic phenotyping for diagnosis and prognosis of human colorectal cancer. *Scientific Reports, 6*.
32. Wang, Z. N., Lin, Y., Liang, J. H., et al. (2017). NMR-based metabolomic techniques identify potential urinary biomarkers for early colorectal cancer detection. *Oncotarget, 8*(62), 105819–105831.
33. Lecuyer, L., Bala, A. V., Deschasaux, M., et al. (2018). NMR metabolomic signatures reveal predictive plasma metabolites associated with long-term risk of developing breast cancer. *International Journal of Epidemiology, 47*(2), 484–494.
34. Ishikawa, S., Sugimoto, M., Kitabatake, K., et al. (2016). Identification of salivary metabolomic biomarkers for oral cancer screening. *Scientific Reports, 6*, 31520.
35. Locasale, J. W., Melman, T., Song, S. S., et al. (2012). Metabolomics of human cerebrospinal fluid identifies signatures of malignant glioma. *Molecular & Cellular Proteomics, 11*(6).
36. Kline, E. E., Treat, E. G., Averna, T. A., et al. (2006). Citrate concentrations in human seminal fluid and expressed prostatic fluid determined via H-1 nuclear magnetic resonance spectroscopy outperform prostate specific antigen in prostate cancer detection. *Journal of Urology, 176*(5), 2274–2279.
37. Morelli, M. A. C., Iuliano, A., Schettini, S. C. A., et al. (2018). NMR metabolomics study of follicular fluid in women with cancer resorting to fertility preservation. *Journal of Assisted Reproduction and Genetics, 35*(11), 2063–2070.
38. Hu, J. Z., Rommereim, D. N., Minard, K. R., et al. (2008). Metabolomics in lung inflammation: A high-resolution H-1 NMR study of mice exposed to silica dust. *Toxicology Mechanisms and Methods, 18*(5), 385–398.
39. Montuschi, P., Paris, D., Melck, D., et al. (2012). NMR spectroscopy metabolomic profiling of exhaled breath condensate in patients with stable and unstable cystic fibrosis. *Thorax, 67*(3), 222–228.
40. Anderson, J. R., Chokesuwattanaskul, S., Phelan, M. M., et al. (2018). H-1 NMR metabolomics

identifies underlying inflammatory pathology in osteoarthritis and rheumatoid arthritis synovial joints. *Journal of Proteome Research, 17*(11), 3780–3790.
41. Liu, Z. G., Wang, L. M., Zhang, L. M., et al. (2016). Metabolic characteristics of 16HBE and A549 cells exposed to different surface modified gold Nanorods. *Advanced Healthcare Materials, 5*(18), 2363–2375.
42. Ruiz-Aracama, A., Peijnenburg, A., Kleinjans, J., et al. (2011). An untargeted multi-technique metabolomics approach to studying intracellular metabolites of HepG2 cells exposed to 2,3,7,8-tetrachlorodi benzo-p-dioxin. *BMC Genomics, 12*, 251.
43. Zhang, L. M., Wang, L. M., Hu, Y. L., et al. (2013). Selective metabolic effects of gold nanorods on normal and cancer cells and their application in anticancer drug screening. *Biomaterials, 34*(29), 7117–7126.
44. Kim, K., Aronov, P., Zakharkin, S. O., et al. (2009). Urine metabolomics analysis for kidney cancer detection and biomarker discovery. *Molecular & Cellular Proteomics, 8*(3), 558–570.
45. Nishiumi, S., Kobayashi, T., Ikeda, A., et al. (2012). A novel serum metabolomics-based diagnostic approach for colorectal cancer. *PLoS One, 7*(7), e40459.
46. Slupsky, C. M., Steed, H., Wells, T. H., et al. (2010). Urine metabolite analysis offers potential early diagnosis of ovarian and breast cancers. *Clinical Cancer Research, 16*(23), 5835–5841.
47. Zhang, X. Y., Wang, Y. L., Hao, F. H., et al. (2009). Human serum metabonomic analysis reveals progression axes for glucose intolerance and insulin resistance statuses. *Journal of Proteome Research, 8*(11), 5188–5195.
48. Tian, Y., Nichols, R. G., Cai, J. W., et al. (2018). Vitamin A deficiency in mice alters host and gut microbial metabolism leading to altered energy homeostasis. *Journal of Nutritional Biochemistry, 54*, 28–34.
49. Zhang, L. M., Ye, Y. F., An, Y. P., et al. (2011). Systems responses of rats to aflatoxin B1 exposure revealed with metabonomic changes in multiple biological matrices. *Journal of Proteome Research, 10*(2), 614–623.
50. Gowda, G. A. N., Gowda, Y. N., & Raftery, D. (2015). Expanding the limits of human blood metabolite quantitation using NMR spectroscopy. *Analytical Chemistry, 87*(1), 706–715.
51. Jiang, L. M., Huang, J., Wang, Y. L., et al. (2012). Eliminating the dication-induced intersample chemical-shift variations for NMR-based biofluid metabonomic analysis. *Analyst, 137*(18), 4209–4219.
52. Rocha, C. M., Barros, A. S., Goodfellow, B. J., et al. (2015). NMR metabolomics of human lung tumours reveals distinct metabolic signatures for adenocarcinoma and squamous cell carcinoma. *Carcinogenesis, 36*(1), 68–75.
53. Schmahl, M. J., Regan, D. P., Rivers, A. C., et al. (2018). NMR-based metabolic profiling of urine, serum, fecal, and pancreatic tissue samples from the Ptf1a-Cre; LSL-KrasG12D transgenic mouse model of pancreatic cancer. *PLoS One, 13*(7), e0200658.
54. Wu, H. F., Southam, A. D., Hines, A., et al. (2008). High-throughput tissue extraction protocol for NMR- and MS-based metabolomics. *Analytical Biochemistry, 372*(2), 204–212.
55. Tian, Y., Zhang, L. M., Wang, Y. L., et al. (2012). Age-related topographical metabolic signatures for the rat gastrointestinal contents. *Journal of Proteome Research, 11*(2), 1397–1411.
56. Allen, J., Zhang, J. T., Quickel, M. D., et al. (2018). Ron receptor signaling ameliorates hepatic fibrosis in a diet-induced nonalcoholic steatohepatitis mouse model. *Journal of Proteome Research, 17*(9), 3268–3280.
57. Zhang, L. M., Hatzakis, E., Nichols, R. G., et al. (2015). Metabolomics reveals that aryl hydrocarbon receptor activation by environmental chemicals induces systemic metabolic dysfunction in mice. *Environmental Science & Technology, 49*(13), 8067–8077.
58. Wan, Q. F., Wang, Y. L., & Tang, H. R. (2017). Quantitative C-13 traces of glucose fate in hepatitis B virus -infected hepatocytes. *Analytical Chemistry, 89*(6), 3293–3299.
59. Blundell, C. D., DeAngelis, P. L., Day, A. J., et al. (2004). Use of N-15-NMR to resolve molecular details in isotopically-enriched carbohydrates: Sequence-specific observations in hyaluronan oligomers up to decasaccharides. *Glycobiology, 14*(11), 999–1009.
60. Merchant, T. E., Degraaf, P. W., Minsky, B. D., et al. (1993). Esophageal cancer phospholipid characterization by P-31 NMR. *NMR in Biomedicine, 6*(3), 187–193.
61. Dai, H., Xiao, C. N., Liu, H. B., et al. (2010a). Combined NMR and LC-DAD-MS analysis reveals comprehensive metabonomic variations for three phenotypic cultivars of Salvia miltiorrhiza Bunge. *Journal of Proteome Research, 9*(3), 1565–1578.
62. Dai, H., Xiao, C. N., Liu, H. B., et al. (2010b). Combined NMR and LC-MS analysis reveals the metabonomic changes in Salvia miltiorrhiza Bunge induced by water depletion. *Journal of Proteome Research, 9*(3), 1460–1475.
63. Wishart, D. S., Tzur, D., Knox, C., et al. (2007). HMDB: The human metabolome database. *Nucleic Acids Research, 35*, D521–D526.
64. Cui, Q., Lewis, I. A., Hegeman, A. D., et al. (2008). Metabolite identification via the madison metabolomics consortium database. *Nature Biotechnology, 26*(2), 162–164.
65. Ulrich, E. L., Akutsu, H., Doreleijers, J. F., et al. (2008). BioMagResBank. *Nucleic Acids Research, 36*, D402–D408.

66. Ludwig, C., Easton, J. M., Lodi, A., et al. (2012). Birmingham metabolite library: A publicly accessible database of 1-D H-1 and 2-D H-1 J-resolved NMR spectra of authentic metabolite standards (BML-NMR). *Metabolomics: Official journal of the Metabolomic Society, 8*(1), 8–18.
67. Ellinger, J. J., Chylla, R. A., Ulrich, E. L., et al. (2013). Databases and software for NMR-based metabolomics. *Current Metabolomics, 1*, 28–40.
68. Brennan, L. (2014). NMR-based metabolomics: From sample preparation to applications in nutrition research. *Progress in Nuclear Magnetic Resonance Spectroscopy, 83*, 42–49.
69. Lever, J., Krzywinski, M., & Atman, N. (2017). Points of significance principal component analysis. *Nature Methods, 14*(7), 641–642.
70. Trygg, J., & Wold, S. (2002). Orthogonal projections to latent structures (O-PLS). *Journal of Chemometrics, 16*(3), 119–128.
71. Duan, Y. X., An, Y. P., Li, N., et al. (2013). Multiple univariate data analysis reveals the inulin effects on the high-fat-diet induced metabolic alterations in rat myocardium and testicles in the preobesity state. *Journal of Proteome Research, 12*(7), 3480–3495.
72. Xu, S., Tian, Y., Hu, Y. L., et al. (2016). Tumor growth affects the metabonomic phenotypes of multiple mouse non-involved organs in an A549 lung cancer xenograft model. *Scientific Reports, 6*, 28057.
73. Rodriguez-Martinez, A., Posma, J. M., Ayala, R., et al. (2018). MWASTools: An R/bioconductor package for metabolome-wide association studies. *Bioinformatics, 34*(5), 890–892.
74. Chong, J., Soufan, O., Li, C., et al. (2018). MetaboAnalyst 4.0: Towards more transparent and integrative metabolomics analysis. *Nucleic Acids Research, 46*(W1), W486–W494.
75. Xia, J. G., & Wishart, D. S. (2011). Web-based inference of biological patterns, functions and pathways from metabolomic data using MetaboAnalyst. *Nature Protocols, 6*(6), 743–760.
76. Sun, L. C., Song, L. B., Wan, Q. F., et al. (2015). cMyc-mediated activation of serine biosynthesis pathway is critical for cancer progression under nutrient deprivation conditions. *Cell Research, 25*(4), 429–444.
77. Abrantes, A. M., Tavares, L. C., Pires, S., et al. (2014). Metabolic effects of hypoxia in colorectal cancer by C-13 NMR isotopomer analysis. *BioMed Research International, 2014*, 1–10.
78. Harris, T., Degani, H., & Frydman, L. (2013). Hyperpolarized C-13 NMR studies of glucose metabolism in living breast cancer cell cultures. *NMR in Biomedicine, 26*(12), 1831–1843.
79. Pavlova, N. N., & Thompson, C. B. (2016). The emerging hallmarks of cancer metabolism. *Cell Metabolism, 23*(1), 27–47.
80. Hu, J. M., & Sun, H. T. (2018). Serum proton NMR metabolomics analysis of human lung cancer following microwave ablation. *Radiation Oncology, 13*, 40.
81. Rocha, C. M., Carrola, J., Barros, A. S., et al. (2011). Metabolic signatures of lung cancer in biofluids: NMR-based metabonomics of blood plasma. *Journal of Proteome Research, 10*(9), 4314–4324.
82. Weljie, A. M., Newton, J., Mercier, P., et al. (2006). Targeted profiling: Quantitative analysis of H-1 NMR metabolomics data. *Analytical Chemistry, 78*(13), 4430–4442.
83. Farshidfar, F., Weljie, A. M., Kopciuk, K., et al. (2012). Serum metabolomic profile as a means to distinguish stage of colorectal cancer. *Genome Medicine, 4*, 42.
84. Gu, J. P., Xiao, Y. Q., Shu, D., et al. (2019). Metabolomics analysis in serum from patients with colorectal polyp and colorectal cancer by H-1-NMR spectrometry. *Disease Markers*.
85. Singh, A., Sharma, R. K., Chagtoo, M., et al. (2017). H-1 NMR metabolomics reveals association of high expression of inositol 1, 4, 5 trisphosphate receptor and metabolites in breast cancer patients. *PLoS One, 12*, 1.
86. Michalkova, L., Hornik, S., Sykora, J., et al. (2018). Diagnosis of pancreatic cancer via(1)H NMR metabolomics of human plasma. *Analyst, 143*(24), 5974–5978.
87. Wojtowicz, W., Zabek, A., Deja, S., et al. (2017). Serum and urine H-1 NMR-based metabolomics in the diagnosis of selected thyroid diseases. *Scientific Reports, 7*, 1–13.
88. Gomez-Cebrian, N., Rojas-Benedicto, A., Albors-Vaquer, A., et al. (2019). Metabolomics contributions to the discovery of prostate cancer biomarkers. *Metabolites, 9*(3), 48.
89. Yonezawa, K., Nishiumii, S., Kitamoto-Matsuda, J., et al. (2013). Serum and tissue metabolomics of head and neck cancer. *Cancer Genomics & Proteomics, 10*(5), 233–238.
90. Fan, T. W. M., Lane, A. N., Higashi, R. M., et al. (2009). Altered regulation of metabolic pathways in human lung cancer discerned by C-13 stable isotope-resolved metabolomics (SIRM). *Molecular Cancer, 8*, 41.
91. Ganti, S., & Weiss, R. H. (2011). Urine metabolomics for kidney cancer detection and biomarker discovery. *Urologic Oncology-Seminars and Original Investigations, 29*(5), 551–557.
92. Lima, A. R., Bastos, M. D., Carvalho, M., et al. (2016). Biomarker discovery in human prostate cancer: An update in metabolomics studies. *Translational Oncology, 9*(4), 357–370.
93. Cao, M., Zhao, L. C., Chen, H. G., et al. (2012). NMR-based metabolomic analysis of human bladder cancer. *Analytical Sciences, 28*(5), 451–456.
94. Cheng, X. M., Liu, X. Y., Liu, X., et al. (2018). Metabolomics of non-muscle invasive bladder cancer: Biomarkers for early detection of bladder cancer. *Frontiers in Oncology, 8*, 494.

95. Turkoglu, O., Zeb, A., Graham, S., et al. (2016). Metabolomics of biomarker discovery in ovarian cancer: A systematic review of the current literature. *Metabolomics: Official journal of the Metabolomic Society, 12*(4).
96. Cartlidge, C. R., Abellona, U. M. R., Alkhatib, A. M. A., et al. (2017). The utility of biomarkers in hepatocellular carcinoma: Review of urine-based H-1-NMR studies – What the clinician needs to know. *International Journal of General Medicine, 10*, 431–442.
97. Srivastava, S., Roy, R., Singh, S., et al. (2010). Taurine – a possible fingerprint biomarker in non-muscle invasive bladder cancer: A pilot study by H-1 NMR spectroscopy. *Cancer Biomarkers, 6*(1), 11–20.
98. Tian, Y., Cai, J. W., Gui, W., et al. (2019). Berberine directly affects the gut microbiota to promote intestinal farnesoid X receptor activation. *Drug Metabolism and Disposition, 47*(2), 86–93.
99. Lee, S. H., An, J. H., Park, H. M., et al. (2012). Investigation of endogenous metabolic changes in the urine of pseudo germ-free rats using a metabolomic approach. *Journal of Chromatography B, Analytical Technologies in the Biomedical and Life Sciences, 887*, 8–18.
100. Bezabeh, T., Somorjai, R., Dolenko, B., et al. (2009). Detecting colorectal cancer by H-1 magnetic resonance spectroscopy of fecal extracts. *NMR in Biomedicine, 22*(6), 593–600.
101. Weir, T. L., Manter, D. K., Sheflin, A. M., et al. (2013). Stool microbiome and metabolome differences between colorectal cancer patients and healthy adults. *PLoS One, 8*(8), e70803.
102. Osman, M. A., Neoh, H. M., Ab Mutalib, N. S., et al. (2018). 16S rRNA gene sequencing for deciphering the colorectal cancer gut microbiome: Current protocols and workflows. *Frontiers in Microbiology, 9*, 767.
103. Wang, Z., Zolnik, C. P., Qiu, Y. P., et al. (2018). Comparison of fecal collection methods for microbiome and metabolomics studies. *Frontiers in Cellular and Infection Microbiology, 8*, 301.
104. Van Gulik, W. M., Canelas, A. B., Taymaz-Nikerel, H., et al. (2012). Fast sampling of the cellular metabolome. *Methods in Molecular Biology (Clifton, NJ), 881*, 279–306.
105. Nittoli, A. C., Costantini, S., Sorice, A., et al. (2018). Effects of alpha-zearalenol on the metabolome of two breast cancer cell lines by 1H-NMR approach. *Metabolomics: Official journal of the Metabolomic Society, 14*(3), 33.
106. Lauri, I., Savorani, F., Iaccarino, N., et al. (2016). Development of an optimized protocol for NMR metabolomics studies of human Colon Cancer Cell lines and first insight from testing of the protocol using DNA G-Quadruplex ligands as novel anti-cancer drugs. *Metabolites, 6*(1), 4.
107. Lima, A. R., Pinto, J., Bastos, M. D., et al. (2018). NMR-based metabolomics studies of human prostate cancer tissue. *Metabolomics: Official Journal of the Metabolomic Society, 14*(7), 88.
108. Martinez-Lopez, F. J., Banuelos-Hernandez, A. E., Becerra-Martinez, E., et al. (2017). H-1 NMR metabolomic signatures related to giant cell tumor of the bone. *RSC Advances, 7*(72), 45385–45392.
109. Wang, H. J., Zhang, H. L., Deng, P. C., et al. (2016). Tissue metabolic profiling of human gastric cancer assessed by H-1 NMR. *BMC Cancer, 16*, 371.
110. Hofmann, M., & Braumann, E. U. (2004). *NMR microsample holder which allows safe and simple exchanges of the sample tube*. Google Patents.
111. Martin, G. E. (2005). Small-volume and high-sensitivity NMR probes. In G. A. Webb (Ed.), *Annual reports on NMR spectroscopy* (Annual Reports on NMR Spectroscopy) (Vol. 56, pp. 1–96). San Diego: Elsevier Academic Press Inc. https://doi.org/10.1016/s0066-4103(05)56001-0.
112. Hoult, D. I., & Richards, R. E. (1976). Signal-to-noise ratio of nuclear magnetic-resonance experiment. *Journal of Magnetic Resonance, 24*(1), 71–85.
113. Wu, N. A., Peck, T. L., Webb, A. G., et al. (1994). H-1-NMR spectroscopy on the nanoliter scale for static and online measurements. *Analytical Chemistry, 66*(22), 3849–3857.
114. Webb, A. G. (1997). Radiofrequency microcoils in magnetic resonance. *Progress in Nuclear Magnetic Resonance Spectroscopy, 31*, 1–42.
115. Lacey, M. E., Subramanian, R., Olson, D. L., et al. (1999). High-resolution NMR spectroscopy of sample volumes from 1 nL to 10 μL. *Chemical Reviews, 99*(10), 3133–3152.
116. Molinski, T. F. (2009). Nanomole-scale natural products discovery. *Current Opinion in Drug Discovery & Development, 12*(2), 197–206.
117. Anklin, C. (2016). Chapter 3 Small-volume NMR: Microprobes and cryoprobes. In *Modern NMR approaches to the structure elucidation of natural products: Volume 1: Instrumentation and software* (Vol. 1, pp. 38–57). The Royal Society of Chemistry. https://doi.org/10.1039/9781849735186-00038.
118. Bayer, E., Albert, K., Nieder, M., et al. (1982). On-line coupling of liquid chromatography and high-field nuclear magnetic resonance spectrometry. *Analytical Chemistry, 54*(11), 1747–1750.
119. Albert, K. (1999). Liquid chromatography-nuclear magnetic resonance spectroscopy. *Journal of Chromatography A, 856*(1–2), 199–211.
120. Spraul, M., Hofmann, M., Dvortsak, P., et al. (1993). High-performance liquid chromatography coupled to high-field proton nuclear magnetic resonance spectroscopy: Application to the urinary metabolites of ibuprofen. *Analytical Chemistry, 65*(4), 327–330.
121. Akira, K., Mitome, H., Imachi, M., et al. (2010). LC-NMR identification of a novel taurine-related metabolite observed in 1H NMR-based metabonomics of genetically hypertensive rats. *Journal of Pharmaceutical and Biomedical Analysis, 51*(5), 1091–1096.

122. Smith, C. A., Want, E. J., O'Maille, G., et al. (2006). XCMS: Processing mass spectrometry data for metabolite profiling using nonlinear peak alignment, matching, and identification. *Analytical Chemistry, 78*(3), 779–787.
123. Xi, Y. X., & Rocke, D. M. (2008). Baseline correction for NMR spectroscopic metabolomics data analysis. *BMC Bioinformatics, 9*, 10.
124. Zhang, Z. M., Chen, S., & Liang, Y. Z. (2010). Baseline correction using adaptive iteratively reweighted penalized least squares. *Analyst, 135*(5), 1138–1146.
125. Alonso, A., Marsal, S., & Julia, A. (2015). Analytical methods in untargeted metabolomics: State of the art in 2015. *Frontiers in Bioengineering and Biotechnology, 3*, 23.
126. Jiang, B., Luo, F., Ding, Y., et al. (2013). NASR: An effective approach for simultaneous noise and artifact suppression in NMR spectroscopy. *Analytical Chemistry, 85*(4), 2523–2528.
127. Chaubey, Y. P. (2000). Resampling methods: A practical guide to data analysis. *Technometrics, 42*(3), 311–311.
128. Puchades-Carrasco, L., Palomino-Schatzlein, M., Perez-Rambla, C., et al. (2016). Bioinformatics tools for the analysis of NMR metabolomics studies focused on the identification of clinically relevant biomarkers. *Briefings in Bioinformatics, 17*(3), 541–552.
129. Xia, J. G., Bjorndahl, T. C., Tang, P., et al. (2008). MetaboMiner – Semi-automated identification of metabolites from 2D NMR spectra of complex biofluids. *BMC Bioinformatics, 9*, 16.
130. Ludwig, C., & Gunther, U. L. (2011). MetaboLab–advanced NMR data processing and analysis for metabolomics. *BMC Bioinformatics, 12*, 366.
131. Tulpan, D., Leger, S., Belliveau, L., et al. (2011). MetaboHunter: An automatic approach for identification of metabolites from H-1-NMR spectra of complex mixtures. *BMC Bioinformatics, 12*, 22.
132. Jiang, B., Jiang, X. W., Xiao, N., et al. (2010). Gridding and fast Fourier transformation on non-uniformly sparse sampled multidimensional NMR data. *Journal of Magnetic Resonance, 204*(1), 165–168.
133. Osullivan, J. D. (1985). A fast sinc function gridding algorithm for fourier inversion in computer-tomography. *IEEE Transactions on Medical Imaging, 4*(4), 200–207.

Regulation of Glycolysis in Head and Neck Cancer

Sibi Raj, Ashok Kumar, and Dhruv Kumar

1 Introduction

Head and neck squamous cell carcinoma (HNSCC) is currently the sixth leading cancer worldwide [1]. Most head and neck cancers arise in the epithelial cells of the oral cavity, larynx, oropharynx, and hypopharynx mainly associated with the lifestyle risk factors like alcohol and tobacco [2, 3]. Several strains of human papilloma virus are also known to induce HNSCCs in human population [4]. Metabolic reprogramming in HNSCC, specifically glucose metabolism, is a key feature in oncogenesis [5]. A classic example of metabolic reprogramming in cancer cells was explained by Otto Warburg in the 1920s with the term aerobic glycolysis [6]. Majority of cancer cells depend on high rate of glycolysis because of impaired mitochondria for their survival and growth [7]. The mitochondrial damage and hypoxia condition in cancer cells lead to activation of glycolytic genes such as glucose transporter-1 and hexokinase-II which alter the normal cellular metabolism [8, 9]. Under normal conditions cells undergo aerobic glycolysis and produce two adenosine triphosphates (ATPs), and the end-product of glycolysis, pyruvate, is utilized in mitochondrial respiration (OXPHO) to produce 36 ATPs [10, 11]. While the HNSCCs exposed to hypoxia increase the import of glucose from the tumor microenvironment so that the cancer cells could maintain a balance of energy and aggressively perform glycolysis, it generates less ATPs than OXPHOS [12].

The conversion of glucose into pyruvate by various glycolytic enzymes in HNSCC helps the cancer cells to meet major cellular needs by building intermediates for anabolic reactions, such as the formation of fatty acids, amino acids, and nucleotides. In glycolysis, the key reactions catalyzed by the enzymes hexokinase, phosphofructokinase, and pyruvate kinase are majorly upregulated in cancer cells, leading to the generation of intermediate metabolites for the biosynthetic pathways such as pentose phosphate pathway, serine biosynthesis, glutaminolysis, and glyceraldyhyde-3phosphate pathway for the production of amino acids, nucleotides, and lipids for the growth and survival of cancer cells [13, 14].

Several mutations in genes such as *EGFR*, *NOTCH*, *PI3K*, *PTEN*, and *Akt* have been commonly reported in HNSCC. Mutations in these pathway create abnormal metabolic and mitogenic signaling in HNSCC [15]. Tweardy et al. reported that EGFR is most commonly overexpressed and mutated in HNSCC, and 91%

S. Raj · D. Kumar (✉)
Amity Institute of Molecular Medicine & Stem Cell Research, Amity University,
Noida, Uttar Pradesh, India
e-mail: dkumar13@amity.edu

A. Kumar
Department of Biochemistry, All India Institute of Medical Sciences (AIIMS),
Bhopal, Madhya Pradesh, India

S. Hu (ed.), *Cancer Metabolomics*, Advances in Experimental Medicine and Biology 1280,
https://doi.org/10.1007/978-3-030-51652-9_15

of HNSCC have increased levels of transforming growth factor-α (TGF-α), an EGFR ligand [16]. EGFR-VIII, a constitutively active mutant, increased cell movement and invasion. Activated EGFR leads to activation of several downstream signaling pathways which include RAS/RAF/MEK (MAPK), PI3K/Akt, and JAK/STAT-3 [17]. Studies by Makinoshima et al. showed that EGFR signaling induces increased glucose metabolism by producing metabolites in glycolysis pathway and pentose phosphate pathway (PPP) by regulating glucose transport via GLUT3 expression [18]. Mutation in p53 gene is one of the first detected and highly found in 50–80% cases of HNSCC. P53 controls the cellular metabolism by regulating glycolysis and mitochondrial respiration by transcriptional regulation of its downstream gene TP53-induced glycolysis regulator (TIGAR) [19]. TP53 mutation is found in high rates in HNSCC and is associated with the increased use of tobacco and alcohol leading to increased risk of progression to cancer [20, 21]. Studies by Agrawal et al. [22] showed from whole-exome sequencing that NOTCH 1 gene as the second most mutated gene in HNSCC [22]. Recent studies have shown that 60–70% of HNSCC patients have aberrant NOTCH pathway. Hyper-activated Notch signaling upregulates glycolysis by the activation of the PI3K/Akt serine/threonine kinase pathway, whereas hypo-activated NOTCH signaling weakens the mitochondrial activity and induces glycolysis in a p53-dependent manner [23]. Genetic aberrations in PI3K are most common in HNSCC. The PI3K/Akt pathway is a growth factor signaling network which can regulate tumor cell metabolism [24]. Dysregulated PI3K/Akt pathway enhances the glucose catabolism via the localization of hexokinase to the mitochondrial membrane and activating citrate lyase, a major enzyme required for fatty acid synthesis. Elstrom et al. reported that activated Akt targets certain downstream targets such as mTOR which affects the cell survival and proliferation and cytoskeletal organization in HNSCC [25].

Mutations in Ras gene have been found in 4–5% of HNSCC cases [22]. Phosphorylation of Ras gene leads to the activation of downstream signaling factors like MEK and ERK which target genes that are responsible for cell growth and survival [26]. It can also activate the PI3K signaling cascade.

Seiwert et al. [27] reported that MET and HGF are overexpressed in 80% of HNSCC cases [27]. MET overexpression in HNSCC leads to enhanced cell motility, angiogenesis, and invasion/metastases [28, 29]. Kumar et al. [5] reported that c-Met/HGF signaling induces metabolic alterations in HNSCC cells via the cross signaling through stromal cells such as CAFs [5].

STAT-3 is reported to be constitutively activated in HNSCC. STAT-3 pathway triggers the cellular proliferation and suppresses apoptosis in HNSCC [30]. Phosphorylation of JAKs can occur directly by receptor tyrosine kinases (RTKs) such as EGFR subsequently activating RAS and PI3K pathways. JAK/STAT pathway promotes cell growth and survival, angiogenesis, and suppression of immune supervision. STAT proteins are important factors that mediate EGFR signaling which can trigger increased glycolysis in cancer cells via upregulation of key enzymatic factors involved in glycolysis [31].

Over the past few decades there has been growing interest in tumor microenvironment and to know its role in tumor progression. The mutual signaling between tumor and stroma has been reported in several cancers and is known to facilitate tumor metabolism, growth invasion, and resistance [32].

Currently treatment of HNSCC is typically determined in a multifaceted way, with the histological subtype, subsite, staging information, patient fitness, baseline swallow, and airway function guiding management decisions. Patients with early stage diseases are treated with surgery or radiotherapy based on primary tumor subtype with 70–90% cure rate.

Understanding the oncogenic factors that lead to metabolic alterations in HNSCC would pave a novel way for HNSCC treatment by targeting the key factors involved in glycolysis and other metabolic pathways.

2 Glucose Metabolism in HNSCC

Since Otto Warburg in the 1920s demonstrated that cancer cells are exceptionally glycolytic when compared to normal cells, it has been clear that the metabolism in cancer cells differ from that of normal cells [33]. This phenomenon was later known as aerobic glycolysis or Warburg effect (Fig. 1). Tumor cells undergo a metabolic shift from mitochondrial oxidation to glycolysis generating two molecules of pyruvate [34]. Pyruvate generated is converted to lactate by the enzyme lactate dehydrogenase A (LDH-A). Fantin et al. [35] reported that the NAD^+ generated through the transformation of pyruvate to lactate helps in maintaining the glycolytic flux in cancer cells [35].

The possible reasons why cancer cells highly depend on glycolysis is: (1) ATP generation through glycolysis is much faster than OXPHOS; (2) increased glycolytic flux produce enough intermediates for the biosynthesis of amino acids, nucleic acids, lipid bilayers, and fatty acids for the cell growth; and (3) NADPH produced by pentose phosphate pathway (PPP) maintains glutathione levels in cells, emerging in the resistance of cancer cells to chemotherapeutic molecules [36].

The advantageous use of glycolysis by cancer cells involves defects in mitochondria, adaptation to hypoxic tumor microenvironment, and abnormal signaling and expression of enzymes. The known key players that are involved in glucose metabolism in HNSCC are GLUT-1, HK-II, HIF-1, MCTs, TKTL-1, PKM2, and PFKFB [37].

2.1 Hypoxia Inducible Factor-1

Hypoxia inducible factor-1 (HIF-1) is a transcription factor that responds to decreased oxygen availability in cancer cells (hypoxia) [38]. It is a dimer made up of alpha and beta subunit. At normoxic conditions, the alpha subunit of HIF is hydroxylated at conserved prolyl residues by HIF-prolyl hydroxylases and subsequently is ubiquitinated by the VHL E3 ubiquitin ligase [9].

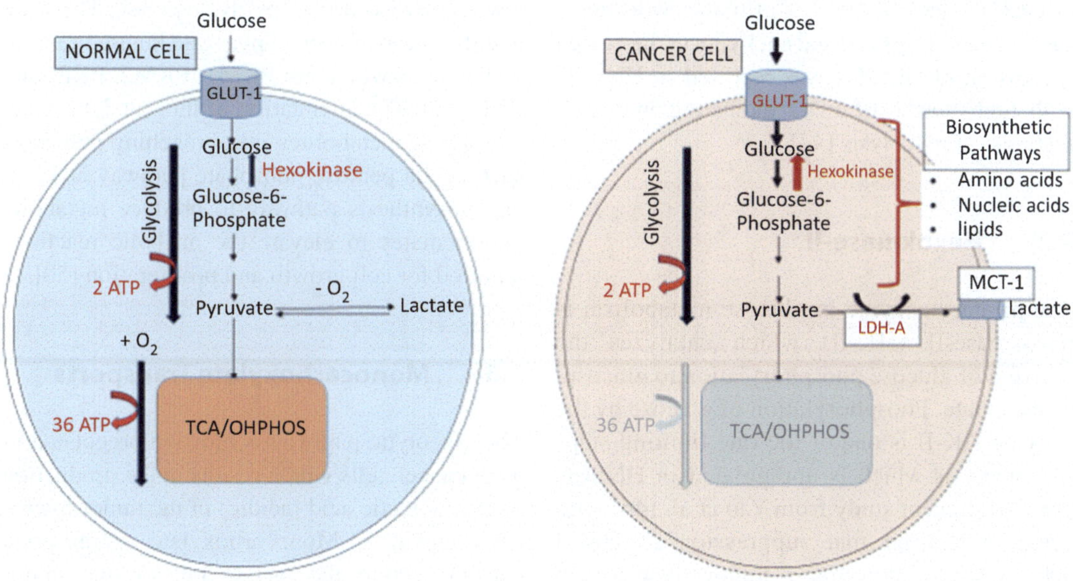

Fig. 1 Glycolysis in normal and cancer cells. Normal cells metabolize glucose to pyruvate followed by mitochondrial oxidation of pyruvate to CO_2 through the TCA cycle and the oxidative phosphorylation process, generating 36 ATPs per glucose. O_2 is essential as it is required as the final acceptor of electrons. When O_2 is limited, pyruvate is metabolized to lactate. Cancer cells metabolize most glucose to lactate despite the availability of O_2 (the Warburg effect), forwarding glucose metabolites from energy production to anabolic process to accelerate cell proliferation, at the expense of generating only two ATPs per glucose

Due to uncontrolled proliferation of cancer cells, hypoxic conditions are developed leading to the activation of HIF-1 alpha which upregulates several genes that include glycolytic enzymes such as hexokinase, phosphoglycerate kinase, lactate dehydrogenase A (LDH-A), and glucose transporters (GLUT-1, GLUT-3) [39].

Activation of HIF-1 in tumor cells can promote the uptake of glucose by overexpression of the glycolytic enzymes such as HK-II, glucose transporters, and LDH-A, resulting in increased glycolysis in tumor cells [40].

2.2 Glucose Transporter-1

Glucose is taken inside the cells with the help of solute transporters GLUTs. GLUT-1 is encoded by SLC2A1 gene which facilitates the transport of glucose across the plasma membrane of mammalian cells [41]. Kunkel et al. showed that uncontrolled proliferation of tumor cells leads to hypoxic condition in HNSCC leading to activation of GLUT transporters [42]. Overexpression of GLUT-1 and GLUT-3 is affiliated with many cancers including head and neck cancer. Increased expression of GLUT-1 was reported in HNSCC with high uptake of FDG indicating increased high rate of glycolysis [42].

2.3 Hexokinase-II

The primary enzyme in glucose metabolism is hexokinase-II (HK-II) which catalyzes the reaction of glucose phosphorylation to glucose-6-phosphate. Phosphorylation of glucose by the enzyme HK-II is one of the rate limiting steps in glycolysis which is upregulated in HNSCC [43, 44]. Recent study from Yao et al. [45] with Limonin showed that suppression of HK-II activity led to inhibition of tumor glycolysis in hepatocellular carcinoma, demonstrating that glycolysis inhibition was attributed to the decrease of HK-II activity [45]. These studies demonstrate that HK-II plays a key role in tumor progression by elevating glycolysis in cancer cells.

2.4 Lactate Dehydrogenase A

Lactate dehydrogenase A regulates glycolysis by catalyzing the final step of anaerobic glycolysis, that is, conversion of pyruvate to lactate, along with oxidation of NADH to NAD^+ [46, 47]. LDH consists of five active isoenzymes which are tetrametric metabolic enzymes made of two subunits M and H encoded by *Ldh-A* and *Ldh-B*, respectively, in human tissue. In cancer cells, NAD^+ released is utilized to sustain the glycolytic flux to different pathways [35, 48].

2.5 Pyruvate Kinase M2

The third committed step of glucose metabolism is the conversion of phosphoenol pyruvate (PEP) to pyruvate by enzyme pyruvate kinase (PK). Cancer cells utilize diverse mechanisms to elevate the flux of glucose in glycolysis except the last step [49]. Last step is commonly attenuated in cancer cells. Attenuation is mainly achieved by using PKM2 to catalyze the reaction which is a low affinity isoform of pyruvate kinase. There are mainly four isoforms of pyruvate kinase in mammalian cells which are PKM1, PKM2, PKR, and PKL [49]. The attenuation of this catalytic reaction averts metabolites into branching pathways such as the pentose phosphate pathway and serine biosynthesis pathway to produce metabolic intermediates to elevate the anabolic reactions required for cell growth and proliferation [50].

2.6 Monocarboxylate Transports

The glycolytic pathway is mostly upregulated in most cancer cells which results in the production of excess lactic acid (acidic) in the tumor microenvironment. Monocarboxylate transports (MCT) secrete the lactate outside the tumor microenvironment and prevent highly acidic environment [51]. In cancer cells MCT-1 acts as a unidirectional lactate transporter while MCT-4 is a bidirectional transporter [52]. Ullah MS et al. [53] has reported that MCT-4 is overexpressed in most of the cancer cells with high glycolytic activity [53]. MCTs play an important task in the metabolic stability of the tumor microenvironment; they are responsible for the maintenance of glycolytic and acid-resistant phenotypes thus granting the malignant behavior of cancer cells [54]. MCTs manage high rate of glycolysis by facilitating lactate export and are also involved in pH regulation via co-transport of protons.

3 Signaling Pathways in HNSCC Glucose Metabolism

Mammalian cells start cell growth by entering cell cycle which requires receptor-mediated signal transduction initiated by extracellular growth factors. The beginning of cell growth and division initiates a metabolic requirement for sufficient carbon, nitrogen, and free energy for the synthesis of new proteins, lipids, and nucleic acids required by a proliferating cell. Aerobic glycolysis in tumor cells is regulated by abnormal signaling pathways, including PI3K/Akt, EGFR, NOTCH, and c-Met.

3.1 Akt Signaling

Amornphimoltham et al. reported that Akt is overexpressed in 60% cases of HNSCC with elevated rate of glycolysis [55]. Akt signaling employs immediate influence on glycolysis in cancer cells by various mechanisms. Akt has been reported to localize GLUT-1 to the plasma membrane and regulate hexokinase expression and mitochondrial expression [56]. Akt indirectly activates the enzyme phosphofructokinase-1 (PFK-1), which is the one of the rate controlling enzymes in glycolysis pathway. It activates PFK-1 by administering phosphorylating phosphofructokinase-2 (PFK-2), which ends in the production of fructose-2,6-bisphosphate (F-1,6P2), the most powerful allosteric activator of PFK-1 [57]. These findings were supported by the activity of Akt correlated with the increase in glycolysis in glioblastoma cells, concluding that Akt plays a major role in upregulation of glycolysis in cancer cells [58].

3.2 EGFR Signaling

Epidermal growth factor receptor (EGFR) is a transmembrane cell surface receptor that belongs to the human epidermal growth factor receptor family of tyrosine kinases. Increased expression of EGFR occurs in more than 90% of HNSCC [59]. EGFR VIII is the most common mutation seen in 42% of HNSCC cases. Activation of EGFR induces translocation of PKM2 into the nucleus through the EGFR/Erk-1/2 pathway. Erk-2 which is present in the downstream of EGFR phosphorylates PKM-2 at ser-37, which in turn is localized to the nucleus. The nuclear PKM-2 contributes to the Warburg effect in cancer cells [60]. PKM-2 upregulates the glycolytic genes GLUT-1 and LDH-A. Studies by Babic et al. revealed that in brain cancer, activated EGFRVIII mutation results in enhanced glycolysis by promoting glycolytic gene expression [61].

3.3 HIF-1 Signaling

Hypoxia-induced factor-1 (HIF) is a transcription factor, having two subunits HIF-1α and HIF-1β. HIF-1α is an oxygen sensitive subunit and activated under hypoxia conditions [9]. Under normoxic conditions HIF-1α is negatively regulated by von Hippel-Lindauprotein (pVHL), a tumor suppressor protein resulting in subsequent degradation of HIF-1α by ubiquitination [62].

In cancer cells due to rapid proliferation there is lack of oxygen availability in the cell environment which subsequently activates HIF-1α, which results in the activation of glycolytic genes like GLUT-1 and hexokinase-II mediating high levels of glucose metabolism in cancer cells [39].

3.4 NOTCH Signaling

Mammals possess four different notch receptors, NOTCH-1, NOTCH-2, NOTCH-3, and NOTCH-4, which are single transmembrane domain receptors consisting of an extracellular domain (NECD), transmembrane domain (TD), and an intracellular domain (NICD) [63]. NOTCH-1 is the second most mutated gene found in 10–15% of HNSCC tumors [64]. The effect of NOTCH signaling on hepatocytic glycolysis has been reported to be majorly arbitrated via synergy of NICD with transcription factor forkhead box protein O1 (FOXO1) [65]. FOXO1 consequently activates the transcription of the catalytic subunit of glucose-6-phosphatase and phosphoenol pyruvate carboxy kinase, a rate-limiting enzyme involved in glycolysis. Elevated NOTCH signaling leads to increased glycolytic phenotype via PI3K/Akt signaling pathway in several types of cancer cells [23].

3.5 JAK/STAT Signaling

Janus kinases (JKs) belong to a family of non-receptor tyrosine kinases which gets activated by several cytokine bound receptors. Cytokine receptors do not contain intrinsic tyrosine kinase activity but is activated by transphosphorylation through constantly bound JAK molecules. Activation of cytokine receptors phosphorylates and dimerizes the STAT proteins and translocates them to the nucleus where they act as transcription factors. Ras-MAPK and PI3K-Akt pathways are also activated by JAKs. Increased levels of STAT-3 are found to be associated with patients having tobacco-induced HNSCC. Increased STAT-3 levels have been reported in HNSCC tumors which are attributed to increase in Ras and EGFR signaling. STAT-3 activation in tumor cells support cell survival and growth, angiogenesis, and suppression of immune system.

3.6 Hepatocyte Growth Factor/c-Met Signaling

Hepatocyte growth factor (HGF) is a protein secreted by mesenchymal stem cells that stimulates cell growth, cell motility, and morphogenesis through its receptor c-Met [66]. In HNSCC, HGF is mainly secreted by the cancer-associated fibroblasts in the microenvironment. c-Met is a receptor tyrosine kinase encoded by the proto-oncogene MET located on the long arm of chromosome 7 at position 7q31.2 [67]. Overexpression of c-Met protein is the mostly seen alteration in about 90% of the HNSCC cases. Knowles et al. had reported that in HNSCC the abnormal c-Met signaling contributes to the tumor progression and promotes the metastasis of HNSCC tumor cells to distant organs [28]. Studies by Kumar et al. revealed that HGF/c-Met axis prompts the morphogenesis of epithelial cells via EMT [68]. HGF activation by c-Met results in reduced E-cadherin expression in HNSCC cells which leads to the translocation of the protein to the cytoplasm and reduced expression is associated with distant metastasis and recurrent disease [69]. The HGF/c-Met pathway induces cell invasion and migration via multiple mechanisms among which is increased expression of matrix metalloproteinases (MMP) in HNSCC. MMPs are proteases that are accountable for the degradation and remodeling of extracellular matrix. In HNSCC cancer cell lines exposed to HGF stimulate increased expression of MMP-2 and MMP-9, resulting in the degradation of extracellular matrix and increased invasion [70]. Lui et al. had reported that HGF/c-Met signaling promotes tumor progression and cell survival by TP53-induced glycolysis and apoptosis regulator (TIGAR) [71]. Targeted inhibition of c-Met led to significant decrease in the expression of TIGAR in nasopharyngeal cells subsequently declining the intracellular nicotinamide adenine dinucleotide phosphate (NADPH) levels necessary for escaping apoptosis [71]. Lui et al. reported that increased expression of TIGAR in HNSCC cells eliminated the growth inhibitory effects of c-Met inhibitors [71].

4 Role of Tumor Microenvironment in HNSCC Metabolism

Over the last few decades there has been an increase in interest over tumor microenvironment studies as there have been findings that tumor microenvironment plays an important role in tumor progression, aggressivity, and metastasis process [72]. Tumor microenvironment is the environment around the tumor that includes blood vessels, immune cells, fibroblast, signaling molecules, and extracellular matrix (ECM) [73]. Spill et al. reported that cancer cells majorly affect the tumor microenvironment by releasing extracellular signals, promoting tumor angiogenesis, tumor metastasis affecting the growth, and evolution of cancer cells [74]. In HNSCC, cancer-associated fibroblasts (CAF) are abundant in the stroma and are critical to tumor metabolism [75, 5].

Studies from Curry et al. indicate that epithelial cancer cells derive nutrients from CAFs by maintaining a coupled metabolism. Cancer cells activate glycolysis in nearby stroma and utilize the by-products such as lactate and pyruvate as energy source [76].

Studies from Knowles et al. have reported that CAFs secrete hepatocyte growth factor which binds and activates c-Met tyrosine kinase receptor on HNSCC cells triggering tumor cell proliferation, invasion, and metastasis [28]. HNSCC cells modulate the microenvironment CAFs by secreting basic fibroblast growth factor (bFGF), which binds to fibroblast growth factor receptor (FGFR) expressed on various cell surfaces that mediate cell proliferation and migration [77]. Hitosugi et al. reported that FGFR activation upregulates mitochondrial pyruvate dehydrogenase kinase-1 (PDK-1) and promotes the cellular metabolism [78]. CAFs and HNSCC cells cross regulates cellular metabolism via c-Met/HGF signaling. Studies from Kumar et al. showed that HGF secreted by CAFs regulates HNSCC metabolism and HNSCC cells secrete bFGF and lactate to regulate CAF proliferation and mitochondrial OXPHOS [5]. Also, bFGF stimulation in CAFs leads to increased transcription of p53 inducible regulator of glycolysis and apoptosis (TIGAR) in CAFs enhancing the mitochondrial OXPHOS [5]. Understanding the cross pathway signaling between tumor and tumor microenvironment, which modulates the tumor metabolism leading to tumor progression, can lead to new therapeutic targets for efficient treatment of HNSCC.

5 Therapeutic Interventions for Targeting HNSCC Metabolism

Currently there are very limited treatment options available for head and neck cancer due to poor prognosis and recurrence of the disease. HNSCC is commonly treated via surgery, radiotherapy, chemotherapy, or combination of these approaches [79]. As far, only epidermal growth factor receptor inhibitors have been approved for HNSCC and several other therapies are under clinical trial (Table 1). Bonner et al. for the first time had reported a positive effect with the anti-EGFR antibody Cetixumab combined with radiotherapy in primarily advanced head and neck cancer patients [80]. Silybin (SIL) is a GLUT inhibitor which induces G1 cell cycle arrest, inhibits EGFR, and suppresses angiogenesis [81]. A phase I trial was done with prostate cancer patients [82]. Lonidamide, a derivate of indazole-3-carboxylic acid, is an inhibitor of hexokinase, and also binds to adenine nucleotide translocator leading to tumor cell death via apoptosis [83]. 2-Deoxy glucose (2DG), an analog of glucose, acts as a competitive inhibitor for glucose-6-phosphate isomerase. 2DG is phosphorylated by hexokinase and accumulated inside the cells inhibiting glycolysis [84]. Dichloroacetate is a pyruvate kinase inhibitor. Whitehouse et al. provided evidence that dichloroacetate is an inhibitor of pyruvate kinase and results in in vivo inactivation of pyruvate dehydrogenase kinase and pyruvate oxidation [85]. VLX-600 an electron transport chain inhibitor drug together with dichloroacetate has shown significant anticancer effect in HNSCC murine models [86]. Dichloroacetate inhibits the production and transport of lactate and has also been

Table 1 Drugs targeting cancer metabolism under clinical trials

Drug	Target	Status	Clinical trial no.
Silybin	GLUT	I	NCT03440164
Lonidamine	HK	III	NCT00435448
2- Deoxyglucose	G6P isomerase	I	NCT00633087
TLN-232	PKM2 dimers	II	NCT00735332
Dichloroacetate	PDK	II	NCT01111097
AZD-3965	MCT1	I	NCT01791595
CPI-613	Pyruvate dehydrogenase	I	NCT03699319
Gossypol	LDH-A	II	NCT00540722
Galloflavin	LDH-A	Pre-clinical studies	
Daunorubicin	GLUT-1	I	NCT02914977
Cisplatin ± Cetuximab	EGFR	III	NCT00004865
Carboplalin ± 5-FU ± Panitumumab	EGFR	II	NCT00122460
Dacominitinib	Tyrosine kinase	III	NCT01858389
Gefitinib	Tyrosine kinase	II	NCT00049543
Erlotinib	Tyrosine kinase	II	NCT02013206

tested for metabolic therapy [87]. A combination of this drug with cisplatin and radiation is under clinical trial stage III–IV for HNSCC. Therapies that are in development include panitumumab an IgG2 monoclonal antibody that functions to prevent ligand binding [88]. Nivolumab is another drug which is under phase II clinical trial in combination with chemoradiation for locally advanced cancer [89]. Buparlisib, an PI3K inhibitor, is being studied in combination with cetuximab in metastatic disease and in patients with platinum- and cetuximab-refractory disease as monotherapy [90]. Everolimus and temsirolimus are mTOR inhibitors that are also being studied to disrupt PI3K pathway signaling [91, 92].

6 Conclusion and Future Prospective

Reprogramming of metabolic pathways is an important hallmark in cancer development, which allows cancer cells to grow continuously, even under stress conditions such as hypoxia, where nutrients and oxygen are poor. Several key factors play important role in metabolic regulation in HNSCC such as the regulatory enzymes in glycolysis HK-II, PKM-2, and LDHA and other genes such as GLUT-1, MCT, and HIF-1. Also, aberrant signaling pathways such as PI3K/Akt, EGFR, JAK/STAT, and HGF/c-Met have been associated with HNSCC. Tumor microenvironment has been reported to play a major role in HNSCC metabolic reprogramming. A large portion of HNSCC tumor contains tumor-associated fibroblasts. Cross signaling between tumor and stroma has been shown to facilitate tumor growth and invasion in HNSCC cells. Despite recent advances in cancer treatment, current therapies for HNSCC are associated with poor survival and high morbidity. Innovative therapeutic strategies are needed for improved treatment of this disease. Understanding the metabolic factors supporting tumor progression and invasion might pave a new path for developing novel inhibitors for the cancer treatment.

Tumor cell metabolism is being intensively studied as a novel area for the discovery of new biomarkers and therapeutic interventions. New metabolic targets is continuously being identified in different types of tumors. Altogether, there is convincing evidence that HNSCC requires elevated rate of glucose uptake and conversion for cell survival and progression. This appears to make HNSCC susceptible to targeted therapies employing inhibitors to glycolytic genes or enzymes. Understanding of increased glycolysis and related secondary energetic pathways such as glutaminolysis, pentose phosphate pathway, and serine biosynthetic pathway will lead to new targets to be inhibited for disease treatment.

Meanwhile, due to the role of tumor microenvironment in the disease progression and invasion, a better understanding of how the tumor microenvironment affects HNSCC progression via metabolic alterations might also provide new insight for the cancer therapy.

References

1. Bray, F., et al. (2018). Global cancer statistics 2018: GLOBOCAN estimates of incidence and mortality worldwide for 36 cancers in 185 countries. *CA: a Cancer Journal for Clinicians*. https://doi.org/10.3322/caac.21492.
2. Franceschi, S., et al. (1999). Comparison of the effect of smoking and alcohol drinking between oral and pharyngeal cancer. *International Journal of Cancer*. https://doi.org/10.1002/(SICI)1097-0215(19990924)83:1<1::AID-IJC1>3.0.CO;2-8.
3. Sanderson, R. J., & Ironside, J. A. D. (2002). Squamous cell carcinomas of the head and neck. *BMJ (Clinical Research ed.), 325*(7368), 822–827. https://doi.org/10.1136/bmj.325.7368.822.
4. Marur, S., et al. (2010). HPV-associated head and neck cancer: A virus-related cancer epidemic. *The Lancet Oncology*. https://doi.org/10.1016/S1470-2045(10)70017-6.
5. Kumar, D., et al. (2018). Cancer-associated fibroblasts drive glycolysis in a targetable signaling loop implicated in head and neck squamous cell carcinoma progression. *Cancer Research*. https://doi.org/10.1158/0008-5472.CAN-17-1076.
6. Warburg, O. (2004). The Metabolism of tumors in the body. *The Journal of General Physiology*. https://doi.org/10.1085/jgp.8.6.519.
7. Liu, X., et al. (2010). Warburg effect revisited: An epigenetic link between glycolysis and gastric carcinogenesis. *Oncogene*. https://doi.org/10.1038/onc.2009.332.
8. Brown, R. S., et al. (2002). Expression of hexokinase II and Glut-1 in untreated human breast cancer. *Nuclear Medicine and Biology*. https://doi.org/10.1016/S0969-8051(02)00288-3.
9. Semenza, G. L., et al. (1994). Transcriptional regulation of genes encoding glycolytic enzymes by hypoxia-inducible factor 1. *Journal of Biological Chemistry*.
10. Lunt, S. Y., & Vander Heiden, M. G. (2011). Aerobic glycolysis: Meeting the metabolic requirements of cell proliferation. *Annual Review of Cell and Developmental Biology*. https://doi.org/10.1146/annurev-cellbio-092910-154237.
11. Pfeiffer, T., Schuster, S., & Bonhoeffer, S. (2001). Cooperation and competition in the evolution of ATP-producing pathways. *Science*. https://doi.org/10.1126/science.1058079.
12. Seagroves, T. N., et al. (2001). Transcription factor HIF-1 is a necessary mediator of the pasteur effect in mammalian cells. *Molecular and Cellular Biology*. https://doi.org/10.1128/MCB.21.10.3436-3444.2001.
13. Ayala, A., Fabregat, I., & Machado, A. (1991). The role of NADPH in the regulation of glucose-6-phosphate and 6-phosphogluconate dehydrogenases in rat adipose tissue. *Molecular and Cellular Biochemistry, 105*, 1–5.
14. Reitzer, L. J., Wice, B. M., & Kennell, D. (1979). Evidence that glutamine, not sugar, is the major energy source for cultured HeLa cells. *Journal of Biological Chemistry*. https://doi.org/10.1007/s00125-007-0708-y.
15. Suh, Y., et al. (2014). Clinical update on cancer: molecular oncology of head and neck cancer. *Cell Death & Disease*. https://doi.org/10.1038/cddis.2013.548.
16. Tweardy, D. J. (1993). Elevated levels of transforming growth factor a and epidermal growth factor receptor messenger RNA are early markers of carcinogenesis in head and neck cancer. *Cancer Research*.
17. Sok, J. C., et al. (2006). Mutant epidermal growth factor receptor (EGFRvIII) contributes to head and neck cancer growth and resistance to EGFR targeting. *Clinical Cancer Research*. https://doi.org/10.1158/1078-0432.CCR-06-0913.
18. Makinoshima, H., et al. (2014). Epidermal growth factor receptor (EGFR) signaling regulates global metabolic pathways in EGFR-mutated lung adenocarcinoma. *Journal of Biological Chemistry*. https://doi.org/10.1074/jbc.M114.575464.
19. Wanka, C., Steinbach, J. P., & Rieger, J. (2012). Tp53-induced glycolysis and apoptosis regulator (TIGAR) protects glioma cells from starvation-induced cell death by up-regulating respiration and improving cellular redox homeostasis. *Journal of Biological Chemistry*. https://doi.org/10.1074/jbc.M112.384578.
20. Brennan, J. A., et al. (2002). Association between cigarette smoking and mutation of the p53 gene in squamous-cell carcinoma of the head and neck. *New England Journal of Medicine*. https://doi.org/10.1056/nejm199503163321104.
21. Poeta, M. L., et al. (2007). TP53 mutations and survival in squamous-cell carcinoma of the head and neck. *New England Journal of Medicine*. https://doi.org/10.1056/nejmoa073770.
22. Agrawal, N., et al. (2011). Exome sequencing of head and neck squamous cell carcinoma reveals inactivating mutations in NOTCH1. *Science*. https://doi.org/10.1126/science.1206923.
23. Landor, S. K.-J., et al. (2011). Hypo- and hyper-activated Notch signaling induce a glycolytic switch through distinct mechanisms. *Proceedings of the National Academy of Sciences*. https://doi.org/10.1073/pnas.1104943108.
24. Rathmell, J. C., et al. (2003). Akt-directed glucose metabolism can prevent Bax conformation change

and promote growth factor-independent survival. *Molecular and Cellular Biology*.
25. Elstrom, R. L., et al. (2004). Akt stimulates aerobic glycolysis in cancer cells. *Cancer Research*. https://doi.org/10.1158/0008-5472.CAN-03-2904.
26. Bos, J. L. (1989). Ras oncogenes in human cancer: A review. *Cancer Research*.
27. Seiwert, T. Y., Beck, T. N., & Salgia, R. (2014). The role of HGF/c-MET in head and neck squamous cell carcinoma. In *Molecular determinants of head and neck cancer*. https://doi.org/10.1007/978-1-4614-8815-6_5.
28. Knowles, L. M., et al. (2009). HGF and c-Met participate in paracrine tumorigenic pathways in head and neck squamous cell cancer. *Clinical Cancer Research*. https://doi.org/10.1158/1078-0432.CCR-08-3252.
29. Sierra, J. R., & Tsao, M. S. (2011). c-MET as a potential therapeutic target and biomarker in cancer. *Therapeutic Advances in Medical Oncology*. https://doi.org/10.1177/1758834011422557.
30. Grandis, J. R., et al. (2002). Constitutive activation of Stat3 signaling abrogates apoptosis in squamous cell carcinogenesis in vivo. *Proceedings of the National Academy of Sciences*. https://doi.org/10.1073/pnas.97.8.4227.
31. Sen, M., et al. (2012). First-in-human trial of a STAT3 decoy oligonucleotide in head and neck tumors: Implications for cancer therapy. *Cancer Discovery*. https://doi.org/10.1158/2159-8290.CD-12-0191.
32. Curry, J. M., et al. (2014). Tumor microenvironment in head and neck squamous cell carcinoma. *Seminars in Oncology*. https://doi.org/10.1053/j.seminoncol.2014.03.003.
33. Warburg, O. (2004). The Metabolism of tumors in the body. *The Journal of General Physiology*. https://doi.org/10.1085/jgp.8.6.519.
34. Sandulache, V. C., et al. (2011). Glucose, not glutamine, is the dominant energy source required for proliferation and survival of head and neck squamous carcinoma cells. *Cancer*. https://doi.org/10.1002/cncr.25868.
35. Fantin, V. R., St-Pierre, J., & Leder, P. (2006). Attenuation of LDH-A expression uncovers a link between glycolysis, mitochondrial physiology, and tumor maintenance. *Cancer Cell*. https://doi.org/10.1016/j.ccr.2006.04.023.
36. Shestov, A. A., et al. (2014). Quantitative determinants of aerobic glycolysis identify flux through the enzyme GAPDH as a limiting step. *eLife*. https://doi.org/10.7554/eLife.03342.
37. Zhao, Y., Butler, E. B., & Tan, M. (2013). Targeting cellular metabolism to improve cancer therapeutics. *Cell Death and Disease*. https://doi.org/10.1038/cddis.2013.60.
38. Brahimi-Horn, M. C., Chiche, J., & Pouysségur, J. (2007). Hypoxia signalling controls metabolic demand. *Current Opinion in Cell Biology*. https://doi.org/10.1016/j.ceb.2007.02.003.
39. Ebert, B. L., Firth, J. D., & Ratcliffe, P. J. (1995). Hypoxia and mitochondrial inhibitors regulate expression of glucose transporter-1 via distinct cis-acting sequences. *Journal of Biological Chemistry*. https://doi.org/10.1074/jbc.270.49.29083.
40. Minchenko, O., Opentanova, I., & J, C. (2003). Hypoxic regulation of the 6-phosphofructo-2-kinase/fructose-2,6-bisphosphatase gene family (PFKFB-1-4) expression in vivo. *FEBS Letters, 554*(3), 264–270.
41. Mueckler, M., et al. (1985). Sequence and structure of a human glucose transporter. *Science*. https://doi.org/10.1126/science.3839598.
42. Kunkel, M., et al. (2003). Overexpression of Glut-1 and increased glucose metabolism in tumors are associated with a poor prognosis in patients with oral squamous cell carcinoma. *Cancer*. https://doi.org/10.1002/cncr.11159.
43. Osawa, H., et al. (1995). Regulation of hexokinase II gene transcription and glucose phosphorylation by catecholamines, cyclic AMP, and insulin. *Diabetes*. https://doi.org/10.2337/diab.44.12.1426.
44. Yamada, T., Uchida, M., Kwang-Lee, K., Kitamura, N., Yoshimura, T., Sasabe, E., & Yamamoto, T. (2012). Correlation of metabolism/hypoxia markers and fluorodeoxyglucose uptake in oral squamous cell carcinomas. *Oral Surgery, Oral Medicine, Oral Pathology, Oral Radiology, 113*(4), 464–471.
45. Yao, J., Liu, J., & Zhao, W. (2018). By blocking hexokinase-2 phosphorylation, limonin suppresses tumor glycolysis and induces cell apoptosis in hepatocellular carcinoma. *Onco Targets and Therapy*. https://doi.org/10.2147/OTT.S165220.
46. Blatt, S., et al. (2016). Lactate as a predictive marker for tumor recurrence in patients with head and neck squamous cell carcinoma (HNSCC) post radiation: a prospective study over 15 years. *Clinical Oral Investigations*. https://doi.org/10.1007/s00784-015-1699-6.
47. Flores, A., et al. (2019). Increased lactate dehydrogenase activity is dispensable in squamous carcinoma cells of origin. *Nature Communications*. https://doi.org/10.1038/s41467-018-07857-9.
48. Le, A., et al. (2010). Inhibition of lactate dehydrogenase A induces oxidative stress and inhibits tumor progression. *Proceedings of the National Academy of Sciences*. https://doi.org/10.1073/pnas.0914433107.
49. Tamada, M., Suematsu, M., & Saya, H. (2012). Pyruvate kinase M2: Multiple faces for conferring benefits on cancer cells. *Clinical Cancer Research*. https://doi.org/10.1158/1078-0432.CCR-12-0859.
50. Kurihara-Shimomura, M., et al. (2018). The multifarious functions of pyruvate kinase M2 in oral cancer cells. *International Journal of Molecular Sciences*. https://doi.org/10.3390/ijms19102907.
51. Pinheiro, C., et al. (2012). Role of monocarboxylate transporters in human cancers: State of the art. *Journal of Bioenergetics and Biomembranes*. https://doi.org/10.1007/s10863-012-9428-1.

52. Halestrap, A. P., & Meredith, D. (2004). The SLC16 gene family – From monocarboxylate transporters (MCTs) to aromatic amino acid transporters and beyond. *Pflugers Archiv European Journal of Physiology*. https://doi.org/10.1007/s00424-003-1067-2.
53. Ullah, M. S., Davies, A. J., & Halestrap, A. P. (2006). The plasma membrane lactate transporter MCT4, but not MCT1, is up-regulated by hypoxia through a HIF-1α-dependent mechanism. *Journal of Biological Chemistry*. https://doi.org/10.1074/jbc.M511397200.
54. Halestrap, A. P., & Wilson, M. C. (2012). The monocarboxylate transporter family-Role and regulation. *IUBMB Life*. https://doi.org/10.1002/iub.572.
55. Amornphimoltham, P., et al. (2004). Persistent activation of the Akt pathway in head and neck squamous cell carcinoma: A potential target for UCN-01. *Clinical Cancer Research*. https://doi.org/10.1158/1078-0432.CCR-03-0249.
56. Kim, D. I., Lim, S. K., & Park, M. (2007b). The involvement of phosphatidylinositol 3-kinase/Akt signaling in high glucose-induced downregulation of GLUT-1 expression in ARPE cells. *Life Sciences, 80*, 626–632.
57. Deprez, J., et al. (1997). Phosphorylation and activation of heart 6-phosphofructo-2-kinase by protein kinase B and other protein kinases of the insulin signaling cascades. *Journal of Biological Chemistry*. https://doi.org/10.1074/jbc.272.28.17269.
58. Agnihotri, S., & Zadeh, G. (2016). Metabolic reprogramming in glioblastoma: The influence of cancer metabolism on epigenetics and unanswered questions. *Neuro-Oncology*. https://doi.org/10.1093/neuonc/nov125.
59. Yang, W., Zheng, Y., Xia, Y., Ji, H., Chen, X., Guo, F., Lyssiotis, C. A., Aldape, K., Cantley, L. C., & Z, L. (n.d.). ERK1/2-dependent phosphorylation and nuclear translocation of PKM2 promotes the Warburg effect. *Nature Cell Biology, 15*(1) 124, pp. 1295–1304.
60. Grandis, J. R., et al. (1998). Levels of TGF-α and EGFR protein in head and neck squamous cell carcinoma and patient survival. *Journal of the National Cancer Institute*. https://doi.org/10.1093/jnci/90.11.824.
61. Babic, I., et al. (2013). EGFR mutation-induced alternative splicing of max contributes to growth of glycolytic tumors in brain cancer. *Cell Metabolism*. https://doi.org/10.1016/j.cmet.2013.04.013.
62. Huang, L. E., et al. (2002). Regulation of hypoxia-inducible factor 1 is mediated by an O2-dependent degradation domain via the ubiquitin-proteasome pathway. *Proceedings of the National Academy of Sciences*. https://doi.org/10.1073/pnas.95.14.7987.
63. Kumar, R., Juillerat-Jeanneret, L., & Golshayan, D. (2016). Notch antagonists: Potential modulators of cancer and inflammatory diseases. *Journal of Medicinal Chemistry*. https://doi.org/10.1021/acs.jmedchem.5b01516.
64. Sun, W., et al. (2014). Activation of the NOTCH pathway in head and neck cancer. *Cancer Research*. https://doi.org/10.1158/0008-5472.CAN-13-1259.
65. Bi, P., & Kuang, S. (2015). Notch signaling as a novel regulator of metabolism. *Trends in Endocrinology and Metabolism*. https://doi.org/10.1016/j.tem.2015.02.006.
66. Bottaro, D. P., et al. (1991). Identification of the hepatocyte growth factor receptor as the c-met protooncogene product. *Science*. https://doi.org/10.1126/science.1846706.
67. Park, M., et al. (2006). Sequence of MET protooncogene cDNA has features characteristic of the tyrosine kinase family of growth-factor receptors. *Proceedings of the National Academy of Sciences*. https://doi.org/10.1073/pnas.84.18.6379.
68. Kumar, D., et al. (2015). Mitigation of tumor-associated fibroblast-facilitated head and neck cancer progression with anti-hepatocyte growth factor antibody ficlatuzumab. *JAMA Otolaryngology – Head and Neck Surgery*. https://doi.org/10.1001/jamaoto.2015.2381.
69. Kim, C. H., et al. (2007a). Change of E-cadherin by hepatocyte growth factor and effects on the prognosis of hypopharyngeal carcinoma. *Annals of Surgical Oncology*. https://doi.org/10.1245/s10434-006-9320-5.
70. Koontongkaew, S., Amornphimoltham, P., & Yapong, B. (2009). Tumor-stroma interactions influence cytokine expression and matrix metalloproteinase activities in paired primary and metastatic head and neck cancer cells. *Cell Biology International*. https://doi.org/10.1016/j.cellbi.2008.10.009.
71. Lui, V. W. Y., et al. (2011). Inhibition of c-Met downregulates TIGAR expression and reduces NADPH production leading to cell death. *Oncogene*. https://doi.org/10.1038/onc.2010.490.
72. Korneev, K. V., et al. (2017). TLR-signaling and proinflammatory cytokines as drivers of tumorigenesis. *Cytokine*. https://doi.org/10.1016/j.cyto.2016.01.021.
73. Joyce, J. A., & Fearon, D. T. (2015). T cell exclusion, immune privilege, and the tumor microenvironment. *Science*. https://doi.org/10.1126/science.aaa6204.
74. Spill, F., et al. (2016). Impact of the physical microenvironment on tumor progression and metastasis. *Current Opinion in Biotechnology*. https://doi.org/10.1016/j.copbio.2016.02.007.
75. Desmoulière, A., Guyot, C., & Gabbiani, G. (2004). The stroma reaction myofibroblast: A key player in the control of tumor cell behavior. *International Journal of Developmental Biology*. https://doi.org/10.1387/ijdb.041802ad.
76. Curry, J. M., et al. (2013). Cancer metabolism, stemness and tumor recurrence : MCT1 and MCT4 are functional biomarkers of metabolic symbiosis in head and neck cancer. *Cell Cycle*. https://doi.org/10.4161/cc.24092.
77. Partridge, M., et al. (1996). Expression of bFGF, KGF and FGF receptors on normal oral mucosa and SCC.

European Journal of Cancer Part B: Oral Oncology. https://doi.org/10.1016/0964-1955(95)00056-9.
78. Hitosugi, T., et al. (2011). Tyrosine phosphorylation of mitochondrial pyruvate dehydrogenase kinase 1 is important for cancer metabolism. *Molecular Cell*. https://doi.org/10.1016/j.molcel.2011.10.015.
79. Vermorken, J. B., et al. (2008). Platinum-based chemotherapy plus cetuximab in head and neck cancer. *The New England Journal of Medicine*. https://doi.org/10.1056/NEJMoa0802656.
80. Bonner, J. A., et al. (2010). Radiotherapy plus cetuximab for locoregionally advanced head and neck cancer: 5-year survival data from a phase 3 randomised trial, and relation between cetuximab-induced rash and survival. *The Lancet Oncology*. https://doi.org/10.1016/S1470-2045(09)70311-0.
81. Singh, R. P., et al. (2005). Silibinin strongly inhibits growth and survival of human endothelial cells via cell cycle arrest and downregulation of survivin, Akt and NF-κB: Implications for angioprevention and antiangiogenic therapy. *Oncogene*. https://doi.org/10.1038/sj.onc.1208276.
82. Flaig, T. W., et al. (2010). A study of high-dose oral silybin-phytosome followed by prostatectomy in patients with localized prostate cancer. *Prostate*. https://doi.org/10.1002/pros.21118.
83. Pelicano, H., et al. (2006). Glycolysis inhibition for anticancer treatment. *Oncogene*. https://doi.org/10.1038/sj.onc.1209597.
84. Dwarakarnath, B. S., & Jain, V. (2009). Targeting glucose metabolism with 2-deoxy-D-glucose for improving cancer therapy. *Future Oncology*. https://doi.org/10.2217/fon.09.44.
85. Whitehouse, S., Cooper, R. H., & Randle, P. J. (2015). Mechanism of activation of pyruvate dehydrogenase by dichloroacetate and other halogenated carboxylic acids. *Biochemical Journal*. https://doi.org/10.1042/bj1410761.
86. Zhang, X., et al. (2014). Induction of mitochondrial dysfunction as a strategy for targeting tumour cells in metabolically compromised microenvironments. *Nature Communications*. https://doi.org/10.1038/ncomms4295.
87. Lucido, C. T., Miskimins, W. K., & Vermeer, P. D. (2018). Propranolol promotes glucose dependence and synergizes with dichloroacetate for anti-cancer activity in HNSCC. *Cancers*. https://doi.org/10.3390/cancers10120476.
88. Voigt, M., et al. (2015). Functional dissection of the epidermal growth factor receptor epitopes targeted by panitumumab and cetuximab. *Neoplasia*. https://doi.org/10.1593/neo.121242.
89. Reddy, B. K. M., et al. (2014). Nimotuzumab provides survival benefit to patients with inoperable advanced squamous cell carcinoma of the head and neck: A randomized, open-label, phase IIb, 5-year study in Indian patients. *Oral Oncology*. https://doi.org/10.1016/j.oraloncology.2013.11.008.
90. Soulieres, D., Faivre, S. J., & R, M. (2017). BERIL-1: a phase II, placebo-controlled study of buparlisib (BKM120) Buparlisib and paclitaxel in patients with platinum-pretreated recurrent or metastatic squamous cell carcinoma of the head and neck (BERIL-1): A randomised, double-blind, placebo-control. *The Lancet Oncology, 18*(3), 323–335.
91. Geiger, J. L., et al. (2016). Phase II trial of everolimus in patients with previously treated recurrent or metastatic head and neck squamous cell carcinoma. *Head and Neck*. https://doi.org/10.1002/hed.24501.
92. Massarelli, E., Lin, H., Ginsberg, L. E., Tran, H. T., Lee, J. J., Canales, J. R., Blumenschein, M. D. W. G. R., Lu, C., Heymach, J. V., Kies, M. S., & Papadimitrakopoulou, V. (2015). Phase II trial of everolimus and erlotinib in patients with platinum-resistant recurrent and/or metastatic head and neck squamous cell carcinoma. *Annals of Oncology, 26*(7), 1476–1480.

Fatty Acid Metabolism and Cancer

Zhenning Jin, Yang D. Chai, and Shen Hu

1 Fatty Acid Metabolism

Metabolism is a fundamental process for all cellular functions [1]. Cancer cells can alter the metabolic pathways for glucose, glutamine, and fatty acids to meet cellular energy demand. In the 1920s, Otto Heinrich Warburg made an important observation that cancer cells appeared to have enhanced utilization of glucose for energy production through aerobic glycolysis. In contrast, normal cells favor energy production through mitochondrial oxidative phosphorylation [2]. Meanwhile, glutamine is an abundant nonessential amino acid, and it is critical for adenosine triphosphate (ATP) production through glutamine-driven oxidative phosphorylation [3]. In normal cells, glutamine provides the carbon sources for synthesis of acetyl-CoA and citrate necessary in anabolic processes of cell proliferation [4]. In proliferating cancer cells, upregulation of glutamine metabolism in response to lower intracellular citrate has been linked to dysregulation of tricarboxylic acid (TCA) cycle and lipogenesis to fulfill energy requirement [1, 5]. Glucose, glutamine, and other substrates are precursors for the production of cytosolic acetyl-CoA. Acetyl-CoA in turn donates two-carbon molecules for fatty acid synthesis [6]. Due to their ability for metabolic reprogramming, cancer cells often display upregulated de novo lipogenesis. Whereas, most nonmalignant counterparts preferentially acquire fatty acids from exogenous sources [7]. Historically, studies have been focused on understanding the glucose and glutamine metabolism in cancer cells, while few ones investigated the role of fatty acid metabolism in cancer cells. In this chapter, we aim to provide a short overview of the known fatty acid mechanisms in cancer cells.

Fatty acid is comprised of a carboxyl terminal group with long chains of hydrocarbons that can be either saturated or unsaturated. Both fatty acid synthesis and fatty acid oxidation are important components in fatty acid metabolism [8]. Depending on cell types or conditions, fatty acid synthesis may favor exogenous synthesis or de novo synthesis. De novo fatty acid synthesis primarily relies on two key rate-limiting enzymes, acetyl-CoA carboxylase (ACC) and fatty acid synthase (FASN). ACC can carboxylate acetyl-CoA into malonyl-CoA, while FASN converts acetyl-CoA and malonyl-CoA into long-chain fatty acids such as 16-carbon palmitate (Fig. 1) [9, 10]. In fatty acid oxidation, the rate-limiting enzyme carnitine palmitoyltransferase I (CPT1) catalyzes the reaction of acyl-CoA and carnitine to form acyl-carnitine and transports the product from the cytosol into the mitochondrial matrix [11]. β-oxidation of fatty acid consists of a cyclical series of reactions in the mitochondria through shortening of the fatty acid chains to generate

Z. Jin · Y. D. Chai · S. Hu (✉)
School of Dentistry and Jonsson Comprehensive Cancer Center, University of California, Los Angeles, CA, USA
e-mail: shenhu@ucla.edu

S. Hu (ed.), *Cancer Metabolomics*, Advances in Experimental Medicine and Biology 1280,
https://doi.org/10.1007/978-3-030-51652-9_16

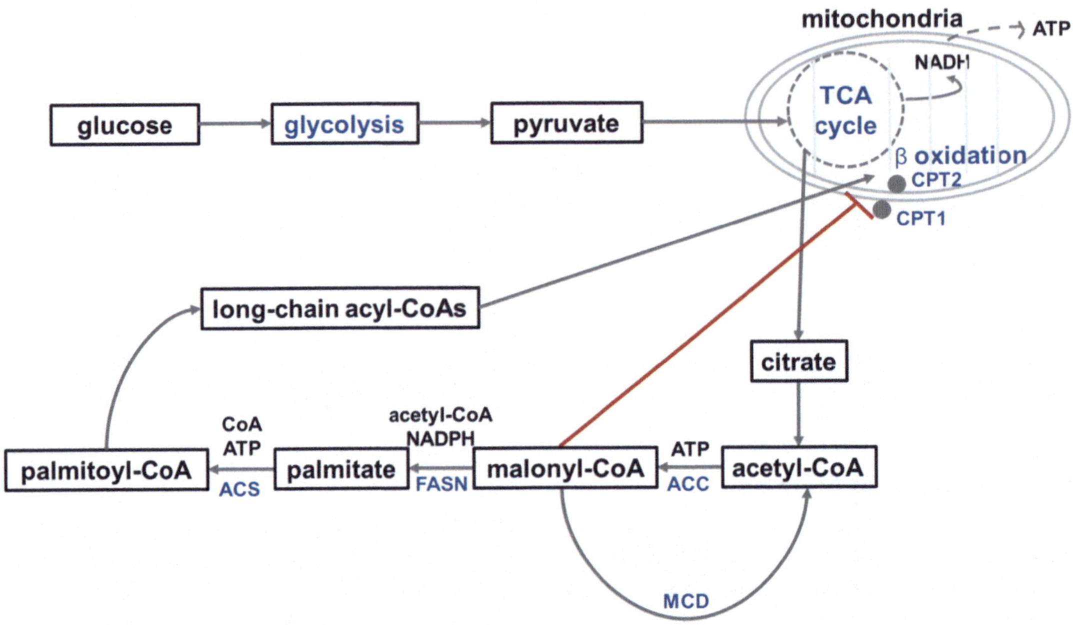

Fig. 1 Fatty acid synthesis pathway. This pathway functions in both cancers and lipogenic tissue such as liver. Extra glucose goes through TCA cycle to produce citrate for fatty acid synthesis. ACC carboxylates acetyl-CoA into malonyl-CoA, while FASN converts malonyl-CoA into long-chain fatty acids, such as palmitate. Malonyl-CoA can also inhibit CPT1, preventing the oxidation of the synthesized palmitoyl-CoA. CPT1 and CPT2 are two mitochondrial enzymes regulating fatty acid oxidation (β-oxidation). CPT1 locates at the outer membrane of mitochondria, while CPT2 locates at the inner membrane of mitochondria. *ACC* acetyl-CoA carboxylase, *FASN* fatty acid synthase, *ACS* fatty acid-CoA ligase, *CPT1* carnitine palmitoyltransferase I, *CPT2* carnitine palmitoyltransferase II. Modified with permission [10]

nicotinamide adenine dinucleotide (NADH), flavin adenine dinucleotide ($FADH_2$), and acetyl-CoA [12]. The collection of NADH and $FADH_2$ further contributes to the production of ATP in the electron transport chain of mitochondrial inner membrane. Fatty acid metabolism allows cells to utilize fatty acids to form cellular membranes, store lipids, and signal with adjacent cells to proliferate and survive. Understanding the mechanisms of fatty acid metabolism and its related pathways may lead to potential targets for therapeutic intervention in human cancers.

2 Fatty Acid Synthesis in Cancer

Fatty acid synthesis refers to the creation of fatty acids from acetyl-CoA and nicotinamide adenine dinucleotide phosphate (NADPH) through the action of FASN enzymes. Proliferating cancer cells require a constant supply of lipids for membrane biogenesis and protein modification [13]. In certain tumor types, significantly enhanced fatty acid synthesis was observed, whereas normal cells depend on exogenous lipogenesis for growth and proliferation. In fact, increased de novo fatty acid synthesis activity has been recognized as a novel metabolic target for therapeutic intervention in human cancers. However, the pathogenesis of de novo fatty acid synthesis in cancer remains largely elusive.

2.1 Regulation of Fatty Acid Synthesis in Cancer

As an important rate-limiting enzyme for the formation of fatty acids, FASN can be regulated at the transcriptional, translational, and the post-translational levels. FASN expression has been shown to be upregulated in various cancer types such as breast and prostate cancer [14, 15]. Endogenous growth factors and steroid hormones can activate phosphatidylinositol-3-kinase (PI3K), protein kinase B (Akt), and mitogen-activated protein kinase (MAPK) signaling cascade through binding interaction with estrogen receptor (ER), androgen receptor (AR), progesterone receptor (PR), epidermal growth factor receptor (EGFR), or human epithelial growth factor receptor 2 (HER2) to activate sterol regulatory element-binding protein 1c (SREBP-1c), which further promotes translational upregulation of FASN and ACC [9, 16]. Mammalian targets of rapamycin (mTOR), p53 family proteins, and lipogenesis-related nuclear protein (SPOT14) transcription factors were found to be overexpressed in breast tumors and are responsible for upregulation of FASN [17–19]. Under hypoxic and low pH conditions, isopeptidase ubiquitin-specific protease-2a (USP2a) helps stabilize stress-induced FASN protein and was also found to be upregulated in prostate cancers [20, 21]. The binding of FASN to HER2 is important to promote tumor growth, survival, and drug resistance [22]. The findings support the idea that tumor-related FASN overexpression may be regulated at translational and transcriptional levels and it serves as a potential therapeutic target of cancer [9].

2.2 Targeting Fatty Acid Synthesis in Cancer

Increased demand of fatty acids for cancer cell survival and proliferation suggests that it might be an anticancer strategy to reduce fatty acids in cancer cells by suppressing fatty acid bioavailability. Several methodologies may be feasible for the suppression of fatty acid bioavailability, for example, blocking fatty acid synthesis, increasing fatty acid degradation by oxidation, converting fatty acids for storage, and limiting fatty acids release from storage [8]. These approaches may take effect independently or combined to limit bioavailability of fatty acids.

Citrate is a critical intermediate that can be converted to bioactivate fatty acids through the action of several metabolic enzymes, including ATP citrate lyase (ACLY), fatty acid synthase (FASN), acetyl-CoA synthetase (ACS, aka, acetate-CoA ligase), and acetyl-CoA carboxylase (ACC). ACLY links the metabolism of carbohydrates, which yield citrate as an intermediate, and the production of acetyl-CoA, which is a precursor for the synthesis of fatty acids. The enzyme is responsible for generating cytosolic acetyl-CoA in many tissue types and involved in multiple biosynthetic pathways such as lipogenesis, cholesterogenesis, and histones acetylation [23]. Downregulation of ACLY in human adenocarcinoma cells and murine lymphoid cells showed suppression in tumor growth, suggesting ACLY may serve as a potential therapeutic target for limiting fatty acid synthesis [24, 25]. The main function of FASN is to catalyze the synthesis of a long-chain saturated fatty acid (e.g., palmitate, C16:0) from acetyl-CoA and malonyl-CoA, in the presence of NADPH. FASN has been reported as a novel therapeutic target, since certain types of cancer cells depend on FASN-mediated de novo fatty acid synthesis for proliferation and survival [8]. Inhibition of FASN induces cell death due to toxic effect of malonyl-CoA accumulation [26].

ACC plays an essential role in regulating fatty acid synthesis because ACC converts acetyl-CoA into malonyl-CoA, which is a required substrate for the biosynthesis of fatty acids. AMP-dependent protein kinase (AMPK) triggers the phosphorylation of ACC and therefore inactivates the enzyme whereas protein phosphatase 2A dephosphorylates ACC, activating the enzyme to produce malonyl-CoA, which is a building block for new fatty acids. In fact, ACC may function either as lipogenic (ACC1 isoform) or oxidative (ACC2 isoform) in mammals. ACC1 is found in the cytoplasm of all cells but is enriched in lipogenic tissue, such as adipose tissue and lactating mammary glands, where fatty acid synthesis is important. However, ACC2 is relatively overexpressed in oxidative tissues, such as the skeletal muscle and the heart tissues. ACC1 and ACC2 are both highly expressed in the liver where both fatty acid oxidation and synthesis are important. The differences in tissue distribution indicate that

ACC1 maintains regulation of fatty acid synthesis whereas ACC2 mainly regulates fatty acid oxidation. Knockdown of ACCs can effectively induce apoptosis in certain types of cancer cells. Silencing of the ACC1 resulted in a significant inhibition of cell proliferation and induction of caspase-mediated apoptosis of highly lipogenic LNCaP prostate cancer cells. In nonmalignant cells with low lipogenic activity, no cytotoxic effects of knockdown of ACC1 were observed. Similar results were also found when knocking down FASN in the prostate cancer cells and nonmalignant cells. These findings indicate that accumulation of malonyl-CoA is not a prerequisite for cytotoxicity induced by inhibition of tumor-associated lipogenesis in prostate cancer cells and suggest that in addition to FASN, ACC1 is a potential target for cancer intervention. In another study of breast cancer cells, silencing of either ACC1 or FASN in cancer cells results in a major decrease in palmitic acid synthesis. Depletion of the cellular pool of palmitic acid is associated with induction of apoptosis concomitant with the formation of reactive oxygen species (ROS) and mitochondrial impairment. Furthermore, supplementation of the culture medium with palmitate or with the antioxidant vitamin E resulted in the complete rescue of cells from both ACC1 and FASN knockdown-induced apoptosis. Finally, human mammary epithelial cells are resistant to RNAi knockdown against either ACC1 or FASN. These data confirm the importance of lipogenesis in cancer cell survival and indicate that this pathway represents a key target for antineoplastic therapy that, however, might require specific dietary recommendation for full efficacy [27, 28].

Studies also suggested that malonyl-CoA was a potential mediator of cytotoxicity induced by FASN inhibition in human breast cancer cells and xenografts, which seems contradicting with the finding discussed above. FASN inhibitors were found to induce a rapid increase in intracellular malonyl-CoA to severalfold above control levels, whereas 5-(tetradecyloxy)-2-furoic acid (TOFA) reduced intracellular malonyl-CoA by 60%. Simultaneous exposure of breast cancer cells to TOFA and an FASN inhibitor resulted in significantly reduced cytotoxicity and apoptosis. Subcutaneous xenografts of MCF7 breast cancer cells in nude mice treated with FASN inhibitor showed fatty acid synthesis inhibition, apoptosis, and inhibition of tumor growth to less than 1/8 of control volumes, without comparable toxicity in normal tissues. The data suggest that malonyl-CoA is a crucial regulatory metabolic intermediate in cellular energy metabolism, and inhibition of FASN may serve as a potential approach to cancer treatment [26].

Malonyl-CoA decarboxylase (MCD) regulates the levels of cellular malonyl-CoA through the decarboxylation of malonyl-CoA to acetyl-CoA. Malonyl-CoA is both a substrate for fatty acid synthesis and an inhibitor of fatty acid oxidation acting as a metabolic switch between anabolic fatty acid synthesis and catabolic fatty acid oxidation. Inhibition of MCD expression and activity was found to reduce ATP levels and cause toxicity to MCF7 breast cancer cells, but not to human fibroblasts. MCD inhibitor also increased cellular malonyl-CoA levels and caused cytotoxicity to a number of human breast cancer cell lines in vitro. These results indicate that MCD knockdown induced cytotoxicity is likely mediated through malonyl-CoA metabolism and MCD is a potential target for cancer therapeutics [29].

Acetyl-CoA synthetase (ACS, aka, acetate-CoA ligase) is an enzyme involved in metabolism of acetate. It is a ligase that catalyzes the formation of acetyl-CoA from acetate and coenzyme A (CoA). Once acetyl-CoA is formed it can be used in the TCA cycle in aerobic respiration to produce energy and electron carriers. This is an alternate route of starting the cycle, as the more common way is producing acetyl-CoA from pyruvate through pyruvate dehydrogenase. As mentioned earlier, acetyl-CoA is a critical precursor for fatty acid synthesis. Therefore, a common function of ACS is to produce acetyl-CoA for this purpose. A functional genomics study revealed that the activity of acetyl-CoA synthetase 2 (ACSS2) contributes to cancer cell growth under low oxygen and lipid-depleted conditions. ACSS2 exhibited copy-number gain in human breast tumors, and ACSS2 expression correlated with the disease progression. ACSS2 expression was upregulated under metabolically stressed conditions, and knockdown of ACSS2 reduced the growth of tumor xenografts. Comparative metabolomic and lipidomic analyses demonstrated that acetate was used as a nutritional source by cancer cells in an ACSS2-dependent manner, and supplied a significant fraction of the carbon within the fatty acid and phospholipid pools. These results demonstrated a critical role for acetate consumption in the production of lipid biomass within the harsh tumor microenvironment [30].

As a key metabolic intermediate, acetyl-CoA may play an important role in transcriptional regulation. In fact, histone acetylation is highly sensitive to the availability of acetyl-CoA. It is an obligate cofactor for histone acetyltransferases (HATs), and the abundance of the nucleocytosolic acetyl-CoA may have a direct impact on the enzymatic activity of HATs [31]. In glioblastoma cells, changes in acetyl-CoA abundance were found to trigger site-specific regulation of histone H3 Lys27 acetylation (H3K27ac). Genes involved in integrin signaling and cell adhesion were identified as acetyl-CoA-responsive, and ACLY-dependent acetyl-CoA production promoted cell migration and adhesion to the extracellular matrix. Mechanistically, the transcription factor NFAT1 (nuclear factor of activated T cells 1) was found to mediate acetyl-CoA-dependent gene regulation and cell adhesion. This study has established that the important role of acetyl-CoA in transcriptional regulation of the cell adhesion gene expression in glioblastoma cells through the impact of H3K27ac and Ca^{2+}–NFAT signaling [32].

Recently, a quantitative analysis of acetate metabolism revealed that ACSS2 fulfills distinct functions depending on its cellular location. Exogenous acetate uptake was controlled by expression of both ACSS2, which supports lipogenesis, and the mitochondrial ACSS1. Interestingly, oxygen and serum limitation increased nuclear localization of ACSS2, and nuclear ACSS2 recaptured acetate released from histone deacetylation for recycling by histone acetyltransferases. This study provided evidence for limited equilibration between nuclear and cytosolic acetyl-CoA and demonstrates that ACSS2 retains acetate to maintain histone acetylation [33].

The long-chain fatty acyl-CoA synthetase (ACSL, aka., long-chain fatty acyl-CoA ligase) is an enzyme of the ligase family that activates the oxidation of complex fatty acids and catalyzes the formation of fatty acyl-CoA. Long-chain acyl-CoAs are substrates for most pathways that use fatty acids for energy production or for the synthesis of complex lipids like phospholipids, cholesteryl esters, ceramide, and triglyceride. Acyl-CoAs are also substrates for β-oxidation in peroxisomes and mitochondria and for ω-oxidation in the endoplasmic reticulum. In addition to these metabolic functions, acyl-CoAs are required for posttranslational protein acylation, and regulation of enzymes, ion channels, membrane potential, protein trafficking, and transcription, as well as cellular budding and fusion. Because most acyl-CoA may be bound to acyl-CoA-binding protein (ACBP), the functional acyl-CoA unit might be bound, rather than free, acyl-CoA [34]. Mammals have five ACSL isoforms (ACSL1, ACSL3, ACSL4, ACSL5, and ACSL6). These isoforms may be differentially upregulated in specific cancer types, and chemical inhibition of ACSL by inhibitors such as Triacsin C (inhibitor of ACSL1, ACSL3, and ACSL4 but not ACSL5 or ACSL6) preferentially induces apoptotic cell death in certain cancer types such as lung, colon, and brain cancer cells. Therefore, when considering treatment through inactivation of ACSL, it is important to note that different drugs have different isoform specificities, so they may have differential effects, as the various isoforms have different tissue specificities, responses to nutritional state, and preferred substrates [8].

Sterol regulatory element binding proteins (SREBPs) are a family of transcription factors that regulate lipid homeostasis by controlling the expression of a range of enzymes required for endogenous cholesterol, fatty acid, triacylglycerol, and phospholipid synthesis. The three SREBP isoforms, SREBP-1a, SREBP-1c, and SREBP-2, have different roles in lipid synthesis.

SREBP-1c is involved in fatty acid synthesis and insulin-induced glucose metabolism (particularly in lipogenesis), whereas SREBP-2 is relatively specific to cholesterol synthesis. The SREBP-1a isoform seems to be implicated in both pathways [35]. EGFR mutations are frequent in glioblastoma. Studies of glioblastomas from patients treated with the EGFR inhibitor lapatinib revealed that EGFR induced the cleavage and nuclear translocation of SREBP-1. This response was mediated by Akt; however, clinical data from rapamycin-treated patients showed that SREBP-1 activation was independent of the mammalian target of rapamycin complex 1, possibly explaining rapamycin's poor efficacy in the treatment of such tumors. Glioblastomas without constitutively active EGFR signaling were resistant to inhibition of fatty acid synthesis, whereas introduction of a constitutively active mutant form of EGFR, EGFRvIII, sensitized tumor xenografts in mice to cell death. These results identify a new EGFR-mediated pro-survival metabolic pathway and suggest new therapeutic approaches to treating EGFR-activated glioblastomas [36].

3 Fatty Acid Oxidation in Cancer

Fatty acid oxidation (aka, β-oxidation) is the catabolic process by which fatty acid molecules are broken down in the mitochondria to generate acetyl-CoA, NADH, and FADH2. It is composed of a cyclical series of reactions that result in the shortening of fatty acids (two carbons per cycle) and that generate in each round NADH, FADH2, and acetyl-CoA, until the last cycle when two acetyl-CoA molecules are originated from the catabolism of a four carbon fatty acid. NADH and FADH2 function as two co-enzymes used in the electron transport chain (ETC) to produce ATP whereas acetyl-CoA enters the TCA cycle to produce citrate. Citrate may leave the mitochondria and enter the cytoplasm to engage NADPH-producing reactions (Fig. 2). Fatty acid oxidation is carried out in energy-demanding tissues (such as the heart and skeletal muscle) and in the liver as a central organ for nutrient supply and conversion [37].

CPT1 is a mitochondrial enzyme responsible for the formation of acyl-carnitines by catalyzing the transfer of the acyl group of a long-chain fatty acyl-CoA to carnitine. The product is often palmitoylcarnitine, but other fatty acids may also be substrates. The carnitine palmitoyltransferase system is an essential step in the beta-oxidation of long-chain fatty acids, and CPT1 is the first component and rate-limiting step of the carnitine palmitoyltransferase system [11]. The acylcarnitine translocase then shuttles the acylcarnitine across the inner mitochondrial membrane where it is converted back into palmitoyl-CoA. Three isoforms of CPT1 are currently known: CPT1A (the liver isoform), CPT1B (the muscle isoform), and CPT1C (the brain isoform) [38]. CPT1C was identified as a potential oncogene, as the frequently upregulated CPT1C expression promotes fatty acid oxidation, ATP production, and tumor growth. AMPK can induce CPT1C expression to protect cancer cells from apoptosis under glucose and oxygen-deprived microenvironment [39].

Carnitine palmitoyltransferase II (CPT2) catalyzes the formation of palmitoyl-CoA from palmitoylcarnitine imported into the mitochondrial inner membrane via the acylcarnitine translocase. The catalytic core of the CPT2 enzyme contains three important binding sites that recognize structural aspects of CoA, palmitoyl, and carnitine. Defects in this gene are associated with mitochondrial long-chain fatty acid oxidation disorders. In obesity-driven and nonalcoholic steatohepatitis (NASH)-driven hepatocellular carcinoma (HCC), the extensive accumulation of acylcarnitine species was seen in HCC tissues and the sera of HCC patients, which could be attributed to the downregulation of CPT2. CPT2 downregulation induced the suppression of fatty acid oxidation, and CPT2 knockdown in HCC cells resulted in their resistance to lipotoxicity by inhibiting the Src-mediated JNK activation. Additionally, oleoylcarnitine enhanced sphere formation by HCC cells via STAT3 activation, suggesting that acylcarnitine accumulation was a surrogate marker of CPT2 downregulation and directly contributed to hepatocarcinogenesis. These results indicate that in obesity-driven and NASH-driven HCC, metabolic reprogramming mediated by the

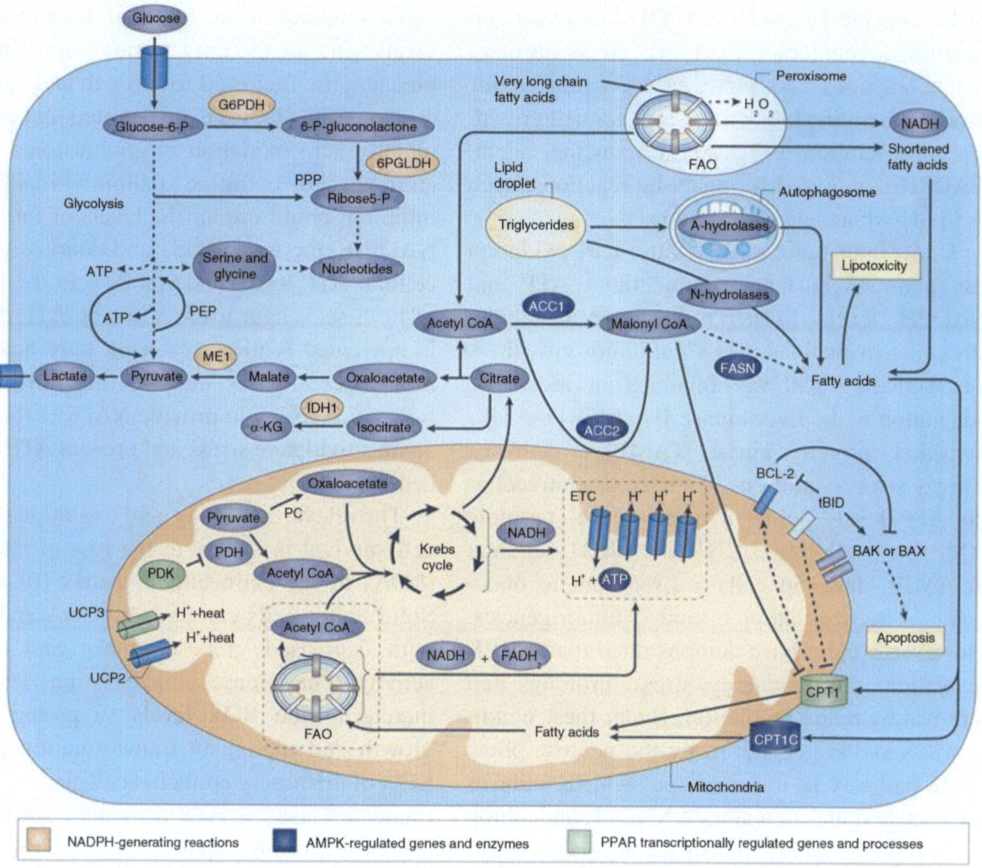

Fig. 2 Effect of fatty acid oxidation on cancer cell metabolism, growth, and survival. The metabolic interactions with fatty acid oxidation (FAO) are as shown. Metabolic routes, including glycolysis, the pentose phosphate pathway (PPP), the Krebs cycle, the electron transport chain (ETC), and FAO are included. FAO main products, acetyl-CoA, NADH, and $FADH_2$, go through various reactions. Acetyl-CoA enters Krebs cycle (TCA cycle) to produce citrate, while generated NADH and $FADH_2$ are oxidized in the ETC for ATP production. Dashed arrows show indirect effects or serial reactions. *G6PDH* glucose-6-phosphate dehydrogenase, *6PGLDH* 6-phosphogluconate dehydrogenase, *ME1* malic enzyme, *IDH1* isocitrate dehydrogenase 1, *α-KG* α-ketoglutarate, *PDH* pyruvate dehydrogenase, *PDK* pyruvate dehydrogenase kinase, *PEP* phosphoenol pyruvate, *PPAR* peroxisome proliferator-activated receptor, *UCP* uncoupling protein. (Reprinted with permission [37])

downregulation of CPT2 enables HCC cells to escape lipotoxicity and promotes hepatocarcinogenesis [40]. Based on the data from the GEO and TCGA databases, we found that the expression level of CPT2 was significantly downregulated in head and neck squamous cell carcinoma (HNSCC) tumor tissues, in comparison with the normal controls, and the patients with high CPT2 expression had better overall survival rate than those with low CPT2 expression. In addition, knockdown of CPT2 significantly promoted the proliferation, migration, and invasion capability of HNSCC cells. On the other hand, overexpression of CPT2 in HNSCC cells significantly impaired the cell proliferation, migration, and invasion ability in HNSCC cells [41].

Fatty acid oxidation is one of the major sources of ATP production. In addition to ATP, fatty acid oxidation is involved in production of cytosolic NADPH, which is the reduced form of NADP+. However, there are other alternative or redundant routes to replenish cytosolic NADPH including the pentose phosphate pathway and the conversion of malate to pyruvate catalyzed by malic enzyme [37, 42]. NAPDH has two main functions, counteract oxidative stress through redox reactions and serve as a co-enzyme for anabolic building block necessary for cell growth and proliferation [43]. As a reducing agent, NADPH is required for anabolic reactions, such as lipid and nucleic acid synthesis.

Under metabolic stress, fatty acid oxidation can maintain sustained intracellular ATP and NADPH levels [44]. Overcoming metabolic stress is a critical step for solid tumor growth. A key signaling pathway involved in metabolic adaptation is the liver kinase B1 (LKB1)–AMP-activated protein kinase (AMPK) pathway. Energy stress conditions that decrease intracellular ATP levels below a certain level promote AMPK activation by LKB1, and LKB1-deficient or AMPK-deficient cells are resistant to oncogenic transformation and tumorigenesis. However, studies have demonstrated that AMPK activation, during energy stress, prolongs cell survival by redox regulation. Under these conditions, NADPH generation by the pentose phosphate pathway is impaired, but AMPK induces alternative routes to maintain NADPH and inhibit cell death. The inhibition of the acetyl-CoA carboxylases ACC1 and ACC2 by AMPK maintains NADPH levels by decreasing NADPH consumption in fatty acid synthesis and increasing NADPH generation by means of fatty acid oxidation. Knockdown of either ACC1 or ACC2 compensates for AMPK activation and facilitates anchorage-independent growth and solid tumor formation in vivo, whereas the activation of ACC1 or ACC2 attenuates these processes. These results suggest that AMPK, in addition to its function in ATP homeostasis, has a key function in NADPH maintenance, which is critical for cancer cell survival under energy stress conditions, such as glucose limitations, anchorage-independent growth, and solid tumor formation in vivo [44].

Normal differentiated cells rely primarily on mitochondrial oxidative phosphorylation to produce ATP to maintain their viability and functions by using three major bioenergetic fuels, glucose, glutamine, and fatty acids. Many cancer cells, however, rely on aerobic glycolysis or elevated glutaminolysis for their growth and survival. In fact, fatty acids are important bioenergetic fuel used for growth and survival of cancer cells. Studies demonstrated that inhibition of fatty acid oxidation in glioblastoma cells by etomoxir, a carnitine palmitoyltransferase 1 inhibitor, could impair the levels of intracellular NADPH, increase ROS, and markedly reduce cellular ATP levels and viability. In the presence of ROS scavenger tiron, however, ATP depletion is prevented without restoring fatty acid oxidation. These results indicate that mitochondrial fatty acid oxidation provide NADPH for defense against oxidative stress and prevent ATP loss and cell death [45].

The relevance of fatty acid oxidation for tumor cell survival is related to the loss of attachment (LOA) to the extracellular matrix (ECM) [11]. Solid tumor cells can undergo LOA and present with decreased glucose uptake and catabolic activity. They sense compensation demand by increasing the ROS levels to promote tumor growth and malignant transformation [37, 46]. LOA of mammary epithelial cells from ECM was found to cause an ATP deficiency owing to the loss of glucose transport, and the ATP deficiency could be rescued by antioxidant treatment without rescue of glucose uptake. This rescue was dependent on stimulation of fatty acid oxidation, which is inhibited by detachment-induced ROS. This study provided evidence of an increase in ROS in matrix-deprived cells in the luminal space of mammary acini, and the discovery that antioxidants facilitate the survival of these cells and enhance anchorage-independent colony formation. The findings show both the importance of matrix attachment in regulating metabolic activity and a mechanism for cell survival in altered matrix environments by antioxidant restoration of ATP generation [47].

Lipogenesis and fatty acid oxidation are mutually exclusive processes coordinated by the level of malonyl-CoA. Malonyl-CoA, an intermediate of fatty acid synthesis, acts as an allosteric inhibitor of CPT1, presumably preventing fatty acid oxidation from occurring simultaneously with active lipogenesis [42]. Decreased activity of ACC, the enzyme that catalyzes the formation of malonyl-CoA from acetyl-CoA, would cause a decreased cellular level of malonyl-CoA. The decreased malonyl-CoA levels in turn prevent inhibition of CPT1 and may cause an ultimate increase in fatty acid oxidation.

Diffuse large B-cell lymphomas (DLBCLs) are a genetically heterogeneous group of tumors and the most common non-Hodgkin lymphomas in adults. Based on DNA microarray analysis of gene expression, DLBCL can be grouped as three discrete subsets: the "B cell receptor/proliferation (BCR-DLBCL)" displaying upregulation of genes encoding BCR signaling components, the "OxPhos-DLBCL" significantly enriched in genes involved in mitochondrial oxidative phosphorylation (OxPhos), and the host response (HR) tumors largely characterized by a brisk host inflammatory infiltrate [48]. The OxPhos-DLBCL subset is actually insensitive to inhibition of BCR survival signaling. Studies showed that, compared with BCR-DLBCLs, OxPhos-DLBCLs display enhanced mitochondrial energy transduction, greater incorporation of nutrient-derived carbons into the TCA cycle, and increased glutathione levels. Moreover, perturbation of the fatty acid oxidation and glutathione synthesis proved selectively toxic to this tumor subset. This study clearly demonstrated the heterogeneity of DLBCL metabolic programs and provided evidence for distinct metabolic fingerprints and associated survival mechanisms in DLBCL, which may have therapeutic implications [48].

Promyelocytic leukemia protein (PML) is a tumor suppressor required for the assembly of a number of nuclear structures, called PML-nuclear bodies, which form among the chromatin of the cell nucleus. PML mutation or loss, and the subsequent dysregulation of these processes, has been implicated in a variety of cancers. Studies have identified that PML–peroxisome proliferator-activated receptor δ (PPAR-δ)–fatty acid oxidation pathway is required for the maintenance of hematopoietic stem cells (HSCs). Loss of PPAR-δ or inhibition of mitochondrial fatty acid oxidation induced loss of HSC maintenance, whereas treatment with PPAR-δ agonists improved HSC maintenance. PML exerts its essential role in HSC maintenance through regulation of PPAR signaling and fatty acid oxidation. Mechanistically, the PML–PPAR-δ–fatty acid oxidation pathway controls the asymmetric division of HSCs. Deletion of Ppard or Pml as well as inhibition of fatty acid oxidation resulted in the symmetric commitment of HSC daughter cells, whereas PPAR-δ activation increased asymmetric cell division. These findings identified a metabolic switch for the control of HSC cell fate with potential therapeutic implications [49].

Recently, a fatty acid oxidation-dependent metabolic shift was found to regulate the activity of hippocampal neural stem/progenitor cells (NSPCs). Quiescent NSPCs showed high levels of CPT1A-dependent fatty acid oxidation, which was downregulated in proliferating NSPCs. Pharmacological inhibition and conditional deletion of CPT1A in vitro and in vivo led to altered NSPC behavior, showing that CPT1A-dependent fatty acid oxidation was required for stem cell maintenance and proper neurogenesis. Interestingly, manipulation of malonyl-CoA, the metabolite that regulates levels of fatty acid oxidation, was sufficient to induce exit from quiescence and to enhance NSPC proliferation. These findings demonstrated an important regulatory role of fatty acid oxidation in governing adult neural stem cell behavior and activity [50].

4 Clinical Perspective

Since de novo fatty acid biosynthesis is significantly enhanced in various types of cancer tissues, it appears to be a promising antineoplastic strategy to inhibit the enzymes that control the fatty acid synthesis in cancer cells. Over the years, a number of fatty acid synthesis inhibitors have been developed for preclinical and clinical studies, including but not limited to TOFA and Soraphen A (ACC inhibitors), Triacscin C (ACSL inhibitor), C75 (4-methylene-2-octyl-5-oxotetrahydrofuran-3-carboxylic acid, FASN inhibitor), and Fatostatin (SREBP inhibitor) [51, 52]. Meanwhile, tumor cells also depend on fatty acid oxidation for extra energy source. There has been growing attention to target the rate-limiting enzyme CPT1 of the fatty acid oxidation for therapeutic intervention. Perhexiline is a CPT1 inhibitor approved for clinical use as an anti-anginal drug in Australia and Asia and currently in clinical trials in the USA [37]. Recently, Perhexiline has been combined with diphenyleneiodonium, an oxidative phosphorylation (OXPHOS) inhibitor, to prevent myeloma tumor xenograft progression [53]. Ranolazine, an inhibitor of the terminal enzyme in fatty acid oxidation, 3-ketoacyl CoA, is an FDA approved piperazine derivative with anti-anginal and potential antineoplastic activities. Ranolazine was found to inhibit breast cancer cell invasion, leukemia cell proliferation, and lung colonization potential [54, 55]. Testing of these compounds, as well as those inhibitors of fatty acid synthesis, may lead to a potential effective anticancer treatment [37, 51]. Inhibition of rate-limiting enzymes responsible for fatty acid metabolism may involve a complex network of signaling cascade that can direct the fate of cellular activity toward survival or programed cell death. Due to cancer cell's ability to metabolic adaption, inhibition of individual enzyme of fatty acid metabolism may not be sufficient as cancer cells are known to rewire alternative metabolic pathways in order to survive [56]. Therefore, a systems approach targeting two or more enzymes of fatty acid metabolism may be needed for a more effective cancer treatment.

References

1. Li, T., & Le, A. (2018). Glutamine metabolism in cancer. *Advances in Experimental Medicine and Biology, 1063*, 13–32.
2. Warburg, O. (1956). On the origin of cancer cells. *Science, 123*(3191), 309–314.
3. Zhdanov, A. V., et al. (2014). Availability of the key metabolic substrates dictates the respiratory response of cancer cells to the mitochondrial uncoupling. *Biochimica et Biophysica Acta, 1837*(1), 51–62.
4. Daye, D., & Wellen, K. E. (2012). Metabolic reprogramming in cancer: unraveling the role of glutamine in tumorigenesis. *Seminars in Cell & Developmental Biology, 23*(4), 362–369.
5. Chen, L., & Cui, H. (2015). Targeting glutamine induces apoptosis: A cancer therapy approach. *International Journal of Molecular Sciences, 16*(9), 22830–22855.
6. Tumanov, S., Bulusu, V., & Kamphorst, J. J. (2015). Analysis of fatty acid metabolism using stable isotope tracers and mass spectrometry. *Metabolic Analysis Using Stable Isotopes, 561*, 197–217.
7. Koundouros, N., Poulogiannis, G. (2020). Reprogramming of fatty acid metabolism in cancer. *British Journal of Cancer, 122*, 4–22.
8. Currie, E., et al. (2013). Cellular fatty acid metabolism and cancer. *Cell Metabolism, 18*(2), 153–161.
9. Mashima, T., Seimiya, H., & Tsuruo, T. (2009). De novo fatty-acid synthesis and related pathways as molecular targets for cancer therapy. *British Journal of Cancer, 100*(9), 1369–1372.
10. Kuhajda, F. P. (2006). Fatty acid synthase and cancer: New application of an old pathway. *Cancer Research, 66*(12), 5977–5980.
11. Qu, Q., et al. (2016). Fatty acid oxidation and carnitine palmitoyltransferase I: Emerging therapeutic targets in cancer. *Cell Death & Disease, 7*, e2226.
12. Quijano, C., et al. (2016). Interplay between oxidant species and energy metabolism. *Redox Biology, 8*, 28–42.
13. Daniels, V. W., et al. (2014). Cancer cells differentially activate and thrive on de novo lipid synthesis pathways in a low-lipid environment. *PLoS One, 9*(9), e106913.
14. Chalbos, D., et al. (1987). Fatty acid synthetase and its mRNA are induced by progestins in breast cancer cells. *The Journal of Biological Chemistry, 262*(21), 9923–9926.
15. Shah, U. S., et al. (2006). Fatty acid synthase gene overexpression and copy number gain in prostate adenocarcinoma. *Human Pathology, 37*(4), 401–409.
16. Kumar-Sinha, C., et al. (2003). Transcriptome analysis of HER2 reveals a molecular connection to fatty acid synthesis. *Cancer Research, 63*(1), 132–139.
17. Yoon, S., et al. (2007). Up-regulation of Acetyl-CoA carboxylase alpha and fatty acid synthase by human epidermal growth factor receptor 2 at the translational level in breast cancer cells. *Journal of Biological Chemistry, 282*(36), 26122–26131.
18. Martel, P. M., et al. (2006). S14 protein in breast cancer cells: Direct evidence of regulation by SREBP-1c, superinduction with progestin, and effects on cell growth. *Experimental Cell Research, 312*(3), 278–288.
19. D'Erchia, A. M., et al. (2006). The fatty acid synthase gene is a conserved p53 family target from worm to human. *Cell Cycle, 5*(7), 750–758.
20. Furuta, E., et al. (2008). Fatty acid synthase gene is up-regulated by hypoxia via activation of Akt and sterol regulatory element binding protein-1. *Cancer Research, 68*(4), 1003–1011.
21. Menendez, J. A., Decker, J. P., & Lupu, R. (2005). In support of Fatty Acid Synthase (FAS) as a metabolic oncogene: Extracellular acidosis acts in an epigenetic fashion activating FAS gene expression in cancer cells. *Journal of Cellular Biochemistry, 94*(1), 1–4.
22. Menendez, J. A., et al. (2004). Inhibition of fatty acid synthase (FAS) suppresses HER2/neu (erbB-2) oncogene overexpression in cancer cells. *Proceedings of the National Academy of Sciences of the United States of America, 101*(29), 10715–10720.

23. Sanchez-Solana, B., Li, D. Q., & Kumar, R. (2014). Cytosolic functions of MORC2 in lipogenesis and adipogenesis. *Biochimica et Biophysica Acta, 1843*(2), 316–326.
24. Hatzivassiliou, G., et al. (2005). ATP citrate lyase inhibition can suppress tumor cell growth. *Cancer Cell, 8*(4), 311–321.
25. Bauer, D. E., et al. (2005). ATP citrate lyase is an important component of cell growth and transformation. *Oncogene, 24*(41), 6314–6322.
26. Pizer, E. S., et al. (1999). Malonyl-coenzyme-A is a potential mediator of cytotoxicity induced by fatty acid synthase inhibition in human breast cancer cells and xenografts. *Clinical Cancer Research, 5*, 3767s–3767s.
27. Brusselmans, K., et al. (2005). RNA interference-mediated silencing of the acetyl-CoA-carboxylase-alpha gene induces growth inhibition and apoptosis of prostate cancer cells. *Cancer Research, 65*(15), 6719–6725.
28. Chajes, V., et al. (2006). Acetyl-CoA carboxylase alpha is essential to breast cancer cell survival. *Cancer Research, 66*(10), 5287–5294.
29. Zhou, W., et al. (2009). Malonyl-CoA decarboxylase inhibition is selectively cytotoxic to human breast cancer cells. *Oncogene, 28*(33), 2979–2987.
30. Schug, Z. T., et al. (2015). Acetyl-CoA synthetase 2 promotes acetate utilization and maintains cancer cell growth under metabolic stress. *Cancer Cell, 27*(1), 57–71.
31. Pietrocola, F., et al. (2015). Acetyl coenzyme A: a central metabolite and second messenger. *Cell Metabolism, 21*(6), 805–821.
32. Li, F., et al. (2018). Discovery and validation of salivary extracellular RNA biomarkers for noninvasive detection of gastric cancer. *Clinical Chemistry, 64*(10), 1513–1521.
33. Bulusu, V., et al. (2017). Acetate recapturing by nuclear acetyl-CoA synthetase 2 prevents loss of histone acetylation during oxygen and serum limitation. *Cell Reports, 18*(3), 647–658.
34. Li, L. O., Klett, E. L., & Coleman, R. A. (2010). Acyl-CoA synthesis, lipid metabolism and lipotoxicity. *Biochimica et Biophysica Acta, 1801*(3), 246–251.
35. Eberlé, D., et al. (2004). SREBP transcription factors: Master regulators of lipid homeostasis. *Biochimie, 86*(11), 839–848.
36. Guo, D. L., et al. (2009). EGFR signaling through an Akt-SREBP-1-dependent, rapamycin-resistant pathway sensitizes glioblastomas to antilipogenic therapy. *Science Signaling, 2*(101), ra82.
37. Carracedo, A., Cantley, L. C., & Pandolfi, P. P. (2013). Cancer metabolism: fatty acid oxidation in the limelight. *Nature Reviews. Cancer, 13*(4), 227–232.
38. Price, N. T., et al. (2002). A novel brain-expressed protein related to carnitine palmitoyltransferase I. *Genomics, 80*(4), 433–442.
39. Zaugg, K., et al. (2011). Carnitine palmitoyltransferase 1C promotes cell survival and tumor growth under conditions of metabolic stress. *Genes & Development, 25*(10), 1041–1051.
40. Fujiwara, N., et al. (2018). CPT2 downregulation adapts HCC to lipid-rich environment and promotes carcinogenesis via acylcarnitine accumulation in obesity. *Gut, 67*(8), 1493–1504.
41. Zhenning Jin, S. H. (2019). *The role of CPT2 in head and neck squamous cell carcinoma.* UCLA thesis ProQuest ID: Jin_ucla_0031N_18007.
42. Ma, Y., et al. (2018). Fatty acid oxidation: An emerging facet of metabolic transformation in cancer. *Cancer Letters, 435*, 92–100.
43. Kumari, S., et al. (2018). Reactive oxygen species: A key constituent in cancer survival. *Biomarker Insights, 13*, 1177271918755391.
44. Jeon, S. M., Chandel, N. S., & Hay, N. (2012). AMPK regulates NADPH homeostasis to promote tumour cell survival during energy stress. *Nature, 485*(7400), 661–665.
45. Pike, L. S., et al. (2011). Inhibition of fatty acid oxidation by etomoxir impairs NADPH production and increases reactive oxygen species resulting in ATP depletion and cell death in human glioblastoma cells. *Biochimica et Biophysica Acta, 1807*(6), 726–734.
46. Panieri, E., & Santoro, M. M. (2016). ROS homeostasis and metabolism: a dangerous liason in cancer cells. *Cell Death & Disease, 7*(6), e2253.
47. Schafer, Z. T., et al. (2009). Antioxidant and oncogene rescue of metabolic defects caused by loss of matrix attachment. *Nature, 461*(7260), 109–113.
48. Caro, P., et al. (2012). Metabolic signatures uncover distinct targets in molecular subsets of diffuse large B cell lymphoma. *Cancer Cell, 22*(4), 547–560.
49. Ito, K., et al. (2012). A PML–PPAR-δ pathway for fatty acid oxidation regulates hematopoietic stem cell maintenance. *Nature Medicine, 18*(9), 1350–1358.
50. Knobloch, M., et al. (2017). A fatty acid oxidation-dependent metabolic shift regulates adult neural stem cell activity. *Cell Reports, 20*(9), 2144–2155.
51. Röhrig, F., & Schulze, A. (2016). The multifaceted roles of fatty acid synthesis in cancer. *Nature Reviews. Cancer, 16*(11), 732–749.
52. Chen, C., et al. (2014, *289*). 4-methylene-2-octyl-5-oxotetrahydrofuran-3-carboxylic acid (C75), an inhibitor of fatty-acid synthase, suppresses the mitochondrial fatty acid synthesis pathway and impairs mitochondrial function. *The Journal of biological chemistry*, (24), 17184–17194.
53. Xu, S., et al. (2019). An HK2 antisense oligonucleotide induces synthetic lethality in $HK1^-$ $HK2^+$ multiple myeloma. *Cancer Research, 79*(10), 2748.
54. Driffort, V., et al. (2014). Ranolazine inhibits NaV1.5-mediated breast cancer cell invasiveness and lung colonization. *Molecular Cancer, 13*, 264.
55. Samudio, I., et al. (2010). Pharmacologic inhibition of fatty acid oxidation sensitizes human leukemia cells to apoptosis induction. *The Journal of Clinical Investigation, 120*(1), 142–156.
56. Zhang, M., et al. (2014). Oral cancer cells may rewire alternative metabolic pathways to survive from siRNA silencing of metabolic enzymes. *BMC Cancer, 14*, 223–223.

HIF-1α Metabolic Pathways in Human Cancer

Naseim Elzakra and Yong Kim

1 Hypoxic Response

Oxygen is directly involved in a wide range of physiological pathways essential for maintaining and promoting homeostasis such as injury response and blood pressure adaptation [2], as well as in pathological processes such as inflammation [3] and tumor formation. A key to understanding such regulations could be accomplished through elucidating the molecular mechanisms by which cells respond and adapt to insufficiency in oxygen supply, a phenomenon known as hypoxic response. Although hypoxia is characterized by suppression in both ATP and protein production as mechanisms to reserve energy, interestingly, there is an abundance of a wide spectrum of genes during the low oxygen status [4, 5]; these genes are referred to as hypoxia-responsive genes. It was reported that 2% of the entire human genome is involved in hypoxia response via interaction with what is known as hypoxia-inducible factors (HIFs), both in a direct and an indirect fashion [6]. Activation of the hypoxia-responsive genes serves to protect cells from the harmful ramifications of oxygen deficiency such as ischemia, particularly that many metabolic and energy-related pathways are controlled by these genes [7, 8]. In addition, hypoxia-responsive genes were found to be heavily involved in the embryonic development. For instance, the deletion of HIF-1α in a mouse embryo leads to death at day 10 [9, 10]. Altogether, hypoxic response is responsible for the activation of a global network of genes that through diverse mechanisms aim to maintain tissue integrity and promote cell survival [6, 11, 12]. Once activated, HIF transcription factors binds to specific DNA sequences unique to their target genes. These DNA regions are called hypoxia-response elements (HREs) [13–16]. Many factors could determine the potential binding between HIFs and HRE, including HIF-1 protein concentration, oxygen tension, availability of cofactors, and posttranslational protein modifications [17, 18].

N. Elzakra (✉)
School of Dentistry, University of California Los Angeles, Los Angeles, CA, USA
e-mail: naseimelzakra@ucla.edu

Y. Kim (✉)
School of Dentistry, University of California Los Angeles, Los Angeles, CA, USA

Laboratory of Stem Cell and Cancer Epigenetics, Center for Oral Oncology Research, UCLA School of Dentistry, Los Angeles, CA, USA

UCLA's Jonsson Comprehensive Cancer Center, Los Angeles, CA, USA

Broad Stem Cell Research Institute, Los Angeles, CA, USA
e-mail: thadyk@ucla.edu

S. Hu (ed.), *Cancer Metabolomics*, Advances in Experimental Medicine and Biology 1280,
https://doi.org/10.1007/978-3-030-51652-9_17

2 Hypoxia-Inducible Factor

Hypoxia-inducible factors (HIFs) are members of a family of transcription factors that are involved in the adaptive responses to hypoxia. Structurally, all HIFs are composed of an alpha and a beta subunit with both subunits belong to the family of basic-helix-loop-helix PAS (Per-Ahr/ ARNT-Sim) family of transcription factors. The three HIF members are named HIF-1, HIF-2, and HIF-3. Both HIF-1 and HIF-2 are heavily involved in the response to hypoxia through their transcriptional activities, whereas the role of HIF-3 in this context remains ill-defined [19]. This family is characterized by its conserved domains for both DNA binding and target specificity [20]. Many characteristics such as heterodimerization, hypoxia-mediated stabilization, and transcriptional activity are shared among all three isoforms [21–24].

HIF-1 transcription factor is a heterodimer consisting of two subunits: an oxygen-labile alpha subunit (HIF-1α) and a stable, constitutively-expressed, oxygen-independent beta subunit (HIF-1β). In hypoxia, HIF-1α is the primary responder, and so, its stability is of greater impact when compared to ARNT [25–29]. Nevertheless, ARNT was shown to be required for the HIF1 overall activity such as binding to other bHLH proteins [30–33].

Structurally, HIF-1α contains two transactivational domains (TADs), the N-terminal (N-TAD) and the C-terminal (C-TAD), that drive the functional interaction with RNA polymerase. TADs also are the sites where the interaction with coactivators is established, a process that has an indispensable role in HIF-1α transcriptional activity. Furthermore, TADs are the domains where post-translational modifications take place [17, 25, 34, 35]. Interestingly, upon hypoxia-mediated HIF1 activation, only its protein levels increase, while mRNA expression remains unchanged. This observation highlights the direct proportional relation between oxygen concentration and protein translation and stability [25, 36]. Lastly, the oxygen-dependent degradation domain (ODD domain) serves as an oxygen sensor site where oxygen-dependent interactions take place [37].

HIF-2 proteins have had many names, such as endothelial PAS protein 1 (EPAS1), HIF-related factor (HRF), HIF-1α-like factor (HLF), and member of PAS family 2 (MOP2) [21–24]. On the level of the protein's primary structure, HIF-2α is very similar to HIF-1α with almost half the amino acids being identical between the two. In particular, the two proteins are sharing 70% and 83% homology in their PAS and bHLH domains, respectively. Moreover, both isoforms are subjected to the same regulatory mechanism owing to the presence of two critical proline residues in their ODD domains [38–40]. Moreover, both HIF-1α and HIF-2α contain N-TAD and C-TAD, while HIF-1β contains only C-TAD (Fig. 1).

HIF-2 expression was thought initially to be exclusive to vascular endothelial cells, specifically in embryonic tissues [35, 42, 43]. Later, HIF-2 protein expression was confirmed in several adult hypoxic tissues [42]. In cancer tissues, HIF-2 expression was also reported to be upregulated, suggesting a potential role in cancer angiogenesis [44] especially with the protein's preference for vascular and stromal tissues [43, 45]. As such, higher levels of HIF-1 are observed in tumor epithelial cells when compared with HIF-2, whereas the opposite is true in macrophages and endothelial cells [46]. In cancer, HIF-2 expression was shown to be directly proportional to the pathological staging of a number of solid cancers such as non-Hodgkin lymphoma [45, 47] and bladder cancer [43]. One explanation for such correlation is that the presence of HIF-2-positive macrophage populations in cancer tissues is beneficial to the tumor microenvironment (TME), therefore inversely affecting patient's survival. Another explanation is related to the role played by HIF-2 in promoting cancer angiogenesis and vascularization [45], since VEGF, the master angiogenic protein, co-reside in stromal tissues as well [48]. Many studies have confirmed the correlation between the HIF-2 and VEGF proteins [43, 49–52].

Noteworthy, many studies reported a contradicting role of HIF-2α in cancer. For example, loss of HIF-2α in KRAS lung tumor increased tumor aggressive behavior [53], whereas overex-

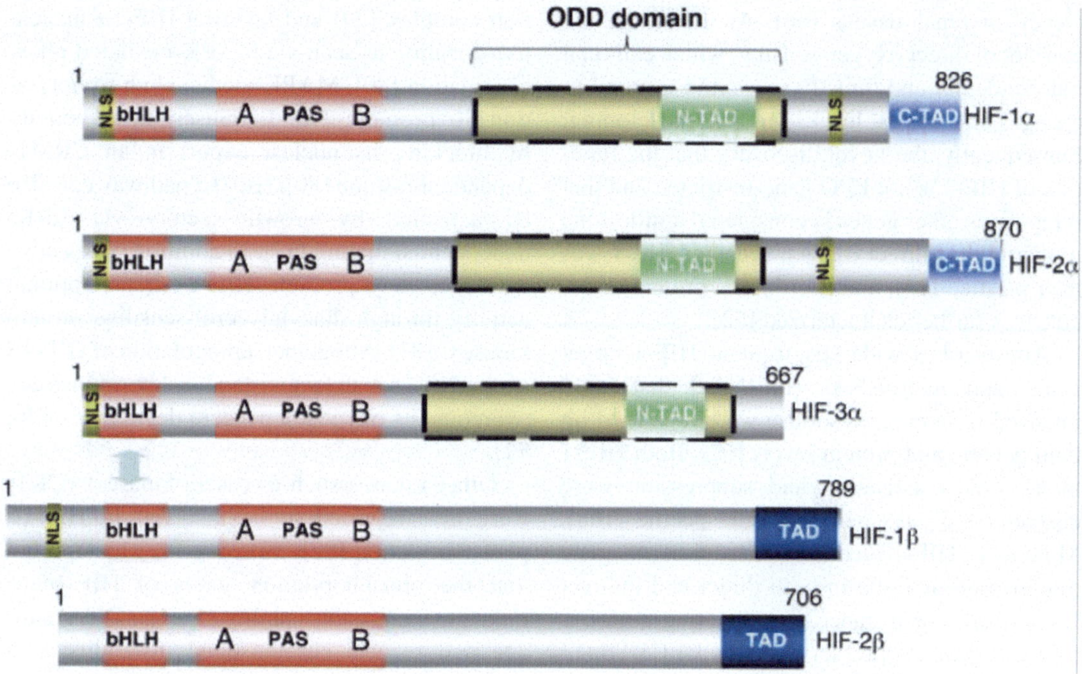

Fig. 1 Schematic of the structure of three HIFα and two HIFβ isoforms. NLS, nuclear localization signal; bHLH, basic helix-loop-helix domain; PAS, per-arnt-sim domain subdivided into PAS A and PAS B; ODD, oxygen-dependent degradation domain; TAD, transactivation domain. HIF-1α and HIF-2α have two distinct TADs, in the C- (C-TAD) and N- (N-TAD) terminal domains. The PAS and bHLH domains are dedicated to dimerization and recognition of target DNA sequences. (Reprinted with permission from [41])

pression and stabilization of HIF-2α protein in an identical tumor model promoted tumor angiogenesis and invasion by increasing the expression of VEGF and SNAIL [54], respectively. The observation that opposite HIF-2α expression profiles mediated tumor growth in the same tumor context, albeit by different mechanisms, suggests that effective targeting of HIF-2α subunit in cancer treatment may be complicated.

The third isoform is referred to as HIF-3 [55], and although it shares a significant structural similarity with the other two isoforms, it is reported that its main function is to inhibit HIF pathway [56]. On the other hand, other studies showed that HIF-3 has a dual action of both stimulating and suppressing other HIF members. Therefore, the role of HIF-3 in hypoxic and cancer tissues in particular is yet to be elucidated [57–60].

HIF β protein was first discovered in the neural tissues where involvement with neural development was assumed [61]. It is also known as the aryl hydrocarbon receptor nuclear translocator (ARNT) [16, 62, 63]. There are two forms of ARNT termed ARNT1 and ARNT2 [64, 65] with both forms are capable of forming a heterodimer with the HIF α isoforms, an interaction crucial for HRE binding and subsequent downstream effector gene activation [65]. Currently, HIF-1α, HIF-2α, and ARNT1 are viewed as the key molecules involved in HIF pathway in response to hypoxia, especially in tumor tissues, while the function of both HIF-3α and ARNT2 is still under investigation. In this review, we will focus on the functional role of HIF-1α in driving hypoxia response in human cancer.

2.1 Discovery of HIF-1

HIF-1 was initially viewed as an essential and exclusive key element in the human erythropoietin (EPO) gene in response to oxygen insufficiency in renal tissues [66]. At that time, the concept of direct oxygen sensing, which cells can independently and directly sense and respond to changes in oxygen level, was still developing. Subsequently, the novel discovery that the function of HIF-1 is not EPO gene-restricted and that it regulates other genes is considered a milestone in the field of direct oxygen sensing. HIF-1 was later purified [14], and shortly, the protein molecule was further characterized [62].

Afterward, a wide spectrum of HIF-1 target genes and microRNAs (miRNAs) that were involved in hypoxic response were identified on both genetic and protein levels [67]. Both HIF-1 target gene's activation and suppression were characterized as being tissue-specific [68]. Moreover, HIF-1-mediated activation of gene transcription may be in both direct and indirect fashion [6]. For instance, by activating miRNAs [67] and gene-suppressors such as DEC1/Stra13 [69], HIF-1 is indirectly silencing certain downstream effector genes. Key biological pathways such as proliferation, energy metabolism, invasion, and metastasis were found to be driven by HIF-1 downstream effector genes [70, 71] (Fig. 2), suggesting the important role of HIF-1-mediated pathways in cancer development and progression.

2.2 Regulation of HIF-1α

It was reported that many oncogenes activate HIF-1α pathway mainly via phosphorylation cascades through upregulating the transcription and translation of HIF-1α mRNA and protein, respectively, and independently of oxygen levels [72]. Similarly, growth factors and cytokines such as epidermal and fibroblast growth factors and insulin-like growth factor could activate HIF-1α through the same phosphorylation mechanism [73–76]. This phosphorylation cascade could promote HIF-1α expression via several pathways. One example is the PI3K/Akt/mTOR-mediated HIF-1α pathway activation as seen in many solid tumors such as in colon [77], prostate [78], and breast cancer [76]. Another mechanism is by enhancing the p300-HIF-1α-C-TAD activation complex [79] and favoring HIF-1α nuclear translocation as seen via MAPK-mediated phosphorylation [80]. MAPK-mediated phosphorylation also promotes HIF-1α transcriptional activity by blocking its nuclear export in an CRM1-dependent fashion [80]. HIF-1α pathway can also be activated by growth factors via ERK-dependent signaling [17]. In addition, vasoactive cytokines may promote HIF-1α transcriptional activity through diacylglycerol-sensitive protein kinase C [81]. Altogether, upregulation of HIF-1α exerted by growth factors and local hormones can overcome its oxygen-dependent degradation [76, 77].

Other kinases such as casein kinase 1 (CK1) were also reported to be involved in HIF-1α phosphorylation [82]. Moreover, it was reported that the phosphorylation status of HIF-1α is linked to the protein's ability to repair DNA damage and reverse chromosomal instability, two characteristics that are extremely important in driving tumor progression and aggressiveness. For instance, dephosphorylation of HIF1α directly leads to repression of NBS1, a DNA mismatch repair gene [83].

In addition to the kinase signaling pathways, loss of function of the gene suppressor von Hippel-Lindau (VHL) results in activation of HIF-1α protein due to the associated lack of protein-degradation suppression [84]. A dysregulation of key carbohydrate metabolic intermediates was also shown to contribute to HIF-1α regulation independently to oxygen levels. For instance, α-ketoglutarate (α-KG) functions as a cofactor for PDH and FIH-1 (factor inhibiting HIF-1) hydroxylates [85] and is therefore directly involved in HIF-1α regulation.

Posttranslational modifications other than phosphorylation are also critical for HIF-1α protein activity. For instance, hydroxylation of HIF-1α protein by prolyl hydroxylase is viewed as the main regulatory mechanism that guards against HIF-1α protein activation in normoxic conditions. HIF hydroxylases exist in two forms: HIF-prolyl hydroxylase, also known as prolyl hydroxylase domain (PHD) proteins, and HIF-asparaginyl hydroxylase, also known as FIH-1 (factor inhibiting HIF-1) [86].

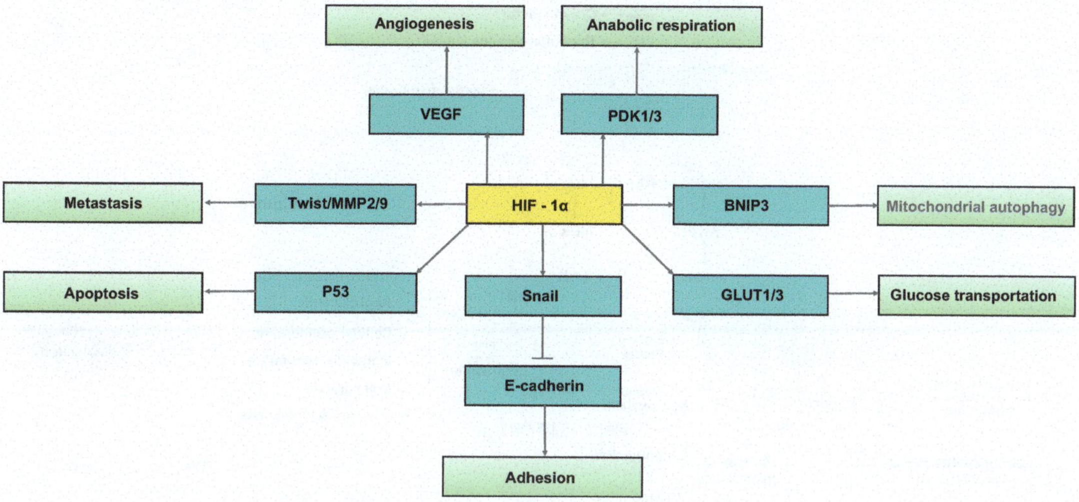

Fig. 2 Representative target genes of HIF-1α and their functions

There are three closely-related isoforms of the PHD protein known as PHD1, PHD2, and PHD3, where PHD2 is considered the most critical under normoxic conditions [87]. PHD enzymes function by hydroxylation of two prolyl segments of HIF-1α protein, where oxygen concentration is an imperative determinant for the reaction initiation [34, 88–90]. This interaction takes place at the ODD domain where the two propyl residues reside. Once hydroxylated, HIF-1α develops a strong binding affinity for a part of an E3 ubiquitin ligase complex VHL protein leading to HIF-1α protein degradation by a proteasome. The reversal of this oxygen-dependent degradation process results in an observed increase in HIF-1α protein levels associated with hypoxia.

A second hydroxylation event targets the asparaginyl residue at the C-TAD of HIF-1α protein by FIH-1. FIH-1 reaction depends exclusively on oxygen availability in the ambient environment [86]. This reaction changes HIF-1α protein's physical properties, such as its water affinity, hindering the interaction between the hydroxylated C-TAD and its coactivators p300/CREB binding protein (CBP) [91, 92]. This reaction will result in C-TAD domain blockage and ultimately HIF-1α transactivation activity inhibition, but not stability, in an oxygen-dependent reversible fashion (Fig. 3).

Redox sensors are equally important to oxygen sensors in the regulation of HIF-1α-mediated hypoxic response. An example is the SIRT1-mediated acetylation process, which is another critical posttranslational modification of HIF-1α. SIRT1 deacetylates HIF-1α by targeting the lysine amino acid leading to the blocking of p300-recruitment and eventually HIF-1α inactivation [94].

2.3 HIF-1α Stability

Although oxygen tension is considered the main factor governing HIF-1α protein stability during hypoxia through the hydroxylation events discussed earlier, mitochondria can also act as a stabilizer of HIF-1α proteins via increased production of reactive oxygen species (ROS) [95–97]. ROS might play a role in protein stabilization mainly through the inactivation of PHD leading to HIF-1α accumulation [98]. Lastly, reports on nitric oxide (NO) effect on HIF are contradictory, with some advocating for HIF-1α stabilization [99–102], whereas others demonstrating an opposite effect on HIF-1α activity [103–105]. Once the protein is stabilized, nuclear translocated, and dimerized with ARNT, hypoxia-responsive genes are activated through HIF-1α binding to a characteristic consensus sequence

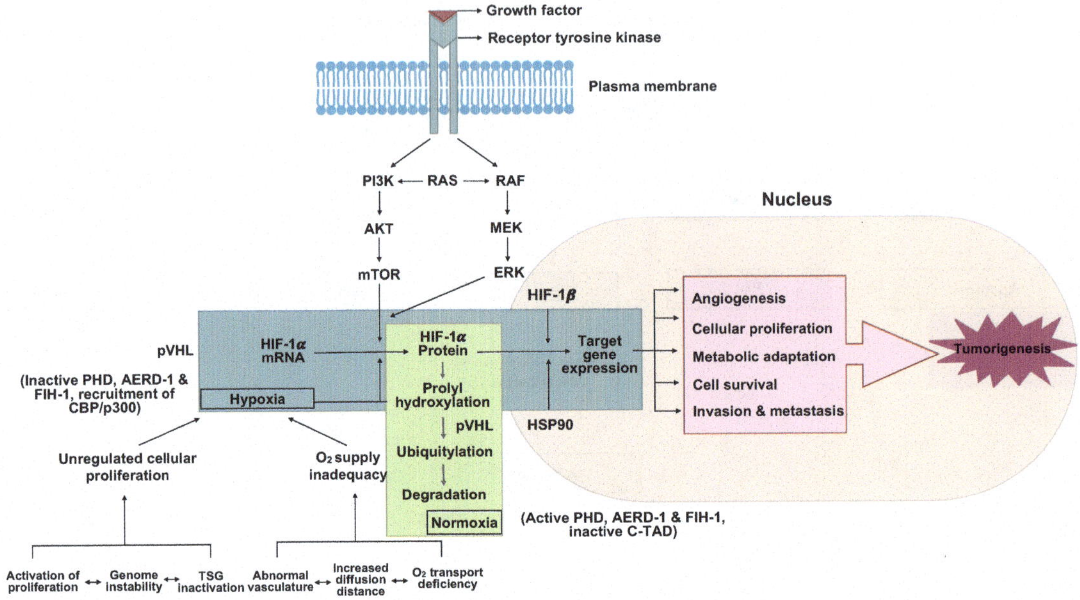

Fig. 3 HIF-1 signaling cascade. Synthesis and constitutive expression of HIF-1α by a cascade involving a series of growth factors and signaling events are indicated. The major differences among the hypoxic and normoxic signaling and sequence of events are also depicted clearly in the flowchart. Normoxia leads to HIF-1α protein degradation whereas hypoxia leads to HIF-1α-regulated target gene expression. The downstream sequence of events leading to tumorigenesis is also portrayed (Modified with permission from [93])

5′-(A/G) CGTG-3 termed HRE [106] located in the upstream region of hypoxia-inducible genes [15, 107, 108].

3 HIF-1α and Metabolic Reprogramming

A shift from glucose metabolism coupled with mitochondrial oxidative to anabolic respiration, known as the Warburg effect, is a hallmark of hypoxia. This metabolic shift takes place through the upregulation of oxygen-independent metabolic pathways, such as glycolysis and downregulation of the oxygen-dependent pathways such as mitochondrial respiration [109]. For instance, overexpression of key glycolytic enzymes such as the rate-limiting enzyme phosphofructokinase [110] and the glycolytic flux regulatory enzymes, 6- phosphofructo-2-kinase and fructose-2,6-bisphosphate, is HIF-1α-mediated in hypoxia [37–40]. Other enzymes such as glucose transporter protein1 (GLUT1) and GLUT3 that are involved in glucose trafficking processes are also the targets of HIF-1α in hypoxia [111, 112]. Noteworthy, there is a positive correlation among cancer pathological staging, GLUT3 and HIF-1α expression and activity levels, a measure that might serve as a prognostic tool [112]. HIF-1α activation also upregulates key enzymes that inhibit acetyl-coenzyme A (acetyl-CoA) production from glucose, therefore inhibiting oxidative phosphorylation. There are two isoforms of the enzyme pyruvate dehydrogenase kinase (PDK) known as PDK1 and PDK3 that directly inhibit acetyl-CoA production and entering into the TCA cycle leading to the shutdown of the oxidative phosphorylation associated with hypoxia. Another approach for cells to shift away from oxidative metabolism is through the activation of mitochondrial autophagy by protein BCL2/adenovirus E1B 19-kDa interacting protein 3 (BNIP3) [113]. BNIP3 functions by activating lactose dehydrogenase A (LDHA) enzyme that converts pyruvate to lactate, therefore promoting the anaerobic respiration.

Similarly, PDK1 and PDK3 were also found to play a role in mitochondrial autophagy [114–116]. In addition, miRNA targets of HIF-1α were found to directly favor the metabolic shift through inhibiting genes that are critical for the mitochondria oxidation machinery and independently of the metabolic enzymes [117]. For instance, miR-210 activation [118] inhibits the iron-sulfur cluster assembly enzyme ISCU, which is essential for the mitochondrial electron transport complex I activity [119, 120]. Noteworthy, due to the scarcity of acetyl-CoA in response to hypoxia, tissues with a high proliferation rate such as cancer will utilize glutamine, instead of glucose, to generate α-ketoglutarate essential for fatty acid synthesis [121, 122]. Glutamine utilization as the main source of energy for such high-energy-demanding cells acts as another repelling force for the pyruvate away from the TCA cycle [121, 122]. HIF-1α-mediated fatty acid metabolism dysregulation in cancer hypoxic tissues was associated with poor survival in many solid tumors such as renal cancer [123]. The high-glycolytic-flux signature in hypoxia serves a unique benefit for cancer tissues, other than solely energy benefit, and that is providing precursors of the pyrimidine/purine pathway needed for DNA synthesis for cell proliferation [124]. For example, it was reported that glucose utilization is directly proportional to increased cancer tissue mass and invasion property [125], suggesting a critical role played by glucose metabolism in tumorigenesis.

HIF-1α significantly contributes to the acidic environment of cancer tissues through the activation of plasma membrane proteins [126] such as monocarboxylate transporter 4 (MCT4), encoded by SLC16A3 gene, through controlling lactic acid transport [127]. Another membranous protein named sodium-hydrogen exchanger 1 (NHE1) that is encoded by the SLC9A gene regulates the pH of the environment through protons pumping [128], and the same mechanism is adopted by carbonic anhydrase 9 (CA9) [129]. In fact, the intracellular alkalinization and extracellular acidification enhance cellular proliferation and invasion [130].

An interesting aspect of HIF-1α regulation lies in its activation loop with pyruvate kinase M2 (PKM2) enzyme. PKM2 is a glycolytic enzyme that may play an important role in cancer progression [131] by promoting glycolysis as well as acting as a coactivator for HIF-1α [132]. HIF-1α also activates the transcription of PKM2 leading to the activation of key oncogenes such as STAT3 and its downstream genes, which further enhances the progression of cancer [133].

4 Hypoxia and Cancer

Tumor hypoxia is an example of a chronic, pathophysiological condition, in which response is insufficient to completely reverse the hypoxic insult [134]. Hypoxia in cancer could be defined on the basis of oxygen and energy levels present in tumors. For instance, a concomitant decrease in both oxygen partial pressure and ATP level occurs in a fibrosarcoma model [135]. A key player in cancer hypoxia dynamics is the hypoxia-induced vascular endothelial growth factor (VEGF). Due to the constant hypoxic insult that cancer tissues are exposed to, VEGF-mediated new blood vessel formation to overcome the oxygen deficiency is slow and disordered. This continuous cycle of defective blood vessel architecture and the activation of hypoxia-mediated pathways is a hallmark for tumor microenvironment (TME) [136] as well as its aggressive phenotype [137]. Many solid tumors such as breast and lung, among others, respond to the decrease in oxygen tension by upregulation of HIF-1α [138–140]. Correlation between hypoxia and tumor malignant transformation had also been observed [141–143].

5 HIF-1α and Immune Cells in Cancer

Many solid tumors are characterized by hypoxia [144] and tumor-associated macrophage (TAM) infiltration [145]. For example, in breast cancer, HIF-1α knockout in TAM caused overstimulation of nitrous oxide (NO) [145, 146], a phenomenon that can put T lymphocytes into anergy status. Hypoxia can also increase the expression of the immune checkpoint programmed death-ligand 1 (PD-L1) on macrophages, dendritic cells, and tumor cells in an HIF-1α-dependent fashion leading to the suppression of effector T-lymphocyte recruitment and activation [147]. Another mechanism that HIF-1α can dampen the antitumor effect of immunity through is the upregulation of regulatory T lymphocytes [148].

6 Role of HIF-1α in Key Cancer Pathways

6.1 Cell Adhesion

Adhesion molecules play a significant role in cancer initiation and progression through promoting its interaction with both intracellular and extracellular environment [149]. HIF-1α is directly involved in the regulation of key adhesion molecules such as β1 integrins and α5β3 and α5β5 expression [150–152]. E-cadherin is also regulated by HIF-1α via its direct regulation of TCF3, ZFHX1A, and ZFHX1B [153] and upregulation of Snail [154] which inhibits E-cadherin gene expression.

6.2 Cell Proliferation

One of the defining characteristics of cancer cells is their uncontrollable proliferation coupled with impairment of cell death pathways and signals awing to overexpression of survival and growth factors; such changes enable cancer cells to adapt to nutritional deprivation or to escape their unfavorable environment. For instance, hypoxia stimulation of VEGF transcription, via the HIF pathway, was shown to be strongly associated with cellular proliferation and metastasis in tumors [155]. Additionally, the expression of hypoxia-mediated telomerase reverse transcriptase (TERT) promotes tumor cells' immortal phenotype [156]. Simultaneously, hypoxia-induced downregulation of membranous integrins was reported to facilitate tumor cell detachment and new tumor growth [157]. A recent study of ARK5 expression in colon cancer showed that it was upregulated in a HIF-1α-dependent manner and that ARK5 serves an important player in cancer proliferation and migration under hypoxic stress [158]; similar effects were also reported in other solid cancers [159–161].

6.3 Metastasis and Invasion

Hypoxia can activate epithelial-to-mesenchymal transition (EMT) via HIF-1α in various types of solid tumors [162–164]. HIF-1α can directly or indirectly regulate key EMT regulators, including TWIST, Snail, carbonic anhydrase IX (CAIX), and GLUT-1 [165–168]. These molecules then trans-activate EMT-related genes, including vimentin, E-cadherin and N-cadherin, to facilitate the progression of the EMT [169, 170]. Matrix metalloproteinase MMP2 and MMP9 have also been reported to be regulated by HIF-1α. The impact of hypoxia-induced MMP-9 expression is extremely central for cellular migration [171, 172]. Besides, two major components of the fibrinolysis system and thus metastasis, named urokinase-type plasminogen activator receptor (uPAR) and plasminogen activator inhibitor-1 (PAI-1), have also been shown to be targets of HIF-1α [173, 174]. TWIST, another essential transcription factor that is involved in hypoxia-mediated EMT and tumor metastasis, is directly regulated by HIF-1α [165]. Other significant HIF-1α target genes directly involved in cancer metastasis are CXC chemokine receptor-4 (CXCR4), c-Met and CC chemokine receptor 7 (CCR7) [175–177], lysyl oxidase (LOX) [6, 178], fibronectin, cathepsin D, and urokinase plasminogen activator [11]. HIF-1α also promotes cell invasion through the upregulation of key invasion-promoting genes such as the autocrine motility factor [179], vimentin, and the receptor tyrosine kinase c-Met [175]. Meanwhile, the stromal-derived factor-1, keratins 14, 18, and 19, the cytokine receptor CXCR4P [180, 181], caveolin-1 (CAV1) [182], uPAR, MMP2, cathepsin D, and fibronectin 1, among others, are transcriptionally upregulated by HIF-1α [183].

6.4 Angiogenesis

Angiogenesis plays an essential role in tumorigenesis. HIF-1α can stimulate an angiogenic response by activating a number of growth factor-encoding genes, including VEGF, angiopoietin1 (ANGPT1) and ANGPT2, placental growth factor (PGF), calcitonin receptor-like receptor (CRLR) [184], and platelet-derived growth factor B (PDGFB) [68, 185]. HIF-1α deletion was reported to be associated with abnormal vasculature [186]. On the other hand, a recent report on pancreatic tumor revealed an alternative mechanism by which cancer cells could maintain angiogenesis in an HIF1α-independent manner [187]. Noteworthy, SUMO-specific protease 1 (SENP1), a HIF-1α target enzyme, is of great importance for HIF-1α stabilization in hypoxia. This positive feedback loop is significant for VEGF activation and angiogenesis [188, 189].

6.5 Apoptosis

Although programmed cell death can be directly triggered by deficiency in oxygen levels in both normal and cancer tissues [190], with accompanying DNA damage [191], the direct effect of HIF pathway on apoptosis is reported to range from apposing cell death [192] to promoting apoptosis [193]. One explanation for this variation in HIF pathway response might be related to the degree for hypoxia and the variation in oxygen tension [194]. A second factor for such fluctuation is the presence of several apoptosis-related proteins, such as cyclin D1, p21, and p27 that are targeted by HIF-1α upon activation, and that apoptosis response depends on the expression profiles of these apoptotic molecules [195]. Lastly, the initial energy level of hypoxic tissues is inevitably a key factor in the apoptosis pathway [196].

Other factors such as the mitochondrial membrane integrity could also trigger an apoptotic response through activating key apoptotic mediators, such as caspase 9, independently of HIF-1α pathway [197]. Wild-type tumor-suppressor gene p53 also plays a critical role in hypoxia-induced apoptosis through caspase 9 and Apaf-1 downstream effector [198, 199]. Other key apoptotic molecules such as BNIP3, a member of the Bcl-2 family [200], and Noxa which is a p53-downstream protein that could sense ROS levels [201] have also been identified as targets of HIF-1α.

7 Clinical Significance and HIF-1α Inhibitors for Cancer Therapy

HIF-1α expression levels were positively correlated with tumor progression in a variety of solid tumors such as glioma and breast cancer, where HIF-1α correlates with tumor pathological grade and invasion in the former [202], and overall poor survival rate in the later [203, 204]. HIF-1α is used as a prognostic marker for different treatment modalities in a variety of solid tumors [205–207].

The combination of HIF-1α expression with oncogenes or tumor suppressor genes is viewed as another powerful prognostic factor. For instance, in ovarian cancer, the coexistence of mutant p53 expression and HIF-1 overexpression was associated with a poor survival rate [208] and resistance to chemotherapy mainly due to p53-mediated activation of RAS signaling that leads to apoptosis impairment [209]. Recently, a correlation between HIF-1α and the tumor suppressor NEDD4L levels in gastric cancer has been proposed as a prognostic marker [210]. In addition, HIF-1α upregulation combined with the antiapoptotic protein Bcl-2 downregulation in esophageal cancer is associated with treatment failure [211].

HIF-1α inhibition provides an innovative approach for modifying tumor niche with promising clinical results. Unfortunately, and awing to the complex network of genes that are regulated by HIF-1α as well as the multilayered HIF-1α regulation mechanisms, it is challenging to develop a specific HIF-1α inhibitor with a high specificity [212]. Another factor that might tremendously affect the drug discovery process is accuracy and sensitivity of the screening methods. Currently, there are several anti-HIF-1α molecules that are classified according to their target site into direct and indirect inhibitors. Direct inhibitors refer to molecules that target the transcriptional activity of HIF-1α, whereas indirect inhibitors are molecules that target HIF-1α transcription and translation on the mRNA and protein levels, respectively [213]. HIF-1α inhibitors are also classified according to the targeted stage of HIF-1α ranging from the mRNA transcription to protein degradation [214]. In conclusion, the continuous search for the specific HIF-1α inhibitor with fewer side effects and better patient tolerance and survival rate is still ongoing. Noteworthy, combination therapy with other target molecules such as antiangiogenic drugs is showing promising results in animal model studies [215, 216]. A comprehensive understanding of the structure, molecular biology, and regulatory machinery of HIF-1α domains will undoubtedly aid in the development of specific HIF-1α inhibitors.

8 Conclusion

It has been nearly three decades since the novel discovery of HIF-1α as a master regulator of hypoxic response as well as its implication in cancer progression and survival in many solid tumors. Since then, HIF-1α was regarded as a significant and promising target in anticancer therapy. A great deal of research in this area as well as the development of HIF-1α inhibitors have clearly translated such impact. Unfortunately, none of these therapies were proven to be precisely and exclusively targeting cancer, leading to undesirable side effects. Indeed, the involvement of HIF-1α in many aspects of physiological pathways seems to be the main obstacle for perfectly targeting it. Therefore, future research may emphasize more on unfolding all the genes and proteins involved in the HIF-1α pathway, elucidating the molecular mechanisms that regulate other HIF members, and finally aim to discover and target a novel cancer-specific molecule from the HIF-1α downstream effectors expanding pool.

References

1. Michiels, C. (2004). Physiological and pathological responses to hypoxia. *The American Journal of Pathology, 164*(6), 1875–1882.
2. Warren, S. M., et al. (2001). Hypoxia regulates osteoblast gene expression. *The Journal of Surgical Research, 99*(1), 147–155.
3. Cramer, T., et al. (2003). HIF-1alpha is essential for myeloid cell-mediated inflammation. *Cell, 112*(5), 645–657.
4. Hochachka, P. W., et al. (1996). Unifying theory of hypoxia tolerance: Molecular/metabolic defense and rescue mechanisms for surviving oxygen lack. *Proceedings of the National Academy of Sciences of the United States of America, 93*(18), 9493–9498.
5. Denko, N., et al. (2003). Hypoxia actively represses transcription by inducing negative cofactor 2 (Dr1/DrAP1) and blocking preinitiation complex assembly. *The Journal of Biological Chemistry, 278*(8), 5744–5749.
6. Manalo, D. J., et al. (2005). Transcriptional regulation of vascular endothelial cell responses to hypoxia by HIF-1. *Blood, 105*(2), 659–669.
7. Semenza, G. L. (1998). Hypoxia-inducible factor 1: Master regulator of O2 homeostasis. *Current Opinion in Genetics & Development, 8*(5), 588–594.
8. Wenger, R. H. (2002). Cellular adaptation to hypoxia: O2-sensing protein hydroxylases, hypoxia-inducible transcription factors, and O2-regulated gene expression. *The FASEB Journal, 16*(10), 1151–1162.
9. Iyer, N. V., et al. (1998). Cellular and developmental control of O2 homeostasis by hypoxia-inducible factor 1 alpha. *Genes & Development, 12*(2), 149–162.
10. Ryan, H. E., Lo, J., & Johnson, R. S. (1998). HIF-1 alpha is required for solid tumor formation and embryonic vascularization. *The EMBO Journal, 17*(11), 3005–3015.
11. Semenza, G. L. (2003). Targeting HIF-1 for cancer therapy. *Nature Reviews. Cancer, 3*(10), 721–732.
12. Schofield, C. J., & Ratcliffe, P. J. (2004). Oxygen sensing by HIF hydroxylases. *Nature Reviews. Molecular Cell Biology, 5*(5), 343–354.
13. Semenza, G. L., et al. (1991). Hypoxia-inducible nuclear factors bind to an enhancer element located 3′ to the human erythropoietin gene. *Proceedings of the National Academy of Sciences of the United States of America, 88*(13), 5680–5684.
14. Semenza, G. L., & Wang, G. L. (1992). A nuclear factor induced by hypoxia via de novo protein synthesis binds to the human erythropoietin gene enhancer at a site required for transcriptional activation. *Molecular and Cellular Biology, 12*(12), 5447–5454.
15. Wang, G. L., & Semenza, G. L. (1993). Characterization of hypoxia-inducible factor 1 and regulation of DNA binding activity by hypoxia. *The Journal of Biological Chemistry, 268*(29), 21513–21518.

16. Wang, G. L., & Semenza, G. L. (1993). General involvement of hypoxia-inducible factor 1 in transcriptional response to hypoxia. *Proceedings of the National Academy of Sciences of the United States of America, 90*(9), 4304–4308.
17. Richard, D. E., et al. (1999). p42/p44 mitogen-activated protein kinases phosphorylate hypoxia-inducible factor 1alpha (HIF-1alpha) and enhance the transcriptional activity of HIF-1. *Journal of Biological Chemistry, 274*(46), 32631–32637.
18. Carrero, P., et al. (2000). Redox-regulated recruitment of the transcriptional coactivators CREB-binding protein and SRC-1 to hypoxia-inducible factor 1alpha. *Molecular and Cellular Biology, 20*(1), 402–415.
19. Duan, C. (2016). Hypoxia-inducible factor 3 biology: Complexities and emerging themes. *American Journal of Physiology. Cell Physiology, 310*(4), C260–C269.
20. Wang, G. L., et al. (1995). Hypoxia-inducible factor 1 is a basic-helix-loop-helix-PAS heterodimer regulated by cellular O2 tension. *Proceedings of the National Academy of Sciences of the United States of America, 92*(12), 5510–5514.
21. Ema, M., et al. (1997). A novel bHLH-PAS factor with close sequence similarity to hypoxia-inducible factor 1alpha regulates the VEGF expression and is potentially involved in lung and vascular development. *Proceedings of the National Academy of Sciences of the United States of America, 94*(9), 4273–4278.
22. Flamme, I., et al. (1997). HRF, a putative basic helix-loop-helix-PAS-domain transcription factor is closely related to hypoxia-inducible factor-1 alpha and developmentally expressed in blood vessels. *Mechanisms of Development, 63*(1), 51–60.
23. Hogenesch, J. B., et al. (1997). Characterization of a subset of the basic-helix-loop-helix-PAS superfamily that interacts with components of the dioxin signaling pathway. *The Journal of Biological Chemistry, 272*(13), 8581–8593.
24. Tian, H., McKnight, S. L., & Russell, D. W. (1997). Endothelial PAS domain protein 1 (EPAS1), a transcription factor selectively expressed in endothelial cells. *Genes & Development, 11*(1), 72–82.
25. Huang, L. E., et al. (1996). Activation of hypoxia-inducible transcription factor depends primarily upon redox-sensitive stabilization of its alpha subunit. *The Journal of Biological Chemistry, 271*(50), 32253–32259.
26. Jiang, B. H., et al. (1997). Transactivation and inhibitory domains of hypoxia-inducible factor 1alpha. Modulation of transcriptional activity by oxygen tension. *The Journal of Biological Chemistry, 272*(31), 19253–19260.
27. Salceda, S., & Caro, J. (1997). Hypoxia-inducible factor 1alpha (HIF-1alpha) protein is rapidly degraded by the ubiquitin-proteasome system under normoxic conditions. Its stabilization by hypoxia depends on redox-induced changes. *The Journal of Biological Chemistry, 272*(36), 22642–22647.
28. Jiang, B. H., et al. (1997). V-SRC induces expression of hypoxia-inducible factor 1 (HIF-1) and transcription of genes encoding vascular endothelial growth factor and enolase 1: Involvement of HIF-1 in tumor progression. *Cancer Research, 57*(23), 5328–5335.
29. Chilov, D., et al. (1999). Induction and nuclear translocation of hypoxia-inducible factor-1 (HIF-1): Heterodimerization with ARNT is not necessary for nuclear accumulation of HIF-1alpha. *Journal of Cell Science, 112*(Pt 8), 1203–1212.
30. Wood, S. M., et al. (1996). The role of the aryl hydrocarbon receptor nuclear translocator (ARNT) in hypoxic induction of gene expression. Studies in ARNT-deficient cells. *The Journal of Biological Chemistry, 271*(25), 15117–15123.
31. Maltepe, E., et al. (1997). Abnormal angiogenesis and responses to glucose and oxygen deprivation in mice lacking the protein ARNT. *Nature, 386*(6623), 403–407.
32. Swanson, H. I., & Bradfield, C. A. (1993). The AH-receptor: Genetics, structure and function. *Pharmacogenetics, 3*(5), 213–230.
33. Rowlands, J. C., & Gustafsson, J. A. (1997). Aryl hydrocarbon receptor-mediated signal transduction. *Critical Reviews in Toxicology, 27*(2), 109–134.
34. Bruick, R. K., & McKnight, S. L. (2001). A conserved family of prolyl-4-hydroxylases that modify HIF. *Science, 294*(5545), 1337–1340.
35. Jeong, J. W., et al. (2002). Regulation and destabilization of HIF-1alpha by ARD1-mediated acetylation. *Cell, 111*(5), 709–720.
36. Gradin, K., et al. (1996). Functional interference between hypoxia and dioxin signal transduction pathways: Competition for recruitment of the Arnt transcription factor. *Molecular and Cellular Biology, 16*(10), 5221–5231.
37. Huang, L. E., et al. (1998). Regulation of hypoxia-inducible factor 1alpha is mediated by an O2-dependent degradation domain via the ubiquitin-proteasome pathway. *Proceedings of the National Academy of Sciences of the United States ofAmerica, 95*(14), 7987–7992.
38. Pugh, C. W., et al. (1997). Activation of hypoxia-inducible factor-1; definition of regulatory domains within the alpha subunit. *The Journal of Biological Chemistry, 272*(17), 11205–11214.
39. O'Rourke, J. F., et al. (1999). Oxygen-regulated and transactivating domains in endothelial PAS protein 1: Comparison with hypoxia-inducible factor-1α. *Journal of Biological Chemistry, 274*(4), 2060–2071.
40. Srinivas, V., et al. (1999). Characterization of an oxygen/redox-dependent degradation domain of hypoxia-inducible factor alpha (HIF-alpha) proteins. *Biochemical and Biophysical Research Communications, 260*(2), 557–561.
41. Dayan, F., et al. (2008). A dialogue between the hypoxia-inducible factor and the tumor microenvironment. *Cancer Microenvironment, 1*(1), 53–68.

42. Wiesener, M. S., et al. (2003). Widespread hypoxia-inducible expression of HIF-2alpha in distinct cell populations of different organs. *The FASEB Journal, 17*(2), 271–273.
43. Onita, T., et al. (2002). Hypoxia-induced, perinecrotic expression of endothelial per-ARNT-Sim domain protein-1/hypoxia-inducible factor-2alpha correlates with tumor progression, vascularization, and focal macrophage infiltration in bladder cancer. *Clinical Cancer Research, 8*(2), 471–480.
44. Keith, B., Johnson, R. S., & Simon, M. C. (2011). HIF1alpha and HIF2alpha: Sibling rivalry in hypoxic tumour growth and progression. *Nature Reviews. Cancer, 12*(1), 9–22.
45. Leek, R. D., et al. (2002). Relation of hypoxia-inducible factor-2 alpha (HIF-2 alpha) expression in tumor-infiltrative macrophages to tumor angiogenesis and the oxidative thymidine phosphorylase pathway in human breast cancer. *Cancer Research, 62*(5), 1326–1329.
46. Wiesener, M. S., et al. (1998). Induction of endothelial PAS domain protein-1 by hypoxia: Characterization and comparison with hypoxia-inducible factor-1alpha. *Blood, 92*(7), 2260–2268.
47. Stewart, M., et al. (2002). Expression of angiogenic factors and hypoxia inducible factors HIF 1, HIF 2 and CA IX in non-Hodgkin's lymphoma. *Histopathology, 40*(3), 253–260.
48. Fukumura, D., et al. (1998). Tumor induction of VEGF promoter activity in stromal cells. *Cell, 94*(6), 715–725.
49. Flamme, I., Krieg, M., & Plate, K. H. (1998). Up-regulation of vascular endothelial growth factor in stromal cells of hemangioblastomas is correlated with up-regulation of the transcription factor HRF/HIF-2alpha. *The American Journal of Pathology, 153*(1), 25–29.
50. Giatromanolaki, A., et al. (2001). Relation of hypoxia inducible factor 1 alpha and 2 alpha in operable non-small cell lung cancer to angiogenic/molecular profile of tumours and survival. *British Journal of Cancer, 85*(6), 881–890.
51. Xia, G., et al. (2001). Regulation of vascular endothelial growth factor transcription by endothelial PAS domain protein 1 (EPAS1) and possible involvement of EPAS1 in the angiogenesis of renal cell carcinoma. *Cancer, 91*(8), 1429–1436.
52. Favier, J., et al. (2002). Angiogenesis and vascular architecture in pheochromocytomas: Distinctive traits in malignant tumors. *The American Journal of Pathology, 161*(4), 1235–1246.
53. Mazumdar, J., et al. (2010). HIF-2alpha deletion promotes Kras-driven lung tumor development. *Proceedings of the National Academy of Sciences of the United States of America, 107*(32), 14182–14187.
54. Kim, W. Y., et al. (2009). HIF2alpha cooperates with RAS to promote lung tumorigenesis in mice. *The Journal of Clinical Investigation, 119*(8), 2160–2170.
55. Makino, Y., et al. (2002). Inhibitory PAS domain protein (IPAS) is a hypoxia-inducible splicing variant of the hypoxia-inducible factor-3alpha locus. *The Journal of Biological Chemistry, 277*(36), 32405–32408.
56. Hara, S., et al. (2001). Expression and characterization of hypoxia-inducible factor (HIF)-3alpha in human kidney: Suppression of HIF-mediated gene expression by HIF-3alpha. *Biochemical and Biophysical Research Communications, 287*(4), 808–813.
57. Maynard, M. A., et al. (2003). Multiple splice variants of the human HIF-3 alpha locus are targets of the von Hippel-Lindau E3 ubiquitin ligase complex. *The Journal of Biological Chemistry, 278*(13), 11032–11040.
58. Maynard, M. A., et al. (2007). Dominant-negative HIF-3 alpha 4 suppresses VHL-null renal cell carcinoma progression. *Cell Cycle, 6*(22), 2810–2816.
59. Tanaka, T., et al. (2009). The human HIF (hypoxia-inducible factor)-3alpha gene is a HIF-1 target gene and may modulate hypoxic gene induction. *The Biochemical Journal, 424*(1), 143–151.
60. Heikkila, M., et al. (2011). Roles of the human hypoxia-inducible factor (HIF)-3alpha variants in the hypoxia response. *Cellular and Molecular Life Sciences, 68*(23), 3885–3901.
61. Michaud, J. L., et al. (2000). ARNT2 acts as the dimerization partner of SIM1 for the development of the hypothalamus. *Mechanisms of Development, 90*(2), 253–261.
62. Wang, G. L., & Semenza, G. L. (1995). Purification and characterization of hypoxia-inducible factor 1. *The Journal of Biological Chemistry, 270*(3), 1230–1237.
63. Keith, B., Adelman, D. M., & Simon, M. C. (2001). Targeted mutation of the murine arylhydrocarbon receptor nuclear translocator 2 (Arnt2) gene reveals partial redundancy with Arnt. *Proceedings of the National Academy of Sciences of the United States of America, 98*(12), 6692–6697.
64. Drutel, G., et al. (1996). Cloning and selective expression in brain and kidney of ARNT2 homologous to the Ah receptor nuclear translocator (ARNT). *Biochemical and Biophysical Research Communications, 225*(2), 333–339.
65. Hirose, K., et al. (1996). cDNA cloning and tissue-specific expression of a novel basic helix-loop-helix/PAS factor (Arnt2) with close sequence similarity to the aryl hydrocarbon receptor nuclear translocator (Arnt). *Molecular and Cellular Biology, 16*(4), 1706–1713.
66. Wang, G. L., & Semenza, G. L. (1996). Molecular basis of hypoxia-induced erythropoietin expression. *Current Opinion in Hematology, 3*(2), 156–162.
67. Camps, C., et al. (2014). Integrated analysis of microRNA and mRNA expression and association with HIF binding reveals the complexity of microRNA expression regulation under hypoxia. *Molecular Cancer, 13*, 28.

68. Kelly, B. D., et al. (2003). Cell type-specific regulation of angiogenic growth factor gene expression and induction of angiogenesis in nonischemic tissue by a constitutively active form of hypoxia-inducible factor 1. *Circulation Research, 93*(11), 1074–1081.
69. Yun, Z., et al. (2002). Inhibition of PPAR gamma 2 gene expression by the HIF-1-regulated gene DEC1/Stra13: A mechanism for regulation of adipogenesis by hypoxia. *Developmental Cell, 2*(3), 331–341.
70. Balamurugan, K. (2016). HIF-1 at the crossroads of hypoxia, inflammation, and cancer. *International Journal of Cancer, 138*(5), 1058–1066.
71. Liu, W., et al. (2012). Targeted genes and interacting proteins of hypoxia inducible factor-1. *International Journal of Biochemistry and Molecular Biology, 3*(2), 165–178.
72. Pouyssegur, J., Dayan, F., & Mazure, N. M. (2006). Hypoxia signalling in cancer and approaches to enforce tumour regression. *Nature, 441*(7092), 437–443.
73. Zelzer, E., et al. (1998). Insulin induces transcription of target genes through the hypoxia-inducible factor HIF-1alpha/ARNT. *The EMBO Journal, 17*(17), 5085–5094.
74. Feldser, D., et al. (1999). Reciprocal positive regulation of hypoxia-inducible factor 1alpha and insulin-like growth factor 2. *Cancer Research, 59*(16), 3915–3918.
75. Hellwig-Burgel, T., et al. (1999). Interleukin-1beta and tumor necrosis factor-alpha stimulate DNA binding of hypoxia-inducible factor-1. *Blood, 94*(5), 1561–1567.
76. Laughner, E., et al. (2001). HER2 (neu) signaling increases the rate of hypoxia-inducible factor 1alpha (HIF-1alpha) synthesis: Novel mechanism for HIF-1-mediated vascular endothelial growth factor expression. *Molecular and Cellular Biology, 21*(12), 3995–4004.
77. Fukuda, R., et al. (2002). Insulin-like growth factor 1 induces hypoxia-inducible factor 1-mediated vascular endothelial growth factor expression, which is dependent on MAP kinase and phosphatidylinositol 3-kinase signaling in colon cancer cells. *The Journal of Biological Chemistry, 277*(41), 38205–38211.
78. Zhong, H., et al. (2000). Modulation of hypoxia-inducible factor 1alpha expression by the epidermal growth factor/phosphatidylinositol 3-kinase/PTEN/AKT/FRAP pathway in human prostate cancer cells: Implications for tumor angiogenesis and therapeutics. *Cancer Research, 60*(6), 1541–1545.
79. Sang, N., et al. (2003). MAPK signaling up-regulates the activity of hypoxia-inducible factors by its effects on p300. *The Journal of Biological Chemistry, 278*(16), 14013–14019.
80. Mylonis, I., et al. (2006). Identification of MAPK phosphorylation sites and their role in the localization and activity of hypoxia-inducible factor-1alpha. *The Journal of Biological Chemistry, 281*(44), 33095–33106.
81. Page, E. L., et al. (2002). Induction of hypoxia-inducible factor-1alpha by transcriptional and translational mechanisms. *The Journal of Biological Chemistry, 277*(50), 48403–48409.
82. Kalousi, A., et al. (2010). Casein kinase 1 regulates human hypoxia-inducible factor HIF-1. *Journal of Cell Science, 123*(Pt 17), 2976–2986.
83. To, K. K., et al. (2006). The phosphorylation status of PAS-B distinguishes HIF-1alpha from HIF-2alpha in NBS1 repression. *The EMBO Journal, 25*(20), 4784–4794.
84. Maxwell, P. H., et al. (1999). The tumour suppressor protein VHL targets hypoxia-inducible factors for oxygen-dependent proteolysis. *Nature, 399*(6733), 271–275.
85. Mailloux, R. J., Puiseux-Dao, S., & Appanna, V. D. (2009). Alpha-ketoglutarate abrogates the nuclear localization of HIF-1alpha in aluminum-exposed hepatocytes. *Biochimie, 91*(3), 408–415.
86. Lando, D., et al. (2002). FIH-1 is an asparaginyl hydroxylase enzyme that regulates the transcriptional activity of hypoxia-inducible factor. *Genes & Development, 16*(12), 1466–1471.
87. Berra, E., et al. (2003). HIF prolyl-hydroxylase 2 is the key oxygen sensor setting low steady-state levels of HIF-1alpha in normoxia. *The EMBO Journal, 22*(16), 4082–4090.
88. Jaakkola, P., et al. (2001). Targeting of HIF-alpha to the von Hippel-Lindau ubiquitylation complex by O2-regulated prolyl hydroxylation. *Science, 292*(5516), 468–472.
89. Schofield, C. J., & Ratcliffe, P. J. (2005). Signalling hypoxia by HIF hydroxylases. *Biochemical and Biophysical Research Communications, 338*(1), 617–626.
90. Koivunen, P., et al. (2007). An endoplasmic reticulum transmembrane prolyl 4-hydroxylase is induced by hypoxia and acts on hypoxia-inducible factor alpha. *The Journal of Biological Chemistry, 282*(42), 30544–30552.
91. Hewitson, K. S., et al. (2002). Hypoxia-inducible factor (HIF) asparagine hydroxylase is identical to factor inhibiting HIF (FIH) and is related to the cupin structural family. *The Journal of Biological Chemistry, 277*(29), 26351–26355.
92. Lee, C., et al. (2003). Structure of human FIH-1 reveals a unique active site pocket and interaction sites for HIF-1 and von Hippel-Lindau. *The Journal of Biological Chemistry, 278*(9), 7558–7563.
93. Soni, S., & Padwad, Y. S. (2017). HIF-1 in cancer therapy: Two decade long story of a transcription factor. *Acta Oncologica, 56*(4), 503–515.
94. Lim, J. H., et al. (2010). Sirtuin 1 modulates cellular responses to hypoxia by deacetylating hypoxia-inducible factor 1alpha. *Molecular Cell, 38*(6), 864–878.
95. Chandel, N. S., et al. (1998). Mitochondrial reactive oxygen species trigger hypoxia-induced transcription. *Proceedings of the National Academy of*

Sciences of the United States of America, 95(20), 11715–11720.
96. Chandel, N. S., et al. (2000). Reactive oxygen species generated at mitochondrial complex III stabilize hypoxia-inducible factor-1alpha during hypoxia: A mechanism of O2 sensing. *The Journal of Biological Chemistry, 275*(33), 25130–25138.
97. Schroedl, C., et al. (2002). Hypoxic but not anoxic stabilization of HIF-1alpha requires mitochondrial reactive oxygen species. *American Journal of Physiology. Lung Cellular and Molecular Physiology, 283*(5), L922–L931.
98. Gerald, D., et al. (2004). JunD reduces tumor angiogenesis by protecting cells from oxidative stress. *Cell, 118*(6), 781–794.
99. Kimura, H., et al. (2000). Hypoxia response element of the human vascular endothelial growth factor gene mediates transcriptional regulation by nitric oxide: Control of hypoxia-inducible factor-1 activity by nitric oxide. *Blood, 95*(1), 189–197.
100. Palmer, L. A., Gaston, B., & Johns, R. A. (2000). Normoxic stabilization of hypoxia-inducible factor-1 expression and activity: Redox-dependent effect of nitrogen oxides. *Molecular Pharmacology, 58*(6), 1197–1203.
101. Sandau, K. B., Faus, H. G., & Brune, B. (2000). Induction of hypoxia-inducible-factor 1 by nitric oxide is mediated via the PI 3K pathway. *Biochemical and Biophysical Research Communications, 278*(1), 263–267.
102. Sandau, K. B., Fandrey, J., & Brune, B. (2001). Accumulation of HIF-1alpha under the influence of nitric oxide. *Blood, 97*(4), 1009–1015.
103. Liu, Y., et al. (1998). Carbon monoxide and nitric oxide suppress the hypoxic induction of vascular endothelial growth factor gene via the 5′ enhancer. *The Journal of Biological Chemistry, 273*(24), 15257–15262.
104. Sogawa, K., et al. (1998). Inhibition of hypoxia-inducible factor 1 activity by nitric oxide donors in hypoxia. *Proceedings of the National Academy of Sciences of the United States of America, 95*(13), 7368–7373.
105. Yin, J. H., et al. (2000). iNOS expression inhibits hypoxia-inducible factor-1 activity. *Biochemical and Biophysical Research Communications, 279*(1), 30–34.
106. Wenger, R. H., Stiehl, D. P., & Camenisch, G. (2005). Integration of oxygen signaling at the consensus HRE. *Science's STKE, 2005*(306), re12.
107. Semenza, G. L., et al. (1994). Transcriptional regulation of genes encoding glycolytic enzymes by hypoxia-inducible factor 1. *The Journal of Biological Chemistry, 269*(38), 23757–23763.
108. Jiang, B. H., et al. (1996). Dimerization, DNA binding, and transactivation properties of hypoxia-inducible factor 1. *The Journal of Biological Chemistry, 271*(30), 17771–17778.
109. Wenger, R. H. (2000). Mammalian oxygen sensing, signalling and gene regulation. *The Journal of Experimental Biology, 203*(Pt 8), 1253–1263.
110. Minchenko, A., et al. (2002). Hypoxia-inducible factor-1-mediated expression of the 6-phosphofructo-2-kinase/fructose-2,6-bisphosphatase-3 (PFKFB3) gene. Its possible role in the Warburg effect. *The Journal of Biological Chemistry, 277*(8), 6183–6187.
111. Hayashi, M., et al. (2004). Induction of glucose transporter 1 expression through hypoxia-inducible factor 1alpha under hypoxic conditions in trophoblast-derived cells. *The Journal of Endocrinology, 183*(1), 145–154.
112. Liu, Y., et al. (2009). The expression and significance of HIF-1alpha and GLUT-3 in glioma. *Brain Research, 1304*, 149–154.
113. Zhang, H., et al. (2008). Mitochondrial autophagy is an HIF-1-dependent adaptive metabolic response to hypoxia. *The Journal of Biological Chemistry, 283*(16), 10892–10903.
114. Sowter, H. M., et al. (2001). HIF-1-dependent regulation of hypoxic induction of the cell death factors BNIP3 and NIX in human tumors. *Cancer Research, 61*(18), 6669–6673.
115. Lu, C. W., et al. (2008). Induction of pyruvate dehydrogenase kinase-3 by hypoxia-inducible factor-1 promotes metabolic switch and drug resistance. *The Journal of Biological Chemistry, 283*(42), 28106–28114.
116. Bellot, G., et al. (2009). Hypoxia-induced autophagy is mediated through hypoxia-inducible factor induction of BNIP3 and BNIP3L via their BH3 domains. *Molecular and Cellular Biology, 29*(10), 2570–2581.
117. Ivan, M., et al. (2008). Hypoxia response and microRNAs: No longer two separate worlds. *Journal of Cellular and Molecular Medicine, 12*(5A), 1426–1431.
118. Devlin, C., et al. (2011). miR-210: More than a silent player in hypoxia. *IUBMB Life, 63*(2), 94–100.
119. Chan, S. Y., et al. (2009). MicroRNA-210 controls mitochondrial metabolism during hypoxia by repressing the iron-sulfur cluster assembly proteins ISCU1/2. *Cell Metabolism, 10*(4), 273–284.
120. Favaro, E., et al. (2010). MicroRNA-210 regulates mitochondrial free radical response to hypoxia and Krebs cycle in cancer cells by targeting iron sulfur cluster protein ISCU. *PLoS One, 5*(4), e10345.
121. Metallo, C. M., et al. (2011). Reductive glutamine metabolism by IDH1 mediates lipogenesis under hypoxia. *Nature, 481*(7381), 380–384.
122. Wise, D. R., et al. (2011). Hypoxia promotes isocitrate dehydrogenase-dependent carboxylation of alpha-ketoglutarate to citrate to support cell growth and viability. *Proceedings of the National Academy of Sciences of the United States of America, 108*(49), 19611–19616.
123. Du, W., et al. (2017). HIF drives lipid deposition and cancer in ccRCC via repression of fatty acid metabolism. *Nature Communications, 8*(1), 1769.

124. Griffiths, J. R., et al. (2002). Metabolic changes detected by in vivo magnetic resonance studies of HEPA-1 wild-type tumors and tumors deficient in hypoxia-inducible factor-1beta (HIF-1beta): Evidence of an anabolic role for the HIF-1 pathway. *Cancer Research, 62*(3), 688–695.
125. Younes, M., Lechago, L. V., & Lechago, J. (1996). Overexpression of the human erythrocyte glucose transporter occurs as a late event in human colorectal carcinogenesis and is associated with an increased incidence of lymph node metastases. *Clinical Cancer Research, 2*(7), 1151–1154.
126. Semenza, G. L. (2009). Regulation of cancer cell metabolism by hypoxia-inducible factor 1. *Seminars in Cancer Biology, 19*(1), 12–16.
127. Pinheiro, C., et al. (2012). Role of monocarboxylate transporters in human cancers: State of the art. *Journal of Bioenergetics and Biomembranes, 44*(1), 127–139.
128. Chiche, J., Brahimi-Horn, M. C., & Pouyssegur, J. (2010). Tumour hypoxia induces a metabolic shift causing acidosis: A common feature in cancer. *Journal of Cellular and Molecular Medicine, 14*(4), 771–794.
129. Swietach, P., et al. (2008). Tumor-associated carbonic anhydrase 9 spatially coordinates intracellular pH in three-dimensional multicellular growths. *The Journal of Biological Chemistry, 283*(29), 20473–20483.
130. Gatenby, R. A., et al. (2007). Cellular adaptations to hypoxia and acidosis during somatic evolution of breast cancer. *British Journal of Cancer, 97*(5), 646–653.
131. Christofk, H. R., et al. (2008). The M2 splice isoform of pyruvate kinase is important for cancer metabolism and tumour growth. *Nature, 452*(7184), 230–233.
132. Luo, W., et al. (2011). Pyruvate kinase M2 is a PHD3-stimulated coactivator for hypoxia-inducible factor 1. *Cell, 145*(5), 732–744.
133. Gao, X., et al. (2012). Pyruvate kinase M2 regulates gene transcription by acting as a protein kinase. *Molecular Cell, 45*(5), 598–609.
134. Dvorak, H. F. (1986). Tumors: Wounds that do not heal. Similarities between tumor stroma generation and wound healing. *The New England Journal of Medicine, 315*(26), 1650–1659.
135. Vaupel, P., Schaefer, C., & Okunieff, P. (1994). Intracellular acidosis in murine fibrosarcomas coincides with ATP depletion, hypoxia, and high levels of lactate and total pi. *NMR in Biomedicine, 7*(3), 128–136.
136. Denko, N. C., & Giaccia, A. J. (2001). Tumor hypoxia, the physiological link between Trousseau's syndrome (carcinoma-induced coagulopathy) and metastasis. *Cancer Research, 61*(3), 795–798.
137. Vaupel, P., & Mayer, A. (2014). Hypoxia in tumors: Pathogenesis-related classification, characterization of hypoxia subtypes, and associated biological and clinical implications. *Advances in Experimental Medicine and Biology, 812*, 19–24.
138. Zhong, H., et al. (1999). Overexpression of hypoxia-inducible factor 1alpha in common human cancers and their metastases. *Cancer Research, 59*(22), 5830–5835.
139. Talks, K. L., et al. (2000). The expression and distribution of the hypoxia-inducible factors HIF-1alpha and HIF-2alpha in normal human tissues, cancers, and tumor-associated macrophages. *The American Journal of Pathology, 157*(2), 411–421.
140. Koshikawa, N., et al. (2003). Constitutive upregulation of hypoxia-inducible factor-1alpha mRNA occurring in highly metastatic lung carcinoma cells leads to vascular endothelial growth factor overexpression upon hypoxic exposure. *Oncogene, 22*(43), 6717–6724.
141. Hockel, M., et al. (1996). Hypoxia and radiation response in human tumors. *Seminars in Radiation Oncology, 6*(1), 3–9.
142. Hockel, M., et al. (1998). Tumor hypoxia in pelvic recurrences of cervical cancer. *International Journal of Cancer, 79*(4), 365–369.
143. Hockel, M., et al. (1999). Hypoxic cervical cancers with low apoptotic index are highly aggressive. *Cancer Research, 59*(18), 4525–4528.
144. Semenza, G. L. (2011). Oxygen sensing, homeostasis, and disease. *The New England Journal of Medicine, 365*(6), 537–547.
145. Doedens, A. L., et al. (2010). Macrophage expression of hypoxia-inducible factor-1 alpha suppresses T-cell function and promotes tumor progression. *Cancer Research, 70*(19), 7465–7475.
146. Takeda, N., et al. (2010). Differential activation and antagonistic function of HIF-{alpha} isoforms in macrophages are essential for NO homeostasis. *Genes & Development, 24*(5), 491–501.
147. Noman, M. Z., et al. (2014). PD-L1 is a novel direct target of HIF-1α, and its blockade under hypoxia enhanced MDSC-mediated T cell activation. *The Journal of Experimental Medicine, 211*(5), 781–790.
148. Lee, J. H., et al. (2015). E3 ubiquitin ligase VHL regulates hypoxia-inducible factor-1α to maintain regulatory T cell stability and suppressive capacity. *Immunity, 42*(6), 1062–1074.
149. Okegawa, T., et al. (2004). The role of cell adhesion molecule in cancer progression and its application in cancer therapy. *Acta Biochimica Polonica, 51*(2), 445–457.
150. Cowden Dahl, K. D., et al. (2005). Hypoxia-inducible factor regulates alphavbeta3 integrin cell surface expression. *Molecular Biology of the Cell, 16*(4), 1901–1912.
151. Ryu, M. H., et al. (2010). Hypoxia-inducible factor-1alpha mediates oral squamous cell carcinoma invasion via upregulation of alpha5 integrin and fibronectin. *Biochemical and Biophysical Research Communications, 393*(1), 11–15.
152. Lee, S. H., Lee, Y. J., & Han, H. J. (2011). Role of hypoxia-induced fibronectin-integrin beta1 expression in embryonic stem cell proliferation and migration: Involvement of PI3K/Akt and FAK. *Journal of Cellular Physiology, 226*(2), 484–493.

153. Krishnamachary, B., et al. (2006). Hypoxia-inducible factor-1-dependent repression of E-cadherin in von Hippel-Lindau tumor suppressor-null renal cell carcinoma mediated by TCF3, ZFHX1A, and ZFHX1B. *Cancer Research, 66*(5), 2725–2731.
154. Zhang, Y., Fan, N., & Yang, J. (2015). Expression and clinical significance of hypoxia-inducible factor 1alpha, snail and E-cadherin in human ovarian cancer cell lines. *Molecular Medicine Reports, 12*(3), 3393–3399.
155. Barak, V., et al. (2011). VEGF as a biomarker for metastatic Uveal melanoma in humans. *Current Eye Research, 36*(4), 386–390.
156. Semenza, G. L. (2012). Hypoxia-inducible factors: Mediators of cancer progression and targets for cancer therapy. *Trends in Pharmacological Sciences, 33*(4), 207–214.
157. Hasan, N. M., et al. (1998). Hypoxia facilitates tumour cell detachment by reducing expression of surface adhesion molecules and adhesion to extracellular matrices without loss of cell viability. *British Journal of Cancer, 77*(11), 1799–1805.
158. Peng, J. K., et al. (2018). Etaypoxia-inducible factor 1-alpha promotes colon cell proliferation and migration by upregulating AMPK-related protein kinase 5 under hypoxic conditions. *Oncology Letters, 15*(3), 3639–3645.
159. Suzuki, A., et al. (2003). ARK5 suppresses the cell death induced by nutrient starvation and death receptors via inhibition of caspase 8 activation, but not by chemotherapeutic agents or UV irradiation. *Oncogene, 22*(40), 6177–6182.
160. Suzuki, A., et al. (2004). Regulation of caspase-6 and FLIP by the AMPK family member ARK5. *Oncogene, 23*(42), 7067–7075.
161. Lu, S., et al. (2013). ARK5 promotes glioma cell invasion, and its elevated expression is correlated with poor clinical outcome. *European Journal of Cancer, 49*(3), 752–763.
162. Lester, R. D., et al. (2005). Erythropoietin promotes MCF-7 breast cancer cell migration by an ERK/mitogen-activated protein kinase-dependent pathway and is primarily responsible for the increase in migration observed in hypoxia. *The Journal of Biological Chemistry, 280*(47), 39273–39277.
163. Cannito, S., et al. (2008). Redox mechanisms switch on hypoxia-dependent epithelial-mesenchymal transition in cancer cells. *Carcinogenesis, 29*(12), 2267–2278.
164. Matsuoka, J., et al. (2013). Hypoxia stimulates the EMT of gastric cancer cells through autocrine TGFbeta signaling. *PLoS One, 8*(5), e62310.
165. Yang, M. H., et al. (2008). Direct regulation of TWIST by HIF-1alpha promotes metastasis. *Nature Cell Biology, 10*(3), 295–305.
166. Lendahl, U., et al. (2009). Generating specificity and diversity in the transcriptional response to hypoxia. *Nature Reviews Genetics, 10*(12), 821–832.
167. Tsai, Y. P., & Wu, K. J. (2012). Hypoxia-regulated target genes implicated in tumor metastasis. *Journal of Biomedical Science, 19*, 102.
168. Chu, C. Y., et al. (2016). CA IX is upregulated in CoCl2-induced hypoxia and associated with cell invasive potential and a poor prognosis of breast cancer. *International Journal of Oncology, 48*(1), 271–280.
169. Evans, A. J., et al. (2007). VHL promotes E2 box-dependent E-cadherin transcription by HIF-mediated regulation of SIP1 and snail. *Molecular and Cellular Biology, 27*(1), 157–169.
170. de Herreros, A. G., et al. (2010). Snail family regulation and epithelial mesenchymal transitions in breast cancer progression. *Journal of Mammary Gland Biology and Neoplasia, 15*(2), 135–147.
171. Luo, Y., et al. (2006). Over-expression of hypoxia-inducible factor-1alpha increases the invasive potency of LNCaP cells in vitro. *BJU International, 98*(6), 1315–1319.
172. O'Toole, E. A., et al. (2008). Hypoxia induces epidermal keratinocyte matrix metalloproteinase-9 secretion via the protein kinase C pathway. *Journal of Cellular Physiology, 214*(1), 47–55.
173. Lin, M. T., et al. (2008). Involvement of hypoxia-inducing factor-1alpha-dependent plasminogen activator inhibitor-1 up-regulation in Cyr61/CCN1-induced gastric cancer cell invasion. *The Journal of Biological Chemistry, 283*(23), 15807–15815.
174. Buchler, P., et al. (2009). Transcriptional regulation of urokinase-type plasminogen activator receptor by hypoxia-inducible factor 1 is crucial for invasion of pancreatic and liver cancer. *Neoplasia, 11*(2), 196–206.
175. Pennacchietti, S., et al. (2003). Hypoxia promotes invasive growth by transcriptional activation of the met protooncogene. *Cancer Cell, 3*(4), 347–361.
176. Ishikawa, T., et al. (2009). Hypoxia enhances CXCR4 expression by activating HIF-1 in oral squamous cell carcinoma. *Oncology Reports, 21*(3), 707–712.
177. Li, Y., et al. (2009). Hypoxia induced CCR7 expression via HIF-1alpha and HIF-2alpha correlates with migration and invasion in lung cancer cells. *Cancer Biology & Therapy, 8*(4), 322–330.
178. Erler, J. T., et al. (2006). Lysyl oxidase is essential for hypoxia-induced metastasis. *Nature, 440*(7088), 1222–1226.
179. Funasaka, T., et al. (2005). Regulation of phosphoglucose isomerase/autocrine motility factor expression by hypoxia. *The FASEB Journal, 19*(11), 1422–1430.
180. Staller, P., et al. (2003). Chemokine receptor CXCR4 downregulated by von Hippel-Lindau tumour suppressor pVHL. *Nature, 425*(6955), 307–311.
181. Pan, J., et al. (2006). Stromal derived factor-1 (SDF-1/CXCL12) and CXCR4 in renal cell carcinoma metastasis. *Molecular Cancer, 5*, 56.

182. Castillo Bennett, J., et al. (2018). Hypoxia-induced Caveolin-1 expression promotes migration and invasion of tumor cells. *Current Molecular Medicine, 18*(4), 199–206.
183. Krishnamachary, B., et al. (2003). Regulation of colon carcinoma cell invasion by hypoxia-inducible factor 1. *Cancer Research, 63*(5), 1138–1143.
184. Nikitenko, L. L., et al. (2003). Transcriptional regulation of the CRLR gene in human microvascular endothelial cells by hypoxia. *The FASEB Journal, 17*(11), 1499–1501.
185. Pugh, C. W., & Ratcliffe, P. J. (2003). Regulation of angiogenesis by hypoxia: Role of the HIF system. *Nature Medicine, 9*(6), 677–684.
186. Kotch, L. E., et al. (1999). Defective vascularization of HIF-1alpha-null embryos is not associated with VEGF deficiency but with mesenchymal cell death. *Developmental Biology, 209*(2), 254–267.
187. Maruggi, M., et al. (2019). Absence of HIF1A leads to glycogen accumulation and an inflammatory response that enables pancreatic tumor growth. *Cancer Research, 79*(22), 5839–5848.
188. Cheng, J., et al. (2007). SUMO-specific protease 1 is essential for stabilization of HIF1alpha during hypoxia. *Cell, 131*(3), 584–595.
189. Xu, Y., et al. (2010). Induction of SENP1 in endothelial cells contributes to hypoxia-driven VEGF expression and angiogenesis. *The Journal of Biological Chemistry, 285*(47), 36682–36688.
190. Riva, C., et al. (1998). Cellular physiology and molecular events in hypoxia-induced apoptosis. *Anticancer Research, 18*(6b), 4729–4736.
191. Hammond, E. M., Dorie, M. J., & Giaccia, A. J. (2003). ATR/ATM targets are phosphorylated by ATR in response to hypoxia and ATM in response to reoxygenation. *The Journal of Biological Chemistry, 278*(14), 12207–12213.
192. Akakura, N., et al. (2001). Constitutive expression of hypoxia-inducible factor-1alpha renders pancreatic cancer cells resistant to apoptosis induced by hypoxia and nutrient deprivation. *Cancer Research, 61*(17), 6548–6554.
193. Carmeliet, P., et al. (1998). Role of HIF-1alpha in hypoxia-mediated apoptosis, cell proliferation and tumour angiogenesis. *Nature, 394*(6692), 485–490.
194. Santore, M. T., et al. (2002). Anoxia-induced apoptosis occurs through a mitochondria-dependent pathway in lung epithelial cells. *American Journal of Physiology. Lung Cellular and Molecular Physiology, 282*(4), L727–L734.
195. Kumar, H., & Choi, D. K. (2015). Hypoxia inducible factor pathway and physiological adaptation: A cell survival pathway? *Mediators of Inflammation, 2015*, 584758.
196. McClintock, D. S., et al. (2002). Bcl-2 family members and functional electron transport chain regulate oxygen deprivation-induced cell death. *Molecular and Cellular Biology, 22*(1), 94–104.
197. Yoo, B. H., et al. (2009). Hypoxia-induced downregulation of autophagy mediator Beclin 1 reduces the susceptibility of malignant intestinal epithelial cells to hypoxia-dependent apoptosis. *Autophagy, 5*(8), 1166–1179.
198. Soengas, M. S., et al. (1999). Apaf-1 and caspase-9 in p53-dependent apoptosis and tumor inhibition. *Science, 284*(5411), 156–159.
199. Li, F., et al. (2015). Curcumin induces p53-independent necrosis in H1299 cells via a mitochondria-associated pathway. *Molecular Medicine Reports, 12*(5), 7806–7814.
200. Shimizu, S., et al. (1995). Prevention of hypoxia-induced cell death by Bcl-2 and Bcl-xL. *Nature, 374*(6525), 811–813.
201. Kim, J. Y., et al. (2004). BH3-only protein Noxa is a mediator of hypoxic cell death induced by hypoxia-inducible factor 1alpha. *The Journal of Experimental Medicine, 199*(1), 113–124.
202. Zagzag, D., et al. (2000). Expression of hypoxia-inducible factor 1alpha in brain tumors: Association with angiogenesis, invasion, and progression. *Cancer, 88*(11), 2606–2618.
203. Schindl, M., et al. (2002). Overexpression of hypoxia-inducible factor 1alpha is associated with an unfavorable prognosis in lymph node-positive breast cancer. *Clinical Cancer Research, 8*(6), 1831–1837.
204. Bos, R., et al. (2003). Levels of hypoxia-inducible factor-1alpha independently predict prognosis in patients with lymph node negative breast carcinoma. *Cancer, 97*(6), 1573–1581.
205. Aebersold, D. M., et al. (2001). Expression of hypoxia-inducible factor-1alpha: A novel predictive and prognostic parameter in the radiotherapy of oropharyngeal cancer. *Cancer Research, 61*(7), 2911–2916.
206. Beasley, N. J., et al. (2002). Hypoxia-inducible factors HIF-1alpha and HIF-2alpha in head and neck cancer: Relationship to tumor biology and treatment outcome in surgically resected patients. *Cancer Research, 62*(9), 2493–2497.
207. Koukourakis, M. I., et al. (2002). Hypoxia-inducible factor (HIF1A and HIF2A), angiogenesis, and chemoradiotherapy outcome of squamous cell head-and-neck cancer. *International Journal of Radiation Oncology, Biology, Physics, 53*(5), 1192–1202.
208. Birner, P., et al. (2001). Expression of hypoxia-inducible factor 1alpha in epithelial ovarian tumors: Its impact on prognosis and on response to chemotherapy. *Clinical Cancer Research, 7*(6), 1661–1668.
209. Zhang, X., et al. (2019). Interaction between p53 and Ras signaling controls cisplatin resistance via HDAC4- and HIF-1alpha-mediated regulation of apoptosis and autophagy. *Theranostics, 9*(4), 1096–1114.
210. Jiang, X., et al. (2019). The correlation between NEDD4L and HIF-1alpha levels as a gastric cancer prognostic marker. *International Journal of Medical Sciences, 16*(11), 1517–1524.
211. Koukourakis, M. I., et al. (2001). Hypoxia inducible factor (HIF-1a and HIF-2a) expression in early

esophageal cancer and response to photodynamic therapy and radiotherapy. *Cancer Research, 61*(5), 1830–1832.

212. Wigerup, C., Pahlman, S., & Bexell, D. (2016). Therapeutic targeting of hypoxia and hypoxia-inducible factors in cancer. *Pharmacology & Therapeutics, 164*, 152–169.
213. Masoud, G. N., & Li, W. (2015). HIF-1alpha pathway: Role, regulation and intervention for cancer therapy. *Acta Pharmaceutica Sinica B, 5*(5), 378–389.
214. Hu, Y., Liu, J., & Huang, H. (2013). Recent agents targeting HIF-1alpha for cancer therapy. *Journal of Cellular Biochemistry, 114*(3), 498–509.
215. Falchook, G. S., et al. (2014). Targeting hypoxia-inducible factor-1alpha (HIF-1alpha) in combination with antiangiogenic therapy: A phase I trial of bortezomib plus bevacizumab. *Oncotarget, 5*(21), 10280–10292.
216. Ban, H. S., et al. (2016). Hypoxia-inducible factor (HIF) inhibitors: A patent survey (2011–2015). *Expert Opinion on Therapeutic Patents, 26*(3), 309–322.

Metabolomics of Glioma

Sizhe Feng and Yutong Liu

1 Introduction

Glioma is the most common neoplasm of the central nervous system. Based on the classification system defined by the World Health Organization (WHO), gliomas have been divided into I–IV grades according to the degrees of malignancy. Glioblastoma (grade IV) is the most refractory and common brain malignancy that accounts for 56.6% of gliomas with an incidence rate of 3.21 per 100,000 population [1]. It is noteworthy that the incidence of glioblastoma increases with age. The highest incidence is found in individuals aged 75–84, which is 44.47 per 100,000 population. At present, the therapeutic treatment of this disease is not optimistic. Most patients are prone to recurrence after treatment, and the average survival time of glioblastoma is only about one year [2]. Therefore, glioma is a lethal disease that causes huge burden on individuals, families, and the society. It is urgent to upgrade therapeutic strategies and discover new targeted drugs for this devastating disease [3].

Altered cellular metabolism is an important characteristics of gliomas, especially glioblastoma multiforme (GBM). The activities of GBM cells in glycolysis, TCA cycle, pentose phosphate pathway, and amino acid metabolism are different from those in benign or low-grade gliomas. For instance, the metabolic requirement of growth and proliferation of GBM cells is higher than that of normal cells, and cells must maintain sufficient energy to support the metabolic needs of growth and proliferation. On the one hand, glucose is metabolized to pyruvate through glycolysis without oxygen limitation, and pyruvate then enters the cycle of tricarboxylic acid (TCA) in mitochondria to synthesize high-yield ATP by oxidative phosphorylation. On the other hand, in most malignant cells, even if there is enough oxygen, lactic acid is produced by glycolysis and fermentation to enhance the flux [4]. In recent years, breakthroughs have been made in this field regarding the metabolisms of glioblastoma. In the second part of this book chapter, we will discuss the recent advances in altered metabolic pathways in glioma.

Metabolites are closely related to physiological changes within individual phenotypes and direct indicators of many physiological and biochemical reactions or changes in enzyme activities. Metabolomics can directly detect the physiological and biochemical reactions of all small molecule metabolites present in a biological system, such as cells, tissues, and body fluids (e.g., cerebrospinal fluid, plasma, urine, and saliva). In the process of tumorigenesis, some

S. Feng (✉)
Institute of Neuroscience and Division of Neurosurgery, General Hospital of Northern Theater Command, Shenyang, China

Y. Liu
Department of Pharmacology, Shenyang Pharmaceutical University, Shenyang, China

S. Hu (ed.), *Cancer Metabolomics*, Advances in Experimental Medicine and Biology 1280,
https://doi.org/10.1007/978-3-030-51652-9_18

specific metabolic processes are altered, leading to significant metabolomic changes and metabolic reprogramming. By using metabolomics technology to detect these changes in the tumorigenic process, we may discover metabolite biomarkers for early diagnose/prognosis or predict the progression of tumors. At present, the commonly used methods of metabolomics mainly include nuclear magnetic resonance spectroscopy (NMR) and mass spectrometry (MS). NMR spectroscopy has emerged as a high-throughput and useful technique for qualitative and quantitative metabolomics analysis [5]. It is a fast, nondestructive, nonselective and highly reproducible technology that requires minimal sample preparation and provides highly informative structural information. Traditionally, NMR has been used to elucidate metabolic tracers by determining their structures using in vivo and in vitro ^{13}C NMR. Alternatively, a two-dimensional NMR spectrum obtained using a large number of increments in the indirect dimension can provide ^{13}C-^{13}C scalar coupling information, which can be used to determine the exact positional atoms of the label [6]. ^{13}C NMR has been successfully applied to studying the tumor metabolism of primary GBM and IDH mutant gliomas by infusion of ^{13}C-labeled nutrients (glucose, acetate, and glutamine) [7, 8]. Compared to NMR, high-throughput LC-MS technique may be the best method for analyzing metabolites at low concentrations. Both LC-MS and NMR methods can be used to explore characteristic metabolites of gliomas in plasma and brain biopsies. Furthermore, studies of key metabolic pathways, such as cysteine metabolism, GSH synthesis, and lipid metabolism, in brain tumors may help distinguish glioma grades and develop new clinical intervention strategies. In the third part of this book chapter, we will discuss recent metabolomic applications in glioma, which have provided new molecular insights into the pathogenesis of the disease and demonstrated a promising strategy to identify new metabolite biomarkers for the disease diagnosis/prognosis and treatment efficacy.

2 Recent Advances in Metabolic Pathways of Glioma

At present, classical metabolic pathways such as TCA cycle, glycolysis, and arachidonic acid (AA)/inflammation pathway have been well studied in glioma. TCA cycle is the ultimate metabolic pathway of the three major nutrients, carbohydrates, lipids, and amino acids, and it is also the pivot of carbohydrates, lipids, and amino acids metabolism. Studies have shown that the glycolysis rate of cancer cells increases despite the presence of enough oxygen, while their dependence on oxidative phosphorylation decreases. Besides, histamine may interact with receptors in glioma cells, followed by increased AA metabolism and prostaglandin levels in these cells. Thus, the abnormal metabolism of AA and its metabolites may be related to the occurrence of cancer [9]. Nevertheless, in recent years, attention has been paid to the understanding of new metabolic alterations in glioma cells. A number of novel metabolic pathways have been discovered and studied.

2.1 IDH1/2 Gene Mutation

2.1.1 IDH1/2 Mutation and Glioma

Metabolic disturbances are thought to play a critical role in the advancement of tumors. In recent years, various degrees of isocitrate dehydrogenase gene (IDH) mutations have been found in multiple tumors, including acute myeloid leukemia (AML), chondrosarcoma, intrahepatic cholangiocarcinoma (ICC), paraganglioma, colorectal cancer (CRC), prostate cancer, lung cancer, thyroid carcinoma, and melanoma [10]. IDH mutation is considered to alter the mode of cell metabolism and may be related to the occurrence and development of tumors. In 2008, Parsons et al. discovered IDH1/2 gene mutations in patients with malignant glioblastoma [11]. The WHO subsequently classified glioma into IDH mutant and IDH wild types. This is the first time that molecular typing is used as the gold standard for glioma diagnosis, and it has epoch-making significance.

IDH is a crucial rate-limiting enzyme in the TCA cycle. It catalyzes the oxidative decarboxylation of isocitrate, producing alpha-ketoglutarate (α-KG) and CO_2. This process provides energy and precursors for cell metabolism. At present, three IDH isoforms encoded by different genes have been found in human body, namely IDH1, IDH2, and IDH3. IDH1 is present in cytosol and peroxisome, while IDH2 and IDH3 are present in mitochondria [12]. NADP-dependent IDH1 and IDH2 have considerable sequence similarity (70%) and nearly identical protein conformation [13], while IDH3 has a unique sequence and is an NAD-dependent enzyme [14]. IDH3 plays a decisive role in energy production. To the best of our knowledge, there have been no report of tumor-associated mutations in the IDH3 gene. Hence, IDH3 gene is not discussed in this chapter. Recently, abounding studies have found that the mutation of IDH1/2 gene frequently occurred in low-grade gliomas, secondary glioblastomas (84.6%), anaplastic astrocytomas (69.2%), and anaplastic oligodendrogliomas (86.1%). However, they are rare in primary glioblastoma (5.0%). The most common mutation is the R132H IDH1 mutation (90%). The single arginine at the enzyme activity site is replaced by other amino acids (the most common one is histidine), which results in the loss of the original wild-type biological function of IDH, followed by the acquisition of new enzymes activities. Then α-KG produced during energy metabolism is reduced to 2-hydroxyglutaric acid (2-HG), a carcinogenic metabolite [11, 15]. However, it is ambiguous how these enzymatic changes contribute to tumorigenesis. Next, we discuss how IDH1/2 mutations alter glioma metabolism and how these changes may contribute to tumor formation in glioma.

2.1.2 IDH1/2 Mutation and 2-HG

After mutation of IDH 1/2, mutant IDH competes with wild IDH for substrates. On the one hand, the activity of wild-type IDH is inhibited or even lost. On the other hand, the production efficiency of α-KG decreases after mutation of IDH, and the generated α-KG is reduced to 2-HG under the action of new catalytic enzyme. Consequently, 2-HG expression is significantly increased in cancer cells. In clinic, the elevation of 2-HG can be detected in the serum of IDH mutated glioma. Moreover, 2-HG can be used as a biomarker for clinical detection because the level of 2-HG in normal tissues is very low [10]. In view of the important role of 2-HG in tumors, the mechanism of 2-HG-induced glioma has attracted wide attention in recent years (Fig. 1) [10].

Normally, cells metabolize to produce α-KG, which is combined with a variety of dioxygenases to participate in many important life activities, including collagen synthesis, DNA repair, and hypoxia. However, the level of 2-HG increases after IDH mutation. It is noteworthy that the molecular structure of 2-HG is very similar to that of α-KG. Therefore, 2-HG can competently bind to α-KG-dependent dioxygenase and inhibit the activity of enzyme, which is manifested by the increased expression of hypoxia-induced factor-1α (HIF-1α) [16]. HIF-1α can induce the expression of glycolysis-related enzymes, such as glucose transporter 1 (Glut 1) and hexokinase 2 (HK 2) [16, 17], thus turning cells into glycolysis process. For instance, prolyl hydroxylase (PHD) is a member of the dioxygenases family. Chowdhury et al. found that 2-HG could inhibit the activity of PHD in vitro, followed by the accumulation of HIF-1α in cells. Then the expression of downstream target genes of HIF-1α and a variety of signal pathways related to cell differentiation were activated, which ultimately promoted the formation of tumors [18].

In addition, high levels of 2-HG also inhibit DNA demethylase. Ten-eleven translocation (TET) family can demethylate DNA by catalyzing 5-methylcytosine (5-mc) hydroxylation [19]. TET 2 is the main enzyme of TET family. Many studies have shown that 2-HG can inhibit TET2-catalyzed 5-mc hydroxylation and DNA demethylation [20]. In other words, 2-HG can lead to DNA hypermethylation. In addition, 2-HG also inhibits histone demethylase. Xu et al. found that 2-HG could compete with α-KG, thus inhibiting the activity of histone demethylase containing JmjC domain and showed that histone methylation markers were upregulated and DNA meth-

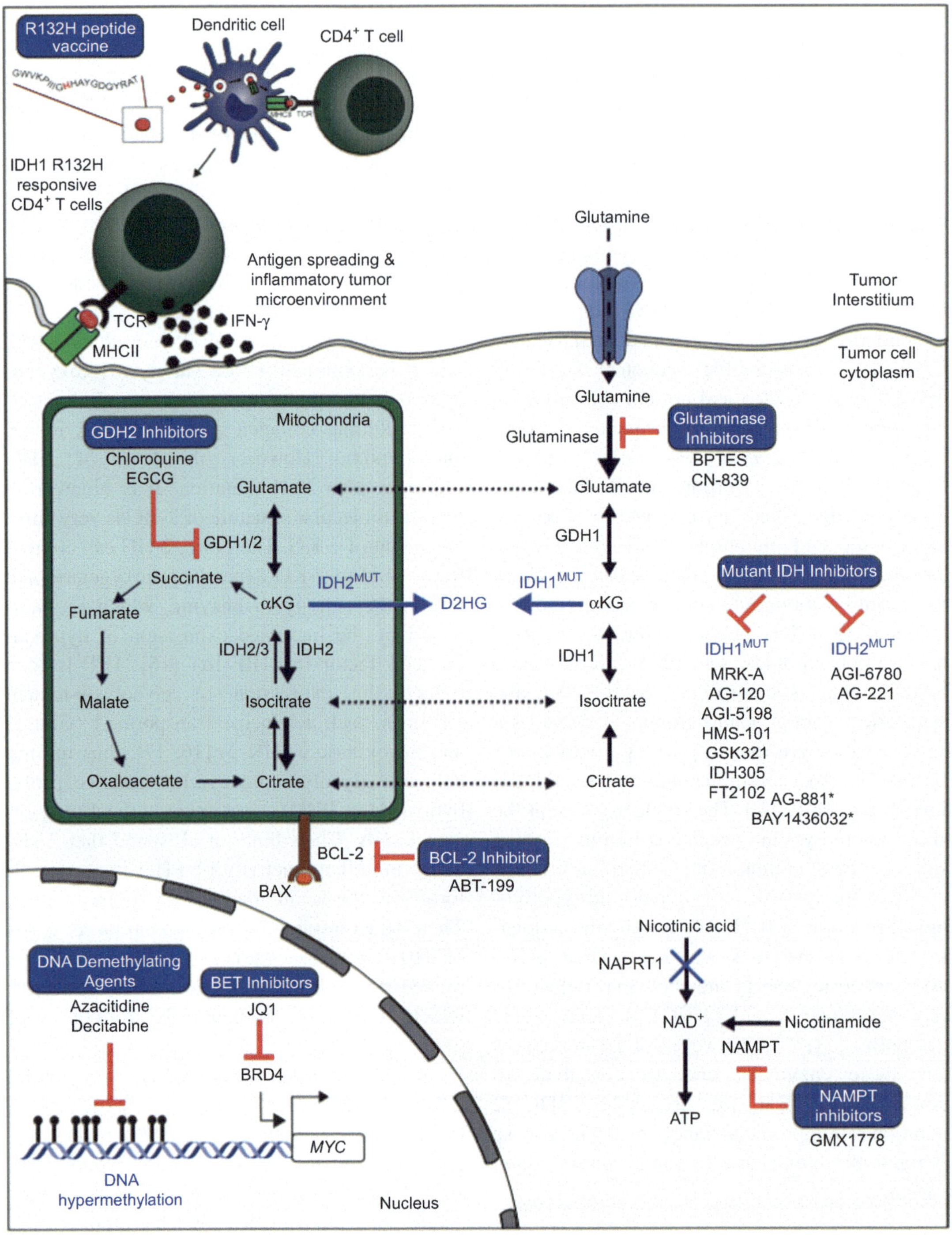

Fig. 1 Potential therapeutic strategies for malignancies that harbor IDH1 or IDH2 mutations. A number of pharmacological inhibitors have been developed to directly inhibit the neomorphic activity of mutant IDH enzymes in an effort to reduce D2HG production and elicit differentiation of malignant progenitor cells. Alternatively, inhibitors of enzymes involved in glutaminolysis, including glutamate dehydrogenases and glutaminase, have been shown to preferentially inhibit the growth of leukemia and glioma cells with IDH mutations. Similarly, NAMPT inhibitors are proposed to exploit the observation that NAPRT1-mediated conversion of nicotinic acid to NAD+ is defective in IDH-mutant gliomas (indicated by an X in the figure). Hypomethylating agents such as azacytidine and decitibine may also promote differentiation of IDH-mutant cells, which exhibit a hypermethylation phenotype that is associated with an inhibition of differentiation. Co-occurring driver alterations, such as MYCN amplification, may be targeted in IDH-mutant tumors using available targeted therapies (e.g., JQ1 for n-Myc overexpression) in a tumor-specific manner. *Indicates pan-mutant IDH inhibitor. Reprinted with permission [10]

ylation finally occurred [21, 22]. It is noteworthy that histone methylation and DNA methylation interact, and the disorder of histone and DNA methylation induced by 2-HG inhibited normal cell differentiation. It promoted the pathological self-renewal of stem cell-like cells, thus transforming them into cancer cells.

2.1.3 Metabolomic Alterations in IDH Mutant Cells

Metabolomics studies of IDH1/2 mutant cells revealed changes in the synthetic pathways of glutamine, fatty acids, and citrate [23]. Reitman et al. analyzed >200 metabolites in IDH1/2-mut oligodendroglioma cells and revealed the changes of amino acids, glutathione metabolites, choline derivatives, and intermediate products of TCA cycle [15]. These changes mimicked the alterations found in cells treated with 2-HG. N-acetyl-aspartyl-glutamic acid (NAAG) was a dipeptide commonly found in the brain, which was reduced by 50-fold in cells expressing IDH1-mut and by 8.3-fold in cells expressing IDH2-mut. A similar reduction in NAAG was detected in the tissues of IDH-mut glioma. Acetyl-CoA (CoA), produced by citrate in the cytoplasm, has been shown to regulate acetylation of cytoplasmic proteins. IDH-mut tumors exhibit disturbed acetyl-CoA metabolism and decreased cytosolic acetyl-CoA concentration, which may result in altered acetylation and activity of many oncogenic proteins [24]. IDH1-mut cells shared a variety of metabolic changes with 2-HG-treated cells, indicating that the production of metabolites was responsible for the observed metabolic effects. IDH1 activity was also an important factor in metabolic adaptation, supporting the maintenance of invasive growth of primary GBM despite difficult metabolic conditions [25].

Besides, IDH1-mut cells produce NADPH, which is involved in lipid metabolism [26]. Studies showed that IDH1/2 participated in protection against oxidative stress by producing molecules with strong reducing properties such as NADPH and α-KG [27, 28]. Those molecules can prevent DNA damage through their interaction with glutathione and thioredoxin production systems [29]. The response driven by IDH1 was the main source of NADPH in the human brain, producing up to 65% of brain NADPH [30]. IDH1/2 were also involved in glutamine metabolism under hypoxia and electron transport chain changes [31]. In addition, Studies revealed that IDH1/2 mutation induced a homologous recombination (HR) defect that renders tumor cells exquisitely sensitive to poly (ADP-ribose) polymerase (PARP) inhibitors [32]. These metabolic changes provided clues to the pathogenesis of tumors associated with IDH gene mutations. Table 1 summarizes the metabolomic alterations in IDH1/2 mutant cells or 2-HG treated cells.

2.2 Other Metabolic Pathways in Glioma

2.2.1 Amino Acid Metabolism

Amino acids are important metabolites in organisms, and metabolic dysregulation of amino acids is a new marker of cancer [34]. Tumor cells absorb amino acids from extracellular environment as carbon and nitrogen sources for protein and nucleotide synthesis [35]. Amino acids ingested from tumor microenvironment also contribute to carbon metabolism and redox maintenance [36, 37]. Tumor cells can also regulate amino acid uptake by regulating the level or activity of specific amino acid transporters [38]. At present, the molecular mechanism of amino acid transporters regulating cancer is still unclear. Below we briefly discuss newly discovered abnormalities in amino acid metabolism pathways in gliomas (Fig. 2) [39].

The first metabolic change observed in tumors is increased glycolysis, which is also known as the Warburg effect, even if there is sufficient oxygen supply. In recent years, the importance of mitochondria and the utilization of oxidizable substrates such as glutamine in the survival and proliferation of cancer cells have been clearly demonstrated [40]. Neurons in normal physiological state metabolize glutamine to glutamic acid and then wrap it into synaptic vesicles for future release. The glutamic acid-glutamine cycle maintains a low extracellular level of glutathione. Disruption of the glutamate-glutamine cycle can

Table 1 Levels of metabolites altered by IDH1/2 mutations in glioma

Sample	Detected signature metabolites		References
	Increased	Decreased	
IDH1 mutant cells	2-Hydroxyglutarate, 5,6-dihydrouracil, acetoacetate, glutamate, glutathione, isoleucine, lactate, maleate, oxaloacetate, oxypurinol, succinate, taurine, threonine, tyramine, valine, xanthine, glycine, serine, sparagine, tyrosine, tryptophan, methionine, glycerol-phosphates, glycerophosphocholine, 4-methyl-2-oxopentanoate and 3-methyl-2-oxopentanoate	Acetate, atrial natriuretic peptide, alanine, betaine, creatine, glycine, leucine, N-Acetylglycine, NAD+, trimethylamine N-oxide, ribulose-5-phosphate, glucose-6-phosphate, aspartate, glutamate, N-acetyl-aspartyl-glutamate, fumarate, malate, α-ketoglutarate, N-acetyl-aspartate, citrate, cis-aconitate, isobutyrylcarnitine, isovalerylylcarnitine, 2-methylbutyroylcarnitine and choline phosphate	[15, 33]
IDH2 mutant cells	2-Hydroxyglutarate, 5,6-dihydrouracil, acetate, acetoacetate, betaine, N-Acetylglycine, NAD+, trimethylamine N-oxide, ribulose-5-phosphate, glycine, serine, threonine, asparagine, tyrosine, tryptophan, methionine, glycerol-phosphates, leucine, isoleucine, valine, 4-methyl-2-oxopentanoate and 3-methyl-2-oxopentanoate	ANP, alanine, glutamate, glutathione, glycine, lactate, maleate, oxaloacetate, oxypurinol, succinate, threonine, tyramine, xanthine, citrate, α-ketoglutarate, aspartate, N-acetyl-aspartyl-glutamate, cis-aconitate, fumarate, and malate, isobutyrylcarnitine, isovalerylylcarnitine, 2-methylbutyroylcarnitine, choline phosphate and glycerophosphocholine	[15, 33]
Cells treated with 2-HG	2-Hydroxyglutarate, glycine, serine, threonine, asparagine, phenylalanine, tyrosine, tryptophan, methionine, glutamate, α-ketoglutarate, leucine, isoleucine, and valine, 4-methyl-2-oxopentanoate, 3-methyl-2-oxopentanoate and glycerophosphocholine	Aspartate, N-acetyl-aspartyl-glutamate, isobutyrylcarnitine, isovalerylylcarnitine, 2-methylbutyroylcarnitine and choline phosphate	[15]

provide neoplastic GBM cells access to glutamine. Cancer cells need glutamine to drive mitochondrial metabolism because the cost of converting glucose to lactic acid is mitochondrial oxidation. In addition to providing carbon for TCA cyclic synthesis, glutamine can also provide a-ketoglutarate to support amino acid catabolism. Glutamine is a direct nitrogen donor for nucleotide biosynthesis and is related to redox balance. Therefore, disruption of the glutamate-glutamine cycle can provide neoplastic GBM cells access to glutamine [41].

It was found that tryptophan and methionine were abnormally metabolized in glioma cells compared with normal astrocytes. GBM cells depend on methionine to proliferate and survive, as well as the maintenance of the S-adenosylmethionine (SAM): S-adenosylhomocysteine (SAH) ratio. When abnormal methionine metabolism occurs, the ratio is changed, which alters the total methylation of DNA, RNA, and protein, and ultimately activates carcinogenic kinases [42]. Similarly, abnormal tryptophan metabolism/indoleamine 2,3-dioxygenase (IDO1) signal is an important metabolic node in GBM. It was found that tryptophan level in GBM cells increased significantly, and tryptophan was converted to kynurenine instead of serotonin catalyzed by IDO enzyme. Kynurenine can activate aromatic hydrocarbon receptors and ultimately immunosuppressive agents, which makes multiple cancer cells escape the immune response and promote the formation of tumors [43].

In recent years, cysteine metabolism, as a new metabolic pathway of glioblastoma, has also attracted wide attention. Normally, cysteine is used to produce glutathione, which has an antioxidant effect. The abnormal metabolic pathway results in the accumulation of cysteine sulfinic acid (CSA) in cells. CSA is one of the major metabolites that differentiate glioblastoma from low-grade glioma. The level of CSA is highly

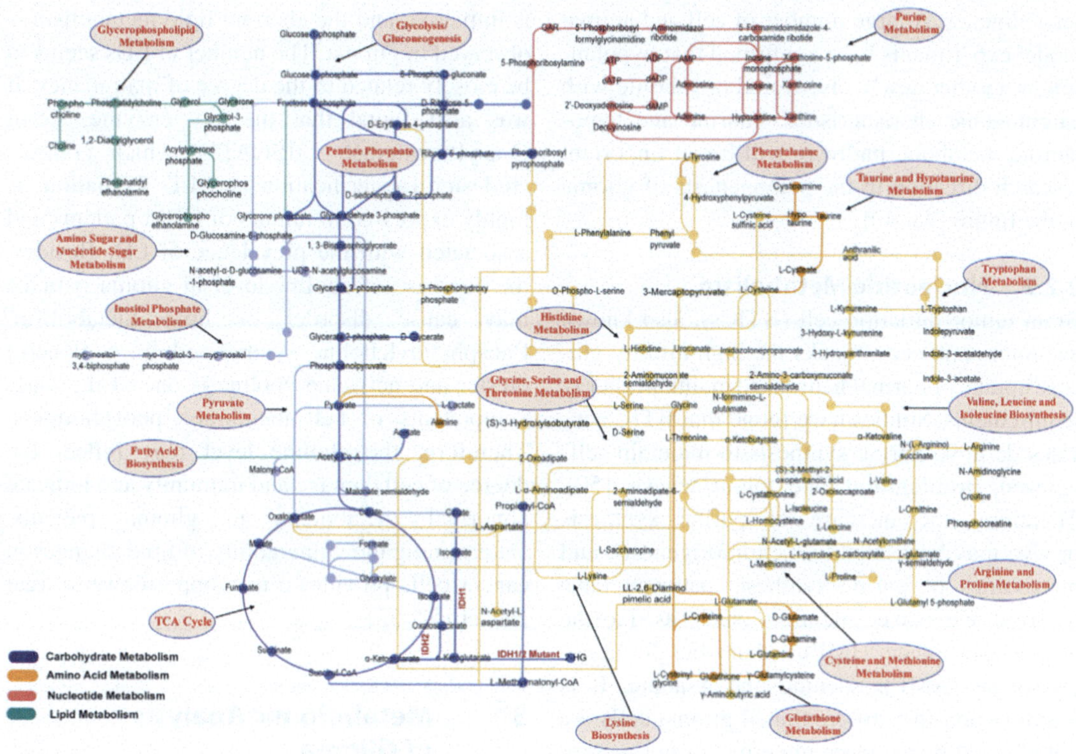

Fig. 2 Major metabolomic pathways involved in brain tumor metabolism. The highlighted boxes represent the metabolic pathways that may be significantly altered in malignant brain tumors. The accumulation of oncometabolite 2-HG resulted from IDH1/2 mutation also contributes to malignancy. *ADP* adenosine diphosphate, *AMP* adenosine monophosphate, *ATP* adenosine triphosphate, *dADP* deoxyadenosine diphosphate, *dAMP* deoxyadenosine monophosphate, *dATP* deoxyadenosine triphosphate, *CoA* coenzyme A, *GAR* glycinamide ribonucleotide, *IDH* isocitrate dehydrogenase, *UDP* uridine diphosphate. Reprinted with permission [39]

consistent with the expression of cysteine dioxygenase 1 (CDO1), a biosynthetic enzyme, in tumors. CAS also has the ability to inhibit oxidative phosphorylation of glioblastoma cells, and the weakening of oxidative phosphorylation is a common metabolic phenotype in carcinogenesis. It has been confirmed that the attenuation of oxidative phosphorylation induced by CSA is attributed to the inhibition of pyruvate dehydrogenase, a regulatory enzyme, and abnormal cysteine metabolism contributes to the growth of invasive high-grade glioma [44].

Studies found that cysteine-glutamate transporter (XCT) encoded by SLC7A11 gene is highly expressed in glioblastoma. XCT, together with its binding partner CD98 (SLC3A2), forms the amino acid transport system X_C^- (SXC). Cystine uptake was carried out through the XC-transporter system, and the main function of SXC is to convert cysteine (oxidative dimerization form of cysteine) into glutamic acid, which promotes tumor growth. Exchange of glutamate during this process also provides a survival advantage for glioma, leading to excitatory death of neurons near the tumor [45–47].

Taurine is an essential amino acid in human body. Hypotaurine, an oxidation product of taurine, can promote the occurrence and development of glioma, and hypotaurine is positively correlated with malignant degree of glioma. Many studies have found that taurine is reduced in plasma of glioma patients. Molecular biology results showed that hypotaurine could competitively inhibit the activity of proline hydroxylase 2, leading to nondegradation of HIF-1α, and then trigger the expression of tumor-related genes. A large number of cell and animal model experiments have confirmed that hypotaurine is another newly discovered metabolite with carcinogenic characteristics. Taurine and hypotaurine metabolic pathway will be an important research direction in the pathogenesis of glioma in the future [48, 49].

2.2.2 Nucleotide Metabolism

Brain tumor initiation cell (BTICs), also known as tumor stem cell, hijacks the high affinity glucose uptake of normal neurons to maintain energy requirements. Studies have found that BTIC activates de novo purine synthesis to maintain self-renewal, proliferation, and tumorigenesis [50]. Therefore, the increase of purine synthesis in vivo may be related to the tumorigenesis, and metabolites of purine synthesis pathway have received extensive attention, such as inosine 5′-monophosphate (IMP), adenosine 5′-monophosphate (AMP), adenine and guanine. It is worth noting that differentiated glioma cells are not affected by the targeting effect of purine biosynthetase, indicating selective dependence on BTIC. Purine synthesis begins with ribonuclease 5-phosphate (R5P). BTICs upregulated the enzymes involved in purine synthesis and effectively introduced glucose-derived R5P into the production of alkaline purine nucleotides. After glucose influx, the carbon flow in BTICs was used to maintain the purine synthesis, which was maintained by the core transcription factor myc. Therefore, the levels of IMP, AMP, and GMP in BTICs increased. In addition, by combining proteomics with intracellular metabolomics, it was found that PTDOH activates Cad through mToR signaling pathway independent of Akt, thereby acutely regulating the production of pyrimidine metabolites. The disorder of purine and pyrimidine metabolism was considered as one of the important factors for the occurrence and development of glioma [51].

2.2.3 Lipid Metabolism

Lipid metabolism reprogramming is a new metabolic feature of malignant tumors. The accumulation of lipid droplets (LD) during the progression of human glioma suggests that lipid metabolism is impaired, and the aberrant lipid metabolism is observed in glioma. The number of LDs seems to be closely related to the degree of malignancy. It was also found that the key enzyme, sterol O-acyltransferase 1 (SOAT1), which controls cholesterol esterification and LD formation, is highly expressed in tumors of GBM patients and associated with the prevalence of LD. Besides, the decrease of choline level in glioma patients may cause disorder of lipid metabolism. Phosphatidylcholine synthesized from glycerol diester and activated choline is one of the main components of cell membrane phospholipids. Therefore, the choline level may reflect the degree of cell damage and immunity and indicate abnormal metabolism in glioma patients. Determining the vulnerability of lipid changes in cancer cells provides a new opportunity to treat cancer [52, 53].

3 Metabolomic Analysis of Glioma

3.1 Cerebrospinal Fluids

Cerebrospinal fluid (CSF) represents an attractive source for monitoring glioma progression because the tissues of CNS are bathed by CSF, and CSF is readily accessible and less invasive compared with traditional pathology [54]. The CSF metabolic alterations are considered as one of the key biomarkers for glioma progression. Due to the availability of high-throughput analytical technologies, metabolomic analysis of CSFs from glioma patients has the potential to monitor glioma progression and the response to therapy [39].

Metabolomic analysis of CSFs have revealed many signature metabolites associated with the development and progression of glioma. Some of these metabolites also vary among the gliomas of different grades. Studies have reported that the levels of citric and isocitric acid in CSFs were remarkably increased in GBM versus the grades I–III gliomas, and the levels of lactic and 2-aminopimelic acids were relatively higher in GBM than the grades I–II gliomas [55, 56]. The report showed that changes in a large number of metabolites in CSFs were associated with the presence of an IDH1 mutation, including acetylcarnitine and shikimate, D-2-HG, malic acid, alanine, glutamate, lactate, phosphocholine, 1-methyl tryptophan, 1-methyl-histidine, arginine, asparagine, N-acetylputrescine, succinic acid semialdehyde, malonate, betaine aldehyde, and pantothenic acid. The levels of D-2-HG, malic acid, succinic acid, alanine, lactic acid, and aminohexanedioic acid were increased, while the levels of glutamic acid, acetylcarnitine, and shikimic acid were decreased significantly in IDH mutant gliomas [57–59].

3.2 Plasma and Serum

There has been an increasing interest of using blood metabolite biomarkers for cancer diagnostics and prognostics. Compared with tumor tissue, plasma is a matrix rich in metabolites, which can be easily obtained by the minimally invasive sampling. Therefore, plasma metabolomic analysis may be more suitable than actual glioma tissues for biomarker discovery, especially when it is difficult to harness normal brain tissues for comparison. Through the metabolomic analysis of high-grade and low-grade gliomas, 18 metabolites were found to be significantly different, and five metabolites, namely uracil, arginine, lactic acid, cysteine, and ornithine, were significantly different between patients with high-grade glioma and low-grade glioma. Ascorbate and aldarate metabolites were associated with high-grade glioma, while glycolysis/gluconeogenesis/pyruvate, eicosanoid, and glutamate metabolites were related to lower-grade disease [60].

In addition, lower levels of arginine were observed in high-grade glioma when compared to low-grade glioma, suggesting greater arginine dependence of the high-grade glioma. Two arginine/proline metabolic pathway intermediates, 2-oxoarginine, which is a guanidino metabolite of arginine, and argininate, which is the conjugate base of arginine, were substantially lower in men years in advance, especially nine or more years, of being diagnosed with glioma when compared with healthy controls (without diagnosis of glioma). In fact, studies have indicated that arginine/proline metabolites are involved in tumorigenesis (including glioblastoma), exogenous arginine is required for tumor growth, and arginine deprivation leads to impairment of glioma cell motility, invasiveness, and adhesion [61–64]. Tumor cells have a high demand for arginine. However, a subset of glioblastomas has a defect in the arginine biosynthetic pathway due to epigenetic silencing of the rate-limiting enzyme argininosuccinate synthetase (ASS1). The metabolism of amino acids such as citrulline, arginine, alanine, and glycine were significantly altered between the two subtypes of ASS1 positive and ASS1 negative GBMs [65]. Metabolomics profiling in plasma samples from glioma patients also correlated with tumor phenotypes. Uridine and guanine were found to be significantly different between patients with GBM and non-GBM, and six metabolites, N-acetylputrescine, trimethylamine-N-oxide (TMAO), nicotinate (niacin), arginine, glucosamine, and methionine, were found to be associated with IDH mutation. Those six significant metabolites separated IDH1 mutation positive from negative glioma patients with 94.4% accuracy. Within arginine and proline metabolism, levels of intermediate metabolites in creatine pathway were all significantly lower in IDH mutation positive than in IDH mutation negative patients, suggesting an increased activity of creatine pathway in IDH mutation positive tumors [66].

Serum metabolomic analysis of GBM patient during the initial phase of radiotherapy revealed that 68 metabolites were lowered in concentration following treatment while 16 metabolites were elevated in concentration. All detected and identified amino acids and fatty acids together with myo-inositol, creatinine, and urea were among the metabolites that decreased in concentration after treatment, while citric acid was among the metabolites that increased in concentration [67]. Another serum study also found that cysteine levels in GBM patients were higher than those in oligodendroglioma patients, while lysine and 2-oxisohexanoic acid were more abundant in the sera of oligodendroglioma patients [39].

3.3 Glioma Tissues

For cancer research, metabolomic analysis of tumor tissues possesses a unique advantage that it can gain more direct insight into disease-specific pathogenesis. Owing to the fact that precancerous tissue is not easily acquired from patients, pair-wise metabolomics analysis of malignant and corresponding normal brain tissues was performed relatively scarcely. C6 cell lines were the rat origin glioma cells, and, genetically, C6 glioma-bearing rats were good models for glioma studies [68]. A recent study found that nine metabolites increased in the rat tumor tissues [69]. Among them, hypotaurine was the only metabolite enriched in the malignant tissues as what had been reported in the metabolomics analysis of human tissues. Except hypotaurine, the other eight metabolites were not found to be different in human glioma tissue metabolomic analysis. It was reported that hypotaurine increased the stability of HIF-1α in human glioma cells in vitro, and hypotaurine was reported as a competitive inhibitor of PHD2 [48]. Besides, 4-aminobutyric acid (GABA), an important inhibitory neurotransmitter, was found at low level in tumors of high-grade glioma patients, while it can be detected in normal brain. Another neurotransmitter, glutamate, is the substrate of GABA and participates in energy supply. The level of glutamate was found to be higher in glioma when compared with normal brain [70].

Although there are relatively few paired metabolomic analyses of malignant and corresponding normal brain tissues, 12 distinct metabolic features were found by comparing the metabolic characteristics of GBM and oligodendroglioma tissues. In high-grade gliomas, blood-brain barrier defects may occur. Therefore, the level of mannitol, a molecule that normally may not be able to cross the blood brain barrier, was found to be higher in high-grade glioma. 2-Hydroxyglutaric acid, GABA, creatinine, glycerol-2-phosphoric acid, glycerol-3-phosphoric acid, libitol, and inositol were higher in oligodendroglioma than those in GBM. Creatinine, a decomposition product of creatine phosphate, converts ADP into ATP. Metabonomic analysis revealed that creatinine level in GBM tumors was lower than that in oligodendroglioma. Glycerol-3-phosphoric acid is the skeleton of triglycerides and glycerol phosphatides. It also participates in the oxidation cycle of fatty acids and produces NADH. Glycerol-3-phosphate levels in GBM were lower than those in oligodendroglioma [70]. Table 2 summarizes some of the significantly altered metabolites identified by metabolomic analysis of CSF, serum/plasma, and glioma tissues.

4 Application of Metabolomics in Glioma

4.1 Diagnosis of Glioma

Considering the high fatality rate of glioma, early diagnosis is the key to patients' survival and positive prognosis. However, due to the variable clinical manifestations of glioma and the lack of reliable screening tools, glioma remains difficult to diagnose. Therefore, an accurate, effective, and noninvasive technique of early diagnosis is needed to improve the prognosis of glioma patients. Metabolomics studies of some key metabolic pathways in brain tumors, such as cysteine metabolism and lipid metabolism, can identify potential biomarkers, which may help to classify gliomas and develop new clinical diagnostic strategies. Given that the published results of metabolomic analysis, different gliomas display different metabolites in cerebrospinal fluid (CSF), tumor tissue, serum, and plasma, which may be of diagnostic value in GBM [39].

In addition, IDH mutation is an early event of glioma, which is closely related to the classification of glioma and can be used as one of the markers of diagnosis and classification. This marker not only makes the diagnosis of glioma more timely and comprehensive but also has significance for further study of the pathogenesis and biological characteristics of glioma. In addition, the important biochemical indicator of mutations in IDH1 and IDH2 were abnormal elevation of 2-HG level. Therefore, the appropriate range of 2-HG reference value can be used as

Table 2 Signature metabolites detected in gliomas by metabolomics

Sample	Detected signature metabolites		References
	Increased	Decreased	
Plasma sample of gliomas patients vs healthy volunteers	Creatinine, histidine, citric acid, very low density lipoprotein (VLDL), low density lipoprotein (LDL), unsaturated lipid, and pyruvate	Taurine, isoleucine, leucine, valine, lactate, alanine, glycoprotein, glutamate, citrate, creatine, myo-inositol, choline, tyrosine, phenylalanine, 1-methylhistidine, α-glucose, and β-glucose	[71]
Plasma sample of high-grade glioma patients vs low-grade glioma patients	Lactate, uridine, and uracil	Arginine	[66]
Plasma samples of glioma patients (Mut-IDH vs WT-IDH)	Sarcosine	Guanidoacetic, N-acetyl putrescine, acid, creatine, creatinine, and trimethylamine-N-oxide	[66]
Serum samples from GBM patients vs healthy volunteers	α-Tocopherol, γ-tocopherol, erythritol, MI, erythronic acid, 2-keto-L-gluconic acid, cysteine, hypoxantine, vitronectin, and aconitate	Xanthine, secondary bile acids glycocholenate sulfate, 3β-hydroxy-5-cholenoic acid, xenobiotic methyl, 4-hydroxybenzoate sulfate, sex steroid 5alpha-pregnan-3beta, 20beta-diol monosulfate, cofactor/vitamin, and oxalate (ethanedioate)	[60, 72, 73]
Serum samples from glioma patients vs healthy volunteers	Serum acylcarnitines stearoylcarnitine, margaroylcarnitine, eicosenoylcarnitine, 1-methylurate, 1-methylxanthine, paraxanthine, theobromine, 5-acetylamino-6-amino-3-methyluracil, theophylline, and 7-methylxanthine	Amino acids 2-oxoarginine, cysteine, argininate, alpha-ketoglutarate, lipid chenodeoxycholate, N-acetyl tyrosine, N-acetyl phenylalanine, phenyl lactate and tyrosine, N-acetyl kynurenine, N-acetyl tryptophan, and xanthurenate	[60]
Serum samples from GBM vs oligodendrogliomas	Cysteine	Lysine and 2-oxoisocaproic acid	[70]
GBM cells and GBM tissues vs normal human astrocytes	Tryptophan, methionine, kynurenine, 5-methylthioadenosine, glutamate, and mannitol	4-Aminobutyric acid (GABA)	[42]
Tissue samples from GBM vs oligodendrogliomas	Mannitol, phenylalanine and choline	2-Hydroxyglutaric acid, 4-aminobutyric acid (GABA), creatinine, glycerol-2-phosphate, glycerol-3-phosphate, ribitol, myo-inositol, creatinine, and cysteine sulfinic acid	[60, 70, 74]
CSF samples from GBM vs oligodendrogliomas	Citric acid, isocitric acid, lactic acid, and 2-aminopimelic acid	Indole, indoleacrylic acid, anthranilic acid, histidine, Pyruvate, oxaloacetic acid, and myo-inositol	[54, 55]
CSF samples of glioma patients (Mut-IDH vs WT-IDH)	Citric acid, isocitric acid, lactic acid, succinate, malic acid, phosphoenol pyruvate, amino adipic acid, and D-2-HG	Pyruvate, oxaloacetic acid, and alanine	[55, 57, 58]
CSF samples of glioma patients vs healthy volunteers	Glycine, serine threonine, alanine, aspartate, glutamate, acetylcarnitine, and shikimate		[57]
Cells from grades I–III gliomas (Mut-IDH vs WT-IDH)	Lactate/choline, 2-hydroxyglutarate, and glycerophosphocholine	Fumarate, malate, glutamate, lactate, phosphocholine, glutathione, glutamine, and myo-inositol	[59, 75]

a sensitive and specific predictor. Metabolomics is more closely related to physiology than genomics and proteomics. Cancer diseases cause the changes of pathophysiological processes and metabolites. By using metabolomics technology for a comprehensive analysis of metabolites in body fluids or tumor tissues, we may find sensitive and specific biomarkers that will provide a better method for diagnosis of glioma [76].

4.2 Prognosis of Glioma

In clinical practice, the survival rates of patients with glioblastoma and low-grade glioma are quite different. Biomarkers are needed for a more reliable prognosis of gliomas. Majos et al. used metabonomic analysis to detect glioma metabolites and pointed out the possibility of using metabolic characteristics for prognosis [77]. In GBM, the metabolic characteristics of tumor samples from patients who survived longer (>3 years) after diagnosis were compared with those of patients who died less than 4 months after diagnosis. The results showed that glycerol-3-phosphate, inositol, libitol, and fructose increased with the prolongation of survival time. High levels of glycine, aminopropanedioic acid, and most likely unknown sterols are associated with short-term survival [70]. Metabonomic analysis of metabolites in serum samples showed that inositol and hexadecanoic acid were associated with longer survival time [78, 79]. In high-grade gliomas, high level of glycine was detected and associated with poor prognosis [80]. Besides, a recent study has found that mutations in IDH1/2 were associated with a good prognosis in patients with glioma (especially GBM) [81]. The proliferation and migration ability of glioma cells expressing mutant IDH1 R132H is weakened, and the survival time of transplanted mice is longer [82].

4.3 Treatment of Glioma

The administration with temozolomide (TMZ), a DNA alkylating agent of the imidazotetrazine class, alongside adjuvant radiation after surgical resection is currently the standard regimen to treat GBM patients. However, the median survival remains 12–15 months because of limited surgical treatment and TMZ-related inherent and acquired resistance [83]. Hence, it is urgently that current therapies are upgraded in order to increase patient survival. Metabolomic analysis is a sensitive and effective approach for monitoring phenotypic changes and verifying pathways that are disturbed when glioma occurs. It certainly can help to identify critical pathways that can be targeted for fighting against glioma drug resistance [39]. Studies have showed that the radioresistance of glioma cells could in part be due to the deregulation of the PI3K/mTOR pathway [84]. Hence, inhibition of the PI3K/mTOR pathway makes adult and pediatric glioma cells more sensitive to radiation [85], and a dual blockade of IGFR1 and PDGFR or mTOR and AKT could be used along with traditional treatment to improve patient survival [86, 87]. Furthermore, application of metabolomics may be used to monitor and assess the therapeutic response to treatment, and to form follow-up treatment plans. In other words, the application of metabonomics may help achieve personalized treatment [88, 89].

5 Conclusion and Future Prospective

Tumor initiation and development is a complex process triggered by multiple factors. Elucidation of the complex mechanisms of tumorigenesis remains the key to effective prevention and treatment of cancer diseases. Numerous evidences have recently shown that tumor is a metabolic disease, and anticancer therapy targeting at tumor metabolism could be a valuable treatment approach. Based on this notion, the research direction of glioma has been partially adjusted, and nutrition and metabolic regulation-based therapies have become one of the main battlefields of gliomas treatment. Many signature metabolites have been discovered in glioma, such as 2-HG, fumaric acid, succinic acid, sarcosine, glycine, glutamine, aspartic acid, choline, serine, glucose, lactic acid, and polyamines, which suggest many metabolic pathways (e.g., glycolysis, TCA, glutaminolysis, pentose phosphate pathway, fatty acid metabolism, amino acid metabolism) may be dysregulated in this disease. Due to their high metabolic adaptability when facing any stress injury, cancer cells may rewire alternative metabolite pathways in order to survive and proliferate. Therefore, a systematic therapy should be used to target multiple metabolic pathways in cancer cells. It is noteworthy that the findings detailed in this chapter are mainly attributed to the increased applications of metabolomics. With additional improvement of related technologies, metabolomics will become a powerful tool to discover truly meaningful biomarkers for new clinical applications in malignant gliomas. Metabolomic studies of gliomas will also facilitate a better understanding of the molecular targets/pathways and the development of new therapeutic treatments in this devastating disease.

References

1. Ostrom, Q. T., et al. (2018). CBTRUS statistical report: Primary brain and other central nervous system tumors diagnosed in the United States in 2011–2015. *Neuro-Oncology, 20*, iv1–iv86.
2. Weller, M., et al. (2017). European Association for Neuro-Oncology (EANO) guideline on the diagnosis and treatment of adult astrocytic and oligodendroglial gliomas. *The Lancet Oncology, 18*, e315–e329.
3. Miller, J. J., Shih, H. A., Andronesi, O. C., & Cahill, D. P. (2017). Isocitrate dehydrogenase-mutant glioma: Evolving clinical and therapeutic implications. *Cancer, 123*, 4535–4546.
4. Clark, P. M., Mai, W. X., Cloughesy, T. F., & Nathanson, D. A. (2016). Emerging approaches for targeting metabolic vulnerabilities in malignant glioma. *Current Neurology and Neuroscience Reports, 16 (2), 17*.
5. Bharti, S. K., & Roy, R. (2012). Quantitative 1H NMR spectroscopy. *TrAC Trends in Analytical Chemistry, 35*, 5–26.
6. Goudar, C., et al. (2010). Metabolic flux analysis of CHO cells in perfusion culture by metabolite balancing and 2D [13C, 1H] COSY NMR spectroscopy. *Metabolic Engineering, 12*, 138–149.
7. Marin-Valencia, I., et al. (2012). Analysis of tumor metabolism reveals mitochondrial glucose oxidation in genetically diverse human glioblastomas in the mouse brain in vivo. *Cell Metabolism, 15*, 827–837.
8. Mashimo, T., et al. (2014). Acetate is a bioenergetic substrate for human glioblastoma and brain metastases. *Cell, 159*, 1603–1614.
9. Tseng, C.-L., & Wei, J.-W. (2012). Investigation on signal transduction pathways after H1 receptor activated by histamine in C6 glioma cells: Involvement of phosphatidylinositol and arachidonic acid metabolisms. *Journal of the Chinese Medical Association, 75*, 143–150.
10. Waitkus, M. S., Diplas, B. H., & Yan, H. (2018). Biological role and therapeutic potential of IDH mutations in cancer. *Cancer Cell, 34*, 186–195.
11. Parsons, D. W., et al. (2008). An integrated genomic analysis of human glioblastoma multiforme. *Science, 321*, 1807–1812.
12. Reitman, Z. J., & Yan, H. (2010). Isocitrate dehydrogenase 1 and 2 mutations in cancer: Alterations at a crossroads of cellular metabolism. *Journal of the National Cancer Institute, 102*, 932–941.
13. Xu, X., et al. (2004). Structures of human cytosolic NADP-dependent isocitrate dehydrogenase reveal a novel self-regulatory mechanism of activity. *The Journal of Biological Chemistry, 279*, 33946–33957.
14. Henderson, N. S. (1965). Isozymes of isocitrate dehydrogenase: Subunit structure and intracellular location. *Journal of Experimental Zoology, 158*, 263–273.
15. Reitman, Z. J., et al. (2011). Profiling the effects of isocitrate dehydrogenase 1 and 2 mutations on the cellular metabolome. *Proceedings of the National Academy of Sciences of the United States of America, 108*, 3270–3275.
16. Zhao, S., et al. (2009). Glioma-derived mutations in IDH1 dominantly inhibit IDH1 catalytic activity and induce HIF-1alpha. *Science, 324*, 261–265.
17. Rankin, E. B., & Giaccia, A. J. (2008). The role of hypoxia-inducible factors in tumorigenesis. *Cell Death and Differentiation, 15*, 678–685.
18. Chowdhury, R., et al. (2011). The oncometabolite 2-hydroxyglutarate inhibits histone lysine demethylases. *EMBO Reports, 12*, 463–469.
19. Losman, J. A., & Kaelin, W. G., Jr. (2013). What a difference a hydroxyl makes: Mutant IDH, (R)-2-hydroxyglutarate, and cancer. *Genes & Development, 27*, 836–852.
20. Figueroa, M. E., et al. (2010). Leukemic IDH1 and IDH2 mutations result in a hypermethylation phenotype, disrupt TET2 function, and impair hematopoietic differentiation. *Cancer Cell, 18*, 553–567.
21. Sasaki, M., et al. (2012). IDH1(R132H) mutation increases murine haematopoietic progenitors and alters epigenetics. *Nature, 488*, 656–659.
22. Xu, W., et al. (2011). Oncometabolite 2-hydroxyglutarate is a competitive inhibitor of alpha-ketoglutarate-dependent dioxygenases. *Cancer Cell, 19*, 17–30.
23. Mardis, E. R., et al. (2009). Recurring mutations found by sequencing an acute myeloid leukemia genome. *The New England Journal of Medicine, 361*, 1058–1066.
24. Ye, D., Guan, K. L., & Xiong, Y. (2018). Metabolism, activity, and targeting of D- and L-2-hydroxyglutarates. *Trends in Cancer, 4*, 151–165.

25. Dang, L., et al. (2009). Cancer-associated IDH1 mutations produce 2-hydroxyglutarate. *Nature, 462*, 739–744.
26. Koh, H. J., et al. (2004). Cytosolic NADP+-dependent isocitrate dehydrogenase plays a key role in lipid metabolism. *The Journal of Biological Chemistry, 279*, 39968–39974.
27. Minard, K. I., & McAlister-Henn, L. (1999). Dependence of peroxisomal beta-oxidation on cytosolic sources of NADPH. *The Journal of Biological Chemistry, 274*, 3402–3406.
28. Lee, S. M., et al. (2002). Cytosolic NADP + –dependent isocitrate dehydrogenase status modulates oxidative damage to cells. *Free Radical Biology and Medicine, 32*, 1185–1196.
29. Metellus, P., et al. (2011). IDH mutation status impact on in vivo hypoxia biomarkers expression: new insights from a clinical, nuclear imaging and immunohistochemical study in 33 glioma patients. *Journal of Neuro-Oncology, 105*, 591–600.
30. Bleeker, F. E., et al. (2010). The prognostic IDH1(R132) mutation is associated with reduced NADP+-dependent IDH activity in glioblastoma. *Acta Neuropathologica, 119*, 487–494.
31. Metallo, C. M., et al. (2011). Reductive glutamine metabolism by IDH1 mediates lipogenesis under hypoxia. *Nature, 481*, 380–384.
32. Sulkowski, P. L., et al. (2017). 2-Hydroxyglutarate produced by neomorphic IDH mutations suppresses homologous recombination and induces PARP inhibitor sensitivity. *Science Translational Medicine, 9, Issue 375*, eaal2463.
33. Wen, H., et al. (2015). Metabolomic comparison between cells over-expressing isocitrate dehydrogenase 1 and 2 mutants and the effects of an inhibitor on the metabolism. *Journal of Neurochemistry, 132*, 183–193.
34. Pavlova, N. N., & Thompson, C. B. (2016). The emerging hallmarks of cancer metabolism. *Cell Metabolism, 23*, 27–47.
35. DeBerardinis, R. J., Lum, J. J., Hatzivassiliou, G., & Thompson, C. B. (2008). The biology of cancer: Metabolic reprogramming fuels cell growth and proliferation. *Cell Metabolism, 7*, 11–20.
36. Altman, B. J., Stine, Z. E., & Dang, C. V. (2016). From Krebs to clinic: Glutamine metabolism to cancer therapy. *Nature Reviews. Cancer, 16*, 619–634.
37. Yang, M., & Vousden, K. H. (2016). Serine and one-carbon metabolism in cancer. *Nature Reviews. Cancer, 16*, 650–662.
38. Bhutia, Y. D., Babu, E., Ramachandran, S., & Ganapathy, V. (2015). Amino Acid transporters in cancer and their relevance to "glutamine addiction": Novel targets for the design of a new class of anticancer drugs. *Cancer Research, 75*, 1782–1788.
39. Pandey, R., Caflisch, L., Lodi, A., Brenner, A. J., & Tiziani, S. (2017). Metabolomic signature of brain cancer. *Molecular Carcinogenesis, 56*, 2355–2371.
40. Oizel, K., et al. (2017). Efficient mitochondrial glutamine targeting prevails over glioblastoma metabolic plasticity. *Clinical Cancer Research: An Official Journal of the American Association for Cancer Research, 23*, 6292–6304.
41. Seyfried, T. N., Flores, R., Poff, A. M., D'Agostino, D. P., & Mukherjee, P. (2015). Metabolic therapy: a new paradigm for managing malignant brain cancer. *Cancer Letters, 356*, 289–300.
42. Palanichamy, K., et al. (2016). Methionine and kynurenine activate oncogenic kinases in glioblastoma, and methionine deprivation compromises proliferation. *Clinical Cancer Research: An Official Journal of the American Association for Cancer Research, 22*, 3513–3523.
43. Kesarwani, P., et al. (2018). Tryptophan metabolism contributes to radiation-induced immune checkpoint reactivation in glioblastoma. *Clinical Cancer Research: An Official Journal of the American Association for Cancer Research, 24*, 3632–3643.
44. Prabhu, A., et al. (2014). Cysteine catabolism: a novel metabolic pathway contributing to glioblastoma growth. *Cancer Research, 74*, 787–796.
45. Gu, Y., et al. (2017). mTORC2 regulates amino acid metabolism in cancer by phosphorylation of the cystine-glutamate antiporter xCT. *Molecular Cell, 67*, 128–138 e127.
46. Shih, A. Y., et al. (2006). Cystine/glutamate exchange modulates glutathione supply for neuroprotection from oxidative stress and cell proliferation. *The Journal of Neuroscience: The Official Journal of the Society for Neuroscience, 26*, 10514–10523.
47. Lewerenz, J., et al. (2013). The cystine/glutamate antiporter system x(c)(−) in health and disease: from molecular mechanisms to novel therapeutic opportunities. *Antioxidants & Redox Signaling, 18*, 522–555.
48. Gao, P., et al. (2016). Hypotaurine evokes a malignant phenotype in glioma through aberrant hypoxic signaling. *Oncotarget, 7*, 15200–15214.
49. Zhao, Y., et al. (2016). A novel strategy for large-scale metabolomics study by calibrating gross and systematic errors in gas chromatography-mass spectrometry. *Analytical Chemistry, 88*, 2234–2242.
50. Wang, X., et al. (2017). Purine synthesis promotes maintenance of brain tumor initiating cells in glioma. *Nature Neuroscience, 20*, 661–673.
51. Mathews, T. P., et al. (2015). Human phospholipase D activity transiently regulates pyrimidine biosynthesis in malignant gliomas. *ACS Chemical Biology, 10*, 1258–1268.
52. Geng, F., et al. (2016). Cbio-07. Lipid droplets, A novel diagnostic biomarker and metabolic target in glioblastoma. *Neuro-Oncology, 18*, vi36–vi36.
53. El Demellawy, D., Saleh, R., Daya, D., & Alowami, S. (2010). Malignant giant cell tumor of the vulva. *International Journal of Gynecological Pathology: Official Journal of the International Society of Gynecological Pathologists, 29*, 93–97.
54. Locasale, J. W., et al. (2012). Metabolomics of human cerebrospinal fluid identifies signatures of malignant glioma. *Molecular & Cellular Proteomics: MCP, 11*, M111 014688.

55. Nakamizo, S., et al. (2013). GC/MS-based metabolomic analysis of cerebrospinal fluid (CSF) from glioma patients. *Journal of Neuro-Oncology, 113*, 65–74.
56. Ahmed, K., & Chinnaiyan, P. (2014). Applying metabolomics to understand the aggressive phenotype and identify novel therapeutic targets in glioblastoma. *Metabolites, 4*, 740–750.
57. Ballester, L. Y., et al. (2018). Analysis of cerebrospinal fluid metabolites in patients with primary or metastatic central nervous system tumors. *Acta Neuropathologica Communications, 6*, 85.
58. Kalinina, J., et al. (2016). Selective detection of the D-enantiomer of 2-hydroxyglutarate in the CSF of glioma patients with mutated isocitrate dehydrogenase. *Clinical Cancer Research: An Official Journal of the American Association for Cancer Research, 22*, 6256–6265.
59. Izquierdo-Garcia, J. L., et al. (2015). Metabolic reprogramming in mutant IDH1 glioma cells. *PLoS One, 10*, e0118781.
60. Huang, J., et al. (2017). A prospective study of serum metabolites and glioma risk. *Oncotarget, 8*, 70366–70377.
61. Allen, M. D., et al. (2014). Prognostic and therapeutic impact of argininosuccinate synthetase 1 control in bladder cancer as monitored longitudinally by PET imaging. *Cancer Research, 74*, 896–907.
62. Delage, B., et al. (2010). Arginine deprivation and argininosuccinate synthetase expression in the treatment of cancer. *International Journal of Cancer, 126*, 2762–2772.
63. Patil, M. D., Bhaumik, J., Babykutty, S., Banerjee, U. C., & Fukumura, D. (2016). Arginine dependence of tumor cells: targeting a chink in cancer's armor. *Oncogene, 35*, 4957–4972.
64. Pavlyk, I., et al. (2015). Arginine deprivation affects glioblastoma cell adhesion, invasiveness and actin cytoskeleton organization by impairment of beta-actin arginylation. *Amino Acids, 47*, 199–212.
65. Moren, L., et al. (2018). Metabolomic profiling identifies distinct phenotypes for ASS1 positive and negative GBM. *BMC Cancer, 18*, 167.
66. Zhao, H., et al. (2016). Metabolomics profiling in plasma samples from glioma patients correlates with tumor phenotypes. *Oncotarget, 7*, 20486–20495.
67. Mörén, L., et al. (2016). Characterization of the serum metabolome following radiation treatment in patients with high-grade gliomas. *Radiation Oncology, 11*, 51–51.
68. Barth, R. F., & Kaur, B. (2009). Rat brain tumor models in experimental neuro-oncology: the C6, 9L, T9, RG2, F98, BT4C, RT-2 and CNS-1 gliomas. *Journal of Neuro-Oncology, 94*, 299–312.
69. Gao, P., et al. (2017). Capillary electrophoresis - Mass spectrometry metabolomics analysis revealed enrichment of hypotaurine in rat glioma tissues. *Analytical Biochemistry, 537*, 1–7.
70. Moren, L., et al. (2015). Metabolomic screening of tumor tissue and serum in glioma patients reveals diagnostic and prognostic information. *Metabolites, 5*, 502–520.
71. Kelimu, A., et al. (2016). Metabonomic signature analysis in plasma samples of glioma patients based on (1)H-nuclear magnetic resonance spectroscopy. *Neurology India, 64*, 246–251.
72. Bjorkblom, B., et al. (2016). Metabolomic screening of pre-diagnostic serum samples identifies association between alpha- and gamma-tocopherols and glioblastoma risk. *Oncotarget, 7*, 37043–37053.
73. Chen, M. H., et al. (2016). Diagnostic and prognostic value of serum vitronectin levels in human glioma. *Journal of the Neurological Sciences, 371*, 54–59.
74. Chang, S. M., et al. (2009). Integration of preoperative anatomic and metabolic physiologic imaging of newly diagnosed glioma. *Journal of Neuro-Oncology, 92*, 401–415.
75. Lazovic, J., et al. (2012). Detection of 2-hydroxyglutaric acid in vivo by proton magnetic resonance spectroscopy in U87 glioma cells overexpressing isocitrate dehydrogenase-1 mutation. *Neuro-Oncology, 14*, 1465–1472.
76. Borodovsky, A., Seltzer, M. J., & Riggins, G. J. (2012). Altered cancer cell metabolism in gliomas with mutant IDH1 or IDH2. *Current Opinion in Oncology, 24*, 83–89.
77. Majos, C., et al. (2011). Proton MR spectroscopy provides relevant prognostic information in high-grade astrocytomas. *AJNR. American Journal of Neuroradiology, 32*, 74–80.
78. Rosel, P., et al. (2000). Altered 5-HT2A binding sites and second messenger inositol trisphosphate (IP3) levels in hippocampus but not in frontal cortex from depressed suicide victims. *Psychiatry Research: Neuroimaging, 99*, 173–181.
79. da Rocha, A. B., Mans, D. R., Regner, A., & Schwartsmann, G. (2002). Targeting protein kinase C: new therapeutic opportunities against high-grade malignant gliomas? *The Oncologist, 7*, 17–33.
80. Peeling, J., & Sutherland, G. (1992). High-Resolution 1H NMR spectroscopy studies of extracts of human cerebral neoplasms. *Magnetic Resonance in Medicine, 24*, 123–136.
81. Watanabe, T., Nobusawa, S., Kleihues, P., & Ohgaki, H. (2009). IDH1 mutations are early events in the development of astrocytomas and oligodendrogliomas. *The American Journal of Pathology, 174*, 1149–1153.
82. Houillier, C., et al. (2010). IDH1 or IDH2 mutations predict longer survival and response to temozolomide in low-grade gliomas. *Neurology, 75*, 1560–1566.
83. Stupp, R., et al. (2009). Effects of radiotherapy with concomitant and adjuvant temozolomide versus radiotherapy alone on survival in glioblastoma in a randomised phase III study: 5-year analysis of the EORTC-NCIC trial. *The Lancet Oncology, 10*, 459–466.
84. Begg, A. C., Stewart, F. A., & Vens, C. (2011). Strategies to improve radiotherapy with targeted drugs. *Nature Reviews. Cancer, 11*, 239–253.
85. Agliano, A., et al. (2017). Pediatric and adult glioblastoma radiosensitization induced by PI3K/mTOR inhibition causes early metabolic alterations

detected by nuclear magnetic resonance spectroscopy. *Oncotarget, 8*, 47969–47983.
86. Szerlip, N. J., et al. (2012). Intratumoral heterogeneity of receptor tyrosine kinases EGFR and PDGFRA amplification in glioblastoma defines subpopulations with distinct growth factor response. *Proceedings of the National Academy of Sciences of the United States of America, 109*, 3041–3046.
87. Little, S. E., et al. (2012). Receptor tyrosine kinase genes amplified in glioblastoma exhibit a mutual exclusivity in variable proportions reflective of individual tumor heterogeneity. *Cancer Research, 72*, 1614–1620.
88. Ahmed, K. A., & Chinnaiyan, P. (2014). Applying metabolomics to understand the aggressive phenotype and identify novel therapeutic targets in glioblastoma. *Metabolites, 4*, 740–750.
89. St-Coeur, P. D., Touaibia, M., Cuperlovic-Culf, M., & Morin, P., Jr. (2013). Leveraging metabolomics to assess the next generation of temozolomide-based therapeutic approaches for glioblastomas. *Genomics, Proteomics & Bioinformatics, 11*, 199–206.

Metabolomics of Oral/Head and Neck Cancer

Gaofei Yin, Junwei Huang, Wei Guo, and Zhigang Huang

1 Introduction

1.1 Oral/Head and Neck Cancer

Oral/head and neck cancer is the sixth most common malignant tumors in the world. Statistical data have shown that the annual cost of treating oral and head and neck tumors in the United States amounts to $3.2 billion, and there are more than 500,000 new cases of oral/head and neck squamous cell carcinoma (OSCC/HNSCC) worldwide every year [1]. In the United States, 40,000 new cases and 7890 deaths are reported annually [2]. HNSCC may occur in the oral cavity, oropharynx, hypopharynx, larynx, nasopharynx, and other mucosal areas. Continuous exposure to tobacco, tobacco products, and alcohol stimulation is known to increase the risk of HNSCC. Over the past decade, with the steady increase of oropharyngeal squamous cell carcinoma (OPSCC), the incidence of laryngeal and hypopharyngeal cancer has declined, and the distribution of primary sites has changed. This change is associated with reduced smoking and alcohol consumption in the population and increased exposure to high-risk carcinogenic human papillomavirus (HPV) [3]. The clinical manifestations vary with the location of the disease. However, most of the HNSCC patients were diagnosed in advanced stages, and more than 40% of the patients had regional lymph node involvement [4]. This contributes to a high mortality rate for HNSCC, and the 5-year survival rate from diagnosis can be as high as 45%. Late-stage visits are mostly due to lack of national cancer screening program and public awareness. If early diagnosis and treatment intervention are implemented, the survival rate of HNSCC patients can reach 80–90% [5].

1.1.1 Symptoms

The most common signs and symptoms associated with oral/head and neck cancer are oral pain, nonunion of oral wounds, persistent pain, oral mass or plaque (white or red lesion), pain around teeth, hoarseness, foreign body sensation in pharynx, sore throat, and neck mass [6]. Because of the special location of oral/head and neck cancer, breathing, diet, speech, and appearance problems often occur. Monitoring these specific signs and symptoms can improve the accuracy of diagnosis and prognosis.

1.1.2 Diagnosis

For first-time visit patients, local endoscopy, and imaging of the corresponding sites are needed. Ultrasound is used to determine the extent of the lesion. The gold standard for the diagnosis of

G. Yin · J. Huang · W. Guo · Z. Huang (✉)
Department of Otolaryngology Head and Neck Surgery, Beijing Tongren Hospital, Key Laboratory of Otolaryngology Head and Neck Surgery, Ministry of Education, Capital Medical University, Beijing, China

S. Hu (ed.), *Cancer Metabolomics*, Advances in Experimental Medicine and Biology 1280,
https://doi.org/10.1007/978-3-030-51652-9_19

OSCC/HNSCC is still based on pathological biopsy, and pathology can determine the degree of tumor differentiation. Risk stratification of the disease is carried out according to the condition of auxiliary examination. Staging is important for the prognosis and treatment of OSCC/HNSCC. TNM staging remains to be the most widely used staging system in OSCC/HNSCC. Differentiation is another common component of diagnosis, because it describes the degree of abnormality between cancer and normal cells. X-ray technologies such as computed tomography (CT), magnetic resonance imaging (MRI), and positron emission tomography (PET) can be used to determine the location, size, and presence of suspected tumor masses and metastases. Laboratory tests can be performed on tissue biopsies and body fluids such as blood, saliva, and urine. Detection with specific tumor markers may help to provide cancer-specific information, which is the main focus of recent individualized diagnosis and treatment.

1.1.3 Treatment

At present, surgery, radiotherapy, chemotherapy, targeted therapy, and immunotherapy constitute a comprehensive treatment system for oral/head and neck tumors. According to the TNM stage and the degree of differentiation of the tumors, treatment options are selected. Early diseases (stage I and II) are usually treated only by surgery or radiotherapy. Locally advanced diseases (stage III and IVA/B), which make up more than 50% of all cases, can be treated with a combined preoperative induction chemotherapy and surgery, whereas metastatic diseases may be treated with targeted immunotherapy. The treatment of locally recurrent disease depends on the site of recurrence, tumor burden, and previous treatment and may include salvage surgery or adjuvant therapy. With the development of new treatment technology, tailored therapy has been gradually applied to treat head and neck cancer patients.

Local surgical treatment can be selected for early-stage patients. The primary lesion can be resected to obtain negative margin and preserve all or part of the organ function. Traditional open surgery or minimally invasive surgery, such as transoral robotic surgery (TOR) or laser surgery, is selected according to the anatomical structure and tumor location [7]. The experience of the surgeon should be considered, and the adjuvant treatment should be combined for the pathological condition. For the treatment of locally advanced diseases, radiotherapy (RT) is used as an adjuvant treatment of surgery or concurrent chemotherapy. According to the treatment time and adjuvant therapy, the radiation dose varies from 60 Gy to 70 Gy [8]. However, when the dose exceeded 55 Gy, the risk of long-term toxicity of radiotherapy to salivary glands and pharyngeal constrictors increased [9]. Recently, the application of intensity-modulated radiation therapy (IMRT) can help with salivary gland preservation, reduce dry mouth, and improve the quality of life of patients.

Chemotherapy is also the choice of treatment for advanced patients. In patients at advanced stages whose tumors are not resectable, induction chemotherapy can be used to control tumors, and patients with high risk of recurrence and metastasis can also benefit from chemotherapy. Meta-analysis of chemotherapy for head and neck cancer shows that the absolute benefit rate of chemotherapy for 2 years is 7%, and the absolute benefit rate for 5 years is 8%, and the risk ratio is 0.81 (95% CI, 0.76–0.88; $P < 0.0001$) [10]. Five years of long-term follow-up showed that OPSCC, patients under 65 years of age, and those receiving intensive radiation therapy at the same time were the main beneficiaries.

Targeted treatment has been mainly focused on mutated genes and related signal pathway genes in HNSCC. Based on comprehensive genomic characterization of somatic genomic alterations in HNSCC, HPV-associated tumors were dominated by helical domain mutations of the oncogene PIK3CA, novel alterations involving loss of TRAF3, and amplification of the cell cycle gene E2F1. Smoking-related HNSCCs demonstrated near universal loss-of-function TP53 mutations and CDKN2A inactivation with frequent copy number alterations. A subgroup of oral cavity tumors with favorable clinical outcomes displayed infrequent copy number alterations in conjunction with activating mutations of HRAS or PIK3CA, coupled with inactivating mutations of CASP8, NOTCH1, and TP53.

Laryngeal tumors contained loss-of-function alterations of the chromatin modifier NSD1, WNT pathway genes AJUBA and FAT1, and activation of oxidative stress factor NFE2L2 [11, 12]. The therapeutic effects of drugs targeting NOTCH1, HER2, MET, EGFR, and WNT/beta-catenin pathways were also studied [13]. So far, however, there is limited progress in targeted therapies for OSCC/HNSCC. The response rate of available single-dose targeted therapy ranges from 10% to 15%, and the clinical efficacy is not ideal [14]. Nevertheless, recent studies have shown immunotherapies are potentially effective for HNSCC treatment. Anti-PD1/PD-L1 agents may be combined with conventional therapeutics to improve treatment results [15].

1.2 Metabolomics

Metabolomics refers to large-scale, systemic study of small molecules, commonly known as metabolites, within cells, biofluids, tissues, or organisms. Collectively, these small molecules and their interactions within a biological system are known as the metabolome. The concept of metabolomics was defined 20 years ago by Nicholson and Fiehn et al. [16, 17]. Compared to genomics and proteomics, metabolomics has its own characteristics. The small changes of gene and protein expression are amplified at the level of metabolites, and the changes of metabolites may reflect the phenotype of an organism more directly than those alterations at gene/protein levels. From this point of view, the study of metabolomics may have higher sensitivity and accuracy when characterizing a phenotype [18, 19].

Metabolomic analysis in cancer research is usually performed on body fluids (e.g., plasma, serum, saliva, urine, ascites and bile, etc.), cultured cells, and tissues. Pretreatment of biological samples is a critical step in metabolomic analysis because the removal of impurities and interfering substances may significantly affect the identification and quantification of metabolites in the sample. Organic solvents such as methanol, acetonitrile, and chloroform are commonly used to extract metabolites from biological samples. In addition to the organic solvents, solid-phase microextraction (SPME) may be used for enrichment of metabolites from biological samples for metabolomic analysis [20].

Nuclear magnetic resonance (NMR) spectroscopy is a commonly used analytical technique for metabolomic analysis [21, 22]. Sample pretreatment for NMR is simple and the cost of analysis is low. However, NMR has relatively low sensitivity and narrow dynamic range, causing problem with metabolite quantification. High-resolution NMR may help solve the problem of low sensitivity. Somashekar et al. successfully distinguished normal and HNSCC tissues using high-resolution magic angle spinning nuclear magnetic resonance (HR-MAS NMR) spectroscopy [23].

Compared to NMR spectroscopy, mass spectrometry (MS) has higher sensitivity, and its resolving power can be improved by combining MS with separation techniques, such as gas chromatography (GC), liquid chromatography (LC), and capillary electrophoresis (CE) [24]. GC-MS is suitable for the separation and identification of volatile compounds, while LC-MS fits for the analysis of low volatile or nonvolatile metabolites. CE-MS, on the other hand, can be effective for analysis of polar or ionic compounds [25]. The method has the advantages of small sample volume, fast speed, low mass detection limit, and high-resolution separation. Busch et al. cross-compared GC-MS, LC-MS, and CE-MS platforms for metabolomic analysis. Using 91 known metabolites covering glycolysis, pentose phosphate pathway, the tricarboxylic acid (TCA) cycle, redox metabolism, amino acids, and nucleotides to test the three different platforms, they found that LC-MS offers a better performance for metabolomic analysis than other single platforms because it is suitable for all strong polar, weak polar, and nonpolar compounds. LC-MS provides the best combination of both versatility and robustness, and if a second platform can be used, it is best complemented by GC-MS. They also suggested that internal standards, such as 13C-labeled biomass extracts, are mandatory for quantitative metabolomics with any methods [26].

Data analysis represents a critical component in metabolomics. An integrated data analysis process may include a number of steps, such as data denoising and processing, peak alignment, metabolite identification (database searching), data normalization, metabolite quantification, classification and discriminant analysis, pathway analysis, and ultimately linking to biological significance. Both identified metabolites (known identities) and unknown metabolic features can be used for classification of phenotypes. A core technology for such analysis is pattern recognition tools, including unsupervised learning methods such as principal component analysis (PCA), nonlinear mapping, cluster analysis, and supervised learning methods such as independent modeling classification, partial least squares, and artificial neural network.

1.3 Application of Metabolomics in Cancer Research

Understanding cancer metabolism requires systematic application of MS or NMR-based analytical techniques for a comprehensive analysis of metabolites in biological samples from healthy and diseased tissues. Metabolomics has emerged as a powerful platform to assess metabolomic anomalies in cancer cells or body fluid samples (e.g., serum, urine, or saliva) of patients. Currently, metabolomics is being used to discover metabolite biomarkers that may aid in patients' diagnosis or prognosis in the clinic, to better understand the complex mechanisms underlying metabolic reprogramming in cancer cells, and to discover novel metabolic pathways and target genes involved in carcinogenesis or cancer progression that could be used for therapeutic interventions. Applications of metabolomics are also emerging in areas such as tumor staging and assessment of treatment efficacy [27].

2 Body Fluid Metabolomics in OSCC/HNSCC

2.1 Saliva Metabolomics

Saliva is a complex body fluid secreted by parotid, submandibular, sublingual, and minor glands. It is a clear, slightly acidic (pH 6.0–7.0) liquid composed of water (99%), protein (0.3%), inorganic (0.2%), and organic compounds. The most abundant proteins in saliva include amylase, cystatin, lactoferrin, mucin, lysozyme, transferrin, and various secretarial immunoglobulins. Sodium, potassium, calcium, magnesium, and chlorides, as well as carbonates and bicarbonates, are the most common inorganic substances in saliva, whereas organic compounds mainly include metabolites, hormones, and growth factors (e.g., epidermal growth factor and vascular endothelial growth factor) [28–31]. Human saliva is an attractive body fluid for disease diagnosis and prognosis because saliva testing is simple, safe, low cost, and noninvasive [28, 29]. Salivary protein biomarkers have been demonstrated for detection of multiple human diseases including oral cancer, Sjögren's syndrome, systemic lupus erythematosus (SLE), and burning mouth syndrome (BMS) [32–37]. Recently, salivary metabolite biomarkers have been developed for gout, a metabolic disease, using a metabolomic approach based on capillary ion chromatography with mass spectrometry. A panel of three metabolite biomarkers, uric acid, oxalic acid, and l-homocysteic acid, were successfully validated among gout and hyperuricemia patients with enzymatic assays and may have potential applications in the disease diagnosis and prognosis [38]. Another reason for salivary diagnostics is that there is efficient substance exchange between saliva and circulation system by active transport and active or passive diffusion. Circulation biomarkers may be well present in saliva for disease diagnosis and prognosis. In addition, the protein levels in saliva are lower than those in plasma or serum, and the possibility of nonspecific interference for metabolite analysis is much lower. Saliva metabolomic analysis may be effective to develop metabolite biomarkers for local diseases such as oral/head and neck cancer, Sjögren's syndrome, and BMS or even systemic conditions such as lung/gastric cancers, metabolic diseases (e.g., gout and diabetes), and autoimmune diseases (e.g., rheumatoid arthritis and SLE).

Sample collection and processing are important aspects of saliva metabolomic analysis. Saliva can be collected in different ways as needed. For example, unstimulated saliva is usually collected by passive flow to calibration tubes or pre-weighed vials to measure the flow rate per unit time. When volumetric measurements are not required, saliva may be collected with cotton swabs, gauze, or filter strips and then washed, centrifuged, or sucked directly from the mouth with a plastic suction tube. When large amounts of saliva are needed for analysis, stimulated saliva can be collected for metabolomic analysis. These aspects may directly or indirectly interfere with data quality and ultimately biological interpretation. Samples should be collected as soon as possible and stored in deep freezer (80 °C). If possible, the freezing and thawing cycles should be minimized.

In 2008, Yan et al. demonstrated that LC-MS profiles of salivary metabolites with hierarchical principal component analysis (HPCA) could be used to build a diagnostic model to discriminate OSCC, oral lichen planus (OLP), and oral leukoplakia (OLK). HPCA combined with kernel fisher discriminant analysis achieved high accuracy in diagnosis of test samples, suggesting that salivary metabolomic profiles may be used for early detection of oral cancer and precancer [39]. Using CE-MS-based metabolomic analysis of saliva samples from oral cancer patients, Sugimoto et al. identified a number of candidate metabolite biomarkers for oral cancer, including polyamine, ornithine, and putrescine. Potential metabolite biomarkers were also found in whole saliva of patients with pancreatic or breast cancer [40]. Similar CE-MS-based metabolomic approach was also applied to investigate the effect of timing of sample collection on salivary metabolite biomarker discovery [41], identify a set of 17 potential salivary metabolite biomarkers for OSCC screening [42], and develop a set of 25 potential salivary biomarkers for Japanese OSCC patients, including choline, p-hydroxyphenylacetic acid, and 2-hydroxy-4-methylvaleric acid ($P < 0.001$); valine, 3-phenyllactic acid, leucine, hexanoic acid, octanoic acid, terephthalic acid, γ-butyrobetaine, and 3-(4-hydroxyphenyl)propionic acid ($P < 0.01$); and isoleucine, tryptophan, 3-phenylpropionic acid, 2-hydroxyvaleric acid, butyric acid, cadaverine, 2-oxoisovaleric acid, N6,N6,N6-trimethyllysine, taurine, glycolic acid, 3-hydroxybutyric acid, heptanoic acid, alanine, and urea [43]. Wei et al. profiled the salivary metabolites from 37 OSCC patients, 32 OLK patients, and 34 healthy subjects using UPLC with quadrupole/time-of-flight mass spectrometry (qTOF MS). A panel of five salivary metabolites including γ-aminobutyric acid, phenylalanine, valine, n-eicosanoic acid, and lactic acid were selected to build prediction models, and valine, lactic acid, and phenylalanine in combination yielded satisfactory sensitivity, specificity, and positive predictive value in distinguishing OSCC from the controls or OLK [44]. Wang et al. adopted an integrated separation approach of RPLC and hydrophilic interaction chromatography combined with TOF MS for saliva metabolomic analysis. Using this approach, they identified 14 (eight upregulated and six downregulated) potential salivary metabolite biomarkers for OSCC. Receiver operating characteristic (ROC) analysis indicated that five salivary biomarkers (propionylcholine, N-acetyl-L-phenylalanine, sphinganine, phytosphingosine, and S-carboxymethyl-L-cysteine) in combination yielded high accuracy, sensitivity, and specificity in distinguishing early stage of OSCC from the control [45]. Using NMR and LC-MS/MS-based metabolomic analyses of 159 OSCCs and 35 normal controls, Lohavanichbutr et al. discovered four metabolites, glycine, proline, citrulline, and ornithine, were associated with early-stage OCC in both discovery and validation sets [46]. Shigeyama et al. demonstrated zeolite-based thin-film microextraction coupled with GC-MS for profiling of volatile organic compounds (VOCs) in human saliva samples of OSCC patients and found 27 VOCs depicted significant differences between OSCC and healthy control groups. Among them, 12 salivary VOCs that were characteristic of OSCC patients were identified for pattern recognition analyses to detect oral cancer [47]. In addition, NMR spectroscopy has been used to identify significantly altered saliva metabolites in patients with HNSCC or parotid gland tumors [48, 49]. Finally, saliva metabolomic analysis has been applied to discovery of salivary metabolite biomarkers for breast and pancreatic cancers [50–53]. Particularly, the CE-MS-based metabolomic analysis revealed elevated levels of polyamines such as spermine, N_1-acetylspermidine, and N_1-acetylspermine in the saliva samples of pancreatic cancer patients. The combination of four metabolites including N_1-acetylspermidine showed high accuracy in discriminating pancreatic cancer from chronic pancreatitis and healthy control [53].

2.2 Serum Metabolomics

Serum metabolomics has been applied to the discovery of signature metabolite biomarkers for clinical applications in OSCC/HNSCC. NMR-based metabolomic analysis showed that the patients with OSCC had a distinct signature of altered energy metabolism in blood serum, including altered lipolysis (an accumulation of ketone bodies), a distorted Krebs cycle, and amino acid catabolism [54], as well as abnormal choline metabolism (downregulation of choline with concomitant upregulation of its breakdown product in the form of trimethylamine N-oxide) [55]. Similar approach was used to identify four biomarkers (glutamine, propionate, acetone, and choline) to differentiate OSCCs from healthy controls and four biomarkers (glutamine, acetone, acetate, and choline) to discriminate OLK cases from OSCCs with considerable sensitivity and specificity [56], as well as metabolite signatures (lipid metabolism, amino acid metabolism, glycolysis, ketogenesis, TCA cycle, and energy metabolism) for esophageal squamous cell carcinoma (ESCC) [57, 58] and thyroid disease [59]. Recently, NMR-based metabolomic analysis followed by PCA and partial least squares discriminate analysis (PLS-DA) was used to compare the serum metabolomic alterations after two different surgeries in the patients with papillary thyroid carcinoma (PTC). Compared to unilateral thyroidectomy, total thyroidectomy reversed some highly increased metabolite levels (e.g., taurine and betaine). More significant variations in abnormal metabolites were noted after total thyroidectomy than after unilateral thyroidectomy (e.g., alanine, choline, hippurate, and formic acid). This information suggests that the choice of surgical method for PTC patients should be based not only on the tumor condition but also on the potential consequences of metabolic variations. Total thyroidectomy reversed some increased metabolite levels but led to accumulation of some other metabolites due to the loss of thyroid function; thus, metabolic disturbances caused by thyroid hormone deficiency should be prevented in advance [60]. Serum metabolomic analysis has also been demonstrated for real-time monitoring of treatment-induced toxicity and cachexia in HNSCC patients and serve as a method for early detection of high-risk patients. By using NMR-based metabolomic analysis of 170 HNSCC patients undergoing radio-/chemoradiotherapy (RT/CHRT) followed by PCA and orthogonal partial least squares discriminant analysis (OPLS-DA), Boguszewicz et al. detected a group of distinct outliers corresponding to ketone bodies (3-hydroxybutyrate, acetone, and acetoacetate), which are useful to identify the individuals at high risk of weight loss. Particularly, 3-hydroxybutyrate is a relatively sensitive marker that allows earlier identification of the patients at higher risk of $> 10\%$ weight loss. These findings indicate that metabolic alterations, characteristic for malnutrition or cachexia, can be detected at the beginning of the treatment, making it possible to monitor the patients with a higher risk of weight loss [61].

MS-based serum metabolomic analysis has been used to discover potential metabolite biomarkers, including 1-palmitoyl-sn-glycero-3-phosphocholine, 1-o-hexadecyl-2-acetyl-sn-glycero-3-phosphocholine, and 12-dipalmitoyl-sn-glycero-3-phosphocholine, for laryngeal cancer. These metabolites are mainly involved in phospholipids catabolism, linoleic acid metabolism, α-linoleic acid metabolism, and arachidonic acid metabolism [62]. Significant upregulation of estradiol-17-beta-3-sulfate, L-carnitine, 5-methylthioadenosine (MTA), 8-hydroxyadenine, 2-methylcitric acid, putrescine, and estrone-3-sulfate was found in OLKs and OSCCs versus normal controls, whereas significant upregulation of 5,6-dihydrouridine, 4-hydroxypenbutolol glucuronide, 8-hydroxyadenine, and putrescine was evident in OSCCs versus OLKs [63]. A total of 37 serum metabolite signatures were discovered by using GC-TOF MS with PCA and OPLS-DA analyses for distant metastasis in

PTC. These potential biomarkers are related to amino acid, lipid, glucose, vitamin metabolism, and diet/gut microbiota interaction. Pathway analysis showed "alanine, aspartate and glutamate metabolism" and "inositol phosphate metabolism" were the most relevant pathways [64]. Lastly, serum metabolomic analysis has revealed significantly altered phosphatidylcholine metabolism in ESCC [65] and led to the discovery of prognostic biomarker, d-mannose, in esophageal adenocarcinoma [66], as well as potential metabolite biomarkers, including valine, γ-aminobutyric acid, and pyrrole-2-carboxylic acid, for lymph node metastasis in ESCC [67].

2.3 Urine Metabolomics

Urine metabolomic analysis has led to potential metabolite biomarkers, including d-pantothenic acid, palmitic acid, myristic acid, oleamide, sphinganine, and phytosphingosine, for laryngeal cancer. These metabolites may play roles in sphingolipid metabolism, fatty acid biosynthesis, fatty acid elongation in mitochondria, pantothenate and coenzyme A biosynthesis, beta-alanine metabolism, and fatty acid metabolism and, as a combination, reached a high ROC value, sensitivity, and specificity to distinguish laryngeal cancer from healthy controls [68]. Urinary metabolomic analysis has also been used to identify potential metabolite biomarkers for thyroid diseases [59] and ESCC [69]. The results showed that ESCC patients had altered acylcarnitines, amino acids, nucleosides, and steroid derivative levels when compared to healthy controls.

Standardized protocols are critical to generate highly robust and reproducible metabolomics data for cancer metabolite biomarker discovery. Previous reports have detailed the procedures for large-scale metabolic profiling of serum and plasma samples using GC-MS or LC-MS [70], global urinary metabolomic analysis with GC-MS or LC-MS [71, 72], and NMR-based metabolomic profiling of urine, plasma, serum, and tissue extracts [73]. These well-prepared protocols may allow a meaningful comparison and cross-validation of metabolomic analysis results and metabolite biomarker discovery/validation among different research laboratories.

3 Metabolomic Analysis of OSCC/HNSCC Cell Lines and Tissues

A new platform coupling capillary ion chromatography (CIC) with Orbitrap MS has been demonstrated for metabolomic analysis of HNSCC cells. CIC allowed an excellent separation of anionic polar metabolites, including isomeric metabolites, and the sensitivities increased by up to 100-fold compared to RPLC. The detection limits for a panel of standard metabolites were between 0.04 and 0.5 nmol/L (0.2–3.4 fmol). This platform was applied to differential metabolomic analysis of highly and low invasive HNSCC cells as well as cancer stem cells (CSCs) and non-stem cancer cells (non-CSCs); a single metabolomic analysis could quantify more than 4000 metabolites [74]. Using similar platform combined with stable isotope-labeled internal standards, Hu et al. demonstrated a targeted metabolomics approach to quantitative analysis of metabolites in a specific metabolic pathway in HNSCC cells. This methodology acquires both targeted and global metabolomic data in a same analytical run, and the use of stable isotope-labeled standards facilitates accurate quantitation of targeted metabolites in large-scale metabolomics analysis. Their findings suggest that the metabolic phenotypes are distinct between high and low invasive head and neck cancer cells and between CSCs and non-SCCs [75].

By using a lipidomic approach, Zhao et al. revealed a consistent elevation of glycosphingolipids and particularly the accumulation of gangliosides in HNSCC cells. Repression of this same class of lipids was observed upon genetic correction of fanconi anemia (FA) patient-derived HNSCC cells. Functional studies demonstrated that ganglioside upregulation was required for HNSCC cell invasion driven by FA pathway loss and inhibition of glycosphingolipid biosynthesis attenuated the invasive characteristics of

FA-deficient HNSCC cells [76]. Tan et al. conducted a combined metabolomic/proteomic study and demonstrated that fatty acid oxidation (FAO) was active in radiation-resistant nasopharyngeal cancer (NPC) cells, and the rate-limiting enzyme of FAO, carnitine palmitoyl transferase 1 A (CPT1A), was consistently upregulated in these cells. The protein level of CPT1A was significantly associated with poor overall survival of NPC patients following radiotherapy, and inhibition of CPT1A re-sensitized NPC cells to radiation therapy by activating mitochondrial apoptosis both in vitro and in vivo. These findings suggest that targeting CPT1A could be a beneficial approach to improving the therapeutic effects of radiotherapy in NPC patients [77]. Cystine-glutamate antiporter (xCT) present in CD44 variant (CD44v)-expressing cancer cells contributes to the resistance to oxidative stress and cancer therapy through promoting glutathione (GSH)-mediated antioxidant defense. xCT and glutamine transporter ASCT2 were found to be correlated with undifferentiation and diminished along with cell differentiation in HNSCC. The cytotoxicity of the xCT inhibitor sulfasalazine relied on ASCT2-dependent glutamine uptake and glutamate dehydrogenase (GLUD)-mediated α-ketoglutarate (α-KG) production. Metabolome analysis revealed that sulfasalazine treatment triggered the increase of glutamate-derived tricarboxylic acid cycle intermediate α-KG, in addition to the decrease of cysteine and GSH content. Furthermore, ablation of GLUD markedly reduced the sulfasalazine cytotoxicity in CD44v-expressing stemlike HNSCC cells. These findings establish a rationale for the use of glutamine metabolism (glutaminolysis)-related genes, including ASCT2 and GLUD, as biomarkers to predict the efficacy of xCT-targeted therapy for HNSCC tumors [78]. Comparative metabolomic analysis of radiosensitive and radioresistant cell lines also led to interesting findings about the intracellular metabolisms. Both UM-SCC-74B and UM-SCC-74A were established from the same cancer patient. However, UM-SCC-74B is clearly more radioresistant than UM-SCC-74A. LC-MS-based metabolic profiling demonstrated significant differences in the nicotinic acid and nicotinamide metabolism and purine metabolism between the two cell lines before irradiation. In the more radiosensitive UM-SCC-74A cells, the most significant alterations after irradiation were linked to tryptophan metabolism. In the more radioresistant UM-SCC-74B cells, the major alterations after irradiation were connected to nicotinic acid and nicotinamide metabolism, purine metabolism, the methionine cycle as well as the serine, and glycine metabolism. The data suggest that the more radioresistant cell line UM-SCC-74B altered the metabolism to control redox status, manage DNA-repair, and change DNA methylation after irradiation. This provides new insights on the mechanisms of radiation response, which may aid future identification of biomarkers associated with radioresistance of HNSCC cells [79].

Sandulache et al. investigated glucose and glutamine dependence and sensitivity to metabolic inhibitors of a panel of 15 HNSCC cell lines and used LC-MS-based metabolomic analysis combined with individual measurements of reducing potential, adenosine triphosphate, and lactate production to characterize cellular metabolic phenotypes. Their results indicated that HNSCC energy and reducing potential levels closely mirrored extracellular glucose concentrations. Glucose starvation induced cell death despite the activation of secondary energetic pathways. Conversely, glutamine was not required for HNSCC survival and did not serve as a significant source of energy. 2-Deoxyglucose (2-DG) and its fluorinated derivative decreased glycolytic and Krebs cycle activity, cellular energy, and reducing potential and inhibited HNSCC cell proliferation. 2-DG effects were potentiated by the addition of metformin, but not by inhibitors of the pentose phosphate pathway or glutaminolysis. Despite dependence on glucose catabolism, the authors identified a subset of cell lines with relative resistance to starvation and found that the presence of wild-type p53 can partially protect tumor cells from glucose starvation. Based on these findings, they concluded that HNSC cells are dependent on glucose, not glutamine, for energy production and survival, providing a rationale for treatment strategies that target glucose catabolism. However, antimetabolic strategies may need to be tailored to the tumor background, more specifically, p53 status [80].

In addition, metabolome analysis showed that nuclear factor erythroid 2-related factor 2 (Nrf2) strongly promoted metabolic reprogramming to glutathione metabolism, which synthesizes the essential fuels for cancer progression in ESCC. Furthermore, metabolome analysis of ESCC tissue specimens confirmed that samples displaying high Nrf2 expression promoted glutathione synthesis. Metabolic reprogramming to glutathione metabolism, and ROS detoxification by activation of Nrf2, enhanced cancer progression and led to a poor clinical outcome in ESCC patients [81]. In addition, hyperactive Nrf2 was found to cause metabolic reprogramming and upregulation of metabolic genes in the mouse esophagus. One of the glycolytic enzymes pyruvate kinase M2 was not only differentially upregulated, but also glycosylated and oligomerized, resulting in increased ATP biosynthesis. Blocking glycolysis inhibited cell proliferation and may therefore have therapeutically beneficial effects on Nrf2-expressing ESCC in humans [82]. Recently, a spatially resolved metabolomics approach was demonstrated to discover tumor-associated metabolites and metabolic enzymes directly in their native state in ESCC tissues by using airflow-assisted desorption electrospray ionization mass spectrometry imaging (AFADESI-MSI). This in situ metabolomics analysis provided insights into the understanding of ESCC metabolic reprogramming, particularly the ESCC-associated metabolic pathways, including proline biosynthesis, glutamine metabolism, uridine metabolism, histidine metabolism, fatty acid biosynthesis, and polyamine biosynthesis [83].

A main application of tissue metabolomic analysis is to discover metabolite biomarkers for oral/head and neck cancer. Since thyroid gland produces hormones that control the speed of body metabolism, there has been a growing interest in metabolomics studies of PTC. A number of studies have reported new signature metabolites in PTC, which include acetate, taurine, and succinic acid (upregulated in malignant versus benign tumor); choline, phosphocholine, myo-inositol, and scyllo-inositol (downregulated in malignant versus benign tumor); citrate, glucose, fructose, galactose, mannose, 2-keto-D-gluconic acid, arachidonic acid, malonic acid, and rhamnose (downregulated in PTC versus normal thyroid tissue); and lactic acid, inosine, cholesterol, and hydroxyproline (upregulated in PTC versus normal thyroid tissues) [84–90]. However, a recent metabolomic study of 1540 serum-plasma matched samples and 114 tissues from healthy volunteers, benign thyroid nodule (BTN), and PTC patients enrolled from six independent centers concluded that BTN and PTC showed no significant differences but rather overlap in circulating metabolic signatures. Six metabolite biomarkers, namely, myo-inositol, α-N-phenylacetyl-L-glutamine, proline betaine, L-glutamic acid, LysoPC(18:0), and LysoPC(18:1), were highly accurate for differential diagnosis of healthy controls versus thyroid nodules (BTN + PTC) [91]. Nevertheless, these published studies revealed abnormalities of energy metabolism (glycolysis, lipid, and TCA cycle), nucleotide/phosphatidylcholine biosynthesis, amino acid metabolism, one carbon metabolism and tryptophan metabolism, purine/pyrimidine metabolism, and taurine/hypotaurine metabolism [87, 89].

CE-MS analysis of OSCC and adjacent normal tissues for the metabolome profiles, including the Embden-Meyerhof-Parnas pathway (EMPP), the pentose phosphate pathway, TCA cycle, and amino acids, revealed an increased glucose consumption and lactate production in OSCC tissues. The decrease of glucose along with the decrease of the downstream intermediates in the EMPP implied that incorporated glucose was mainly consumed for biosynthesis. Glutamine consumption with the increase of the intermediates in the last half of the TCA indicated the involvement of glutaminolysis, in which glutamine was converted to lactate via the last half of the TCA. These observations suggest that the Warburg effect, which stems from the combined enhancement of glucose consumption and glutaminolysis, exists in OSCC [92]. A combined LC-MS and GC-MS analysis of HNSCC and adjacent normal tissues revealed a set of upregulated metabolites, including 2-hydroxyglutarate (2-HG) and 3-GMP in HNSCCs. Meanwhile, metabolomic analysis of the oral washes from HNSCC patients (presurgical) and healthy controls identified elevated levels of beta-alanine, alpha-hydroxyisovalerate, tryptophan, and hexanoylcarnitine in HNSCCs (range 7.8–12.2-fold). Among the identified metabolite signatures, acylcarnitine and 2HG may have potential as noninvasive biomarkers for HNSCC [93]. Similarly, a GC-MS analysis of preneoplastic and neoplastic lesions of oral cavity revealed a number of metabolite signatures that could distinguish among oral cancer, precancerous, and control group samples. The aminoacyl-tRNA biosynthesis, cyanoamino acid metabolism, and glycine, serine, and threonine biosynthesis were significantly dysregulated pathways found in oral cancer and precancer. Downregulated amino acid levels might be the result of enhanced energy metabolism or upregulation of the appropriate biosynthetic pathways and required cell proliferation in cancer tissues [94].

Although it is well known that cancer cells use alternate energetic pathways, the metabolic pathways underlying the energy production in CSCs remain largely unknown. Kamarajan et al. characterized the metabolic characteristics of HNSCC and head and neck CSCs using a combination of UPLC-MS/MS, GC-MS, and in vitro/in vivo models [95]. They identified metabolite biomarker panels that distinguish head and neck cancer from healthy controls and confirmed involvement of glutamate and glutaminolysis. Glutaminase, which catalyzes glutamate formation from glutamine, and aldehyde dehydrogenase (ALDH), a stemness marker, were highly expressed in primary and metastatic HNSCC tissues, tumorspheres, and CSC when compared to controls. Exogenous glutamine induced stemness via glutaminase, whereas inhibiting glutaminase suppressed stemness in vitro and tumorigenesis in vivo. It was found head and neck CSC (CD44(hi)/ALDH(hi)) exhibited higher glutaminase, glutamate, and sphere levels than CD44(lo)/ALDH(lo) cells. Glutaminase drove transcriptional and translational ALDH expression, and glutamine could direct CD44(lo)/ALDH(lo) cells toward stemness. These findings suggest that glutaminolysis regulates tumorigenesis and CSC metabolism via ALDH, and glutamate is an important biomarker of cancer metabolism whose regulation via glutaminase works in concert with ALDH to mediate cancer stemness [95].

4 Conclusion

Despite the rapid advancement of MS- and NMR-based metabolomics technologies, the metabolomics studies of oral/head and neck cancer remain in its infancy. Although metabolomic analyses of body fluid and tissue samples from OSCC/HNSCC patients have identified many potential metabolite biomarkers, there seem to be contradicting results in the published studies and the identified metabolite biomarkers are certainly warranted for further validation with large patient populations. The metabolic mechanisms underlying the cancer cell proliferation, invasion and metastasis, sustained angiogenesis, and evasion of apoptosis in OSCC/HNSCC remain largely unknown. Metabolomics can facilitate our understanding the metabolic reprogramming and associated metabolic pathways during HNSCC/OSCC carcinogenesis and progression. It will not only lead to the discovery of highly sensitive and specific metabolite biomarkers for clinical applications (e.g., early diagnosis, prognosis, and treatment efficacy), but may also reveal metabolic target genes for therapeutic interventions in oral/head and neck cancer.

Acknowledgments The authors thank for the financial support from the National Natural Science Foundation of China (81670946).

References

1. Torre, L. A., et al. (2012). Global cancer statistics, 2012. *CA: A Cancer Journal for Clinicians, 65*(2), 87–108.
2. Siegel, R. L., Miller, K. D., & Jemal, A. (2015). Cancer statistics, 2015. *CA: A Cancer Journal for Clinicians, 65*(1), 5–29.
3. Gillison, M. L., Broutian, T., Pickard, R. K., et al. (2012). Prevalence of oral HPV infection in the

United States, 2009–2010. *Journal of the American Medical Association, 307*(7), 693–703.

4. Marur, S., & Forastiere, A. A. (2008). Head and neck cancer: Changing epidemiology, diagnosis, and treatment. *Mayo Clinic Proceedings, 83*(4), 489–501.
5. Tiziani, S., Lopes, V., & Gunther, U. L. (2009). Early stage diagnosis of oral cancer using 1H NMR-based metabolomics. *Neoplasia, 11*(3), 269–276.
6. Ahlberg, A., Engström, T., Nikolaidis, P., et al. (2011). Early self-care rehabilitation of head and neck cancer patients. *Acta Oto-Laryngologica, 131*(5), 552–561.
7. Kofler, B., Laban, S., Busch, C. J., Lörincz, B., & Knecht, R. (2014). New treatment strategies for HPV-positive head and neck cancer. *European Archives of Oto-Rhino-Laryngology, 271*(7), 1861–1867.
8. Pfister, D. G., Ang, K. K., Brizel, D. M., et al. (2013). National Comprehensive Cancer Network. Head and neck cancers, version 2.2013: Featured updates to the NCCN guidelines. *Journal of the National Comprehensive Cancer Network, 11*(8), 917–923.
9. Langendijk, J. A., Doornaert, P., Verdonck-de Leeuw, I. M., Leemans, C. R., Aaronson, N. K., & Slotman, B. J. (2008). Impact of late treatment-related toxicity on quality of life among patients with head and neck cancer treated with radiotherapy. *Journal of Clinical Oncology, 26*(22), 3770–3776.
10. Pignon, J. P., Bourhis, J., Domenge, C., Designé, L., & MACH-NC Collaborative Group. (2000). Chemotherapy added to locoregional treatment for head and neck squamous-cell carcinoma: Three meta-analyses of updated individual data. *Lancet, 355*(9208), 949–955.
11. Cancer Genome Atlas Network. (2015). Comprehensive genomic characterization of head and neck squamous cell carcinomas. *Nature, 517*(7536), 576–582.
12. Lechner, M., Frampton, G. M., Fenton, T., et al. (2013). Targeted next-generation sequencing of head and neck squamous cell carcinoma identifies novel genetic alterations in HPV+ and HPV− tumors. *Genome Medicine, 5*(5), 49.
13. Burtness, B., Bauman, J. E., & Galloway, T. (2013). Novel targets in HPV-negative head and neck cancer: Overcoming resistance to EGFR inhibition. *The Lancet Oncology, 14*(8), e302–e309.
14. Cohen, E. E., Kane, M. A., List, M. A., et al. (2005). Phase II trial of gefitinib 250 mg daily in patients with recurrent and/or metastatic squamous cell carcinoma of the head and neck. *Clinical Cancer Research, 11*(23), 8418–8424.
15. Alfieri, S., Cavalieri, S., & Licitra, L. (2018). Immunotherapy for recurrent/metastatic head and neck cancer. *Current Opinion in Otolaryngology & Head and Neck Surgery, 26*(2), 152–156.
16. Nicholson, J. K., Lindon, J. C., & Holmes, E. (1999). Metabonomics: Understanding the metabolic responses of living systems to pathophysiological stimuli via multivariate statistical analysis of biological NMR spectroscopic data. *Xenobiotica, 29*(11), 1181–1189.
17. Fiehn, O. (2001). Combining genomics, metabolome analysis, and biochemical modelling to understand metabolic networks. *Comparative and Functional Genomics, 2*(3), 155–168.
18. Taylor, J., King, R. D., Altmann, T., & Fiehn, O. (2002). Application of metabolomics to plant genotype discrimination using statistics and machine learning. *Bioinformatics, 18*(Suppl 2), S241–S248.
19. Nicholson, J. K., Connelly, J., Lindon, J. C., & Holmes, E. (2002). Metabolomics: A platform for studying drug toxicity and gene function. *Nature Reviews Drug Discovery, 1*(2), 153–161.
20. Chetwynd, A. J., Abdul-Sada, A., & Hill, E. M. (2015). Solid-phase extraction and nanoflow liquid chromatography-nanoelectrospray ionization mass spectrometry for improved global urine metabolomics. *Analytical Chemistry, 87*(2), 1158–1165.
21. Dunn, W. B., Bailey, N. J., & Johnson, H. E. (2005). Measuring the metabolome: Current analytical technologies. *The Analyst, 130*(5), 606–625.
22. O'Connell, T. M. (2012). Recent advances in metabolomics in oncology. *Bioanalysis, 4*(4), 431–451.
23. Somashekar, B. S., Kamarajan, P., Danciu, T., Kapila, Y. L., Chinnaiyan, A. M., Rajendiran, T. M., & Ramamoorthy, A. (2011). Magic angle spinning NMR-based metabolic profiling of head and neck squamous cell carcinoma tissues. *Journal of Proteome Research, 10*(11), 5232–5241.
24. Drexler, D. M., Reily, M. D., & Shipkova, P. A. (2011). Advances in mass spectrometry applied to pharmaceutical metabolomics. *Analytical and Bioanalytical Chemistry, 399*(8), 2645–2653.
25. Asiago, V. M., Alvarado, L. Z., Shanaiah, N., et al. (2010). Early detection of recurrent breast cancer using metabolite profiling. *Cancer Research, 70*(21), 8309–8318.
26. Büscher, J. M., Czernik, D., Ewald, J. C., Sauer, U., & Zamboni, N. (2009). Cross-platform comparison of methods for quantitative metabolomics of primary metabolism. *Analytical Chemistry, 81*(6), 2135–2143.
27. Kaushik, A. K., & DeBerardinis, R. J. (2018). Applications of metabolomics to study cancer metabolism. *Biochimica Et Biophysica Acta. Reviews on Cancer, 1870*(1), 2–14.
28. Hu, S., Loo, J. A., & Wong, D. T. (2006). Human body fluid proteome analysis. *Proteomics, 6*(23), 6326–6353.
29. Hu, S., Loo, J. A., & Wong, D. T. (2007). Human saliva proteome analysis and disease biomarker discovery. *Expert Review of Proteomics, 4*(4), 531–538.
30. Aps, J. K., & Martens, L. C. (2005). Review: The physiology of saliva and transfer of drugs into saliva. *Forensic Science International, 150*, 119–131.
31. Soini, H. A., Klouckova, I., Wiesler, D., Oberzaucher, E., Grammer, K., Dixon, S. J., et al. (2010). Analysis of volatile organic compounds in human saliva by a static sorptive extraction method and gas chromatography-mass spectrometry. *Journal of Chemical Ecology, 36*, 1035–1042.

32. Cui, L., Zhao, X., & Hu, S. (2019). Determination of autoantibodies to salivary gland antigens. *Methods in Molecular Biology, 1901*, 103–112.
33. Ji, E. H., Diep, C., Liu, T., et al. (2017). Potential protein biomarkers for burning mouth syndrome discovered by quantitative proteomics. *Molecular Pain, 13*, 1744806916686796.
34. Hu, S., Vissink, A., Arellano, M., et al. (2011). Identification of autoantibody biomarkers for primary Sjögren's syndrome using protein microarrays. *Proteomics, 11*(8), 1499–1507.
35. Hu, S., Gao, K., Pollard, R., et al. (2010). Preclinical validation of salivary biomarkers for primary Sjögren's syndrome. *Arthritis Care Res (Hoboken), 62*(11), 1633–1638.
36. Hu, S., Wang, J., Meijer, J., et al. (2007). Salivary proteomic and genomic biomarkers for primary Sjögren's syndrome. *Arthritis and Rheumatism, 56*(11), 3588–3600.
37. Hu, S., Arellano, M., Boontheung, P., et al. (2008). Salivary proteomics for oral cancer biomarker discovery. *Clinical Cancer Research, 14*(19), 6246–6252.
38. Cui, L., Liu, J., Yan, X., & Hu, S. (2017). Identification of metabolite biomarkers for gout using capillary ion chromatography with mass spectrometry. *Analytical Chemistry, 89*(21), 11737–11743.
39. Yan, S. K., Wei, B. J., Lin, Z. Y., et al. (2008). A metabonomic approach to the diagnosis of oral squamous cell carcinoma, oral lichen planus and oral leukoplakia. *Oral Oncology, 44*(5), 477–483.
40. Sugimoto, M., Wong, D. T., Hirayama, A., et al. (2010). Capillary electrophoresis mass spectrometry – based saliva metabolomics identified oral, breast and pancreatic cancer – specific profiles. *Metabolomics, 6*(1), 78–95.
41. Ishikawa, S., Sugimoto, M., Kitabatake, K., et al. (2017). Effect of timing of collection of salivary metabolomic biomarkers on oral cancer detection. *Amino Acids, 49*(4), 761–770.
42. Ishikawa, S., Sugimoto, M., Kitabatake, K., et al. (2016). Identification of salivary metabolomic biomarkers for oral cancer screening. *Scientific Reports, 6*, 31520.
43. Ohshima, M., Sugahara, K., Kasahara, K., & Katakura, A. (2017). Metabolomic analysis of the saliva of Japanese patients with oral squamous cell carcinoma. *Oncology Reports, 37*(5), 2727–2734.
44. Wei, J., Xie, G., Zhou, Z., et al. (2011). Salivary metabolite signatures of oral cancer and leukoplakia. *International Journal of Cancer, 129*(9), 2207–2217.
45. Wang, Q., Gao, P., Wang, X., & Duan, Y. (2014). The early diagnosis and monitoring of squamous cell carcinoma via saliva metabolomics. *Scientific Reports, 4*, 6802.
46. Lohavanichbutr, P., Zhang, Y., Wang, P., et al. (2018). Salivary metabolite profiling distinguishes patients with oral cavity squamous cell carcinoma from normal controls. *PLoS One, 13*(9), e0204249.
47. Shigeyama, H., Wang, T., Ichinose, M., Ansai, T., & Lee, S. W. (2019). Identification of volatile metabolites in human saliva from patients with oral squamous cell carcinoma via zeolite-based thin-film microextraction coupled with GC-MS. *Journal of Chromatography. B. Analytical Technologies in the Biomedical and Life Sciences, 1104*, 49–58.
48. Mikkonen, J. J. W., Singh, S. P., Akhi, R., et al. (2018). Potential role of nuclear magnetic resonance spectroscopy to identify salivary metabolite alterations in patients with head and neck cancer. *Oncology Letters, 16*(5), 6795–6800.
49. Grimaldi, M., Palisi, A., Rossi, G., et al. (2018). Saliva of patients affected by salivary gland tumour: An NMR metabolomics analysis. *Journal of Pharmaceutical and Biomedical Analysis, 160*, 436–442.
50. Zhong, L., Cheng, F., Lu, X., Duan, Y., & Wang, X. (2016). Untargeted saliva metabonomics study of breast cancer based on ultra performance liquid chromatography coupled to mass spectrometry with HILIC and RPLC separations. *Talanta, 158*, 351–360.
51. Takayama, T., Tsutsui, H., Shimizu, I., et al. (2016). Diagnostic approach to breast cancer patients based on target metabolomics in saliva by liquid chromatography with tandem mass spectrometry. *Clinica Chimica Acta, 452*, 18–26.
52. Cavaco, C., Pereira, J. A. M., Taunk, K., et al. (2018). Screening of salivary volatiles for putative breast cancer discrimination: An exploratory study involving geographically distant populations. *Analytical and Bioanalytical Chemistry, 410*(18), 4459–4468.
53. Asai, Y., Itoi, T., Sugimoto, M., et al. (2018). Elevated polyamines in saliva of pancreatic cancer. *Cancers (Basel), 10*(2), 43.
54. Tiziani, S., Lopes, V., & Günther, U. L. (2009). Early stage diagnosis of oral cancer using 1H NMR-based metabolomics. *Neoplasia, 11*(3), 269.
55. Bag, S., Banerjee, D. R., Basak, A., et al. (2015). NMR ((1)H and (13)C) based signatures of abnormal choline metabolism in oral squamous cell carcinoma with no prominent Warburg effect. *Biochemical and Biophysical Research Communications, 459*(4), 574–578.
56. Gupta, A., Gupta, S., & Mahdi, A. A. (2015). ^{1}H NMR-derived serum metabolomics of leukoplakia and squamous cell carcinoma. *Clinica Chimica Acta, 441*, 47–55.
57. Zhang, J., Bowers, J., Liu, L., et al. (2012). Esophageal cancer metabolite biomarkers detected by LC-MS and NMR methods. *PLoS One, 7*(1), e30181.
58. Zhang, X., Xu, L., Shen, J., et al. (2013). Metabolic signatures of esophageal cancer: NMR-based metabolomics and UHPLC-based focused metabolomics of blood serum. *Biochimica et Biophysica Acta, 1832*(8), 1207–1216.
59. Wojtowicz, W., Zabek, A., Deja, S., et al. (2017). Serum and urine 1H NMR-based metabolomics in the diagnosis of selected thyroid diseases. *Scientific Reports, 7*(1), 9108.
60. Wang, B., Zhang, L. Y., Wang, S. S., Yang, Y. H., & Zhao, W. X. (2018). NMR-based metabolomics to

select a surgical method for treating papillary thyroid carcinoma. *Clinics (São Paulo, Brazil), 73*, e333.
61. Boguszewicz, Ł., Bieleń, A., Mrochem-Kwarciak, J., et al. (2019). NMR-based metabolomics in real-time monitoring of treatment induced toxicity and cachexia in head and neck cancer: A method for early detection of high risk patients. *Metabolomics, 15*(8), 110.
62. Zhang, X., Hou, H., Chen, H., Liu, Y., Wang, A., & Hu, Q. (2018). Serum metabolomics of laryngeal cancer based on liquid chromatography coupled with quadrupole time-of-flight mass spectrometry. *Biomedical Chromatography, 32*(5), e4181.
63. Sridharan, G., Ramani, P., & Patankar, S. (2017). Serum metabolomics in oral leukoplakia and oral squamous cell carcinoma. *Journal of Cancer Research and Therapeutics, 13*(3), 556–561.
64. Shen, C. T., Zhang, Y., Liu, Y. M., et al. (2017). A distinct serum metabolic signature of distant metastatic papillary thyroid carcinoma. *Clinical Endocrinology, 87*(6), 844–852.
65. Mir, S. A., Rajagopalan, P., Jain, A. P., et al. (2015). LC-MS-based serum metabolomic analysis reveals dysregulation of phosphatidylcholines in esophageal squamous cell carcinoma. *Journal of Proteomics, 127*(Pt A), 96–102.
66. Gu, J., Liang, D., Pierzynski, J. A., et al. (2017). D-mannose: A novel prognostic biomarker for patients with esophageal adenocarcinoma. *Carcinogenesis, 38*(2), 162–167.
67. Jin, H., Qiao, F., Chen, L., Lu, C., Xu, L., & Gao, X. (2014). Serum metabolomic signatures of lymph node metastasis of esophageal squamous cell carcinoma. *Journal of Proteome Research, 13*(9), 4091–4103.
68. Chen, J., Hou, H., Chen, H., et al. (2019). Urinary metabolomics for discovering metabolic biomarkers of laryngeal cancer using UPLC-QTOF/MS. *Journal of Pharmaceutical and Biomedical Analysis, 167*, 83–89.
69. Xu, J., Li, J., Zhang, R., et al. (2019). Development of a metabolic pathway-based pseudo-targeted metabolomics method using liquid chromatography coupled with mass spectrometry. *Talanta, 192*, 160–168.
70. Dunn, W. B., Broadhurst, D., Begley, P., et al. (2011). Procedures for large-scale metabolic profiling of serum and plasma using gas chromatography and liquid chromatography coupled to mass spectrometry. *Nature Protocols, 6*(7), 1060–1083.
71. Want, E. J., Wilson, I. D., Gika, H., et al. (2010). Global metabolic profiling procedures for urine using UPLC-MS. *Nature Protocols, 5*(6), 1005–1018.
72. Chan, E. C., Pasikanti, K. K., & Nicholson, J. K. (2011). Global urinary metabolic profiling procedures using gas chromatography-mass spectrometry. *Nature Protocols, 6*(10), 1483–1499.
73. Beckonert, O., Keun, H. C., Ebbels, T. M., et al. (2007). Metabolic profiling, metabolomic and metabonomic procedures for NMR spectroscopy of urine, plasma, serum and tissue extracts. *Nature Protocols, 2*(11), 2692–2703.
74. Wang, J., Christison, T. T., Misuno, K., et al. (2014). Metabolomic profiling of anionic metabolites in head and neck cancer cells by capillary ion chromatography with Orbitrap mass spectrometry. *Analytical Chemistry, 86*(10), 5116–5124.
75. Hu, S., Wang, J., Ji, E. H., Christison, T., Lopez, L., & Huang, Y. (2015). Targeted metabolomic analysis of head and neck cancer cells using high performance ion chromatography coupled with a Q exactive HF mass spectrometer. *Analytical Chemistry, 87*(12), 6371–6379.
76. Zhao, X., Brusadelli, M. G., Sauter, S., et al. (2018). Lipidomic profiling links the Fanconi Anemia pathway to glycosphingolipid metabolism in head and neck cancer cells. *Clinical Cancer Research, 24*(11), 2700–2709.
77. Tan, Z., Xiao, L., Tang, M., et al. (2018). Targeting CPT1A-mediated fatty acid oxidation sensitizes nasopharyngeal carcinoma to radiation therapy. *Theranostics, 8*(9), 2329–2347.
78. Okazaki, S., Umene, K., Yamasaki, J., et al. (2019). Glutaminolysis-related genes determine sensitivity to xCT-targeted therapy in head and neck squamous cell carcinoma. *Cancer Science, 110*(11), 3453–3463.
79. Lindell Jonsson, E., Erngren, I., Engskog, M., et al. (2019). Exploring radiation response in two head and neck squamous carcinoma cell lines through metabolic profiling. *Frontiers in Oncology, 9*, 825.
80. Sandulache, V. C., Ow, T. J., Pickering, C. R., et al. (2011). Glucose, not glutamine, is the dominant energy source required for proliferation and survival of head and neck squamous carcinoma cells. *Cancer, 117*(13), 2926–2938.
81. Kitano, Y., Baba, Y., Nakagawa, S., et al. (2018). Nrf2 promotes oesophageal cancer cell proliferation via metabolic reprogramming and detoxification of reactive oxygen species. *The Journal of Pathology, 244*(3), 346–357.
82. Fu, J., Xiong, Z., Huang, C., et al. (2019). Hyperactivity of the transcription factor Nrf2 causes metabolic reprogramming in mouse esophagus. *The Journal of Biological Chemistry, 294*(1), 327–340.
83. Sun, C., Li, T., Song, X., et al. (2019). Spatially resolved metabolomics to discover tumor-associated metabolic alterations. *Proceedings of the National Academy of Sciences of the United States of America, 116*(1), 52–57.
84. Miccoli, P., Torregrossa, L., Shintu, L., et al. (2012). Metabolomics approach to thyroid nodules: A high-resolution magic-angle spinning nuclear magnetic resonance-based study. *Surgery, 152*(6), 1118–1124.
85. Torregrossa, L., Shintu, L., Nambiath Chandran, J., et al. (2012). Toward the reliable diagnosis of indeterminate thyroid lesions: A HRMAS NMR-based metabolomics case of study. *Journal of Proteome Research, 11*(6), 3317–3325.
86. Chen, M., Shen, M., Li, Y., et al. (2015). GC-MS-based metabolomic analysis of human papillary thyroid carcinoma tissue. *International Journal of Molecular Medicine, 36*(6), 1607–1614.

87. Tian, Y., Nie, X., Xu, S., et al. (2015). Integrative metabonomics as potential method for diagnosis of thyroid malignancy. *Scientific Reports, 5*, 14869.
88. Wojakowska, A., Chekan, M., Marczak, Ł., et al. (2015). Detection of metabolites discriminating subtypes of thyroid cancer: Molecular profiling of FFPE samples using the GC/MS approach. *Molecular and Cellular Endocrinology, 417*, 149–157.
89. Xu, Y., Zheng, X., Qiu, Y., Jia, W., Wang, J., & Yin, S. (2015). Distinct metabolomic profiles of papillary thyroid carcinoma and benign thyroid adenoma. *Journal of Proteome Research, 14*(8), 3315–3321.
90. Rezig, L., Servadio, A., Torregrossa, L., et al. (2018). Diagnosis of post-surgical fine-needle aspiration biopsies of thyroid lesions with indeterminate cytology using HRMAS NMR-based metabolomics. *Metabolomics, 14*(10), 141.
91. Huang, F. Q., Li, J., Jiang, L., et al. (2019). Serum-plasma matched metabolomics for comprehensive characterization of benign thyroid nodule and papillary thyroid carcinoma. *International Journal of Cancer, 144*(4), 868–876.
92. Ogawa, T., Washio, J., Takahashi, T., Echigo, S., & Takahashi, N. (2014). Glucose and glutamine metabolism in oral squamous cell carcinoma: Insight from a quantitative metabolomic approach. *Oral Surgery, Oral Medicine, Oral Pathology, Oral Radiology, 118*(2), 218–225.
93. Mukherjee, P. K., Funchain, P., Retuerto, M., et al. (2016). Metabolomic analysis identifies differentially produced oral metabolites, including the oncometabolite 2-hydroxyglutarate, in patients with head and neck squamous cell carcinoma. *BBA Clinical, 7*, 8–15.
94. Musharraf, S. G., Shahid, N., Naqvi, S. M. A., Saleem, M., Siddiqui, A. J., & Ali, A. (2016). Metabolite profiling of Preneoplastic and neoplastic lesions of oral cavity tissue samples revealed a biomarker pattern. *Scientific Reports, 6*, 38985.
95. Kamarajan, P., Rajendiran, T. M., Kinchen, J., Bermúdez, M., Danciu, T., & Kapila, Y. L. (2017). Head and neck squamous cell carcinoma metabolism draws on Glutaminolysis, and Stemness is specifically regulated by Glutaminolysis via aldehyde dehydrogenase. *Journal of Proteome Research, 16*(3), 1315–1326.

Metabolomics of Gastric Cancer

Wroocha Kadam, Bowen Wei, and Feng Li

1 Introduction

1.1 Metabolomics

Cellular metabolism broadly includes all the processes involved in the production of energy from the nutrients absorbed by a cell from the environment. All the products and intermediates that are generated during the synthesis and utilization of the nutrients could be collectively referred to as metabolites. The expression levels of cellular metabolites have significant effect on gene expression, gene regulation and pathway interactions, ultimately resulting in a meaningful physiological phenotype. Metabolomics is an emerging field of study that measures all the metabolites within a biological sample (metabolome) [1]. This comprehensive profiling of metabolites in a biological sample such as tissues or body fluids provides in-depth understanding of the system's response to environmental or genetic stress and underlying metabolic mechanisms which may discover metabolite biomarkers for clinical applications in human diseases.

Nuclear magnetic resonance (^{1}H NMR) spectroscopy and mass spectrometry (MS) are the primary analytical techniques combined with multivariate statistical methods used to characterize a metabolome and identify major metabolite changes. NMR spectroscopy does not rely on separation of the analytes while MS requires preseparation of the analytes commonly by gas chromatography (GC) or high-performance liquid chromatography (HPLC). Capillary electrophoresis coupled mass spectrometry (CE-MS) also shows great promise for metabolomic analysis [2], due to CE has a higher separation efficiency than HPLC and can separate a wider range of metabolite classes than GC. In the era of personalized medicine, metabolomics is expected to become a routine approach to monitoring a patient's health [3]. The measurement of metabolomics profiles benefits our understanding of the relationship between individual's disease state and molecular mechanisms by monitoring disease development, progression and treatment efficacies from both pharmaceutical and surgical interventions. Periodic screening of metabolite profiles allows to detect any phenotypic changes over a patient's lifetime, thereby monitoring the overall health status [1].

Over the years, we have witnessed numerous genetic underpinnings found in relation to the unique hallmarks of cancer cells, which provide crucial insight of the signalling pathways underlying the cancer diseases. The first two hallmarks lie in that cancer cells are insensitive to anti-growth signals and self-sufficiently produce

W. Kadam · F. Li (✉)
UCLA School of Dentistry, Los Angeles, CA, USA
e-mail: fengli@ucla.edu

B. Wei
UCLA School of Medicine, Los Angeles, CA, USA

S. Hu (ed.), *Cancer Metabolomics*, Advances in Experimental Medicine and Biology 1280,
https://doi.org/10.1007/978-3-030-51652-9_20

growth signals and other factors for sustained angiogenesis needed for cell function and survival. The next two hallmarks are the ability of cancer cells to circumvent senescence and gain self-renewability. Lastly, tissue invasion and metastasis are the most fatal characteristics of cancer [4]. All these physiological changes must need a vast reprogramming of the cancer cell metabolism to provide enough cellular energy required to adapt constantly changing and often hostile systemic conditions. The ability of measuring these metabolic alterations at high-throughput and systemic level could facilitate more in-depth understanding of cancer metabolisms. Meanwhile, the identified signature metabolites and related pathways/genes may serve as biomarkers for cancer diagnosis, prognosis and treatment efficacy or molecular targets for therapeutic interventions [5, 6].

1.2 Gastric Cancer

Gastric cancer develops when the cancer cells formed in the lining of the stomach. Approximately 90% of all gastric neoplasms are adenocarcinomas which originate from the glands of the gastric mucosa. Tumours occurring at oesophagogastric junction (EGJ) may be difficult to distinguish as either a gastric or an oesophageal primary, especially because of increased incidence of adenocarcinoma in the oesophagus. Gastric cancer is the fourth most common cancer worldwide with the highest incidence rates in Asia, Eastern Europe and South America regions [7]. This malignant tumour easily metastasizes to other solid organs within the abdomen, as well as to extra-abdominal sites. Trends in survival rates from the 1970s to now have not shown great improvement. The survival rates for gastric cancer are among the worst of any solid tumours, because early stomach cancer causes few symptoms; the disease is usually advanced with involvement of regional nodes when the diagnosis is made which reduces survival considerably. In this regard, it is critical to develop molecular biomarkers for early detection and screening of gastric cancer [8].

There are many risk factors involved in the development of gastric cancer; important ones are the *Helicobacter pylori* (*H. pylori*) infection, genetic factors, dietary factors, and lifestyle factors which are strongly linked to gastric cancer [9]. *H. pylori* infection has demonstrated its oncogenicity through its direct epigenetic effects on gastric epithelial cells and indirect inflammatory response on the gastric mucosa (Fig. 1) [10]. Gastric adenocarcinoma can be classified into histologic subtypes as adenocarcinoma, papillary adenocarcinoma, tubular adenocarcinoma, mucinous adenocarcinoma, signet ring cell carcinoma, adenosquamous carcinoma, squamous cell carcinoma, small cell carcinoma and undifferentiated carcinoma or classified as intestinal, diffuse and mixed type [11]. Clinical staging is crucial to institute definitive treatment when diagnosed with gastric cancer. Based on evidence from physical examination, radiologic imaging, endoscopy, biopsy, laboratory and histological findings, correct staging of the cancer will determine its prognosis with appropriate treatment modalities. The evaluation of altered metabolism in gastric cancer could provide additional guidance on cancer patients' diagnosis, staging, treatment decision making and prognosis. Some of the altered metabolisms in gastric cancer is summarized in (Fig. 2) [12].

2 Recent Advances in Gastric Cancer Metabolism

2.1 Glucose Metabolism

The metabolism of glucose in gastric cancer cells is augmented differently from that of normal gastric epithelium. There is an upregulation of aerobic glycolysis (a.k.a., Warburg effect) in gastric cancer to meet increased demands of cell proliferation, as evidenced by significantly higher levels of lactate in urine and tissue samples of gastric cancer patients. The accumulated lactic acid provides an acidic microenvironment that exacerbates the decomposition of extracellular matrix by proteolytic activity [13]. Also, this microenvironment is conducive for formation of blood ves-

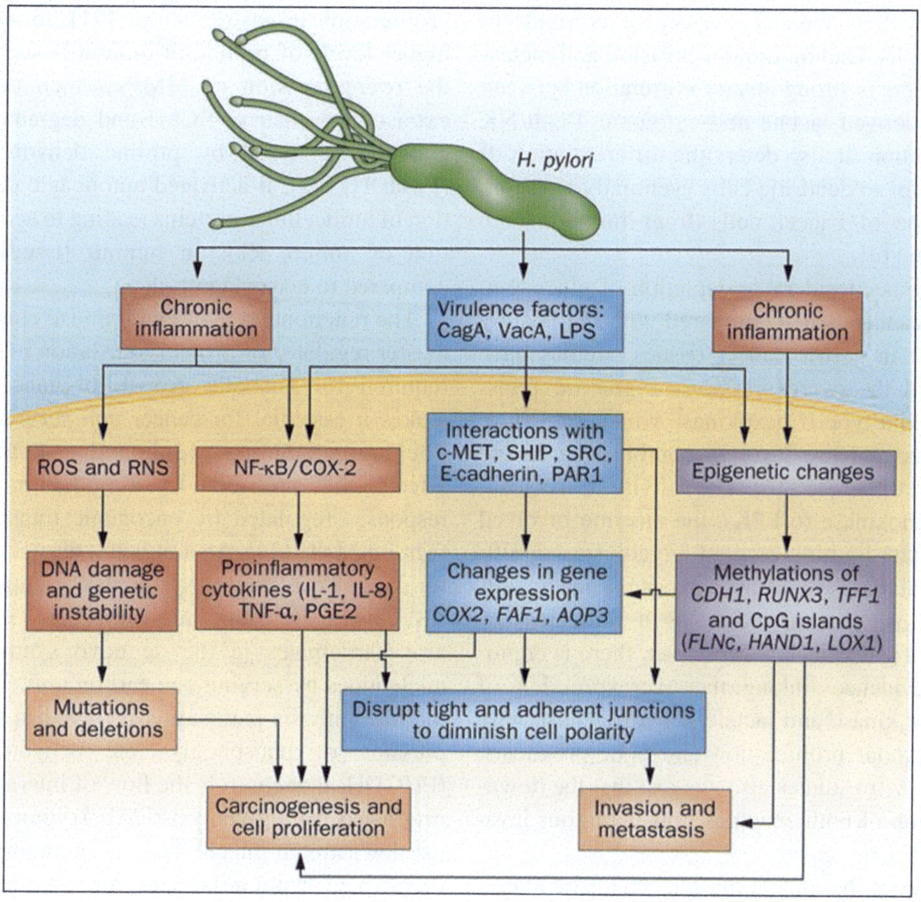

Fig. 1 Involvement of *H. pylori* infection in development and progression of gastric cancer. *H. pylori* and its several virulence factors, such as CagA, interact with gastric epithelial cells to induce chronic inflammation, mucosal damage and multiple alterations in gene expression and genetic/epigenetic changes, eventually leading to gastric carcinogenesis. Abbreviations: *ROS*, reactive oxygen species; *RNS*, reactive nitrogen species; *COX-2*, cyclooxygenase-2; *VacA*, vacuolating cytotoxin A; *LPS*, lipopolysaccharide; *CpG island*, areas of cytosine and guanine repeats (Reprinted with permission from [10])

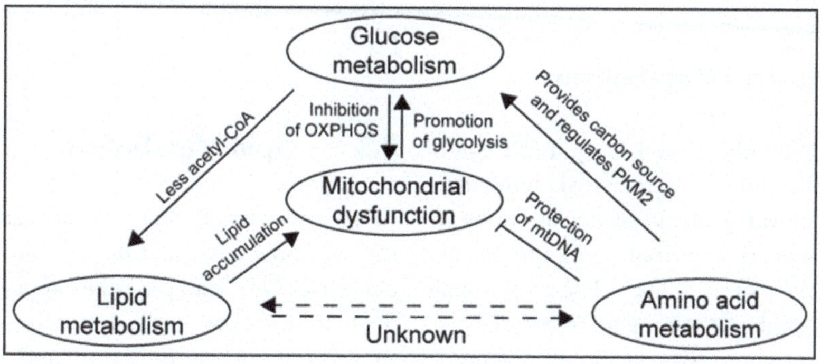

Fig. 2 Altered metabolism observed in gastric cancer. An overview of the metabolic pathways mediating upregulation of glycolysis and mitochondrial dysfunction in gastric cancer. Abbreviations: *mtDNA*, mitochondrial DNA; *OXPHOS*, oxidative phosphorylation; *PKM2*, pyruvate kinase M2 (Reprinted with permission from [12])

sels providing abundant supply of nutrients to cancer cells, leading tumour invasion and metastasis. There is strong inverse correlation between tumour-derived lactate and cytotoxic T-cell/NK cell function. It also deters the differentiation of monocytes to dendritic cells eventually resulting in escape of cancer cells from immunogenic response [14].

There is considerable depletion of glucose in gastric cancers when compared with the healthy controls. In gastric cancer tissues, studies have indicated the overexpression of glucose transporters and type II hexokinase which can cause decreased glucose level in combination to the Warburg effect [15, 16]. The activity of fructose-6-phosphokinase (6-FPK), the enzyme involved in the rate-limiting step of glycolysis, significantly increases in gastric cancer tissues, resulting in low glucose levels, as it regulates the output of glucose [17]. Moreover, there is cumulative evidence linking the overexpression of pyruvate kinase and lactate dehydrogenase with rapid tumour proliferation and poor prognosis, while in vitro studies also suggest that the downregulation of both enzymes impair tumour invasion [17–19].

The contributions of these mechanistic alterations in aerobic glycolysis are crucial for understanding the gastric carcinogenesis and progression (Fig. 3) [20]. Any intervention with the glycolytic switch in cancer cells may provide a new and promising therapeutic strategy for hampering further oncogenic transformation in gastric cancer.

2.2 Amino Acid Metabolism

Amino acids are building blocks required for cellular protein biosynthesis and cytoskeleton formation, while elevated levels of amino acids in microenvironment are contributing factors in carcinogenesis. The amino acids related to tricarboxylic citric acid (TCA) cycle represent an alternative energy source of cancer cell proliferation. The rapid proliferation rate is directly correlated with elevated glycine, and interfering glycine uptake and its biosynthesis impaired the proliferation in gastric cancer [21]. In addition, higher levels of proline in tumour tissues cause the overexpression of MMPs which degrades extracellular matrix (ECM) and degradation of collagen catalysed by proline dehydrogenase (PRODH) [22]. It activated autophagic degradation of intracellular proteins leading to accumulation of amino acids in tumour tissues when compared to normal controls.

The functional role of glutamine to control the master regulator of protein translation mTORC1 required for anabolic growth of cancer cells makes it essential for cancer cell survival [23]. The reprogramming of glutamine metabolism affects the proliferation via the metabolic responses regulated by oncogenic transcription factor c-MYC [24]. Also, it is the nitrogen donor for the de novo synthesis of both nucleotides and several key metabolic enzymes (Fig. 4). Serine also participates in the de novo synthesis of nucleotides by serving one carbon unit. The serine biosynthesis pathway is involved in overexpression of phosphoglycerate dehydrogenase (PHGDH) that controls the flow of intermediates originated from glycolysis [25]. Tryptophan and its downstream metabolites (kynurenine, kynurenic acid, anthranilic acid, nicotinic acid) are related to the pathogenesis and prognosis of gastric cancer. Kynurenine pathway is catalysed by indoleamine-2,3-dioxygenase (IDO), and higher IDO expression plays an immunosuppressive role inhibiting T-cell-mediated cytotoxicity and favouring gastric cancer cell proliferation. 3-Hydroxyanthanilie acid also has suppressive effects on inflammation and immune response [26].

2.3 Lipid Metabolism

In gastric cancer, there is noticeable increased rate of lipogenesis and the upregulation of mitochondrial fatty acid β-oxidation utilizing the fatty acids to meet the demand of cell membrane synthesis, mainly for lipid raft and lipid-modified signalling molecules [27]. The intensive fatty acid degradation via β-oxidation causes significantly larger build-ups of fatty acids such as

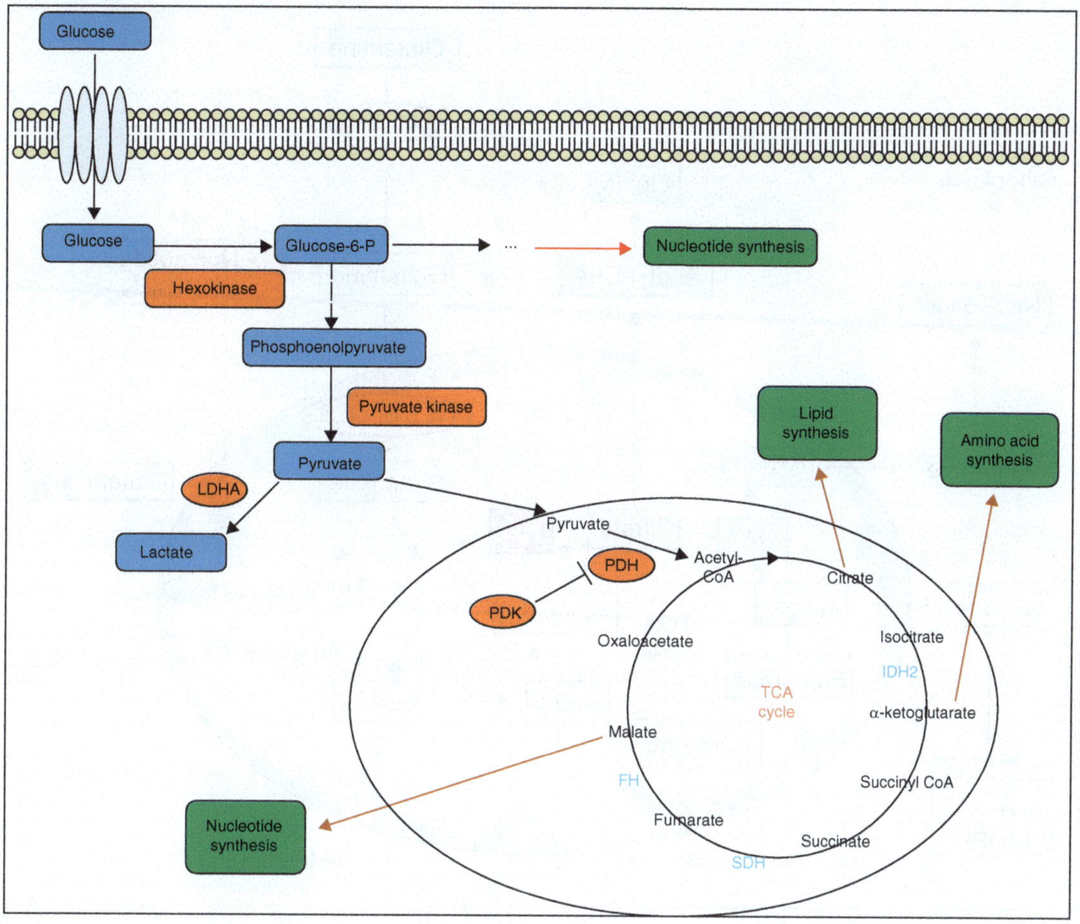

Fig. 3 Alterations in mechanism of aerobic glycolysis in gastric cancer. An outline of glucose metabolism in gastric cancer shows the interplay between glucose and the other three metabolic pathways (Reprinted with permission from [20])

hexadecenoic acid, docosahexaenoic acid, heptanoic acid and especially β-hydroxybutyrate, in cancer tissues, while elevated octadecanoic acid is found in blood of gastric cancer patients [28]. The enhanced fatty acid β-oxidation produces more ATP and acetyl coenzyme-A accelerating the rate of citric acid oxidation, an important metabolic reprogramming in serving as the energy source in early stages. This increased production of polyunsaturated fatty acids is also associated with tumour cell proliferation, apoptosis and angiogenesis [29]. The upregulation of lipid peroxides can be detected by the elevated levels of azelaic acid, which is the end product of linoleic acid undergone peroxide decomposition, in blood [26]. The overall accelerated lipid metabolism thus might explain the severe weight loss observed in patients with late stages of gastric cancer.

The increased demands for fatty acids needed by proliferating tumour cells are largely dependent on de novo synthesis. The cancer cells thus synthesize a large fraction of their membrane lipids rather than acquiring them from extracellular sources. The fatty acid synthase (FAS) enzyme catalyses the synthesis of palmitate from acetyl-CoA or malonyl-CoA in the presence of NADPH as a redox equivalent during de novo lipogenesis. FAS is indeed upregulated in gastric cancer, and the increased FAS expression has been linked to tumour proliferation, chemoresistance and poorer prognosis [30].

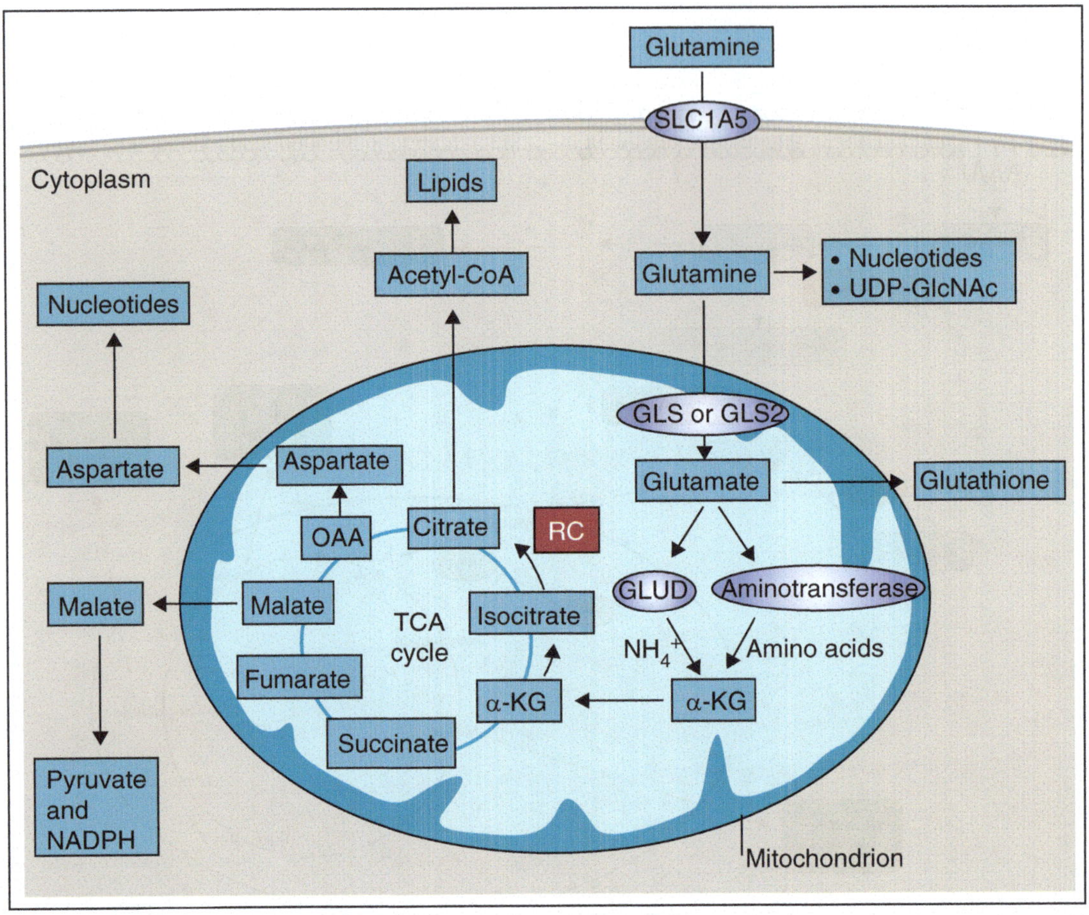

Fig. 4 Role of glutamine metabolism in gastric cancer. This figure depicts how the elevated level of glutamine is incorporated in satisfying the increased energy demands in gastric cancer cells (Reprinted with permission from [34])

2.4 Nucleotide Metabolism

Cancer progression is frequently dependent on nucleotide synthesis and metabolism which are significantly upregulated to supply the energy demands during rapid cancer cell proliferation. The accumulation of uric acid or urate, the end products of nucleotide catabolism, is found in gastric cancer patients [31]. The various purine compounds show different levels such as hypoxanthine and guanosine are increased while there is decrease in uridine levels [26]. Though ATP and GTP are associated with energy metabolism with nucleotides, the cancer cells use small portion of glucose for oxidative phosphorylation or fumarate respiration to generate energy under special conditions of glucose deprivation and severe hypoxia in microenvironment instead of fortifying more ATP to advance its growth compared to their normal counterparts. This can explain why there is no significant difference found in nucleotide phosphate levels (ATP, ADP, GTP and GDP), total adenylate and energy charge between gastric cancer and normal tissues [32].

2.5 Other Metabolisms in Gastric Cancer

Increased levels of five TCA intermediates, α-ketoglutaric acid, malic acid, fumarate, succinate and citric acid, have been noted in gastric cancer [28, 29, 33]. The cancer cells may still use anaerobic glycolysis and possibly fumarate respiration, which explains the accumulation of fumarate and succinate. Some elevated amino acids, such as glutamine [34], threonine, phenylalanine, tyrosine, valine, cysteine or proline, can also be converted into these TCA intermediates to generate energy [26, 35]. In addition, citric acid is often elevated and used for the de novo fatty acid synthesis [28, 29, 33, 36].

The levels of creatinine, a waste product of muscle metabolism, were found to be significantly increased in the urine samples of gastric cancer patients who exhibited lower total body skeletal mass (cachectic patients) [37]. The gastric flora might produce metabolites to affect the cancer cell metabolism. Changes in metabolites in gastric cancer such as butanoic acid, mannitol and p-cresol, which are commonly thought of artificial substances, could be derived from gastric microbiome [38]. Therefore, metabolomics of gastric microbiome and its interactions with cancer cells can be important to understand the metabolic reprogramming in gastric cancer.

3 Metabolomic Analysis of Gastric Cancer

3.1 Diagnosis

Early diagnosis can tremendously change the outcome of cancer treatment, but conventional cancer biomarkers and diagnostic techniques fall short of providing satisfactory early detection. There were 18 metabolites distinctly detected between the malignant tissues and adjacent non-malignant tissues of gastric mucosa with ROC (receiver operating characteristics) value of 0.9629 [39]. Also, there is an obvious distinction in serum metabolic profiles of gastrointestinal cancers including oesophageal, gastric and colorectal when compared to healthy individuals. There are changes in the levels of 3-hydroxypropionic acid and pyruvic acid to sufficiently segregate gastric cancer from oesophageal and colorectal cancer. It also shows high sensitivity (84.6 and 70.0%) and specificity (71.4 and 90.9%) when compared with current serum biomarkers such as CA19-9 and CEA [40]. The diagnostic potential of serum metabolomic profiles between gastric cancer and non-cancer groups has been well demonstrated and even in different pathological subtypes of gastric cancer has different metabolic signatures in early stage of gastric carcinogenesis. Intestinal-type adenocarcinoma of gastric cancer is known to precede by a sequence of gastric lesions known as Correa's cascade [11]. Studies have observed the relative difference in plasma metabolomic profiles (e.g. threonate, glutamate and azelaic acid) between diffuse-type gastric cancer patients and those with Correa's cascade [31].

A recent study demonstrated that 14 out of 17 metabolites altered in urine sample of gastric cancer patients showed a better diagnostic value than classic blood biomarkers. A set of amino acid, L-alanine, L-isoleucine, L-serine, L-threonine, L-proline and L-methionine formed a characteristic biosignature for discrimination of gastric cancer patients from healthy control population [41]. Another study also indicated that gastric cancer patients had a unique urine metabolic profile in contrast to healthy subjects, especially 2-hydroxyisobutyrate, 3-indoxylsulfate and alanine, producing an ROC value of 0.95 [37].

3.2 Prognosis

Most gastric cancer cases are detected in late stages when the cancer cells have already metastasized resulting in poor clinical outcomes. There are no currently available molecular markers for predicting metastasis and prognosis of gastric cancer. Thus, it is important to identify signature metabolite biomarkers for prognostic applications in gastric cancer [41]. Another metabolomics study compared the urinary metabolomes between xenograft mice (transplanted with human gastric cancer cell line SGC-7901) with metastasis and those without metastasis. The results indicated that alanine, butanoic acid, glycerol, L-threonic acid and L-proline were significantly decreased whereas butanedioic acid and myo-inositol were significantly increased in in metastasis group when compared to non-metastasis group [42]. Furthermore, metabolomic analysis of gastric cancer tissues revealed that L-cysteine, hypoxanthine and L-tyrosine were significantly upregulated whereas phenanthrenol and butanoic acid were significantly downregulated in invasive tumours versus non-invasive tumours. These metabolite biomarkers could differentiate invasive from non-invasive gastric cancers with ROC value of 0.969 [39].

Metabolomic analysis of mouse model xenografts identified a number of differentially expressed metabolites between metastasis and non-metastasis groups. Among these metabolites, proline was the most upregulated tissue metabolite in the metastasis group, which was 2.45-fold higher than that in non-metastasis group. Glutamine was the most downregulated tissue metabolite in the metastasis group, which was 1.71-fold lower than that in the non-metastasis group. The lactic acid, L-alanine, L-valine, leucine, malic acid, L-aspartic acid, serine, phosphoserine, dimethylglycine, glycine, L-glutamic acid, L-lysine, myo-inositol, propanedioic acid, docosanoic acid, octadecanoic acid, arginine, pyrrolidine and pyrimidine were significantly upregulated, while the glucose, succinate, L-isoleucine, L-methionine, propanamide, L-threonic acid and butanedioic acid were remarkably downregulated in the metastasis group compared to the non-metastasis group. According to this animal model study, the main metabolic pathways associated with metastasis of gastric cancer included glycolysis (lactic acid, alkaline), serine metabolism (serine, phosphoserine), proline metabolism (proline), TCA cycle (succinate, malic acid), fatty acid metabolism (docosanoic acid and octadecanoic acid) and methylation (glycine) [43]. Also, studies revealed that gastric cancer patients with higher levels of proline, p-cresol and 4-hydroxybenzoic acid had worse prognosis, and the p-cresol concentrations closely correlated with gastric cancer stage, which progressively increased with the late stages [41]. The elevated proline may serve as a promising prognostic biomarker for gastric cancer as accumulation of proline in tumour tissues because of the degradation of collagen. Upregulation of proline also causes the overexpression of MMPs, degrading ECM and enhancing tumour invasion and metastasis [44].

3.3 Treatment

Treatment efficacy regulates the balance between maximizing the therapeutic response and minimizing adverse effects of a novel treatment of cancer. The prediction of treatment efficacy (e.g. chemosensitivity) is a challenging problem in the management of cancer. Previous studies have suggested that metabolomic analysis of human xenograft model of gastric cancer may provide an effective approach to chemosensitivity prediction. BALB/c-nu/nu mice were transplanted with MKN-45 cell line to establish the xenograft model, and then the mice were randomized into treatment group (cisplatin and 5-fluorouracil) (5-FU) and control group (0.9% sodium chloride). Metabolomic analysis of mouse plasma samples after treatment revealed a series of endogenous metabolites, including 1-acyl-lysophosphatidycholines, polyunsaturated fatty acids and their derivatives, as potential indicators of chemosensitivity [45]. The PRODH was identified as a potential biomarker for measuring intracellular dynamic responses to 5-FU. As there is upregulation of PRODH expression after 5-FU administration, which further catalyses the biosynthesis of glutamate from proline, the treatment reduced the level of proline but increased the level of glutamate dramatically [46]. The FAS enzyme implicated in lipogenesis is also a potential target in antineoplastic therapy [30]. Similarly, 1-acyl-lysophosphatidylcholine regulates the activity of enzymes like phospholipase A2 (PLA2), which catalyses the production of arachidonic acid that is likely to promote cell cycle arrest and apoptosis dependent on ceramide pathway, and lysophosphatidylcholine acetyltransferases, which catalyses the phospholipid synthesis linked to tumour cell proliferation. Thus, 1-acyl-lysophosphatidylcholine and related polyunsaturated fatty acid might serve as targets for evaluating gastric cancer chemosensitivity [47].

The investigation of adriamycin (ADR) treatment for gastric adenocarcinoma revealed increased levels of trimethylamine oxide, hippurate and taurine in the urine samples of ADR-treated patient group compared to untreated patient group. These metabolic alterations trigger apoptosis in gastric cancer cells via ADR-induced genotoxic stress, attributing to the pharmacological effect of ADR [48]. In addition, lactate dehydrogenase A (LDH-A) and pyruvate dehydrogenase B (PDH-B) may serve as therapeutic targets in gastric cancer treatment. The downregulation of LDH-A and overexpression of PDH-B inhibits cell growth and migration as there is dysregulation of pyruvate efflux into the Krebs cycle rather than the glycolysis process in gastric cancer [49].

4 Conclusion and Future Perspective

Although gastric cancer is one of the most common malignancies worldwide, its pathogenesis and molecular mechanisms remain largely unknown [50]. Metabolomics represents a powerful tool to study the altered metabolisms in gastric cancer. It not only allows a comprehensive analysis of metabolites and related metabolic pathways in cancer cells but also can study the interactions between cancer cells and tumour microenvironment as well as between tumour cells and gastric microbiome [38]. Metabolomic studies of gastric cancer have harnessed potential metabolite biomarkers for the disease diagnosis, prognosis and treatment efficacy and also demonstrated metabolic pathways/target genes for potential therapeutic interventions. With the improvement of metabolomics technology, data analysis tools and study design [51], we can envision that metabolomics will significantly enhance our understanding of the carcinogenesis and progression process of gastric cancer and may eventually facilitate a tailored management of gastric cancer patients.

References

1. Clish, C. B. (2015). Metabolomics: An emerging but powerful tool for precision medicine. *Cold Spring Harbor Molecular Case Studies, 1*(1), a000588–a000588.
2. Vermeersch, K. A., & Styczynski, M. P. (2013). Applications of metabolomics in cancer research. *Journal of Carcinogenesis, 12*, 9.
3. Riekeberg, E., & Powers, R. (2017). New frontiers in metabolomics: From measurement to insight. *F1000Res, 6*, 1148.
4. Pavlova, N. N., & Thompson, C. B. (2016). The emerging hallmarks of cancer metabolism. *Cell Metabolism, 23*(1), 27–47.
5. Puchades-Carrasco, L., & Pineda-Lucena, A. (2017). Metabolomics applications in precision medicine: An oncological perspective. *Current Topics in Medicinal Chemistry, 17*(24), 2740–2751.
6. Wishart, D. S. (2016). Emerging applications of metabolomics in drug discovery and precision medicine. *Nature Reviews Drug Discovery, 15*, 473. https://doi.org/10.1038/nrd.2016.32.
7. Siegel, R. L., Miller, K. D., & Jemal, A. (2016). Cancer statistics, 2016. *CA: A Cancer Journal for Clinicians, 66*(1), 7–30.
8. Li, F., Yoshizawa, J. M., Kim, K. M., Kanjanapangka, J., Grogan, T. R., Wang, X., Elashoff, D. E., Ishikawa, S., Chia, D., Liao, W., Akin, D., Yan, X., Lee, M. S., Choi, R., Kim, S. M., Kang, S. Y., Bae, J. M., Sohn, T. S., Lee, J. H., Choi, M. G., Min, B. H., Lee, J. H., Kim, J. J., Kim, Y., Kim, S., & Wong, D. T. W. (2018). Discovery and validation of salivary extracellular RNA biomarkers for noninvasive detection of gastric cancer. *Clinical Chemistry, 64*(10), 1513–1521.
9. Cheng, X. J., Lin, J. C., & Tu, S. P. (2016). Etiology and prevention of gastric cancer. *Gastrointestinal Tumors, 3*(1), 25–36.
10. Wadhwa, R., Song, S., Lee, J.-S., Yao, Y., Wei, Q., & Ajani, J. A. (2013). Gastric cancer—Molecular and clinical dimensions. *Nature Reviews Clinical Oncology, 10*, 643.
11. Piazuelo, M. B., & Correa, P. (2013). Gastric cáncer: Overview. *Colombia Médica (Cali), 44*(3), 192–201.
12. Liu, Y., Zhang, Z., Wang, J., Chen, C., Tang, X., Zhu, J., & Liu, J. (2019). Metabolic reprogramming results in abnormal glycolysis in gastric cancer: A review. *Oncotargets and Therapy, 12*, 1195–1204.
13. Jung, J., Jung, Y., Bang, E. J., Cho, S. I., Jang, Y. J., Kwak, J. M., Ryu, D. H., Park, S., & Hwang, G. S. (2014). Noninvasive diagnosis and evaluation of curative surgery for gastric cancer by using NMR-based metabolomic profiling. *Annals of Surgical Oncology, 21*(Suppl 4), S736–S742.
14. Fischer, K., Hoffmann, P., Voelkl, S., Meidenbauer, N., Ammer, J., Edinger, M., Gottfried, E., Schwarz, S., Rothe, G., Hoves, S., Renner, K., Timischl, B., Mackensen, A., Kunz-Schughart, L., Andreesen, R., Krause, S. W., & Kreutz, M. (2007). Inhibitory effect of tumor cell-derived lactic acid on human T cells. *Blood, 109*(9), 3812–3819.
15. Koukourakis, M. I., Pitiakoudis, M., Giatromanolaki, A., Tsarouha, A., Polychronidis, A., Sivridis, E., & Simopoulos, C. (2006). Oxygen and glucose consumption in gastrointestinal adenocarcinomas: Correlation with markers of hypoxia, acidity and anaerobic glycolysis. *Cancer Science, 97*(10), 1056–1060.
16. Pedersen, P. L., Mathupala, S., Rempel, A., Geschwind, J. F., & Ko, Y. H. (2002). Mitochondrial bound type II hexokinase: A key player in the growth

and survival of many cancers and an ideal prospect for therapeutic intervention. *Biochimica et Biophysica Acta, 1555*(1–3), 14–20.
17. Gatenby, R. A., & Gillies, R. J. (2004). Why do cancers have high aerobic glycolysis? *Nature Reviews. Cancer, 4*(11), 891–899.
18. Augoff, K., Hryniewicz-Jankowska, A., & Tabola, R. (2015). Lactate dehydrogenase 5: An old friend and a new hope in the war on cancer. *Cancer Letters, 358*(1), 1–7.
19. Wu, J., Hu, L., Chen, M., Cao, W., Chen, H., & He, T. (2016). Pyruvate kinase M2 overexpression and poor prognosis in solid tumors of digestive system: Evidence from 16 cohort studies. *Oncotargets and Therapy, 9*, 4277–4288.
20. Yuan, L. W., Yamashita, H., & Seto, Y. (2016). Glucose metabolism in gastric cancer: The cutting-edge. *World Journal of Gastroenterology, 22*(6), 2046–2059.
21. Jain, M., Nilsson, R., Sharma, S., Madhusudhan, N., Kitami, T., Souza, A. L., Kafri, R., Kirschner, M. W., Clish, C. B., & Mootha, V. K. (2012). Metabolite profiling identifies a key role for glycine in rapid cancer cell proliferation. *Science (New York, N.Y.), 336*(6084), 1040–1044.
22. Phang, J. M., Donald, S. P., Pandhare, J., & Liu, Y. (2008). The metabolism of proline, a stress substrate, modulates carcinogenic pathways. *Amino Acids, 35*(4), 681–690.
23. Nicklin, P., Bergman, P., Zhang, B., Triantafellow, E., Wang, H., Nyfeler, B., Yang, H., Hild, M., Kung, C., Wilson, C., Myer, V. E., MacKeigan, J. P., Porter, J. A., Wang, Y. K., Cantley, L. C., Finan, P. M., & Murphy, L. O. (2009). Bidirectional transport of amino acids regulates mTOR and autophagy. *Cell, 136*(3), 521–534.
24. Liu, W., Le, A., Hancock, C., Lane, A. N., Dang, C. V., Fan, T. W., & Phang, J. M. (2012). Reprogramming of proline and glutamine metabolism contributes to the proliferative and metabolic responses regulated by oncogenic transcription factor c-MYC. *Proceedings of the National Academy of Sciences of the United States of America, 109*(23), 8983–8988.
25. Possemato, R., Marks, K. M., Shaul, Y. D., Pacold, M. E., Kim, D., Birsoy, K., Sethumadhavan, S., Woo, H. K., Jang, H. G., Jha, A. K., Chen, W. W., Barrett, F. G., Stransky, N., Tsun, Z. Y., Cowley, G. S., Barretina, J., Kalaany, N. Y., Hsu, P. P., Ottina, K., Chan, A. M., Yuan, B., Garraway, L. A., Root, D. E., Mino-Kenudson, M., Brachtel, E. F., Driggers, E. M., & Sabatini, D. M. (2011). Functional genomics reveal that the serine synthesis pathway is essential in breast cancer. *Nature, 476*(7360), 346–350.
26. Xiao, S., & Zhou, L. (2017). Gastric cancer: Metabolic and metabolomics perspectives (Review). *International Journal of Oncology, 51*(1), 5–17.
27. Munoz-Pinedo, C., El Mjiyad, N., & Ricci, J. E. (2012). Cancer metabolism: Current perspectives and future directions. *Cell Death & Disease, 3*, e248.
28. Aa, J., Yu, L., Sun, M., Liu, L., Li, M., Cao, B., Shi, J., Xu, J., Cheng, L., Zhou, J., Zheng, T., Wang, X., Zhao, C., Gu, R., Zhang, F., Shi, R., & Wang, G. J. M. (2012). Metabolic features of the tumor microenvironment of gastric cancer and the link to the systemic macroenvironment. *Metabolomics, 8*(1), 164–173.
29. Song, H., Wang, L., Liu, H. L., Wu, X. B., Wang, H. S., Liu, Z. H., Li, Y., Diao, D. C., Chen, H. L., & Peng, J. S. (2011). Tissue metabolomic fingerprinting reveals metabolic disorders associated with human gastric cancer morbidity. *Oncology Reports, 26*(2), 431–438.
30. Ito, T., Sato, K., Maekawa, H., Sakurada, M., Orita, H., Shimada, K., Daida, H., Wada, R., Abe, M., Hino, O., & Kajiyama, Y. (2014). Elevated levels of serum fatty acid synthase in patients with gastric carcinoma. *Oncology Letters, 7*(3), 616–620.
31. Xu, S., Wu, Q., & Yu, S. (2011). Application of metabonomics in gastrointestinal disease clinical diagnosis. *Sheng Wu Yi Xue Gong Cheng Xue Za Zhi, 28*(3), 645–648.
32. Hirayama, A., Kami, K., Sugimoto, M., Sugawara, M., Toki, N., Onozuka, H., Kinoshita, T., Saito, N., Ochiai, A., Tomita, M., Esumi, H., & Soga, T. (2009). Quantitative metabolome profiling of colon and stomach cancer microenvironment by capillary electrophoresis time-of-flight mass spectrometry. *Cancer Research, 69*(11), 4918–4925.
33. Liang, Q., Wang, C., & Li, B. (2015). Metabolomic analysis using liquid chromatography/mass spectrometry for gastric cancer. *Applied Biochemistry and Biotechnology, 176*(8), 2170–2184.
34. Altman, B. J., Stine, Z. E., & Dang, C. V. (2016). From Krebs to clinic: Glutamine metabolism to cancer therapy. *Nature Reviews. Cancer, 16*(10), 619–634.
35. Chen, Z., Lu, W., Garcia-Prieto, C., & Huang, P. (2007). The Warburg effect and its cancer therapeutic implications. *Journal of Bioenergetics and Biomembranes, 39*(3), 267–274.
36. Costello, L. C., Franklin, R. B. J. M., & Biochemistry, C. (2005). 'Why do tumour cells glycolyse?': From glycolysis through citrate to lipogenesis. *Molecular and Cellular Biochemistry, 280*(1), 1.
37. Chan, A. W., Mercier, P., Schiller, D., Bailey, R., Robbins, S., Eurich, D. T., Sawyer, M. B., & Broadhurst, D. (2015). 1H-NMR urinary metabolomic profiling for diagnosis of gastric cancer. *British Journal of Cancer, 114*, 59.
38. Lertpiriyapong, K., Whary, M. T., Muthupalani, S., Lofgren, J. L., Gamazon, E. R., Feng, Y., Ge, Z., Wang, T. C., & Fox, J. G. (2014). Gastric colonisation with a restricted commensal microbiota replicates the promotion of neoplastic lesions by diverse intestinal microbiota in the *Helicobacter pylori* INS-GAS mouse model of gastric carcinogenesis. *Gut, 63*(1), 54.
39. Wu, H., Xue, R., Tang, Z., Deng, C., Liu, T., Zeng, H., Sun, Y., Shen, X. J. A., & Chemistry, B. (2010). Metabolomic investigation of gastric cancer tissue using gas chromatography/mass spectrometry. *Analytical and Bioanalytical Chemistry, 396*(4), 1385–1395.

40. Ikeda, A., Nishiumi, S., Shinohara, M., Yoshie, T., Hatano, N., Okuno, T., Bamba, T., Fukusaki, E., Takenawa, T., Azuma, T., & Yoshida, M. (2012). Serum metabolomics as a novel diagnostic approach for gastrointestinal cancer. *Biomedical Chromatography, 26*(5), 548–558.
41. Chen, Y., Zhang, J., Guo, L., Liu, L., Wen, J., Xu, L., Yan, M., Li, Z., Zhang, X., Nan, P., Jiang, J., Ji, J., Zhang, J., Cai, W., Zhuang, H., Wang, Y., Zhu, Z., & Yu, Y. (2016). A characteristic biosignature for discrimination of gastric cancer from healthy population by high throughput GC-MS analysis. *Oncotarget, 7*(52), 87496–87510.
42. Hu, J. D., Tang, H. Q., Zhang, Q., Fan, J., Hong, J., Gu, J. Z., & Chen, J. L. (2011). Prediction of gastric cancer metastasis through urinary metabolomic investigation using GC/MS. *World Journal of Gastroenterology, 17*(6), 727–734.
43. Chen, J. L., Tang, H. Q., Hu, J. D., Fan, J., Hong, J., & Gu, J. Z. (2010). Metabolomics of gastric cancer metastasis detected by gas chromatography and mass spectrometry. *World Journal of Gastroenterology, 16*(46), 5874–5880.
44. Brown, G. T., & Murray, G. I. (2015). Current mechanistic insights into the roles of matrix metalloproteinases in tumour invasion and metastasis. *The Journal of Pathology, 237*(3), 273–281.
45. Wang, X., Yan, S.-K., Dai, W.-X., Liu, X.-R., Zhang, W.-D., & Wang, J.-J. (2010). A metabonomic approach to chemosensitivity prediction of cisplatin plus 5-fluorouracil in a human xenograft model of gastric cancer. *International Journal of Cancer, 127*(12), 2841–2850.
46. Sasada, S., Miyata, Y., Tsutani, Y., Tsuyama, N., Masujima, T., Hihara, J., & Okada, M. (2013). Metabolomic analysis of dynamic response and drug resistance of gastric cancer cells to 5-fluorouracil. *Oncology Reports, 29*(3), 925–931.
47. Ganesan, K., Ivanova, T., Wu, Y., Rajasegaran, V., Wu, J., Lee, M. H., Yu, K., Rha, S. Y., Chung, H. C., Ylstra, B., Meijer, G., Lian, K. O., Grabsch, H., & Tan, P. (2008). Inhibition of gastric cancer invasion and metastasis by PLA2G2A, a novel beta-catenin/TCF target gene. *Cancer Research, 68*(11), 4277–4286.
48. Kim, K. B., Yang, J. Y., Kwack, S. J., Kim, H. S., Ryu, D. H., Kim, Y. J., Bae, J. Y., Lim, D. S., Choi, S. M., Kwon, M. J., Bang, D. Y., Lim, S. K., Kim, Y. W., Hwang, G. S., & Lee, B. M. (2013). Potential metabolomic biomarkers for evaluation of adriamycin efficacy using a urinary 1H-NMR spectroscopy. *Journal of Applied Toxicology: JAT, 33*(11), 1251–1259.
49. Cai, Z., Zhao, J. S., Li, J. J., Peng, D. N., Wang, X. Y., Chen, T. L., Qiu, Y. P., Chen, P. P., Li, W. J., Xu, L. Y., Li, E. M., Tam, J. P., Qi, R. Z., Jia, W., & Xie, D. (2010). A combined proteomics and metabolomics profiling of gastric cardia cancer reveals characteristic dysregulations in glucose metabolism. *Molecular & Cellular Proteomics: MCP, 9*(12), 2617–2628.
50. Choi, J.-I., Joo, I., & Lee, J. M. (2014). State-of-the-art preoperative staging of gastric cancer by MDCT and magnetic resonance imaging. *World Journal of Gastroenterology, 20*(16), 4546–4557.
51. Buscher, J. M., Czernik, D., Ewald, J. C., Sauer, U., & Zamboni, N. (2009). Cross-platform comparison of methods for quantitative metabolomics of primary metabolism. *Analytical Chemistry, 81*(6), 2135–2143.

Index

S. Hu (ed.), *Cancer Metabolomics*, Advances in Experimental Medicine and Biology 1280,
https://doi.org/10.1007/978-3-030-51652-9

D

E

F

The manufacturer's authorised representative in the EU is Springer
Nature Customer Service Centre GmbH, Europaplatz 3, 69115 Heidelberg,
Germany. If you have any concerns regarding our products, please
contact ProductSafety@springernature.com

Printed and bound by CPI Group (UK) Ltd, Croydon, CR0 4YY
22/09/2026
02221062-0019